Imaging for **STUDENTS**

Imaging for STUDENTS

FIFTH EDITION

Craig P Hacking
Associate Professor of Radiology and Academic Lead for Clinical Radiology, University of Queensland Medical School; and Consultant Radiologist and Medical Director of Medical Imaging at the Royal Brisbane and Women's Hospital, Brisbane, Australia

David A Lisle
Associate Professor of Medical Imaging, University of Queensland Medical School; Consultant Radiologist, Brisbane Private Hospital, Brisbane, Australia; and examiner for the Royal Australian and New Zealand College of Radiologists

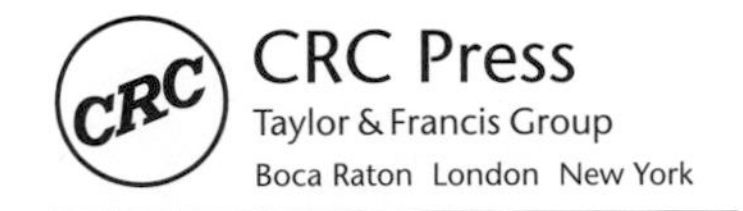

CRC Press is an imprint of the
Taylor & Francis Group, an **informa** business

Fifth edition published 2023
by CRC Press
6000 Broken Sound Parkway NW, Suite 300, Boca Raton, FL 33487-2742

and by CRC Press
4 Park Square, Milton Park, Abingdon, Oxon, OX14 4RN

CRC Press is an imprint of Taylor & Francis Group, LLC

ISBN: 978-1-032-31751-9 (hbk)
ISBN: 978-1-032-31748-9 (pbk)
ISBN: 978-1-003-31113-3 (ebk)

DOI: 10.1201/9781003311133

Typeset in Palatino Lt Std
by Evolution Design & Digital Ltd (Kent)

Access the Companion Website: www.routledge.com/cw/hacking

Printed in Great Britain by Bell and Bain Ltd, Glasgow

To my beautiful smart wife, Deb, our three energetic and intelligent children, Hamish, Bailey and Henrietta, my supportive mother, Liz, and my late father, Peter, who would have been so proud.

CPH

To my beautiful and supportive wife, Lyn, and our three precious daughters, Victoria, Charlotte and Margot.

DAL

Contents

Preface

In the decade since the publication of the fourth edition of *Imaging for Students*, the field of medical imaging has continued to advance. This is due to multiple factors, including more sophisticated and faster imaging techniques, increasing use of evidence-based guidelines and structured reporting systems, and advances in diverse fields such as molecular biology, computer technology and data analysis.

This edition encompasses some of these advances, providing fundamental coverage that will aid medical students and junior healthcare staff alike.

The aims of this fifth edition build on those of the previous four:

1. To introduce the various imaging modalities, including advantages and disadvantages
2. To outline a logical approach to interpretation of radiographs, including the chest X-ray
3. To illustrate important fundamental medical imaging findings of common pathologies
4. To provide an approach to the appropriate requesting of imaging investigations in a range of clinical scenarios.

To fulfil these aims, we have maintained the clinically orientated approach established in previous editions, with some restructuring of content and the addition of new chapters and sections. Chapter 1 gives a brief outline of each of the imaging modalities, including new developments such as spectral CT. Chapter 2 outlines safety issues encountered in current imaging practice, information that we believe is essential for referring clinicians when weighing up the possible benefits of an investigation against its potential risks. Chapter 3 contains new content and discusses current and emerging concepts, such as structured reporting systems and artificial intelligence.

A new chapter entitled 'How to read a chest X-ray' provides greater depth in this important medical skill and comprises lists of differentials for commonly encountered radiographic findings. The chapters covering the different body systems have been updated significantly and many images are either new or updated. 'Non-orthopaedic trauma' is a new amalgamated chapter that has expanded the trauma imaging content from within the body system chapters in previous editions. It focuses on trauma concepts and injury patterns and recognizes the ongoing development of this subspecialty field of radiology. Summary boxes that list investigations of choice and key points are retained in most chapters.

Some content has been transferred to the companion website, which has expanded significantly. This website now incorporates a much larger basic imaging anatomy section, oncology staging systems, trauma grading schema and details on the various Reporting and Data Systems (RADS) that are increasingly featured in radiology reports.

Those of us working in medical imaging continue to respond to the daily challenges of clinical demand, continued advances in technology and the need to contain medical costs. Our ongoing hope is that with this new edition of *Imaging for Students*, medical students and junior doctors may see the central importance of medical imaging in modern clinical diagnosis and intervention. We also hope that some may be inspired to pursue a career in the tremendously diverse and rewarding field of modern medical imaging.

CPH and DAL
Brisbane, May 2022

Acknowledgements

Several people have made contributions to this edition. Our thanks to the following for appropriate case examples: Professor Alan Coulthard, Associate Professor Karin Steinke, Mr Michael Truloff and Drs Avi Chikamartala, Fallon Cominos, Jen Gillespie, Sam Kyle, Kate Mahady, Jane McIniery and Tim Wastney. Thanks also to Dr Kate Mahady for her advice on the interventional neuroradiology section and Dr Debbie Shellshear for her invaluable clinical expertise in reviewing the paediatric chapter.

Author biographies

Craig P Hacking is the Medical Director of Medical Imaging and Lead Emergency Radiologist at the Royal Brisbane and Women's Hospital, Brisbane, Australia. He is the current Academic Lead for Clinical Radiology and an Associate Professor at the University of Queensland. Craig is a contributing editor and previous managing editor of Radiopaedia.org and a lead presenter for the emergency radiology, medical imaging anatomy and trauma radiology Radiopaedia courses, which are offered free online to 119 developing countries. Craig was a founding executive committee member for the Australian and New Zealand Emergency Radiology Group (ANZERG), and a former lead anatomy examiner and viva examiner for the Royal Australian and New Zealand College of Radiologists (RANZCR). He graduated medical school at the University of Queensland and has been teaching anatomy and radiology for over 20 years. It is a privilege for Craig to be asked to co-author the fifth edition of *Imaging for Students* by one of his radiology mentors, David A Lisle.

David A Lisle is a consultant radiologist at Brisbane Private and St Vincent's Northside Hospitals in Brisbane, Australia. David wrote his first book, *Imaging for Surgeons,* while working as a senior registrar in Aberdeen, UK, in 1991. Since then, he has authored a further edition of *Imaging for Surgeons* and four editions of *Imaging for Students.* He is delighted to be co-authoring this latest fifth edition with his friend and colleague, Craig P Hacking. David has worked as a consultant radiologist in Queensland and New Zealand for over 30 years. He is an Associate Professor in Medical Imaging at the University of Queensland Medical School and an examiner in neuroradiology for the Royal Australian and New Zealand College of Radiologists (RANZCR). David is also passionate about outreach work to less well-resourced nations in radiology. He is an active member of the global radiology charity Radiology Across Borders and he provides regular online teaching to colleagues in developing nations.

We will not cease from exploration
and the end of all our exploring
will be to arrive where we started
and know the place for the first time.
TS Eliot

It's human nature to stretch, to go, to see, to understand. Exploration is not a choice, really; it's an imperative.
Michael Collins, Apollo 11 Astronaut

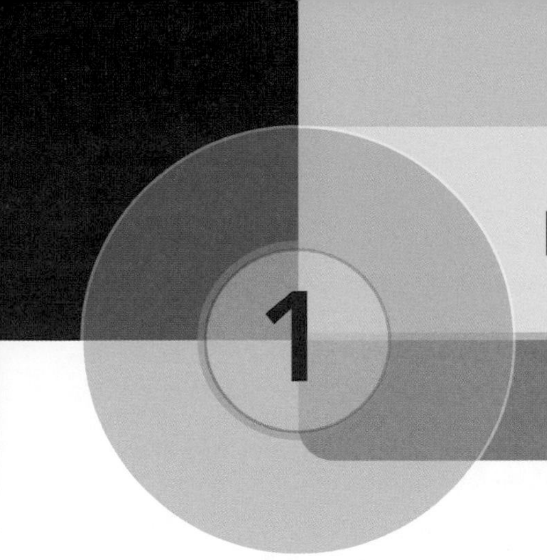

1 Introduction to medical imaging

1.1 RADIOGRAPHY (X-RAY IMAGING)

1.1.1 CONVENTIONAL RADIOGRAPHY (X-RAYS, 'PLAIN FILMS')

X-rays are produced in an X-ray tube by focusing a beam of high-energy electrons onto a tungsten target. X-rays are a form of electromagnetic radiation, able to pass through the human body and produce an image of internal structures. The resulting image is called a radiograph, and is more commonly known as an 'X-ray' or 'plain film'. The common terms 'chest X-ray' and 'abdomen X-ray' are widely accepted and abbreviated to CXR and AXR, respectively.

Three variable components of an X-ray exposure are kVp, mA and time. The kilovoltage peak (kVp) governs the penetrating strength of an X-ray beam, referred to as beam quality. Milliamperes (mA) refers to the tube current, i.e. the number of X-ray photons being produced by the X-ray tube. When multiplied by the time of exposure in seconds, the factor mAs provides a measure of the number of photons in each exposure, i.e. the quantity of the X-ray beam. Technicians balance these two settings, kVp and mAs, to produce X-ray exposures that provide images of diagnostic quality while minimizing the radiation dose to the patient.

As a beam of X-rays passes through the human body some of the X-rays are absorbed or scattered, producing a reduction or attenuation of the beam. Attenuation occurs as a result of two main processes: the photoelectric effect and Compton scatter. The photoelectric effect occurs when an incident X-ray photon removes an electron from an inner orbital shell of an atom. The X-ray photon is absorbed, and the electron is emitted as a photoelectron. The photoelectric effect is most likely to occur when the energy of the X-ray photon is equal to, or just greater than, the binding energy of the electron (K edge) or when the electron is tightly bound in the inner K shell. The photoelectric effect is highly dependent on the atomic number of atoms within tissues, and less so on the physical density. Compton scatter occurs when X-ray photons interact with free electrons that are not bound to atoms or with weakly bound electrons in the outer valence shells of atoms. The X-ray photon changes direction and loses some of its energy to the electron. Compton scatter is highly dependent on the density of tissues, and not on atomic number.

Mainly as a result of these two processes, tissues of high density and/or high atomic number cause more X-ray beam attenuation and are shown as lighter grey or white on a radiograph. Less dense tissues and structures cause less attenuation of the X-ray beam and appear darker on radiographs than tissues of higher density. Five principal densities are

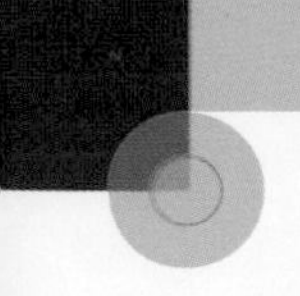

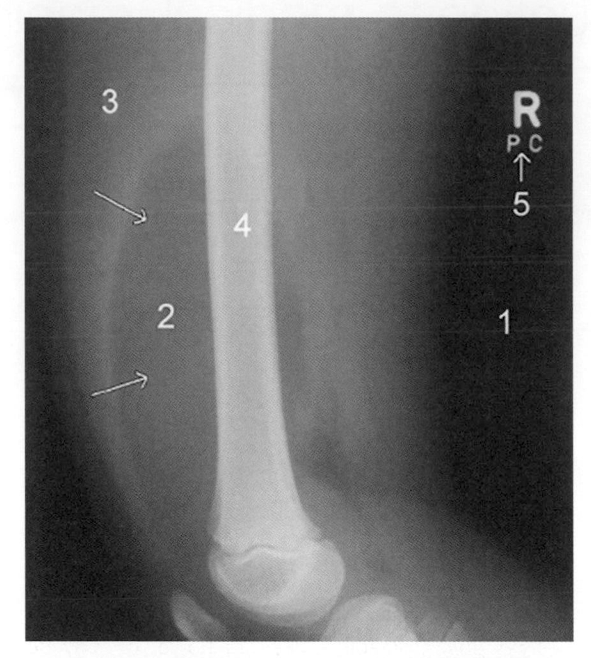

Figure 1.1 The five principal radiographic densities. This radiograph of a benign lipoma (arrows) in a child's thigh demonstrates the five basic radiographic densities: (1) air; (2) fat; (3) soft tissue; (4) bone; (5) metal.

recognized on plain radiographs (Fig. 1.1), listed here in order of increasing density:

1. Air/gas: black, e.g. lungs, bowel and stomach
2. Fat: dark grey, e.g. subcutaneous tissue layer and retroperitoneal fat
3. Soft tissues/water: light grey, e.g. solid organs, heart, blood vessels, muscle and fluid-filled organs such as bladder
4. Bone: off-white
5. Contrast material/metal: bright white.

1.1.2 COMPUTED RADIOGRAPHY, DIGITAL RADIOGRAPHY AND PICTURE ARCHIVING AND COMMUNICATION SYSTEM

In the past, X-ray films were processed in a darkroom or in free-standing daylight processors. In modern practice, radiographic images are produced digitally using one of two processes: computed radiography (CR) and digital radiography (DR). CR employs cassettes that are inserted into a laser reader following X-ray exposure. An analogue–digital converter produces a digital image. DR uses a detector screen containing silicon detectors that produce an electrical signal when directly exposed to X-rays. This signal is analysed to produce a digital image. Digital images obtained by CR and DR are sent to viewing workstations for interpretation, which may include various manipulation tools such as:

- Magnification of areas of interest
- Windowing to manipulate density and contrast
- Measurements of distances and angles.

Medical imaging departments employ large computer storage facilities and networks known as Picture Archiving and Communication Systems (PACS). Images obtained by CR and DR are stored digitally, as are images from other modalities, including computed tomography (CT), magnetic resonance imaging (MRI), ultrasound (US) and scintigraphy. PACS allow instant recall and display of a patient's imaging studies. Monitors throughout the hospital in wards, meeting rooms or operating theatres allow remote access to images.

1.1.3 FLUOROSCOPY

Radiographic examination of the anatomy and motion of internal structures by a constant stream of X-rays in real time is known as fluoroscopy. Uses of fluoroscopy include:

- Angiography and interventional radiology
- Contrast studies of the gastrointestinal tract (Fig. 1.2)
- Hysterosalpingography (HSG)
- Guidance of therapeutic joint injections and arthrograms
- Screening in theatre:
  - General surgery, e.g. operative cholangiography
  - Urology, e.g. retrograde pyelography
  - Orthopaedic surgery, e.g. reduction and fixation of fractures, joint replacements.

Fluoroscopy units fall into two categories: image intensifier and flat panel detector (FPD). Image intensifier units have been in use since the 1950s. An image intensifier is a large vacuum tube that converts X-rays into light. Images are viewed in

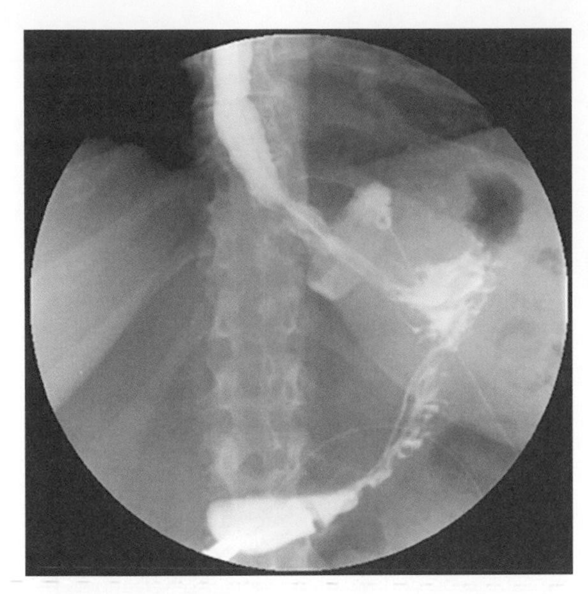

Figure 1.2 Fluoroscopy: Gastrografin swallow. A gastric band applied laparoscopically for weight loss. The Gastrografin swallow shows normal appearances: normal orientation of the gastric band, Gastrografin flowing through the centre of the band and no obstruction or leakage.

real time via a closed-circuit television chain and recorded as required. FPD fluoroscopy units are common in angiography suites and cardiac catheterization laboratories ('cath labs'). The FPD consists of an array of millions of tiny detector elements. Most FPD units work by converting X-ray energy into light and then to an electrical signal. Although they are more expensive, FPD units have several technical advantages over image intensifier systems, including smaller size of equipment, fewer imaging artefacts and reduced radiation exposure.

1.1.4 DIGITAL SUBTRACTION ANGIOGRAPHY

Further utility of fluoroscopy is gained with digital subtraction techniques, whereby a computer removes unwanted information from a radiographic image. Digital subtraction is particularly useful for angiography, referred to as digital subtraction angiography (DSA). The principles of digital subtraction are illustrated in Fig. 1.3.

A relatively recent innovation is rotational three-dimensional fluoroscopic imaging. For this technique the fluoroscopy unit rotates through 180° while acquiring images, producing a cine display that resembles a three-dimensional CT image. This image may be rotated and reorientated to produce a greater understanding of anatomy during complex diagnostic and interventional procedures.

1.2 CONTRAST MATERIALS

The ability of conventional radiography and fluoroscopy to display a range of organs and structures may be enhanced using various contrast materials, also known as contrast media. The most common contrast materials are based on barium or iodine, materials that have a high atomic number, strongly absorb X-rays and are subsequently white on radiography.

For demonstration of the gastrointestinal tract with fluoroscopy, contrast materials may be swallowed or injected via nasogastric tube to outline the oesophagus, stomach and small bowel or may be introduced via an enema tube to delineate the large bowel. Gastrointestinal contrast materials are usually based on barium, which is non-water soluble. Occasionally a water-soluble contrast material based on iodine is used for imaging of the gastrointestinal tract, particularly when aspiration or perforation may be encountered.

Iodinated (iodine containing) water-soluble contrast media may be injected into veins, arteries and various body cavities and systems. Iodinated contrast materials are used in CT (see section 1.3.2), angiography (DSA) (Fig. 1.3) and arthrography (injection into joints).

1.3 COMPUTED TOMOGRAPHY

1.3.1 COMPUTED TOMOGRAPHY PHYSICS AND TERMINOLOGY

CT is an imaging technique whereby cross-sectional images are obtained with the use of X-rays. The patient is passed through a rotating gantry that has an X-ray tube on one side and a set of detectors on the other. The tube and detectors rotate as the patient passes through on the scanning table, thus acquiring a continuous set of data. Modern scanners employ multiple rows of detectors, and CT in current practice may

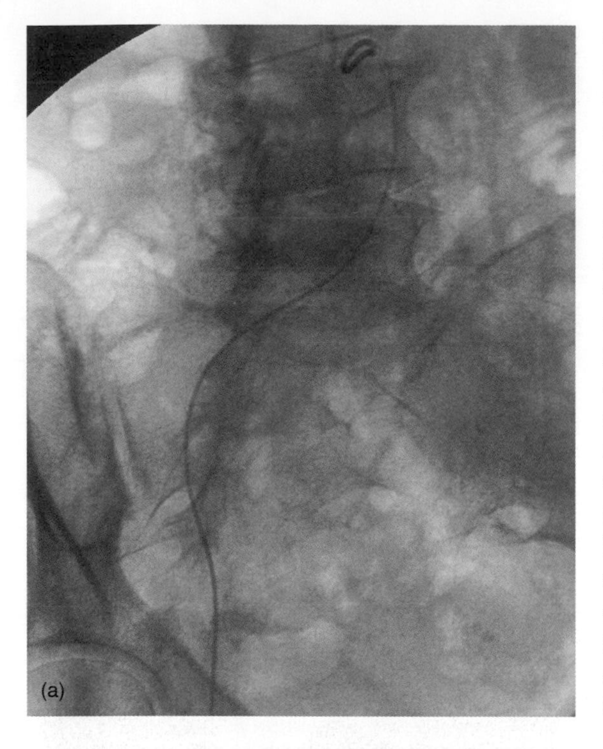

also be referred to as multidetector row CT (MDCT) or multislice CT. The original MDCT scanners in the mid- to late 1990s used two or four rows of detectors, followed by 16- and 64-detector row scanners; 256- and 320-row scanners are now widely available.

Information from the detectors is analysed by computer and displayed as a grey-scale image, with a much greater array of densities displayed than on conventional X-ray studies. This allows accurate depiction of cross-sectional anatomy, differentiation of organs and pathology and increased sensitivity to the presence of specific materials such as fat or calcium. High-density objects and materials with high atomic numbers cause more attenuation of the X-ray beam and are therefore displayed as lighter grey than are objects of lower density. White and light grey objects are therefore said to be of 'high attenuation'; dark grey and black objects are said to be of 'low attenuation'. MDCT allows the acquisition of overlapping fine sections of data, which in turn allows the reconstruction of highly accurate and detailed three-dimensional images as well as sections in any desired plane (Fig. 1.4).

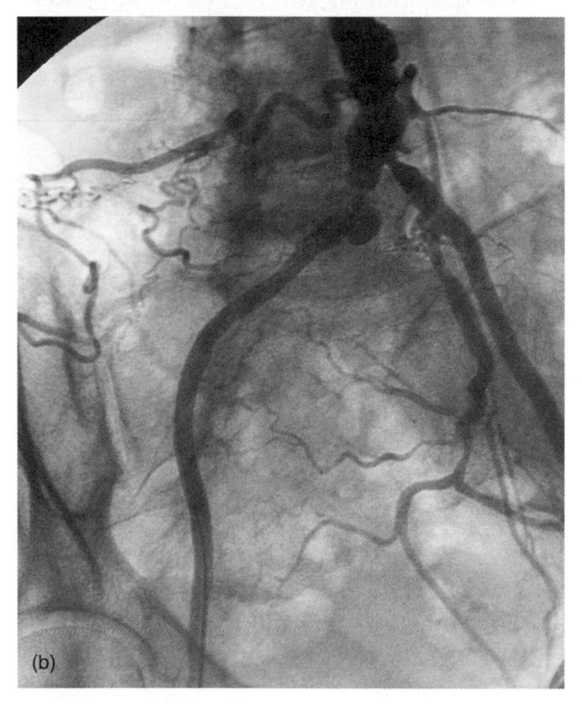

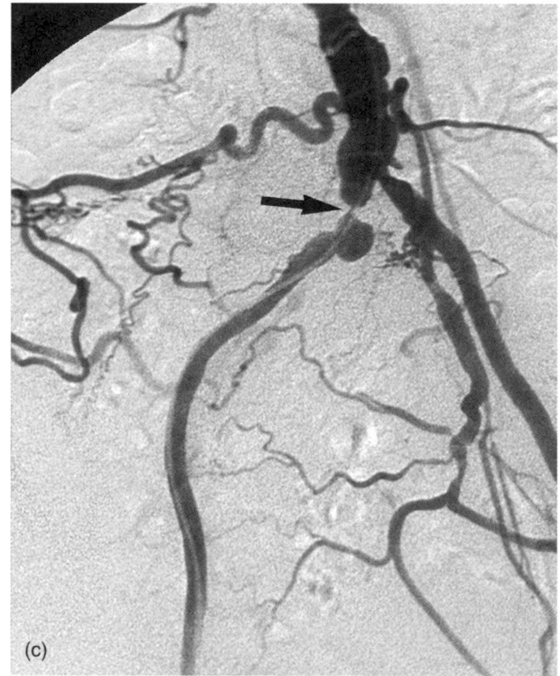

Figure 1.3 Digital subtraction angiography (DSA). (a) Mask image performed prior to injection of contrast material. (b) Contrast material injected, producing opacification of the arteries. (c) Subtracted image. The computer subtracts the mask from the contrast image, leaving an image of contrast-filled arteries unobscured by overlying structures. Note a stenosis of the right common iliac artery (arrow).

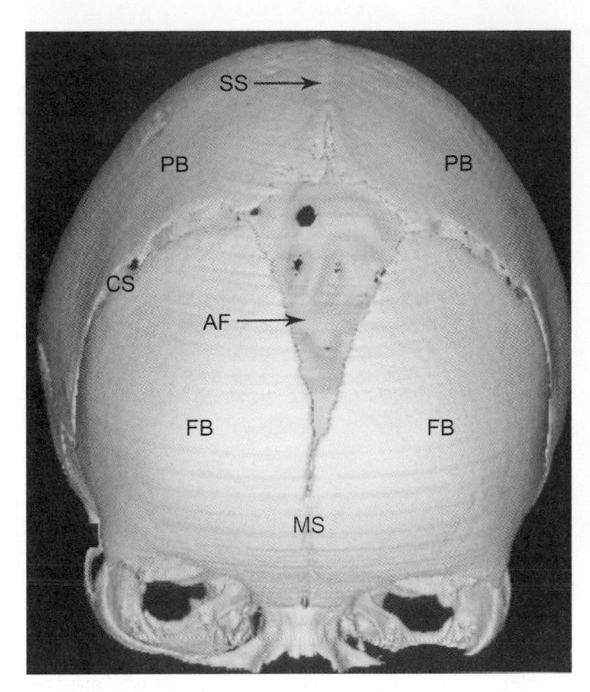

Figure 1.4 Three-dimensional reconstruction of an infant's skull showing a fused sagittal suture. Structures labelled as follows: anterior fontanelle (AF), coronal sutures (CS), frontal bones (FB), metopic suture (MS), parietal bones (PB), fused sagittal suture (SS). Normal sutures are seen on three-dimensional CT as lucent lines between skull bones. Note the lack of a normal lucent line at the position of the sagittal suture, indicating fusion.

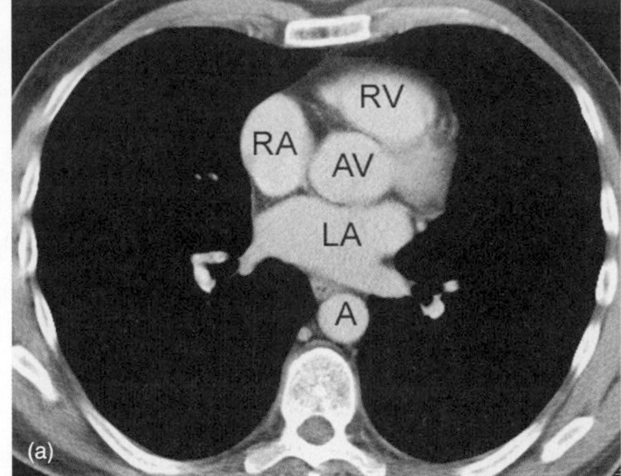

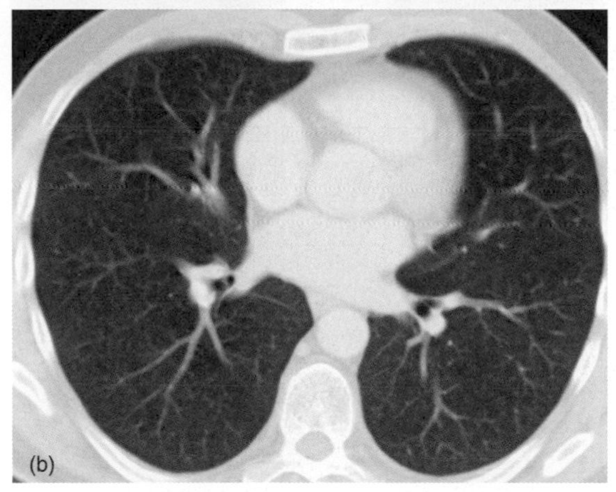

Figure 1.5 CT windows. (a) Mediastinal windows showing mediastinal anatomy: descending aorta (A), aortic valve (AV), left atrium (LA), right atrium (RA), right ventricle (RV). (b) Lung windows showing lung anatomy.

By altering the grey-scale settings the image information can be manipulated to display the various tissues of the body. For example, in chest CT, where a wide range of tissue densities is present, an image depicting the mediastinal structures well shows almost no lung detail. By setting a 'lung window' the lung parenchyma is seen in detail (Fig. 1.5).

The relative density of an area of interest may be measured electronically and is given as an attenuation value, expressed in Hounsfield units (HU) (named for Godfrey Hounsfield, the inventor of CT). In CT, water is assigned an attenuation value of 0 HU. Substances that are less dense than water, including fat and air, have negative values (Fig. 1.6); substances of greater density than water have positive values. Approximate attenuation values for common substances are as follows:

- Water: 0 HU
- Muscle: 40 HU
- Contrast-enhanced artery: 130 HU
- Cortical bone: 500 HU
- Fat: –120 HU
- Air: –1000 HU.

1.3.2 CONTRAST MATERIALS IN COMPUTED TOMOGRAPHY

Intravenous iodinated contrast material is used in CT for several reasons:

- Differentiation of normal blood vessels from abnormal masses, e.g. hilar vessels versus lymph nodes (Fig. 1.7)

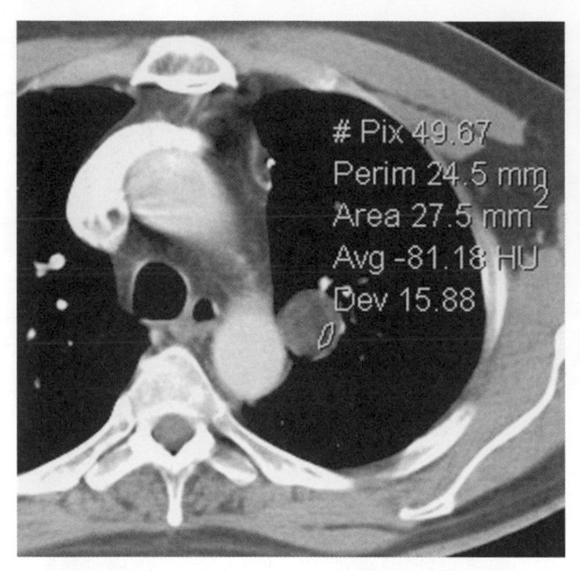

Figure 1.6 CT attenuation measurements. Hounsfield unit (HU) measurements in a lung nodule reveal negative values (–81 HU), indicating fat. This is consistent with a benign pulmonary hamartoma, for which no further follow-up or treatment is required.

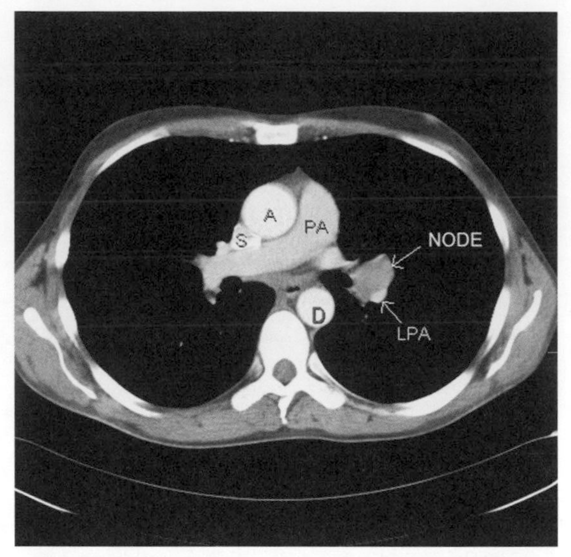

Figure 1.7 Intravenous contrast in CT. An enlarged left hilar lymph node is differentiated from enhancing vascular structures: ascending aorta (A), descending aorta (D), left pulmonary artery (LPA), main pulmonary artery (PA), superior vena cava (S).

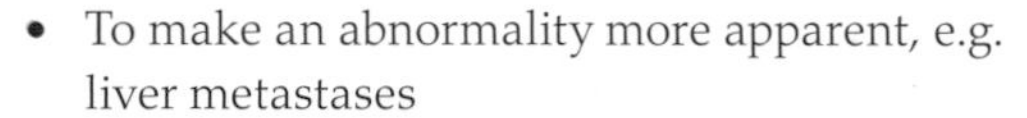

- To make an abnormality more apparent, e.g. liver metastases
- To demonstrate the vascular nature of a mass and thus aid in characterization
- CT angiography.

Oral contrast material may also be used for abdomen CT, though less commonly than in the past and usually for specific indications:

- Diagnosis of leaking surgical anastomoses
- CT enterography.

For detailed examination of the pelvis and distal large bowel, administration of rectal contrast material is occasionally used.

1.3.3 SPECTRAL COMPUTED TOMOGRAPHY

Spectral CT, dual-energy CT and multi-energy CT are terms used interchangeably to describe a range of CT techniques in which advanced scanners can determine material composition by comparing tissue CT attenuation at multiple X-ray photon energy levels. As described above, a beam of X-rays interacts with biological tissues, primarily because of Compton scattering and the photoelectric effect. These two main interactions occur at different rates with different X-ray energies. Spectral CT uses acquisition of images at different energies and/or detection of various energy spectra to differentiate material composition according to the proportional occurrence of Compton scattering and photoelectric absorption.

There are two basic methods of spectral scanning: source-based spectral scanning and detector-based spectral scanning. Source-based scanning is achieved by several means:

- Rapid kVp switching, whereby the X-ray tube can alternate between high and low energies during the gantry rotation
- Dual kVp spin, in which the tube can rotate twice, once with lower energies and again with higher energies
- Dual-source CT, which uses two orthogonal X-ray sources of different energies
- Split or twin beam, in which a conventional X-ray beam is split into two different energies with special filters.

Detector-based scanning uses a conventional X-ray beam analysed by a dual-layer detector (sandwich detector). The inner layer absorbs low-energy photons; higher energy photons that pass through the upper detector are absorbed by the second outer layer.

Photon-counting detector (PCD) CT is an emerging CT technology that offers improved spatial resolution and material differentiation with the use of semiconducting detectors. At the time of writing, PCD CT is still in early clinical trials.

All spectral CT scanners are able to obtain standard (conventional) CT images. Various specialized applications offered by spectral CT are listed below.

- *Virtual mono-energetic (monoE) reconstructions.* MonoE images are computer-generated representations of images that would be derived if the patient was scanned with an X-ray beam at a single, specific energy. Low-energy monoE reconstructions emphasize iodinated contrast within viscera and vessels, giving subtly enhancing structures or suboptimal vascular scans an 'iodine boost'. Patients who require smaller doses of contrast (e.g. renal impairment) may benefit from low-monoE images. High-monoE images are used to reduce artefact from metal or dense calcium, e.g. in atheromatous or stented coronary and cerebral arteries
- *Virtual non-contrast (VNC) reconstructions.* VNC images are obtained by subtracting iodine density from contrast-enhanced scans, thereby potentially reducing the radiation dose by negating the need to perform non-contrast acquisitions in multiphase studies, e.g. gastrointestinal tract bleeding studies
- *Iodine maps.* Iodine perfusion maps are used in CT pulmonary angiogram (CTPA) to demonstrate underperfused regions of lung due to pulmonary emboli. These images also allow differentiation of calcification from contrast enhancement. Iodine concentration can be quantified in mg/mL
- *Z-effective (Z_{eff}) maps.* Pixel values are calculated to represent the effective atomic number (Z) of the imaged material. Z_{eff} maps can act as surrogate perfusion maps, e.g. to display perfusion defects due to pulmonary emboli in the lung (Fig. 1.8). Z_{eff} maps can also identify cholesterol gallstones, which are of similar density to bile, and therefore not visible on conventional CT images

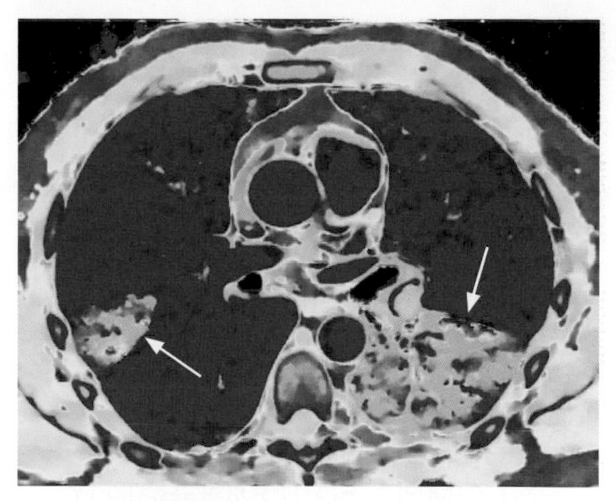

Figure 1.8 Transverse spectral CT *Z*-effective colour map of the chest showing reduced perfusion due to pulmonary emboli as regions of light blue and green in segments of the left lower and right upper lobes (arrows). Normally perfused lung is dark blue.

- *Uric acid.* Uric acid reconstructions can display structures containing uric acid. Two common applications are the diagnosis of sodium urate deposition in gouty arthropathy and characterization of uric acid renal calculi that can be treated with dissolution therapy
- *Calcium suppression.* High attenuation from calcium can be suppressed or removed to reveal subtle bone marrow lesions or bone marrow oedema, or to differentiate calcium from haemorrhage in soft-tissue masses.

1.3.4 APPLICATIONS OF COMPUTED TOMOGRAPHY

Although in many clinical scenarios CT has been replaced by other imaging techniques, it remains a robust technology with many applications, such as:

- Acute cerebral pathologies, including stroke assessment and brain perfusion scanning
- Acute trauma
- Acute abdomen
- Oncology staging and restaging
- CT angiography: coronary, cerebral, carotid, pulmonary, renal, visceral, peripheral

- Cardiac CT, including CT coronary angiography, functional assessment and coronary artery calcium scoring
- CT colonography (virtual colonoscopy)
- Fractures in complex areas: acetabulum, foot and ankle, distal radius and carpus
- Display of complex anatomy for planning of cranial and facial reconstruction surgery
- Protocol-driven CT for planning of joint replacements.

1.3.5 LIMITATIONS AND DISADVANTAGES OF COMPUTED TOMOGRAPHY

- Ionizing radiation (see Chapter 2)
- Hazards of intravenous contrast material (see Chapter 2)
- Lack of portability of equipment
- Relatively high cost.

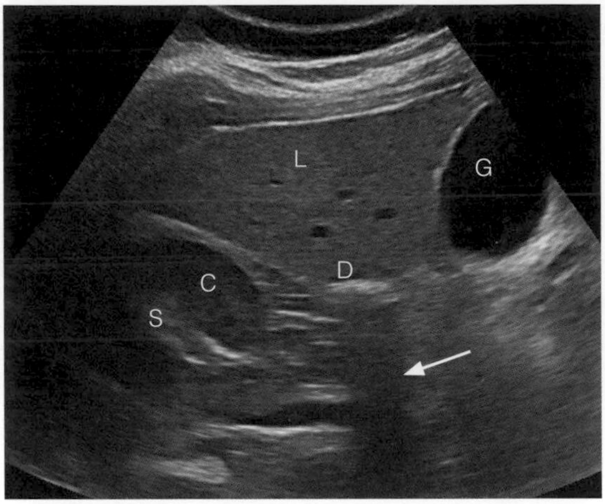

Figure 1.9 Transverse US of the abdomen demonstrates tissues of varying echogenicity. Note the anechoic bile in the gallbladder (G), homogeneous moderate echogenicity of the liver (L), mildly hypoechoic renal cortex (C), hyperechoic fat in the renal sinus (S). Also note the hyperechoic gas in the duodenum (D), causing posterior 'dirty' shadowing (arrow).

1.4 ULTRASOUND

1.4.1 ULTRASOUND PHYSICS AND TERMINOLOGY

US imaging uses ultra-high-frequency sound waves to produce cross-sectional images of the body. The basic component of the US probe is the piezoelectric crystal. Excitation of this crystal by electrical signals causes it to emit ultra-high-frequency sound waves; this is the piezoelectric effect. Sound waves are reflected back to the crystal by the various tissues of the body. These reflected sound waves (echoes) act on the piezoelectric crystal in the US probe to produce an electrical signal, again by the piezoelectric effect. Analysis of this electrical signal by a computer produces a cross-sectional image.

Solid organs, fluid filled structures and tissue interfaces produce varying degrees of sound wave reflection and are said to be of different echogenicity. Tissues that are hyperechoic reflect more sound than tissues that are hypoechoic. In an US image, hyperechoic tissues are shown as white or light grey and hypoechoic tissues are seen as dark grey (Fig. 1.9). Pure fluid is anechoic (reflects virtually no sound) and is black on US images. Furthermore, because virtually all sound is transmitted through a fluid-containing area, tissues distally receive more sound waves and hence appear lighter. This effect is known as 'acoustic enhancement' and is seen in tissues distal to the gallbladder, the urinary bladder and simple cysts. The reverse effect, known as 'acoustic shadowing', occurs with gas-containing bowel, gallstones, renal stones and breast malignancy.

1.4.2 DOPPLER ULTRASOUND

Anyone who has heard a police or ambulance siren speed past will be familiar with the influence of a moving object on sound waves, known as the Doppler effect. An object travelling towards the listener causes sound waves to be compressed, producing a higher frequency; an object travelling away from the listener produces a lower frequency. The Doppler effect has been applied to US imaging. Flowing blood causes an alteration to the frequency of sound waves returning to the US probe. This frequency change or shift is calculated, allowing quantification of blood flow. The combination of conventional two-dimensional US imaging with Doppler US is known as duplex US.

Colour Doppler is an extension of these principles, with blood flowing towards the transducer coloured red and blood flowing away from the transducer coloured blue. The colours are superimposed on the cross-sectional image, allowing instant assessment of the presence and direction of flow. Colour Doppler is used in many areas of US, including echocardiography and vascular US (Fig. 1.10). Colour Doppler is also used to confirm blood flow within organs (e.g. testis to exclude torsion) and to assess the vascularity of tumours.

Power Doppler is another imaging technique that uses the amplitude of the Doppler signal to generate a colour-coded representation of blood flow. The colour map of power Doppler usually ranges from red to yellow, with a paler colour indicating a higher intensity of blood flow. Power Doppler is highly sensitive to the presence, not the direction, of blood flow. It is used in a variety of scenarios, such as renal grafts, the thyroid, the testes and other superficial structures to detect blood flow (Fig. 1.11).

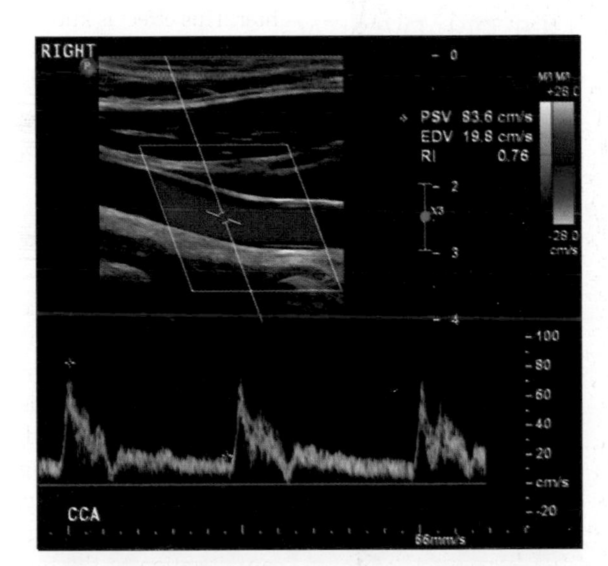

Figure 1.10 Colour Doppler US of the left common carotid artery. Note that the red colour indicating blood flow towards the US probe fills the arterial lumen with no visible plaque or stenosis. A normal arterial waveform is shown, with peak systolic velocity (PSV) of 83.6 cm/s, end-diastolic velocity (EDV) of 19.8 cm/s and a resistive index (RI) of 0.76.

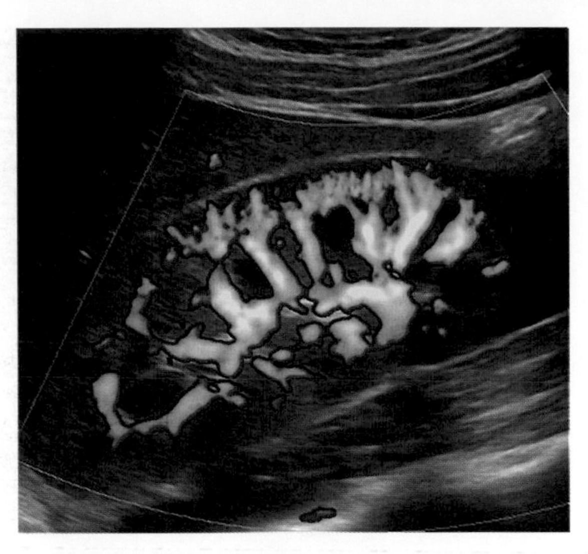

Figure 1.11 Power Doppler image demonstrating normal vascularity in the right kidney. This is a colour representation of Doppler amplitude, showing flowing blood regardless of direction. Note that even small distal arteries in the renal cortex are visualized.

1.4.3 SHEAR WAVE ELASTOGRAPHY

As will be discussed further in Chapter 7, liver diseases that cause hepatic fibrosis and cirrhosis are a major issue in modern practice. The need for non-invasive methods to diagnose potentially reversible changes, prior to the development of end-stage disease, has led to the development of new technologies. One such technique is shear wave elastography (SWE). Elastography refers to the measurement of tissue stiffness, known as the Young modulus (*E*). A modulus is a numerical value that expresses a physical property of a material. The Young modulus of elasticity represents the ability of a material to withstand changes in length when placed under compression or lengthening tension. The unit of *E* is the pascal (N/m^2); this is expressed as kilopascals (kPa) in the case of SWE.

For the performance of SWE, an US transducer emits a focused US pulse, known as the acoustic radiation force impulse (ARFI). This generates shear waves, which travel perpendicular to the impulse. The velocity of these shear waves is measured by the US transducer and recorded in metres per second (m/s). Shear wave velocity increases with tissue stiffness. The Young modulus may be calculated by the following formula: E (kPa) = $3.\rho.v^2$, where ρ is the tissue density and v is shear wave velocity (m/s). Although SWE is mostly used for the assessment of the liver, other applications have been described, including the evaluation of breast and thyroid lesions.

1.4.4 CONTRAST-ENHANCED ULTRASOUND

The accuracy of US in certain applications may be enhanced using intravenously injected microbubble contrast agents. Microbubbles measure 3–5 μm in diameter and consist of spheres of gas (e.g. perfluorocarbon) stabilized by a thin biocompatible shell. When within the US beam, microbubbles rapidly oscillate, which increases the echogenicity of blood for up to 5 minutes following intravenous injection. Beyond this time the biocompatible shell is metabolized, and the gas diffuses into the blood and is absorbed. Microbubble contrast agents are very safe, with a reported incidence of anaphylactoid reaction of around 0.014%. Common uses of contrast-enhanced US (CEUS) include:

- Echocardiography, e.g. improved visualization of intracardiac shunts such as a patent foramen ovale ('bubble study')
- Assessment of liver masses: dynamic blood flow characteristics of liver masses may be visualized with CEUS, similar to dynamic contrast-enhanced CT and MRI
- Assessment of renal and pancreatic masses in patients with contraindications to iodinated contrast and MRI.

1.4.5 APPLICATIONS AND ADVANTAGES OF ULTRASOUND

Advantages of US over other imaging modalities include:

- Lack of ionizing radiation:
  - Particularly relevant in pregnancy and paediatrics
- Relatively low cost
- Portability of equipment.

US scanning is applicable to:

- Solid organs, including liver, kidneys, spleen and pancreas
- Urinary tract
- Obstetrics and gynaecology
- Small organs, including thyroid and testes
- Breast
- Musculoskeletal system.

An assortment of probes is available for imaging and biopsy guidance of various body cavities and organs, including:

- Transvaginal US (TVUS): accurate assessment of gynaecological problems and of early pregnancy up to about 12 weeks' gestation
- Transrectal US (TRUS): guidance of prostate biopsy, staging of rectal cancer
- Endoscopic US (EUS): assessment of tumours of the upper gastrointestinal tract and pancreas
- Transoesophageal echocardiography (TOE): TOE removes the problem of overlying ribs and lung, which can obscure the heart and aorta when performing conventional echocardiography.

1.4.6 DISADVANTAGES AND LIMITATIONS OF ULTRASOUND

- US is highly operator dependent: unlike CT and MRI, which produce cross-sectional images in a reasonably programmed fashion, US relies on the operator to produce and interpret images at the time of examination
- US cannot penetrate gas or bone
- Bowel gas may obscure structures deep in the abdomen, such as the pancreas or renal arteries.

1.5 SCINTIGRAPHY (NUCLEAR MEDICINE)

1.5.1 PHYSICS OF SCINTIGRAPHY AND TERMINOLOGY

Scintigraphy refers to the use of gamma (γ) radiation to form images following the injection of various radiopharmaceuticals. The key word to understanding scintigraphy is 'radiopharmaceutical'. 'Radio' refers to the radionuclide, i.e. the emitter of γ rays.

The most used radionuclide in clinical practice is technetium, written in this text as ^{99m}Tc, where 99 is the atomic mass and the lower case 'm' stands for metastable. Metastable means that the technetium atom has two basic energy states: high and low. As the technetium transforms from the high-energy state to the low-energy state, it emits a quantum of energy in the form of a γ ray, which has energy of 140 keV (Fig. 1.12).

Other commonly used radionuclides include gallium citrate (^{67}Ga), indium (^{111}In) and iodine (^{131}I).

The 'pharmaceutical' part of radiopharmaceutical refers to the compound to which the radionuclide is bound. This compound varies depending on the tissue to be examined.

For some applications such as thyroid scanning, free technetium (referred to as pertechnetate) without a binding pharmaceutical is used. The γ rays emitted by the radionuclides are detected by a gamma camera that converts the absorbed energy of the radiation to an electrical signal. This signal is analysed by a computer and displayed as an image.

1.5.2 SINGLE PHOTON EMISSION COMPUTED TOMOGRAPHY (SPECT) AND SPECT-CT

SPECT is a scintigraphic technique whereby the computer is programmed to analyse data coming from a single depth within the patient. SPECT allows greater sensitivity in the detection of subtle lesions overlain by other active structures (Fig. 1.12). The accuracy of SPECT may be further enhanced by fusion with CT. Scanners that combine SPECT with CT are now widely available. SPECT-CT fuses highly sensitive SPECT findings with anatomically accurate CT images, thus improving sensitivity and specificity.

The main applications of SPECT-CT include bone scintigraphy, cardiac scanning, MIBG staging of neuroblastoma (see Table 1.1) and cerebral perfusion studies.

1.5.3 POSITRON EMISSION TOMOGRAPHY (PET) AND PET-CT

PET utilizes radionuclides (also known as radiotracers or PET tracers) that decay by positron emission.

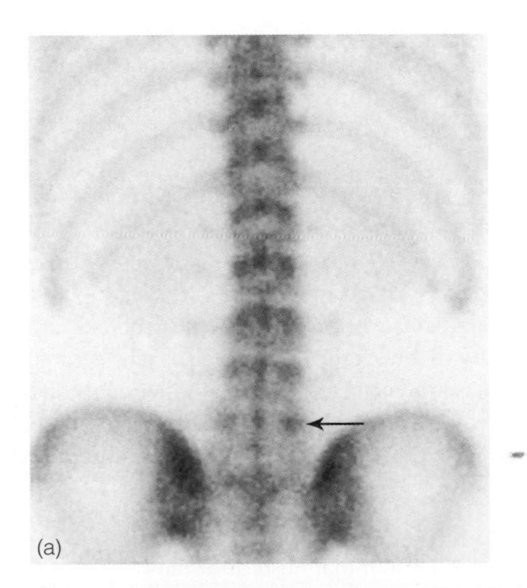

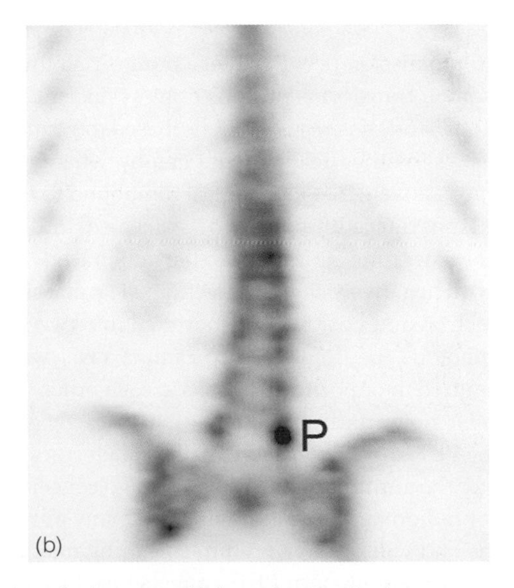

Figure 1.12 Single photon emission CT (SPECT). (a) Scintigraphy in a man with lower back pain shows a subtle area of mildly increased activity (arrow). (b) SPECT scan in the coronal plane shows an obvious focus of increased activity in a pars interarticularis defect (P).

Table 1.1 Radionuclides and radiopharmaceuticals in clinical practice.

Clinical application	Radiopharmaceutical
Bone scintigraphy	^{99m}Tc-methylene diphosphonate (MDP)
	^{99m}Tc-hydroxymethylene diphosphonate (HDP)
Thyroid imaging	^{99m}Tc (pertechnetate)
Parathyroid imaging	^{99m}Tc (pertechnetate)
	^{99m}Tc-sestamibi (MIBI)
Renal scintigraphy	^{99m}Tc-mercaptoacetyltriglycerine (MAG3)
	^{99m}Tc-diethyltriaminepentaacetic acid (DTPA)
Renal cortical scan	^{99m}Tc-dimercaptosuccinic acid (DMSA)
Staging/localization of neuroblastoma or phaeochromocytoma	^{123}I-metaiodobenzylguanidine (MIBG) ^{131}I-MIBG
Myocardial perfusion imaging	^{99m}Tc-MIBI
	^{99m}Tc-tetrofosmin
Cardiac gated blood pool scan	^{99m}Tc-labelled red blood cells
Ventilation/perfusion lung scan (VQ scan)	Ventilation: ^{99m}Tc-Technegas (30-to 60-nm carbon particles) Perfusion: ^{99m}Tc-macroaggregated albumen (MAA)
Hepatobiliary imaging	^{99m}Tc-iminodiacetic acid analogue, e.g. DISIDA or HIDA
Gastrointestinal motility study	^{99m}Tc-sulfur colloid in solid food and liquid
Meckel diverticulum scan	^{99m}Tc (pertechnetate)
Infection imaging	Gallium citrate (^{67}Ga)
	^{99m}Tc-hexamethylpropyleneamine oxime (HMPAO)-labelled white blood cells
Cerebral blood flow imaging (brain SPECT)	^{99m}Tc-HMPAO (Ceretec) ^{99m}Tc-ethinyl cysteinate dimer (ECD)

Abbreviation: SPECT, single photon emission computed tomography.

Positron emission occurs when a proton-rich unstable isotope transforms protons from its nucleus into neutrons and positrons. PET is based on similar principles to other fields of scintigraphy, whereby an isotope is attached to a biological compound to form a radiopharmaceutical, which is injected into the patient. Positrons emitted from the radionuclide collide with negatively charged electrons. The masses of an electron and positron are converted into two 511-keV photons, i.e. high-energy gamma rays, which are emitted in opposite directions to each other. This event is known as annihilation.

The PET camera consists of a ring of detectors that register the annihilations. An area of high concentration of radiopharmaceutical will have many annihilations and will be shown on the resulting image as a 'hot spot'. All modern PET scanners fuse PET with CT or, less commonly, MRI. PET-CT fusion imaging combines the functional and metabolic information of PET with the precise cross-sectional anatomy of CT, thereby greatly increasing the specificity of the technique (Fig. 1.13).

The most commonly used radiopharmaceutical in PET scanning is 2-deoxyglucose labelled with the positron-emitter fluorine-18 (fluorodeoxyglucose, FDG). 2-Deoxyglucose is an analogue of glucose, and therefore FDG accumulates in areas of high glucose metabolism. Normal physiological uptake of FDG occurs in the brain (high level of glucose metabolism), in the myocardium and in the renal collecting systems, ureters and bladder. The commonest roles of FDG-PET-CT imaging may be summarized as follows:

- Oncology:
  - Tumour diagnosis and staging
  - Assessment of tumour response to therapy and tumour recurrence

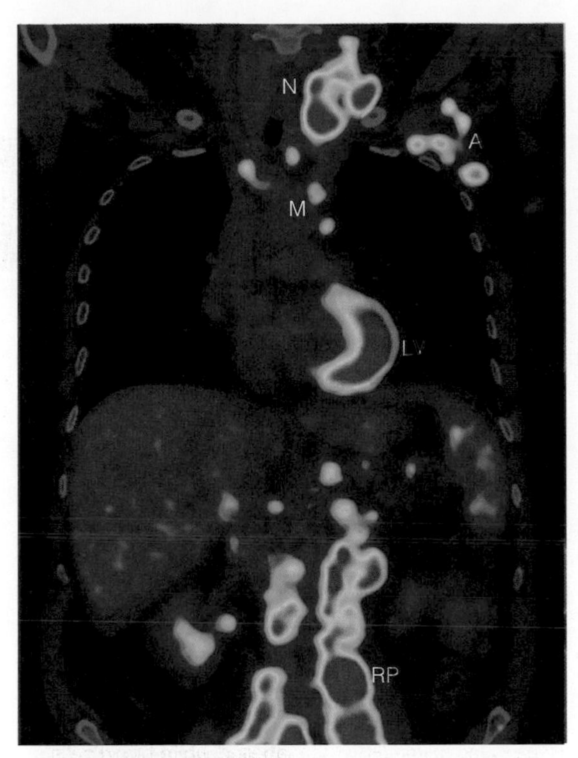

Figure 1.13 Lymphoma: FDG-PET-CT. Enlarged FDG-avid nodes in the left axilla (A), mediastinum (M), left neck (N) and retroperitoneum (RP). Note the normal FDG avidity in the left ventricular myocardium (LV).

- Differentiate benign and malignant masses, e.g. solitary pulmonary nodule
- Cardiac: non-invasive assessment of myocardial viability in patients with coronary artery disease
- Central nervous system:
  - Characterization of dementia disorders
  - Localization of seizure focus in epilepsy.

Other biological compounds that are commonly used in PET-CT are gallium-68 bound to prostate-specific membrane antigen molecules (^{68}Ga-PSMA) and gallium-68 bound to somatostatin analogues, such as tetraazacyclododecane–tetraacetic acid and tyrosine-3-octreotate (^{68}Ga-DOTATATE). PSMA is overexpressed in patients with prostate cancer and PSMA-PET-CT is used in the staging of this disease. Tyrosine-3-octreotate is bound by somatostatin receptors on the surface of neuroendocrine cells and DOTATATE-PET-CT is used in the diagnosis and staging of neuroendocrine tumours (NETs). These include carcinoid tumours, phaeochromocytomas, medullary thyroid tumours and pancreatic NETs such as insulinoma, gastrinoma and vasoactive polypeptide secretory tumour (VIPoma).

Numerous other PET radiopharmaceuticals are undergoing development and clinical trials. These include agents that bind to β-amyloid fibrils that may be used to assess amyloid-related conditions such as Alzheimer disease and agents that bind to tau protein that may find a role in the assessment of Alzheimer disease and other tauopathies such as progressive supranuclear palsy.

1.5.4 THERANOSTICS

The term theranostics, a fusion of therapy and diagnostics, refers to a combination of therapeutic and diagnostic modalities for specific diseases or clinical scenarios. In modern practice, the term theranostics usually refers to applications of scintigraphy in oncology. As discussed above, scintigraphy uses radiopharmaceuticals to transport γ- or positron-emitting radionuclides to specific biological targets. The same, or similar, pharmaceuticals can be used to transport radionuclides that emit particulate radiation. Particulate radiation in the form of alpha (α) particles (two protons and two neutrons) or beta (β) particles (electrons) has a much higher energy than electromagnetic radiation such as γ rays or X-rays.

Theranostics is not a new concept. ^{131}I, a dual-emitting isotope that emits γ and β radiation, has been used to diagnose and treat various thyroid diseases, including differentiated thyroid cancer, since the 1930s. More recent advances in various fields including imaging technology and molecular biology have led to the development of radiopharmaceuticals that include emitters of particulate radiation, such as lutetium-177 (^{177}Lu). Diagnostic and therapeutic radiopharmaceuticals that share the same biological target, referred to as theranostic pairs, can diagnose and stage malignant disease and deliver targeted, high-energy radiation for treatment. Examples of theranostic pairs in current use are:

- ^{68}Ga-PSMA and ^{177}Lu for prostate cancer (see Chapter 8)
- ^{68}Ga-DOTATATE and ^{177}Lu-ocreotate in NETs.

1.5.5 APPLICATIONS AND ADVANTAGES OF SCINTIGRAPHY

Advantages of scintigraphy include:

- Highly sensitive
- Specific functional and metabolic information obtained
- Able to detect and localize pathology not visible on other modalities.

A summary of the more common clinical applications and relevant radionuclides and radiopharmaceuticals is provided in Table 1.1.

1.5.6 DISADVANTAGES AND LIMITATIONS OF SCINTIGRAPHY

Disadvantages of scintigraphy include:

- Longer times for image acquisition
- Relatively poor spatial resolution, overcome by combination with CT or MRI
- Use of ionizing radiation
- Logistic requirements for handling and disposal of radioactive materials.

1.6 MAGNETIC RESONANCE IMAGING

1.6.1 MAGNETIC RESONANCE IMAGING PHYSICS AND TERMINOLOGY

MRI uses the magnetic properties of spinning hydrogen atoms to produce images. The first step in MRI is the application of a strong external magnetic field. For this purpose, the patient is placed within a large powerful magnet. Most current medical MRI machines have field strengths of 1.5 or 3.0 tesla (1.5 T or 3 T). The hydrogen atoms within the patient align in a direction either parallel or antiparallel to the strong external field. A greater proportion aligns in the parallel direction so that the net vector of their alignment, and therefore the net magnetic vector, will be in the direction of the external field. This is known as longitudinal magnetization.

A second magnetic field is applied at right angles to the original external field. This second magnetic field is known as the radiofrequency (RF) pulse because it is applied at a frequency in the same part of the electromagnetic spectrum as radio waves. A magnetic coil known as the RF coil applies the RF pulse. The RF pulse causes the net magnetization vector of the hydrogen atoms to turn towards the transverse plane, i.e. a plane at right angles to the direction of the original strong external field. The component of the net magnetization vector in the transverse plane induces an electrical current in the RF coil. This current is known as the magnetic resonance (MR) signal and is the basis for the formation of an image. Computer analysis of the complex MR signal from the RF receiver coils is used to produce an MR image.

Note that, in viewing MR images, white or light grey areas are referred to as 'high signal'; dark grey or black areas are referred to as 'low signal'. On certain sequences, flowing blood is seen as a black area; this is referred to as a 'flow void'.

Each medical MRI machine consists of multiple magnetic coils:

- 1.5-T or 3-T superconducting magnet to produce the static external field
- Gradient coils, contained in the bore of the superconducting magnet, are used to produce variations to the magnetic field that allow image formation:
  - Rapid switching of these gradients causes the loud noises associated with MRI scanning
- RF coils are applied to, or around, the area of interest and are used to transmit the RF pulse and to receive the RF signal:
  - RF coils come in varying shapes and sizes depending on the part of the body to be examined
  - Larger coils are required for imaging the chest and abdomen, whereas smaller extremity coils are used for small parts such as the wrist or ankle.

1.6.2 TISSUE CONTRAST AND IMAGING SEQUENCES

Much of the complexity of MRI arises from the fact that the MR signal depends on many varied properties of the tissues and structures being examined, including:

- Number of hydrogen atoms present in the tissue (proton density [PD])
- Chemical environment of the hydrogen atoms, e.g. whether in free water or bound by fat
- Flow: blood vessels or cerebrospinal fluid (CSF)
- Magnetic susceptibility
- T1 relaxation time
- T2 relaxation time.

By altering the duration and amplitude of the RF pulse, as well as the timing and repetition of its application, various imaging sequences use these properties to produce image contrast. Terms used to describe the different types of MRI sequences include spin echo, inversion recovery and gradient recalled echo (GRE) (gradient echo).

SPIN ECHO

Spin echo sequences produce images that are T1 weighted and T2 weighted or that display PD. Below is a brief explanation of the terms 'T1' and 'T2'.

Following the application of a 90° RF pulse, the net magnetization vector lies in the transverse plane. Also, all the hydrogen protons are 'in phase', i.e. spinning at the same rate. Upon cessation of the RF pulse, two things begin to happen:

1. The net magnetization vector rotates back to the longitudinal direction: longitudinal or T1 relaxation
2. Hydrogen atoms dephase (spin at slightly varying rates): transverse or T2 relaxation (decay).

A second RF pulse is applied at an angle of 180°. This brings the spinning protons back into phase, producing a refocused echo that is detected and analysed. The time between the initial 90° pulse and the refocused echo is termed the echo time, TE. The pulse sequence is repeated multiple times to obtain sufficient signal to create an image; the time of pulse repetition is termed the repetition time, TR.

The rates at which T1 and T2 relaxation occur are inherent properties of the various tissues. Sequences with short TE and TR values accentuate differences in T1 relaxation rates to produce T1-weighted images. Tissues with long T1 values are shown as low signal while those with shorter T1 values are displayed as higher signal. Gadolinium produces T1 shortening; tissues or structures that enhance with gadolinium-based contrast materials show increased signal on T1-weighted images.

Sequences with long TE and TR values produce T2-weighted images that reflect differences in T2 relaxation rates. Tissues whose protons dephase slowly have a long T2 and are displayed as high signal on T2-weighted images. Tissues with shorter T2 values are shown as lower signal (Fig. 1.14).

PD images are produced by sequences with short TE and long TR that accentuate neither T1 nor T2 differences. The signal strength of PD images mostly reflects the density of hydrogen atoms (protons) in the different tissues. PD images are particularly useful in musculoskeletal imaging for the demonstration of small structures as well as articular cartilage (Fig. 1.15).

Inversion recovery sequences are spin echo sequences that use a 180° preparatory pulse to suppress unwanted signals that may obscure pathology. The two most common inversion recovery sequences are used to suppress fat (STIR) and water (FLAIR). Fat suppression sequences such as STIR (short TI (inversion time) inversion recovery) are used for demonstrating pathology in areas containing a lot of fat, such as the orbits and bone marrow. STIR sequences allow the delineation of bone marrow disorders such as oedema, bruising and infiltration (Fig. 1.16). FLAIR (fluid-attenuated inversion recovery) sequences suppress signal from CSF and are used to image the brain. FLAIR sequences are particularly useful for diagnosing white matter disorders such as multiple sclerosis.

GRADIENT RECALLED ECHO (GRADIENT ECHO)

GRE sequences are widely used in a variety of MRI applications. GRE sequences employ an initial RF pulse with a variable flip angle that partially flips the net magnetization vector towards the transverse plane.

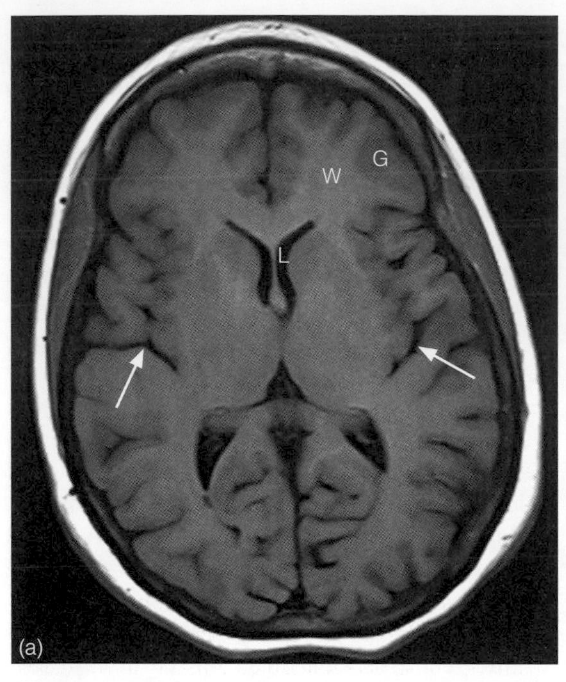

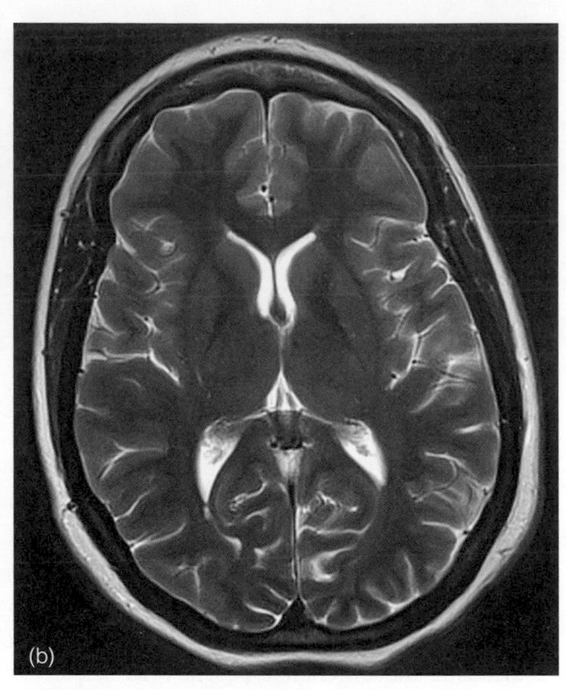

Figure 1.14 MRI of the brain. (a) Transverse T1-weighted image. Note dark cerebrospinal fluid (CSF) in the lateral ventricles (L) and cerebral sulci (arrows). Grey matter (G) is of lower signal than white matter (W). (b) Transverse T2-weighted image. Note that the CSF is bright and the white matter is much darker than the grey matter.

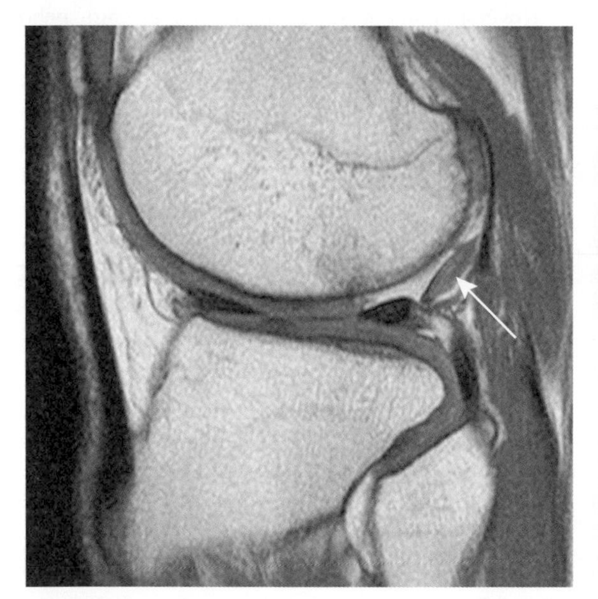

Figure 1.15 Proton density (PD) sequence: articular cartilage tear. Sagittal PD MRI of the knee shows a cartilage fragment detached from the articular surface of the lateral femoral condyle (arrow).

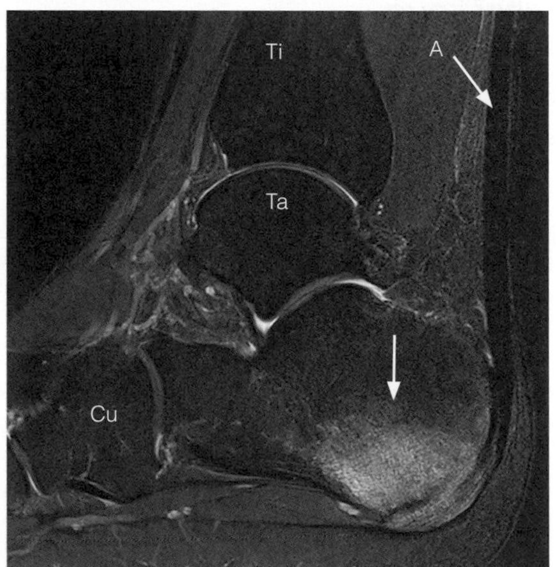

Figure 1.16 Short TI (inversion time) inversion recovery (STIR) sequence: calcaneal stress fracture. Sagittal STIR image of the hindfoot and ankle shows a region of high-signal oedema in the calcaneus (white arrow). A black (sclerotic) line within the bone marrow oedema indicates a calcaneal stress fracture (black arrow). Also note the Achilles tendon (A), cuboid (Cu), talus (Ta), tibia (Ti).

Unlike spin echo, GRE does not include a 180° refocusing pulse. In GRE, local magnetic field inhomogeneities produce signal loss related to magnetic susceptibility, and this signal decay is labelled T2*, as opposed to true T2 weighting in spin echo, where inhomogeneities are removed by the 180° refocusing pulse. Examples of substances with relatively high levels of magnetic susceptibility include iron-containing haemosiderin and ferritin found in chronic blood and deoxyhaemoglobin in venous blood.

1.6.3 ADDITIONAL TECHNIQUES

SUSCEPTIBILITY-WEIGHTED IMAGING

An extension of GRE sequences in the brain, known as SWI, uses subtraction techniques to remove unwanted information and thereby increase sensitivity. SWI is used in neuroimaging to look for chronic blood in patients with suspected vascular tumours, previous trauma or angiopathy. GRE sequences also allow extremely rapid imaging and are used for imaging the heart and abdomen, for high-resolution imaging of the temporal bones and cranial nerves and for obtaining perfusion-weighted images (see section Perfusion-weighted imaging).

DIFFUSION-WEIGHTED IMAGING

Diffusion-weighted imaging (DWI) is sensitive to the random Brownian motion (diffusion) of water molecules within tissue. The greater the amount of diffusion, the greater the signal loss on DWI. Areas of reduced water molecule diffusion show on DWI as relatively high signal. The degree of diffusion may be expressed mathematically by a calculated value known as the apparent diffusion coefficient (ADC). A grey-scale image may be generated to provide a map of ADC values.

An important phenomenon to be aware of when interpreting DWI is T2 shine-through. As the name suggests, this refers to high signal on DWI due to T2 values rather than true restricted diffusion. Areas of reduced diffusion have lower ADC values and are shown as darker grey on ADC maps. By contrast, T2 shine-through shows as light grey on ADC maps.

DWI has many applications. It is the most sensitive imaging modality for the diagnosis of acute cerebral infarction. With the onset of acute ischaemia and cell death there is increased intracellular water (cytotoxic oedema) with restricted diffusion of water molecules. An acute infarct therefore shows on DWI as an area of relatively high signal and on ADC maps as a region of darker grey. DWI is also used for differentiating space-occupying lesions in the brain, e.g. necrotic tumour versus abscess and epidermoid versus arachnoid cyst. It is also used to enhance tumour detection, particularly in the prostate and liver.

DIFFUSION TENSOR IMAGING AND FIBRE TRACTOGRAPHY

An extension of DWI is diffusion tensor imaging (DTI). In CSF, diffusion of water molecules is isotropic, i.e. equal in all directions. In certain tissues, water diffusion may occur more in some directions than in others; this is referred to as anisotropic diffusion. Geometric structures may be described by numeric constructs known as tensors. In the case of DTI, tensors represent numerical expressions of the magnitude and directionality of water molecule diffusion in small volumes of tissue known as voxels. A relevant example is white matter, where diffusion of water molecules occurs preferentially parallel to the long axis of axons. Three-dimensional reconstruction of diffusion tensors can build a representation of white matter tracts in the brain and spine. Known as fibre tractography, this imaging method assigns colour coding depending on the direction of fibres.

The fibre tractography image may be superimposed on conventional MR images to show the relationship of white matter tracts to other structures or pathology (Fig. 1.17). These images may assist in surgical planning, e.g. by assessing whether a tract is displaced or invaded by a tumour. Fibre tractography may also be used to assess disruptions of axons from various pathologies, including traumatic brain injury, infarction and demyelination disorders such as multiple sclerosis.

PERFUSION-WEIGHTED IMAGING

There are currently three commonly used methods for performing perfusion-weighted MRI (PWI). The first of these, dynamic susceptibility contrast-enhanced (DSC) MR perfusion, acquires

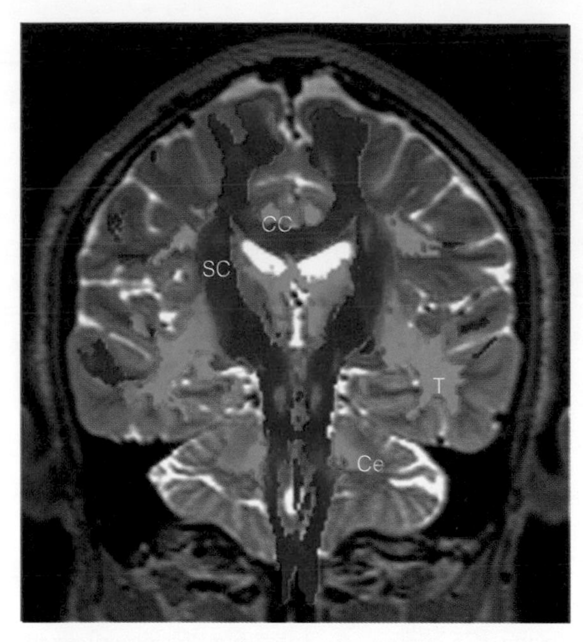

Figure 1.17 Coronal MRI brain tractography. The different colours represent the white matter tracts coursing in different directions: blue for craniocaudal, e.g. spinocortical tracts (SC); red for transverse, e.g. corpus callosum (CC); and green for anteroposterior, e.g. cerebellum (Ce) and deep white matter of temporal lobes (T).

T2*-weighted sequences during passage of an injected bolus of gadolinium-based contrast material. Susceptibility-induced signal loss may be analysed to generate colour maps of various calculated parameters, including regional cerebral blood volume (rCBV), regional cerebral blood flow (rCBF) and mean transit time (MTT) of the contrast bolus.

Another PWI technique is dynamic contrast-enhanced (DCE) MR perfusion, also referred to as permeability MRI. DCE acquires T1-weighted sequences during passage of an injected bolus of gadolinium-based contrast material. Analysis of signal change due to T1 shortening allows the calculation of perfusion parameters. The most common of these is a transfer constant known as k^{trans}, which is a measure of capillary permeability.

A third method of performing PWI is arterial spine labelling (ASL). For ASL, RF pulses are applied to blood proximal to the region to be examined. These pulses reverse the magnetization of protons in blood water (RF labelling). After a short time delay during which the RF-labelled protons flow into the region of interest, images are acquired. Perfusion images in the form of colour maps are generated by the subtraction of labelled images from control (non-labelled) images. In this way, rather than tracking injected contrast material, ASL uses magnetically labelled blood water protons to generate perfusion-weighted images. Until recently, ASL had only very limited clinical applications. Because of various technical advances in image acquisition, ASL is gaining in popularity and, in many centres, is replacing contrast-enhanced perfusion imaging techniques.

PWI has numerous applications. It may be used in patients with cerebral infarct to map out areas of brain at risk of ischaemia that may be salvageable with thrombolysis. PWI also has numerous applications in the imaging of brain tumours, including grading of gliomas, targeting suitable sites for biopsy, assessment of response to therapy as well as helping to differentiate gliomas from non-neoplastic conditions such as infection or demyelination. DCE may be used to assess pathologies associated with increased permeability of brain capillaries, including glioma, metastasis and multiple sclerosis; it is also used in MRI of the prostate.

MAGNETIC RESONANCE SPECTROSCOPY

Magnetic resonance spectroscopy (MRS) uses different frequencies to identify certain molecules in a selected volume of tissue, known as a voxel. Following data analysis, a spectrogram of certain metabolites is created. Metabolites of interest include lipid, lactate, *N*-acetyl-aspartate (NAA), choline, creatinine, citrate and myoinositol. Uses of MRS include characterization of metabolic brain disorders in children, imaging of dementias, differentiation of recurrent cerebral tumour from radiation necrosis and diagnosis of prostatic carcinoma.

BLOOD OXYGEN LEVEL-DEPENDENT IMAGING

Blood oxygen level-dependent (BOLD) imaging is a non-invasive functional MRI (fMRI) technique used for localizing regional brain signal intensity changes in response to task performance. BOLD imaging depends on regional changes in concentration of deoxyhaemoglobin and is therefore a tool to investigate regional cerebral physiology in response to a variety of stimuli. BOLD fMRI may be used prior to surgery for a brain tumour or arteriovenous malformation, as a prognostic indicator of the degree of postsurgical deficit.

1.6.4 MAGNETIC RESONANCE ANGIOGRAPHY AND MAGNETIC RESONANCE VENOGRAPHY

Flowing blood can be shown with different sequences as either signal void (black) or increased signal (white). White blood methods are accompanied by suppression of signal from background stationary tissues, thus increasing the conspicuity of blood vessels. Various MR angiography (MRA) methods are used. These can be subdivided into non-contrast-enhanced and contrast-enhanced methods. Non-contrast-enhanced methods include time of flight, phase contrast and arterial spin labelling. Computer reconstruction techniques allow the display of blood vessels in three dimensions as well as rotation and viewing of these blood vessels from multiple angles. MRA is mostly used to image the arteries of the brain and neck, although it is also commonly used in the imaging of renal and peripheral arteries. MRI of veins is known as MR venography (MRV). MRV is mostly used in neuroimaging to demonstrate the venous sinuses of the brain.

For certain applications, the accuracy of MRA and MRV is increased by contrast enhancement with intravenous injection of gadolinium. Contrast-enhanced methods are generally more sensitive for small vessels and for slower rates of blood flow. A variety of time-resolved methods are also used to allow dynamic angiography with simultaneous display of arterial, mixed and venous phases of blood flow. These are known under various proprietary acronyms such as TWIST or TRICKS.

1.6.5 CONTRAST MATERIAL IN MAGNETIC RESONANCE IMAGING

Gadolinium (Gd) is a paramagnetic substance that causes T1 shortening and therefore increased signal on T1-weighted images. Unbound gadolinium is highly toxic and binding agents such as diethylenetriamine pentaacetic acid (DTPA) are required for *in vivo* use. Gadolinium contrast agents are classified based on two factors:

1. Ionicity (net charge in solution): ionic or non-ionic
2. Molecular structure of the binding agent: linear or cyclic (macrocyclic).

This classification becomes relevant when considering the risks of complications with various agents (see Chapter 2).

Indications for the use of gadolinium enhancement in MRI include:

- Brain:
  - Inflammation: meningitis, encephalitis
  - Tumours: primary (Fig. 1.18), metastases
  - Tumour residuum/recurrence following treatment
- Spine:
  - Postoperative: differentiation of fibrosis from recurrent disc protrusion
  - Infection: discitis, epidural abscess
  - Tumours: primary, metastases
- Musculoskeletal system:
  - Soft-tissue tumours
  - Intra-articular gadolinium: MR arthrography
- Abdomen:
  - Characterization of tumours of liver, kidney and pancreas.

1.6.6 APPLICATIONS AND ADVANTAGES OF MAGNETIC RESONANCE IMAGING

Advantages of MRI in clinical practice include:

- Excellent soft-tissue contrast and characterization
- Lack of artefact from adjacent bones, e.g. pituitary fossa
- Multiplanar capabilities
- Lack of ionizing radiation.

Widely accepted applications of MRI include:

- Imaging modality of choice for most brain and spine disorders

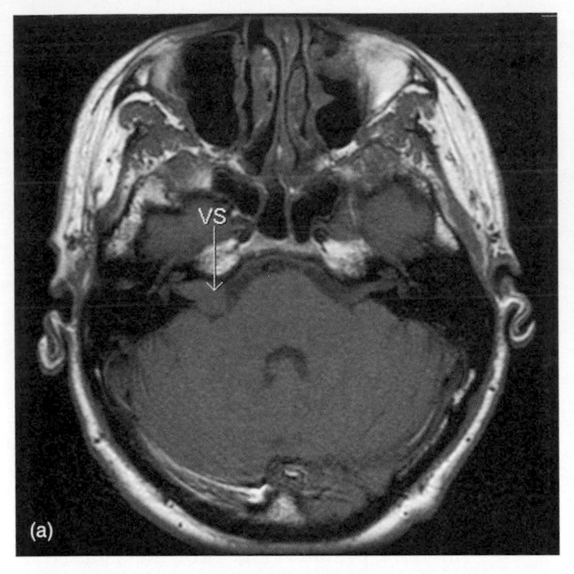

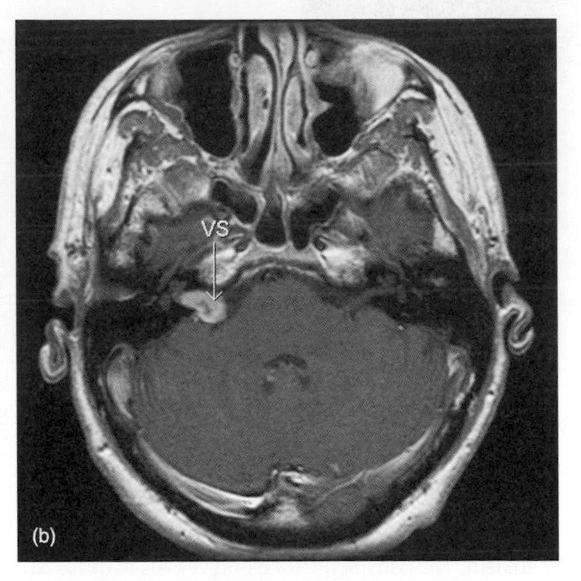

Figure 1.18 Intravenous contrast in MRI: vestibular schwannoma (VS). (a) Transverse T1-weighted image of the posterior fossa shows a right-sided mass. This is of similar signal intensity to adjacent brain. (b) Following injection of gadolinium the mass shows intense enhancement, typical of VS.

- Musculoskeletal disorders, including internal derangements of joints and staging of musculoskeletal tumours
- Cardiac MR is an established technique in specific applications, including assessment of congenital heart disease, myocardial disease and aortic disorders
- MR of the abdomen is used in adults for visualization of the biliary system and for characterization of hepatic, renal, adrenal and pancreatic tumours
- MR enterography assesses bowel wall pathology, such as inflammatory bowel disease
- In children, MR of the abdomen is used for the diagnosis and staging of abdominal tumours
- MRA is used in the imaging of the cerebral circulation; in some centres, it is the initial angiographic method of choice for other areas, including the renal and peripheral circulations.

1.6.7 DISADVANTAGES AND LIMITATIONS OF MAGNETIC RESONANCE IMAGING

- Time taken to complete the examination can be 20–60 minutes:
  - o Young children and infants usually require general anaesthesia
  - o Patients experiencing pain may require intravenous pain relief
  - o For examination of the abdomen, an antispasmodic such as intravenous hyoscine may be required to reduce movement of the bowel
- Safety issues related to ferromagnetic materials within the patient, e.g. surgical clips or electrical devices such as pacemakers (see Chapter 2)
- High auditory noise levels: earplugs should be provided to all patients undergoing MRI examinations
- Claustrophobia:
  - o Modern scanners have a wider bore and claustrophobia is less of a problem than in the past
  - o Intravenous conscious sedation may occasionally be required
- Problems with gadolinium: allergy (extremely rare), brain accumulation and nephrogenic systemic fibrosis (see Chapter 2).

2 Safety in medical imaging

Hazards associated with modern medical imaging are outlined below. They include:

- Exposure to ionizing radiation
- Anaphylactoid reactions to iodinated contrast media
- Contrast-induced nephropathy (CIN)
- Magnetic resonance imaging (MRI) safety issues
- Nephrogenic systemic sclerosis (NSF)
- Gadolinium retention.

2.1 EXPOSURE TO IONIZING RADIATION

2.1.1 RADIATION EFFECTS AND EFFECTIVE DOSE

Radiography, scintigraphy and computed tomography (CT) use ionizing radiation; ultrasound (US) and MRI do not. Radiation effects occur as a result of damage to cells, including cell death and genetic damage. Actively dividing cells such as are found in the bone marrow, lymph glands and gonads are particularly sensitive to radiation effects. In general, two types of effects may result from radiation damage: deterministic effects and stochastic effects. Deterministic effects are due to cell death and include radiation burns, cataracts and decreased fertility. The severity of deterministic effects varies with dose and a dose threshold usually exists below which the effect will not occur. For stochastic effects, the probability of the effect – not its severity – is regarded as a function of dose. Theoretically, there is no dose threshold below which a stochastic effect will not occur. The most discussed stochastic effect is increased cancer risk due to radiation exposure.

The radiation dose from medical imaging is usually expressed as the effective dose. The concept of effective dose considers the susceptibilities of the various tissues and organs, as well as the type of radiation received. The SI unit of effective dose is joules per kilogram and is referred to as the sievert (Sv): 1 Sv = 1.0 J/kg. The effective dose provides a means of calculating the overall risk of radiation effects, especially the risk of cancer.

To try to make sense of quoted effective doses, there is a tendency to compare doses from various imaging tests with the amount of background radiation that is received in normal life. This background radiation comes from minute traces of isotopes in the human body, cosmic radiation from the sun and low-level radiation from the Earth. It varies depending on geographic location but is generally 2–3 mSv/year. Another comparison used is the amount of radiation exposure from flying in an aircraft, which is usually quoted as hours of flying at an altitude of 12,000 metres. A 20-hour flight from Australia to London would result in an exposure of about 0.1 mSv, the equivalent of about five chest radiographs (chest

Table 2.1 Effective doses of some common examinations.

Imaging test	Effective dose (mSv)	Equivalent number of CXRs	Equivalent time of background exposure	Equivalent hours of flying at 12,000 metres
CXR frontal	0.02	1	3 days	4
CXR lateral	0.04	2	6 days	8
Limb X-ray	0.02	1	3 days	4
Lumbar spine X-ray	1.5	75	6 months	300
CT head	2	100	8 months	400
CT pulmonary angiogram	8	400	2 years	1200
CT abdomen	2–10	100–500	8 months–3 years	400–1800
DEXA bone densitometry	0.001	0.05	<1 day	<1
DSA	5–10	250–500	18 months–3 years	900–1800

Abbreviations: DEXA, dual energy X-ray absorptiometry; DSA, digital subtraction angiography.

X-rays, CXRs). Some typical effective doses (mSv) and relevant comparisons are listed in Table 2.1.

2.1.2 MEDICAL RADIATION AND RADIATION PROTECTION

The risks of harm from medical radiation are low and are usually expressed as the increased risk of developing cancer because of exposure. There is public awareness of the possible hazards of medical radiation, and it is important for doctors who refer patients for X-rays, nuclear medicine scans or CT scans to have at least a basic understanding of radiation effects and the principles of radiation protection.

Numerous studies, including those on survivors of the atomic bomb tragedies in Japan in 1945, have shown that ionizing radiation in large doses is harmful. The lifetime risk of developing a cancer from ionizing radiation is estimated at 5% per sievert. International regulatory authorities use these results to assume that there is a small – though definable – risk of developing cancer of 0.005% (1:20,000) per millisievert from medical radiation exposure, with a 5- to 10-year delay before the occurrence of cancer. This would translate to a 1 in 2000 lifetime risk of fatal cancer from a single CT of the abdomen. Opponents of this theory point to a lack of evidence, and believe that there is an as yet undefined threshold below which there is no increased risk attributable to low-level medical radiation.

In any case, most providers and consumers of medical imaging would agree that it is desirable for referring doctors to have some knowledge of the levels of possible radiation exposure associated with common imaging tests. Furthermore, there is widespread acceptance within the medical imaging community that radiation exposure should be minimized. The basic rule of radiation protection is that all justifiable radiation exposure is kept as low as is reasonably achievable (the ALARA principle). This can be done by keeping in mind the following points:

- Each radiation exposure is justified on a case-by-case basis (see Chapter 3)
- Optimize protocols and techniques for specific examinations:
  - Minimum number of radiographs
  - Minimum fluoroscopic screening time used
  - Mobile equipment is only used when the patient is unable to come to the medical imaging department
- Optimize CT protocols:
  - Minimize phases of examination
  - Use image reconstruction algorithms for dose minimization
- US or MRI should be used when possible.

Children are more sensitive to radiation than adults and are at greater risk of developing radiation-induced cancers many decades after the initial exposure. In paediatric radiology, extra measures may be taken to minimize radiation dose, including gonad shields and adjustment of CT scanning parameters.

2.1.3 PREGNANCY

Extra measures should also be taken for the care of women of reproductive age:

- Radiation exposure of the abdomen and pelvis should be minimized
- All females of reproductive age should be asked if they could be pregnant prior to radiation exposure
- Multilingual signs should be posted in the medical imaging department asking patients to notify the radiographer of possible pregnancy.

As organogenesis is unlikely to be occurring in an embryo in the first 4 weeks following the last menstrual period, this is not considered a critical period for radiation exposure. Organogenesis commences soon after the time of the first missed period and continues for the next 3–4 months. During this time the fetus is maximally radiosensitive. Radiographic or CT examination of the abdomen or pelvis should be delayed, if possible, to a time when fetal sensitivity is reduced, i.e. after 24 weeks' gestation or ideally until the baby is born. Where possible, MRI or US should be used. Radiographic exposure to remote areas such as the chest, skull and limbs may be undertaken with minimal fetal exposure at any time during pregnancy. For nuclear medicine studies in the postpartum period, it is advised that breastfeeding be ceased and breast milk discarded for 2 days following the injection of radionuclide.

2.2 ANAPHYLACTOID CONTRAST MEDIUM REACTIONS

Most patients injected intravenously with an iodinated contrast medium experience normal transient phenomena, including a mild warm feeling plus an odd metallic taste in the mouth. With modern iodinated contrast media vomiting at the time of injection is uncommon. More significant adverse reactions to contrast media may be classified as mild, intermediate or severe anaphylactoid reactions.

- Mild anaphylactoid reactions: mild urticaria and pruritus
- Intermediate reactions: more severe urticaria, hypotension and mild bronchospasm
- Severe reactions: more severe bronchospasm, laryngeal oedema, pulmonary oedema, unconsciousness, convulsions, pulmonary collapse and cardiac arrest.

Incidences of mild, intermediate and severe reactions with non-ionic low-osmolar contrast media are 3%, 0.04% and 0.004%, respectively. Fatal reactions are exceedingly rare (1:170,000). All staff working with iodinated contrast materials should be familiar with modern cardiopulmonary resuscitation and emergency procedures should be in place to deal with reactions, including resuscitation equipment and relevant drugs, especially adrenaline. Prior to injection of iodinated contrast medium patients should complete a risk assessment questionnaire to identify predisposing factors known to increase the risk of anaphylactoid reactions, including:

- History of asthma increases the risk by a factor of 10
- History of atopy increases the risk by a factor of 10
- Previous anaphylactoid reaction to iodinated contrast medium: 40% risk of further reactions.

A history of allergy to seafood does not appear to be associated with an increased risk of contrast medium reactions. There is no convincing evidence that pretreatment with steroids or an antihistamine reduces the risk of contrast medium reactions.

2.3 CONTRAST-INDUCED NEPHROPATHY

CIN refers to a reduction in renal function associated with iodinated contrast medium administration. CIN is a controversial topic. Current evidence indicates that other factors such as sepsis are more likely than contrast material to be the cause of renal impairment. In any case, CIN is defined as a 25% or more increase in serum creatine that occurs within 48–72 hours post contrast injection; it is usually transitory and self-limiting.

Several risk factors for the development of CIN have been identified. Principal among these is pre-existing impaired renal function, particularly diabetic nephropathy. CIN is very rare in patients with an estimated glomerular filtration rate (eGFR) of 30 mL/min/1.73 m^2 or higher. Other risk factors include:

- Dehydration
- Sepsis
- Recent organ transplant
- Multiple myeloma.

The risk of developing CIN may be reduced by the following measures:

- eGFR should be measured prior to contrast medium injection if there is a known history of renal disease, but this should not delay contrast-enhanced CT if it is required in an emergency, e.g. trauma or stroke
- The minimum possible dose of contrast medium should be used to provide a diagnostically adequate study
- Patients should be adequately hydrated before and after contrast medium injection; intravenous fluids should be given to dehydrated patients.

2.4 MAGNETIC RESONANCE IMAGING SAFETY ISSUES

Potential hazards associated with MRI predominantly relate to the interaction of the magnetic fields with metallic materials and electronic devices. Reports exist of objects such as spanners, oxygen cylinders and drip poles becoming missiles when placed near an MRI scanner; the hazards to patients and personnel are obvious. Ferromagnetic materials within the patient when inside the magnetic field could possibly heat or move, causing tissue damage. Common potential problems include metal fragments in the eye and various medical devices such as intracerebral aneurysm clips. Patients with a history of penetrating eye injury are at risk for having metal fragments in the eye and should be screened prior to entering the MRI room with orbital radiographs.

MRI-compatible aneurysm clips and other surgical devices have been available for many years. MRI should not be performed until the safety of an individual device has been established. The presence of electrically active implants such as cardiac pacemakers, cochlear implants and neurostimulators is generally a contraindication to MRI unless the safety of an individual device is proven. MRI-compatible pacemakers are now available and are being more commonly used.

A standard questionnaire to be completed by the patient prior to MRI should cover the relevant risk factors outlined above, as well as any history of previous allergic reaction to gadolinium-based contrast media and known renal disease.

2.4.1 NEPHROGENIC SYSTEMIC FIBROSIS

NSF is a rare complication of some gadolinium-based contrast media in patients with renal failure. Initial symptoms consisting of pain, pruritus and lower limb erythema may occur from 1 day to 3 months following injection. As NSF progresses there is thickening of the skin and subcutaneous tissues and fibrosis of internal organs, including the heart, liver and kidneys, similar to systemic sclerosis (scleroderma). Several years ago, the American College of Radiology classified gadolinium-based agents into three groups according to the relative risk of association with NSF. Because of the significantly reduced use of the higher risk agents, plus other factors such as improved clinical guidelines, NSF is now very rare.

2.4.2 GADOLINIUM RETENTION

A recently described phenomenon in patients who have received repeated gadolinium-enhanced MRI studies has been the retention of gadolinium in the brain. Gadolinium retention is characterized by increased signal on T1-weighted images in the globus pallidus and the dentate nucleus of the cerebellum. It is more commonly encountered with linear contrast agents. At the time of writing, despite intensive investigation, there are no known adverse clinical consequences in patients with imaging changes of gadolinium retention. Despite this, many imaging centres are moving to the use of cyclic agents to reduce the risk of any potential harms that may be discovered in the future.

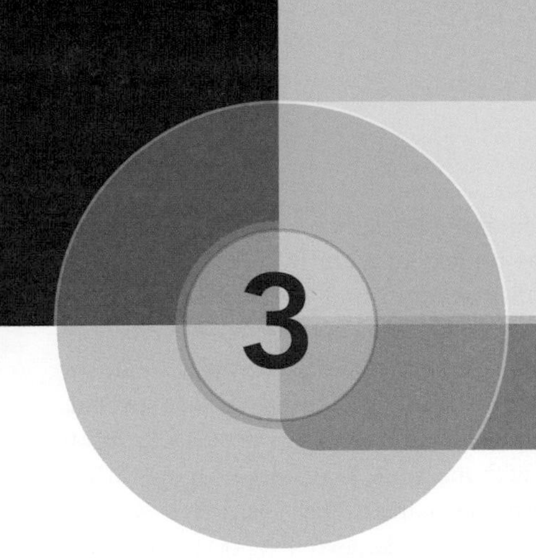

3 Selected concepts in medical imaging

Since the first edition of this book was published in 1996, the field of medical imaging has seen remarkable advances in technology and expertise. These advances have been in parallel with new applications in related clinical specialties, such as oncology, and developments in computer technology. This chapter briefly explores some concepts that are driving the further evolution of medical imaging and enhancing its many applications in modern patient care.

3.1 JUSTIFICATION AND APPROPRIATE IMAGING REQUESTS

The concept of justification consists of assessing the risks of a given medical imaging procedure against its potential benefits. Risks and safety in medical imaging have been discussed in Chapter 2. As outlined in that chapter, the related concept of optimization refers to ensuring that risks, including exposure to ionizing radiation, are minimized. This is the responsibility of medical imaging personnel. On the other hand, the referring clinician is best placed to assess the potential benefits of a medical imaging procedure, including impacts on patient management as well as the exclusion of disease and providing reassurance. Justification is therefore a shared responsibility that highlights the importance of appropriate consultation and adequate communication.

When requesting a medical imaging procedure, the responsibilities of the referring clinician include the provision of adequate and relevant clinical information and notification of previous imaging, particularly when this has been performed in a separate institution. A key responsibility is ensuring that the appropriate imaging test is being requested for a given clinical scenario. This concept informs much of the content of this book. To assist clinicians, there are now multiple evidence-based guidelines published by various colleges and other interested bodies. Many of these are available online and include appropriateness criteria published by the American College of Radiology (ACR) (https://www.acr.org/), the National Institute for Health and Care Excellence in the UK (https://www.nice.org.uk/) and Diagnostic Imaging Pathways in Australia (http://imagingpathways.health.wa.gov.au/). These are supported by various cooperative initiatives such as Image Wisely (imagewisely.org) and Image Gently (imagegently.org).

3.2 STRUCTURED AND CONTEXTUAL REPORTING

As medical imaging has evolved, the difficulty of communicating increasingly complex information in

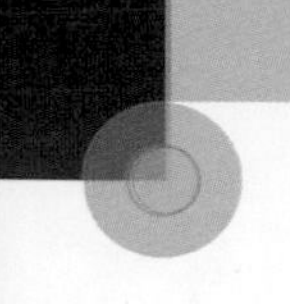

radiology reports has increased. Many radiologists use a free-form style of reporting, which may include an introduction with clinical details and examination technique, followed by a paragraph or more of text describing the findings and ending with a conclusion or impression. There is growing awareness that better communication can be achieved by a more structured reporting style. Structured reports use templates that include standardized headings and language. An excellent example of this style of reporting is used in oncology for staging and restaging of malignancy.

The anatomical extent of most solid tumours is categorized according to the tumour–node–metastasis (TNM) system, which is published and updated by the American Joint Committee on Cancer (AJCC) and the Union for International Cancer Control (UICC). Under the TNM classification system, features of local tumour growth plus the pattern of tumour metastasis are categorized as follows:

- 'T' = primary tumour and local extent
- 'N' = regional lymph nodes
- 'M' = distant metastases, including non-regional lymph nodes.

A structured report based on this system would provide highly relevant data that are individualized for the type of tumour and would include the following headings and information:

- Clinical details
- Imaging technique
- Date and type of previous comparison images
- T: local factors relevant to the tumour, including size, depth of invasion beyond the organ of origin and invasion of adjacent structures
- N: involvement of specific lymph node groups in the primary drainage of the affected organ
- M: distant metastases, including non-regional lymph nodes
- Other findings: findings that are not of direct relevance to the tumour, e.g. incidental gallstones or renal cysts
- Conclusion.

Some structured reporting systems use a checklist approach in which a list of anatomical features is displayed. These features are checked off as either normal or abnormal, with explanation of the nature of any abnormalities. This style of reporting can be quite generic and tedious. An extension of structured reporting known as contextual reporting uses a template-driven style that is much more specifically related to disease and examination type. For example, in imaging of the abdomen, multiple contextual templates may be developed to cover diverse indications such as spectral computed tomography (CT) for renal calculi, staging of rectal cancer with magnetic resonance imaging (MRI) or CT for suspected pancreatitis. Research has indicated that structural and contextual reporting provides more accurate communication of complex imaging data, and this style of reporting is gaining increasing acceptance from referring clinicians.

3.3 USAGE OF REPORTING AND DATA SYSTEMS

An increasingly common type of structured reporting is based on a set of modality- and technique-specific guidelines endorsed by the ACR, known as a Reporting and Data System (RADS). The original RADS method, Breast Imaging RADS (BI-RADS), was published in 1993 to address inconsistencies in the reporting of mammography. The use of BI-RADS in mammography has been mandated by the US Food and Drug Administration, and BI-RADS criteria have been extended to include MRI and ultrasound (US) of the breast.

There are now multiple RADS applied to various organs, pathological conditions and modalities. Most of these ascribe a relative probability of malignancy based on imaging features; CAD-RADS provides a structured categorization of coronary artery disease on CT angiography. Some systems incorporate evidence-based recommendations, including biopsy, further imaging, specialist assessment and follow-up, such as TI-RADS for thyroid lesions. Commonly used RADS are summarized in Table 3.1. Further details of specific RADS may be found in relevant chapters and on the companion website.

3.4 MULTIPARAMETRIC IMAGING

As the name would suggest, multiparametric imaging refers to the use of multiple imaging parameters

Table 3.1 Types of Reporting and Data System (RADS).

System	Modality	Pathological condition
BI-RADS	Mammography, US, MRI	Breast cancer
C-RADS	CT colonography	Colon cancer
CAD-RADS	CT coronary angiography	Coronary artery disease
LI-RADS	CT, MRI, US, CEUS	Liver cancer, especially HCC
Lung-RADS	Low-dose chest CT	Lung cancer screening
NI-RADS	PET-CT, CT, MRI	Head and neck cancer
O-RADS	US	Ovarian cysts and masses
PI-RADS	MRI	Prostate cancer
TI-RADS	US	Cancer in thyroid nodules

Abbreviations: CEUS, contrast-enhanced US; HCC, hepatocellular carcinoma.

to maximize diagnostic accuracy. Conventional imaging provides structural imaging information, including the shape and size of lesions and their relationship to anatomical structures. Chapter 1 includes a description of hybrid imaging in which scintigraphy techniques – single photon emission CT (SPECT) and positron emission tomography (PET) – are combined with CT or MRI to provide a combination of functional and anatomical information. This can be thought of as a type of multifunctional or multiparametric imaging.

Multiparametric MRI uses conventional images combined with other MRI techniques (also described in Chapter 1), such as diffusion-weighted imaging (DWI), perfusion-weighted MRI (PWI), dynamic contrast-enhanced (DCE) and magnetic resonance spectroscopy (MRS). Multiparametric MRI is currently used most in imaging the prostate and brain (Fig. 3.1). In the prostate, a combination of T2-weighted imaging, DWI and DCE is used to detect and monitor prostate cancer. In neuroradiology, conventional anatomical imaging is combined with DWI, PWI and MRS to provide anatomical and other biophysical data such as cellularity, angiogenesis and neovascularity, and metabolite concentrations. Multiparametric MRI is finding multiple applications in imaging of brain tumours, including grading and characterization of neoplasms, assessment of the response to therapy and differentiating neoplasms from non-neoplastic mass-like inflammation and demyelination.

3.5 RADIOMICS

The ability to combine data obtained from multiple imaging modalities has led to the evolving concept of radiomics. The premise of radiomics is that medical images may be analysed quantitatively to obtain information about disease processes that may not be perceptible to the human eye. Most research in radiomics to date has been in oncology and is directed at more accurate classification of tumours and better prediction of clinical outcomes. Radiomics consists of multiple steps in image data analysis. These include the delineation of a region of interest, such as a specific lesion or organ. This is known as image segmentation and is followed by further image processing to extract specific features of interest. Data from multiple imaging modalities may be combined with clinical data such as tissue genomics and protein expression. To date, radiomics has not become established in clinical practice, but that may change with the application of increasingly sophisticated software and with the increasing use of artificial intelligence (AI) techniques.

3.6 ARTIFICIAL INTELLIGENCE

AI is developing into a powerful tool for many medical specialties, and its functions continue to evolve. Medical imaging is one specialty driving the use of AI

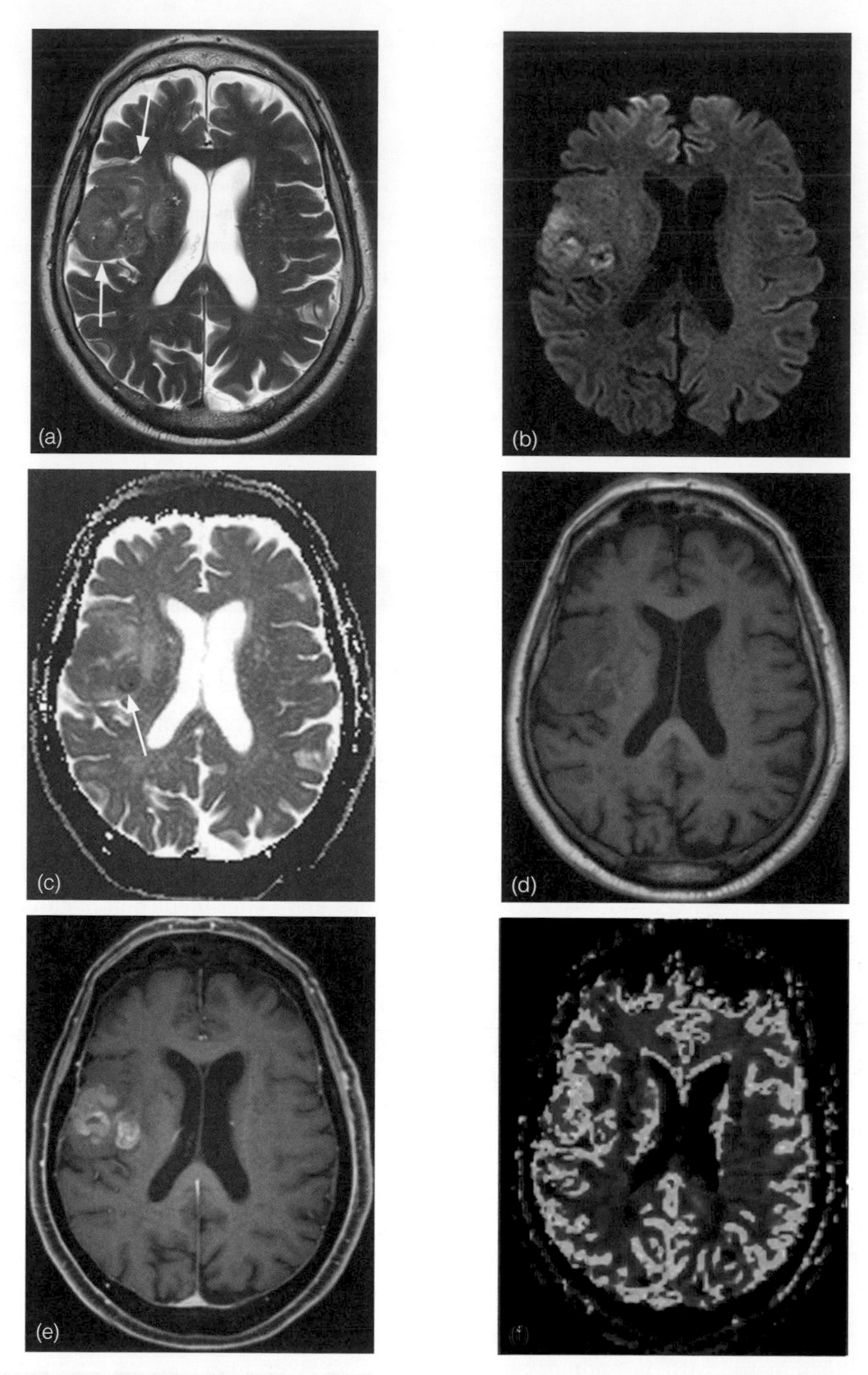

Figure 3.1 Multiparametric MRI: glioblastoma. (a) The T2-weighted image shows a mass of intermediate signal in the right frontal lobe (arrows). (b) The diffusion-weighted image shows increased signal in keeping with diffusion restriction. (c) An apparent diffusion coefficient (ADC) map shows variable reduction in ADC values, which is most marked in the medial aspect of the tumour (arrow). (d) The T1-weighted image shows the mass to be of approximately the same signal as grey matter. (e) The T1 contrast-enhanced image shows heterogeneous enhancement. (f) The perfusion-weighted image shows regions of red colour in the mass corresponding to increased regional blood flow. Note that these correspond to regions of maximum diffusion restriction and contrast enhancement.

and expanding its many applications through extensive research and evaluation. Initially, radiologists were cautious about AI for fear of being displaced or superseded. Instead, AI has evolved in the last decade to augment the role of radiologists in modern clinical practice by optimizing clinical efficiency, improving accuracy and reducing redundancy. Soon all radiologists will use AI in daily medical practice.

3.6.1 TERMINOLOGY

Several terms in AI are used interchangeably in error, so an understanding of basic definitions is important:

- Artificial intelligence (AI) refers to computer informatics systems that have been specifically programmed to perform cognitive functions that would otherwise require human intelligence
- Machine learning (ML) is a subset of AI, in which computer learning involves pattern recognition to improve future performance
- Deep learning (DL) is a subset of ML that involves algorithms that employ deep neural networks. DL is the form of AI most relevant in image interpretation
- Neural networks are multiple layers of nodes (up to millions) that are interconnected and require training with large datasets
- Computer-aided diagnosis/detection (CAD) systems combine elements of AI and digital image processing to highlight possible abnormalities on medical images.

3.6.2 APPLICATIONS

Numerous applications of AI in radiology currently exist and are underpinned by a range of supportive research. These can be broadly categorized into detection, characterization, image quality and workflow.

DETECTION

- Detection of pathology with CAD, e.g. lung nodule detection on a chest radiograph (chest X-ray, CXR) or chest CT; breast lesion identification on mammography.

CHARACTERIZATION

- Probability of disease severity, complications and mortality, e.g. based on the histological subtype of primary brain malignancies as predicted by AI algorithms
- Lesion comparison, e.g. analysing tumour growth or treatment-induced regression between studies at multiple time points
- Tissue volume comparison with equivalent population means, e.g. brain volume in dementia and in neurodegenerative and demyelinating diseases
- Organ segmentation, which refers to the process of analysing individual organs or tissues within complex images, e.g. liver or pancreas on an abdominal CT or structures such as the hippocampus or basal ganglia on an MRI of the brain.

IMAGE QUALITY

- Imaging quality optimization using DL, e.g. correction of motion-degraded cross-sectional images
- Radiation dose optimization, e.g. imaging parameters in CT adjusted for individual patients.

WORKFLOW

- Detection of critical diagnoses to prioritize reporting so that urgent cases are notified to clinicians or radiologists, e.g. flagging a pneumothorax on a CXR
- Standardized report generation and synthesis
- Clinical decision tools, e.g. indicating the most appropriate investigation for a given clinical scenario.

3.6.3 DEVELOPMENT

A detailed description of AI algorithm development in medical imaging is beyond the scope of this book. In simple terms, algorithms are computer-based instructions (code) that calculate an output when applied to medical images. Algorithms are developed by training the system with large volumes of data; in this case, images that have a label (termed a 'ground truth'). For example, an AI algorithm for the detection of pneumothorax on an erect CXR is based on a large dataset of images, some of which have a pneumothorax and have been labelled as such by radiologists. The output generated by AI algorithms aids radiologists in interpreting medical images.

3.6.4 ISSUES WITH ARTIFICIAL INTELLIGENCE IN MEDICINE

There are numerous potential issues associated with the use of AI in humans. These include:

- Ethical concerns around the conduct of companies, software engineers, clinical teams and researchers exploring the use of AI in medicine
- The need for AI products to be exposed to the same level of regulation and safety as medical implants and drugs
- Medicolegal issues pertaining to the ownership of data and the entities responsible for the clinical application of an AI-based medical image assessment
- Consent for large dataset use for training
- Anonymization of images to ensure patient confidentiality
- Intellectual property questions regarding who should benefit financially from medical advances that are reliant on large training datasets
- Economic issues pertaining to AI utilization and resource allocation and the potential for inequalities.

3.6.5 FUTURE DIRECTIONS

Radiology training now incorporates AI to prepare future radiologists for a career in which human interpretation and problem solving are performed in parallel with ML and deep neural networks. Imaging biobanks are large digital storage facilities with increasing potential to provide massive datasets for AI training. Radiomics is a developing method whereby quantitative features from image-based datasets are integrated with established characterization processes to predict disease features such as prognosis and response to treatment. As computer power and storage capabilities grow, non-radiological inputs such as clinical, demographic, pathological and genetic parameters can be integrated into AI datasets, enhancing the predictive power of radiomics in disease management.

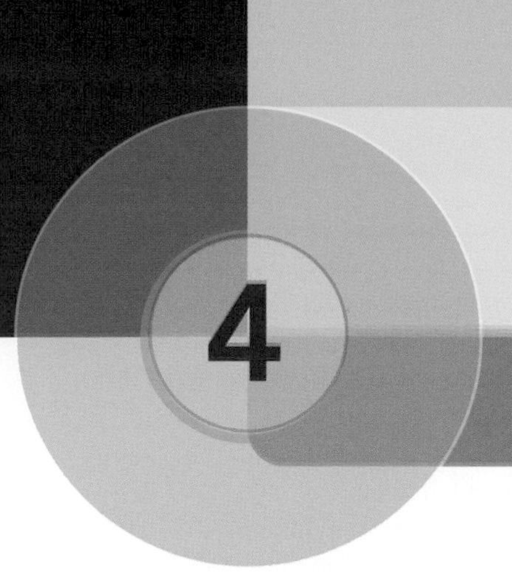

How to read a chest X-ray

This chapter is an introduction to the principles of chest radiograph (chest X-ray, CXR) interpretation. An overview of the standard CXR projections is followed by a brief outline of normal radiographic anatomy. Some notes on the assessment of a few important technical aspects are then provided as well as an outline of a suggested systematic approach. This is followed by more detailed notes on the interpretation of specific findings on a CXR.

4.1 PROJECTIONS PERFORMED

In general, two CXR views, posteroanterior (PA) and lateral, are used in the assessment of most chest conditions. Exceptions where a PA view alone would suffice include:

- Infants and children
- 'Screening' examinations, e.g. for immigration, insurance or diving medicals
- Follow-up of known conditions seen well on the PA view, e.g. pneumonia following antibiotics, metastases following chemotherapy, pneumothorax following drainage.

4.1.1 POSTEROANTERIOR ERECT

To obtain a PA erect CXR the patient is positioned standing with his or her anterior chest wall up against the X-ray detector plate. The X-ray tube lies behind the patient so that X-rays pass through in a posterior to anterior (PA) direction. The PA projection minimizes magnification of anterior structures and therefore provides more accurate assessment of cardiac size.

Reasons for performing the CXR erect:

- Physiological representation of the blood vessels of the mediastinum and lung. In the supine position, mediastinal veins and upper lobe vessels may be distended, leading to misinterpretation. A normal mediastinum may look abnormally wide on a supine CXR
- Gas passes upwards: erect CXR is more accurate for pneumothorax and for free subdiaphragmatic gas
- Fluid passes downwards: pleural effusion is more easily diagnosed.

4.1.2 LATERAL

Reasons for performing a lateral CXR:

- Further view of the lungs, especially those areas obscured on the PA radiograph, including posterior segments of the lower lobes, areas behind the hila and the left lower lobe, which lies behind the heart on the PA radiograph
- Further assessment of cardiac configuration
- Further anatomical localization of lesions
- More sensitive for small pleural effusions
- Lateral view of the thoracic spine.

OTHER PROJECTIONS

In certain circumstances, projections other than those outlined above may be used.

- Anteroposterior (AP)/supine radiograph:
  - Acutely ill or traumatized patients, and patients in intensive care and coronary care units
  - Mediastinum and heart appear wider on an AP supine film owing to venous distension and magnification
- Expiratory radiograph:
  - Increased sensitivity for small pneumothorax: in expiration, the lung is smaller whereas the pneumothorax does not change in volume
  - Suspected bronchial obstruction with air trapping, e.g. inhaled foreign body in a child: in expiration, the normal lung reduces in volume while the lung with an obstructed airway remains inflated
- Decubitus radiograph:
  - Radiograph performed with the patient lying on his or her side
  - Used occasionally in patients too ill to stand where pleural effusion or pneumothorax are suspected and not definitely diagnosed on an AP film
- Oblique radiograph: suspected rib fracture or other chest wall pathologies
- Lateral sternal radiograph: suspected sternal fracture or sternomanubrial dislocation.

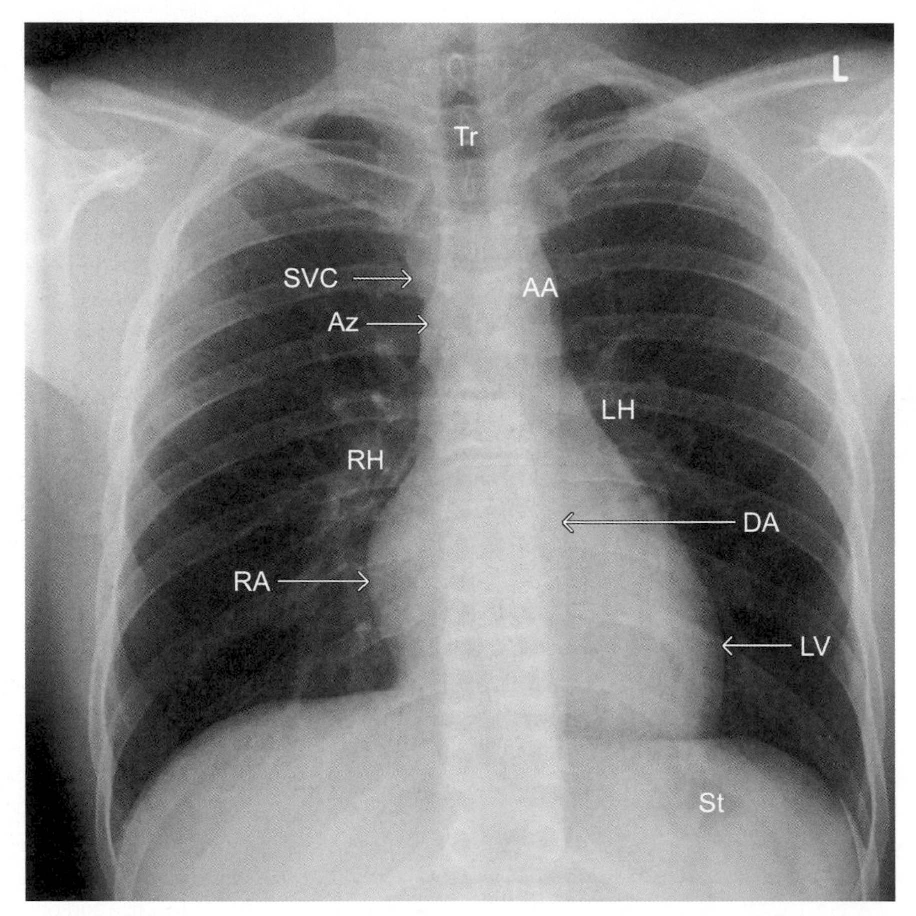

Figure 4.1 Normal posteroanterior CXR. Note the following structures: aortic arch (AA), azygos vein (Az), descending aorta (DA), left hilum (LH), left ventricle (LV), right atrium (RA), right hilum (RH), stomach (St), superior vena cava (SVC), trachea (Tr).

4.2 RADIOGRAPHIC ANATOMY

4.2.1 POSTEROANTERIOR ERECT

Look at a normal PA CXR (Fig. 4.1) and try to identify the following features:

- Trachea in the midline, plus its division into right and left main bronchi
- Right paratracheal stripe: a thin line on the right margin of the trachea:
  - May be lost or thickened in the presence of lymphadenopathy
- Azygos vein: small convex opacity, located in the concavity formed by the junction of the trachea and right main bronchus
- Superior vena cava (SVC): straight border, continuous inferiorly with the right heart border
- Right heart border: formed by the right atrium and outlined by the aerated right middle lobe
- Right hilum: midway between the diaphragm and lung apex:
  - Formed by the right main bronchus and right pulmonary artery, and their lobar divisions
- Aortic arch, sometimes termed the aortic 'knuckle'
- Descending aorta: traced downwards from the aortic arch as a border to the left of the spine:
  - Descending aorta may be obscured by a posterior mediastinal mass or by left lower lobe pathology
- Main pulmonary artery: slightly convex margin between the aortic arch and the left heart border
- Left hilum: posterior to the main pulmonary artery and extending laterally:
  - Formed by the left main bronchus and left pulmonary artery, and their lobar divisions
  - Note that the left hilum is slightly higher than the right
- Left heart border: formed by the left ventricle, except in cases where the right ventricle is enlarged
- Left atrial appendage: lies on the upper left cardiac border; not seen unless it, or the left atrium, is enlarged.

4.2.2 LATERAL

The lateral view is usually performed with the patient's arms held out horizontally. Look at a normal lateral CXR (Fig. 4.2) and try to identify the following features:

- Humeral heads: round opacities projected over the lung apices
- Trachea: air-filled structure in the upper chest, midway between the anterior and posterior chest walls
- Posterior aspect of the aortic arch: convexity posterior to the trachea
- Trachea can be followed inferiorly to the carina, where the right and left main bronchi may be seen end-on as round lucencies
- Left main pulmonary artery forms an opacity posterior and slightly superior to the carina

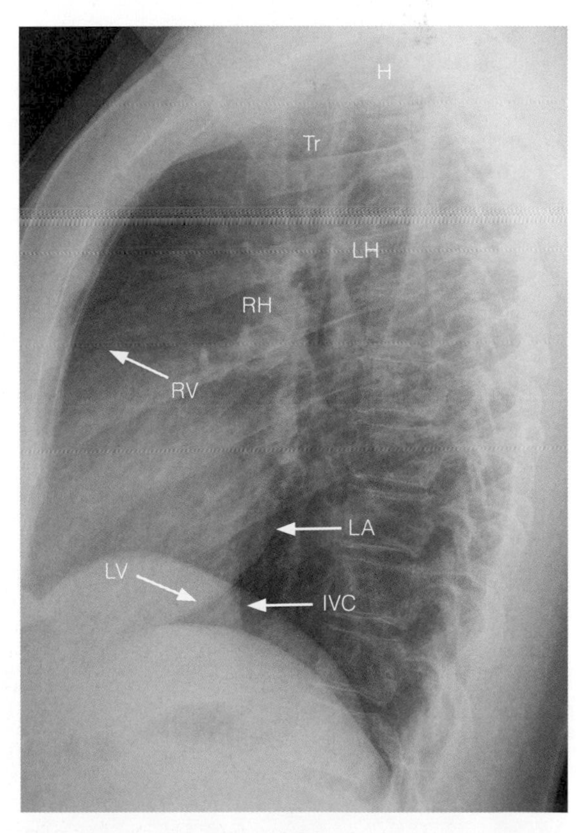

Figure 4.2 Normal lateral CXR. Note the following structures: humeral head (H), inferior vena cava (IVC), left atrium (LA), left hilum (LH), left ventricle (LV), right hilum (RH), right ventricle (RV), trachea (Tr).

- Right pulmonary artery forms an opacity anterior and slightly inferior to the carina
- Posterior cardiac border: formed by the left atrium superiorly and the left ventricle inferiorly
- Anterior cardiac border: formed by the right ventricle
- Main pulmonary artery: forms a convex opacity continuous with the right upper cardiac border.

4.3 TECHNICAL ASSESSMENT

Prior to making a diagnostic assessment it is worthwhile pausing briefly to assess the technical quality of the PA film by assessing centring, rotation and the degree of inspiration.

- Centring of the patient:
  - With proper centring of the patient the lung apices and both costophrenic angles should be visualized
- Rotation:
  - Rotation of the patient may cause anatomical distortion
  - The easiest way to ensure that there is no rotation is to check that the spinous processes of the upper thoracic vertebrae lie midway between the medial ends of the clavicles
- Degree of inspiration:
  - Inadequate inspiration may lead to overdiagnosis of pulmonary opacity or mediastinal widening (Fig. 4.3)
  - With an adequate inspiration, the hemidiaphragms should lie at the level of the fifth or sixth ribs anteriorly, and in children the trachea should be straight.

4.4 DIAGNOSTIC ASSESSMENT

The most important factor in the interpretation of any medical imaging investigation is the clinical context. Accurate interpretation of the CXR may be difficult or impossible in the absence of relevant and accurate clinical information, such as:

- Symptoms: fever, chest pain, shortness of breath, haemoptysis
- Duration of symptoms
- Relevant results from other tests such as spirometry or bronchoscopy

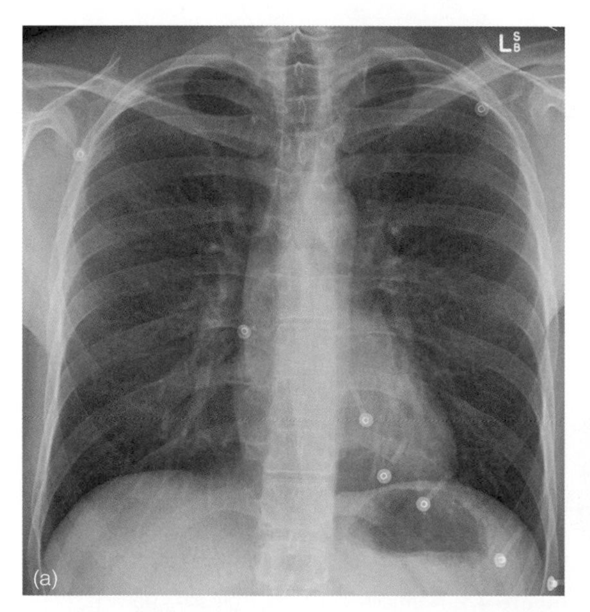

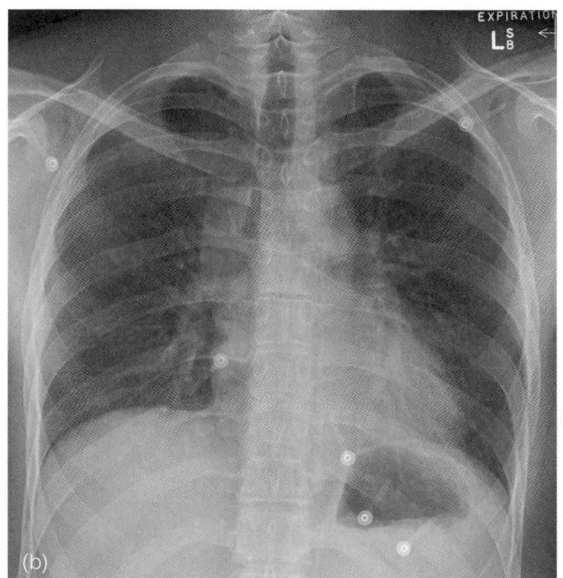

Figure 4.3 Effects of respiration. (a) Inspiratory posteroanterior (PA) CXR. (b) Expiratory PA CXR demonstrates increased apparent mediastinal width and reduced lung volumes. The multiple round opacities on both radiographs are electrocardiogram (ECG) electrodes.

- Relevant past medical history, especially malignancy
- Availability of previous CXRs for comparison to assess whether visible abnormalities are acute or chronic.

When looking at CXRs, use of a systemic checklist approach as outlined in Tables 4.1 and 4.2 will assist in the detection of relevant findings.

4.5 COMMON FINDINGS ON CHEST RADIOGRAPH

The following sections will provide more detailed notes on common findings on a CXR that may be encountered with various pathologies and clinical scenarios. These will be discussed in the order of the systematic approach outlined above, starting with

Table 4.1 Checklist for the posteroanterior view.

Structure/anatomical region	Specific features
Heart	Position, size, configuration, calcification
Mediastinum	Trachea, aorta, SVC, azygos vein
Right and left hilum	Compare relative size, density and position
Pulmonary blood vessels	Compare size of upper and lower lobe vessels
Lungs	Check lungs from top to bottom, and from central to peripheral
'Hidden areas'	• Behind the heart • Behind each hilum • Behind the hemidiaphragms • Lung apices
Lung contours	Mediastinal margins, cardiac borders, hemidiaphragms
Pleural spaces	Check around the periphery of the lung for pleural effusion, pneumothorax, pleural thickening, plaques and calcification
Bones and chest wall	Ribs, clavicles, scapulae and humeri
Other	• Check below the hemidiaphragms for free gas and to ensure that the stomach bubble is in the correct position beneath the left hemidiaphragm • In female patients, check that both breast shadows are present and that there has not been a previous mastectomy • Check the axillae and lower neck for masses or surgical clips

Abbreviation: SVC, superior vena cava.

Table 4.2 Checklist for the lateral view.

Structure/anatomical region	Specific features
Heart	Position, size, configuration, calcification
Mediastinum	Trachea, aorta
Right and left hilum	Compare relative size, density and position
Lungs	• Retrosternal airspace, between the posterior surface of the sternum and the anterior surface of the heart • Identify both hemidiaphragms • Posterior costophrenic angles: very small pleural effusions are seen with greater sensitivity than on the PA film
Bones	Sternum and thoracic spine

Abbreviation: PA, posteroanterior.

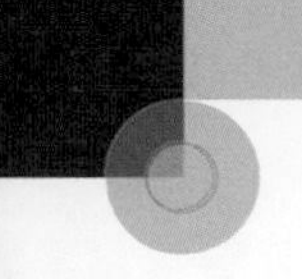

the heart, and progressing through the mediastinum and hila, pulmonary blood vessels, lungs and pleural spaces. Findings related to the lungs will be discussed under separate headings to consider diffuse pulmonary opacity, lobar consolidation and collapse, single and multiple nodules and masses, emphysema and bronchiectasis. For notes on further investigations of respiratory disease, see Chapter 5.

4.5.1 HEART

Assessment of the heart (more correctly referred to as the 'cardiac silhouette') on CXR includes the following features:

- Cardiac position and situs
- Cardiac size
- Specific cardiac chamber enlargement
- Cardiac valve calcification.

CARDIAC POSITION

The normal cardiac apex is directed toward the left chest wall. About two-thirds of the normally positioned heart lies to the left of the midline. Malposition of the heart refers to an abnormally positioned heart, though with normal orientation of the chambers and with the apex still pointing to the left. The heart may be malpositioned to one side by collapse of the ipsilateral lung or by a contralateral space-occupying process such as tension pneumothorax or large pleural effusion. Dextrocardia refers to reversal of the normal orientation of the heart with the cardiac apex directed to the patient's right. With isolated dextrocardia other organs such as the liver and stomach are positioned normally. In situs inversus all the organs are reversed, and the gastric bubble lies beneath the right hemidiaphragm (Fig. 4.4).

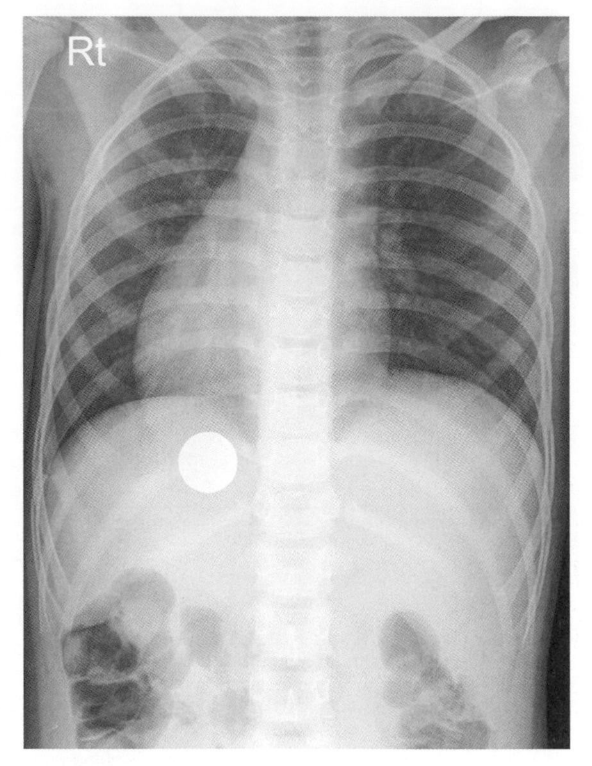

Figure 4.4 Situs inversus: CXR and AXR. Radiograph performed in a 6-year-old girl for a swallowed coin. The orientation of the visible organs is a 'mirror image' of normal, with the heart and stomach to the right and the liver on the left.

CARDIAC SIZE

The cardiothoracic ratio (CTR) refers to the ratio between the maximum transverse diameter of the heart and the maximum transverse diameter of the chest. The CTR is usually expressed as the ratio of these measurements (Fig. 4.5). A CTR of greater than 0.5 on a PA CXR (>0.6 on an AP) is said to indicate cardiac enlargement, although there are several variables, not least of which is the shape of the patient's chest. CTR is unreliable as a one-off measurement; of more significance is changing heart size on serial CXRs.

SIGNS OF SPECIFIC CHAMBER ENLARGEMENT

The signs of specific cardiac chamber enlargement are given in Table 4.3.

CARDIAC VALVE CALCIFICATION

Calcification of the mitral valve annulus is common in elderly patients and may be associated with mitral regurgitation (Fig. 4.6). Calcification of the mitral valve leaflets may occur in rheumatic heart disease or mitral valve prolapse. Mitral valve leaflet or annulus calcification is seen on the lateral CXR inferior to a line from the carina to the anterior costophrenic

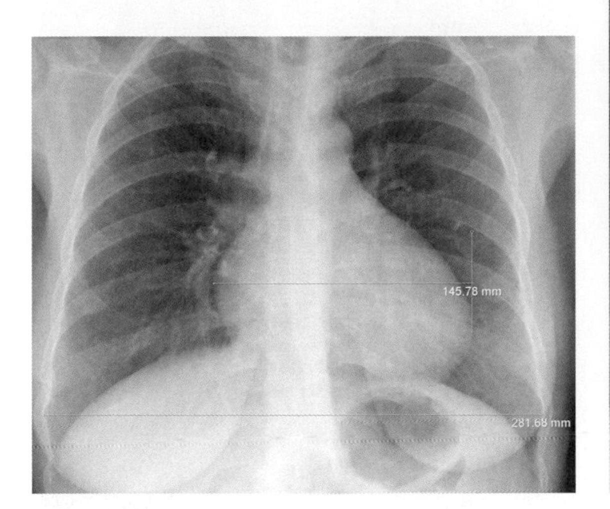

Figure 4.5 Measurement of the cardiothoracic ratio (CTR). CXR shows transverse measurements of the cardiac silhouette and the maximum width of the thorax. The CTR is the ratio calculated between these measurements.

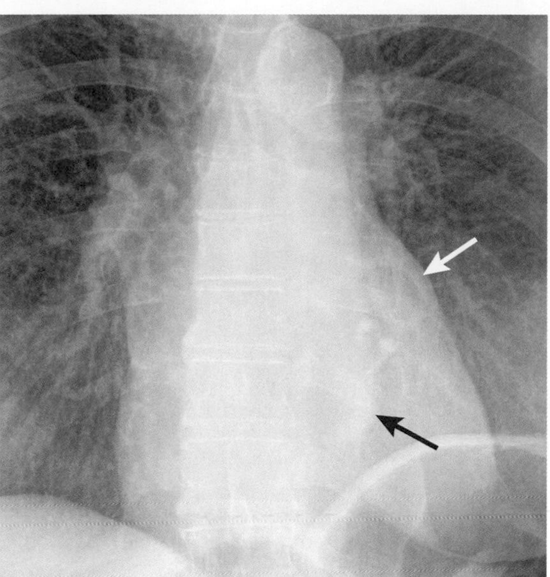

Figure 4.6 Left atrial enlargement and mitral annular calcification. The heart is enlarged with prominence of the left atrial appendage producing a bulge of the upper left cardiac border (white arrow). There is also curvilinear calcification in the mitral valve annulus (black arrow).

Table 4.3 Signs of cardiac chamber enlargement.

Cardiac chamber	Radiological signs of enlargement
Right atrium	Bulging right heart border
Left atrium	• Prominent left atrial appendage on the left heart border (Fig. 4.6) • Double outline of the right heart border • Splayed carina with elevation of the left main bronchus • Bulge of the upper posterior heart border on the lateral view
Right ventricle	• Elevated cardiac apex • Bulging of the anterior upper part of the heart border on the lateral view
Left ventricle	Bulging lower left cardiac border with a depressed cardiac apex

angle, and on the PA CXR inferior to a line from the right cardiophrenic angle to the left hilum.

Aortic valve calcification is associated with aortic stenosis and is seen on the lateral CXR lying above and anterior to a line from the carina to the anterior costophrenic angle.

4.5.2 MEDIASTINAL MASSES

Signs on a CXR that a central opacity or mass lies within the mediastinum rather than the lung include:

- Continuity with the mediastinal outline
- Sharp margin
- Convex margin
- Absence of air bronchograms.

The logical classification and differential diagnosis of mediastinal masses is based on localization to the anterior, middle or posterior mediastinum.

ANTERIOR MEDIASTINAL MASS

CXR signs of an anterior mediastinal mass (Fig. 4.7):

- Merge with the cardiac border

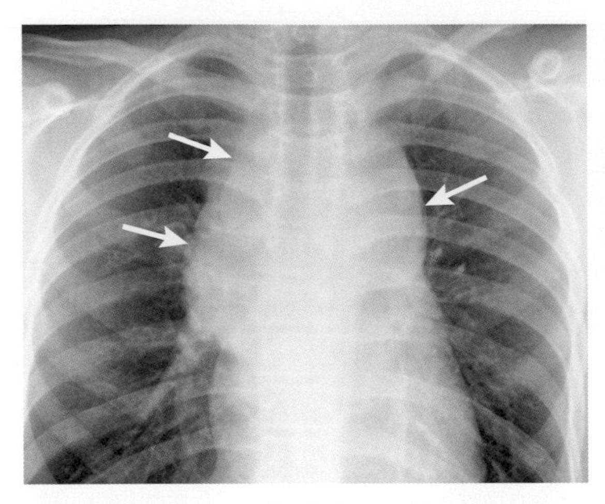

Figure 4.7 Anterior mediastinal mass: Hodgkin disease. A bilateral anterior mediastinal mass merging with the upper cardiac borders (arrows). Note that the mass does not extend above the clavicles.

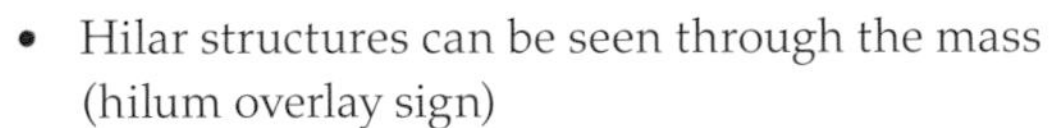

- Hilar structures can be seen through the mass (hilum overlay sign)
- Masses passing upwards into the neck merge radiologically with the soft tissues of the neck and so are not seen above the clavicles:
  - This is known as the cervicothoracic sign; a lesion seen above the clavicles must lie adjacent to aerated lung apices, i.e. posterior and within the thorax
- Displaced trachea.

Causes of an anterior mediastinal mass:

- Retrosternal goitre
- Lymphadenopathy:
  - Lymphoma, especially Hodgkin disease
  - Metastases
- Thymic tumour or cyst
- Germ cell tumour
- Aneurysm of ascending aorta.

MIDDLE MEDIASTINAL MASS

CXR signs of a middle mediastinal mass (Fig. 4.8):

- Opacity that merges with the hilar structures and cardiac borders (loss of the hilum overlay sign).

Causes of a middle mediastinal mass:

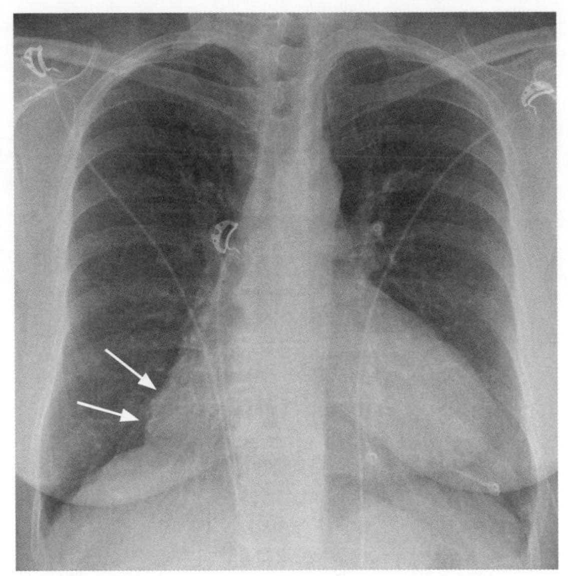

Figure 4.8 Middle mediastinal mass: pericardial cyst. A right middle mediastinal cyst seen as a convex opacity merging with the right cardiac border (arrows).

- Lymphadenopathy, mediastinal or hilar:
  - Bronchogenic carcinoma; less commonly other tumours
  - Lymphoma
- Bronchogenic or pericardial cyst
- Aortic aneurysm.

POSTERIOR MEDIASTINAL MASS

CXR signs of a posterior mediastinal mass (Fig. 4.9):

- Does not obscure the heart and middle mediastinal structures:
  - Cardiac borders and hila clearly seen
- Posterior descending aorta obscured
- May be underlying vertebral changes.

Causes of a posterior mediastinal mass:

- Hiatus hernia:
  - Round opacity located behind the heart
  - May contain a fluid level
- Neurogenic tumour:
  - Well-defined mass in the paravertebral region
  - May be associated with erosion or destruction of vertebral bodies or posterior ribs

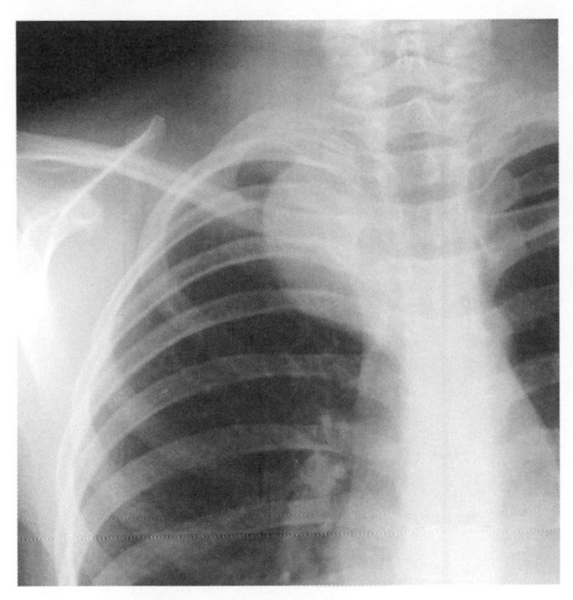

Figure 4.9 Posterior mediastinal mass: neurogenic tumour. A mass can be seen above the clavicle, indicating a posterior position ('cervicothoracic sign').

- Anterior thoracic meningocele:
  - Associated with neurofibromatosis
- Neurenteric cyst:
  - Associated with vertebral abnormalities
- Aneurysm of descending thoracic aorta
- Paravertebral lymphadenopathy or abscess.

4.5.3 HILAR DISORDERS

Each hilar complex, as seen on the PA and lateral CXRs, comprises the proximal pulmonary arteries, bronchus, pulmonary veins and lymph nodes. Hilar lymph nodes are not visualized on a CXR unless enlarged. In assessing hilar enlargement, be it bilateral or unilateral, one must decide whether it is due to enlargement of the pulmonary arteries or to some other cause, such as lymphadenopathy or a mass. If the branching pulmonary arteries are seen to converge into an apparent mass, this is a useful sign of an enlarged main pulmonary artery (hilum convergence sign).

Causes of unilateral hilar enlargement:

- Bronchogenic carcinoma (Fig. 4.10)
- Infection:
  - Tuberculosis (TB)

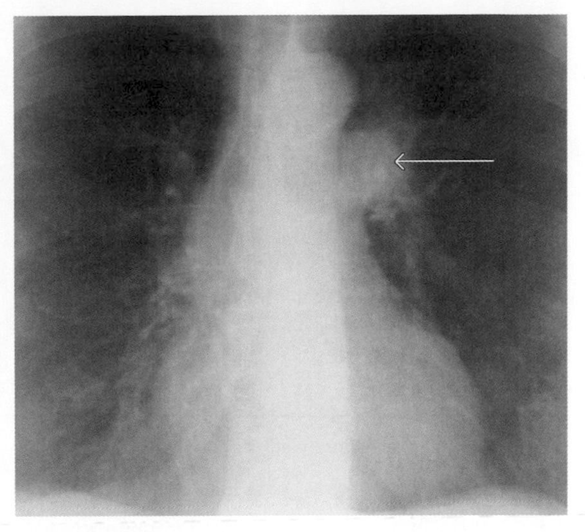

Figure 4.10 Unilateral hilar enlargement (arrow): bronchogenic carcinoma. Note the enlargement of the left hilar opacity, producing an asymmetric appearance compared with the normal right side.

  - Mycoplasma
- Perihilar pneumonia:
  - Pneumonia lying anterior or posterior to the hilum may cause *apparent* hilar enlargement on the PA film
  - Usually obvious on the lateral film
- Other causes of lymphadenopathy (more commonly bilateral):
  - Lymphoma
  - Sarcoidosis
- Causes of enlargement of a single pulmonary artery:
  - Poststenotic dilatation on the left side due to pulmonary stenosis
  - Massive unilateral pulmonary embolus (Fleischner sign)
  - Pulmonary artery aneurysm (often calcified).

Causes of bilateral hilar enlargement:

- Bilateral pulmonary artery enlargement:
  - Pulmonary arterial hypertension
- Lymphoma:
  - Often asymmetrical
- Metastatic malignancy:
  - Bronchogenic carcinoma
  - Non-pulmonary primary, e.g. testis

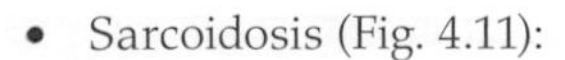

- Sarcoidosis (Fig. 4.11):
    - o Hilar lymphadenopathy is usually symmetrical and lobulated, and associated with right paratracheal lymphadenopathy (1–2–3 sign or Garland triad)
    - o Often accompanied by small interstitial nodules 2–5 mm in diameter spread through both lungs, predominantly in the midzones.

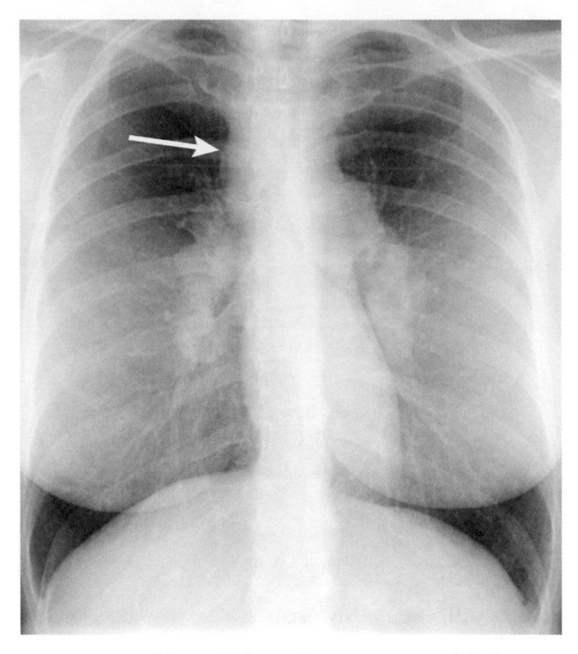

Figure 4.11 Bilateral hilar enlargement: sarcoidosis. Posteroanterior view showing an enlarged and lobulated outline of the right and left hila as a result of lymphadenopathy. Also note focal widening of the right mediastinal outline as a result of lymphadenopathy (arrow).

4.5.4 PULMONARY BLOOD VESSELS

The normal pulmonary vascular pattern has the following features:

- Arteries branching vertically to upper and lower lobes
- Veins running roughly horizontally towards the lower hila
- Upper lobe vessels smaller than lower lobe vessels on erect CXR
- Vessels become difficult to see in the peripheral thirds of the lungs.

Abnormal pulmonary vascular patterns are outlined below:

- Pulmonary venous hypertension:
    - o Associated with cardiac failure and mitral valve disease
    - o Blood vessels in the upper lobes appear larger than those in the lower lobes on erect CXR
    - o Often accompanied on CXR by other signs of cardiac failure: cardiomegaly, pulmonary oedema and pleural effusion.
- Pulmonary arterial hypertension (Fig. 4.12):
    - o Associated with long-standing pulmonary disease, including emphysema, multiple recurrent pulmonary emboli, left-to-right shunts (ventricular septal defect [VSD], atrial septal defect [ASD], patent ductus arteriosus [PDA])
    - o CXR: bilateral hilar enlargement due to enlarged proximal pulmonary arteries with a rapid decrease in the calibre of peripheral vessels ('pruning')

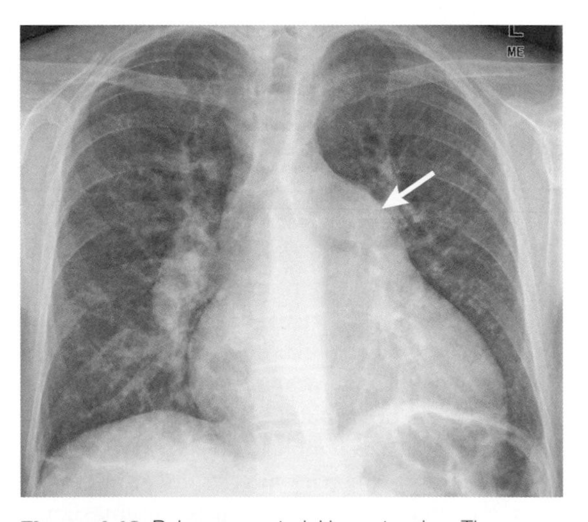

Figure 4.12 Pulmonary arterial hypertension. The dilated main pulmonary artery produces a bulge of the upper left cardiac border (arrow), higher than the left atrial appendage. Also note the prominent hila due to enlarged right and left pulmonary arteries and tapering of the calibre of pulmonary arteries as they extend through the lungs.

- Pulmonary plethora:
  - o Increased pulmonary blood flow caused by left-to-right cardiac shunts (VSD, ASD, PDA)
  - o CXR: increased size and number of pulmonary vessels
- Pulmonary oligaemia:
  - o Reduced pulmonary blood flow associated with pulmonary stenosis/atresia, tetralogy of Fallot, tricuspid atresia, Ebstein anomaly and severe emphysema
  - o CXR: general lucency (blackness) of the lung with a decreased size and number of pulmonary vessels and small main pulmonary arteries.

4.5.5 DIFFUSE PULMONARY SHADOWING

Anatomically, functionally and radiologically the lungs may be divided into two compartments: the alveoli (airspaces) and the interstitium. The interstitium refers to soft-tissue structures between the alveoli, and includes branching distal bronchi and bronchioles and accompanying arteries, veins and lymphatics, plus supporting connective tissue. The most distal small bronchioles are called terminal bronchioles. Distal to each terminal bronchiole, the lung acinus consists of multiple generations of tiny respiratory bronchioles and alveolar ducts. The alveoli, or airspaces, arise from the respiratory bronchioles and alveolar ducts. Disease processes that affect the lung may involve the alveoli or the interstitium, or both. One of the most important factors in narrowing the differential diagnosis of diffuse pulmonary shadowing is the ability to differentiate alveolar from interstitial shadowing.

ALVEOLAR OPACIFICATION

Different causes of alveolar opacification have the same soft-tissue density on CXR. Opacification may be due to oedema, inflammatory fluid, blood, protein or tumour cells. Because appearances are often non-specific, a definite diagnosis is usually only made when the CXR findings correlate with the clinical signs and symptoms.

CXR signs of alveolar shadowing:

- The term 'consolidation' refers to alveolar opacification that obscures pulmonary vessels
- Ground glass opacification refers to hazy alveolar shadowing that does not obscure pulmonary vessels and is better defined on computed tomography (CT)
- Alveolar opacity tends to appear rapidly after the onset of symptoms
- Fluffy, ill-defined areas of opacification
- Air bronchograms (Fig. 4.13): air-filled bronchi can be seen as they are outlined by surrounding consolidated lung; air bronchograms are not seen in pleural or mediastinal processes.

Three patterns of distribution of alveolar shadowing tend to occur:

1. Segmental or lobar distribution
2. Bilateral opacification spreading from the hilar regions into the lungs with relative sparing of the peripheral lungs; sometimes referred to as a 'bat wing' distribution

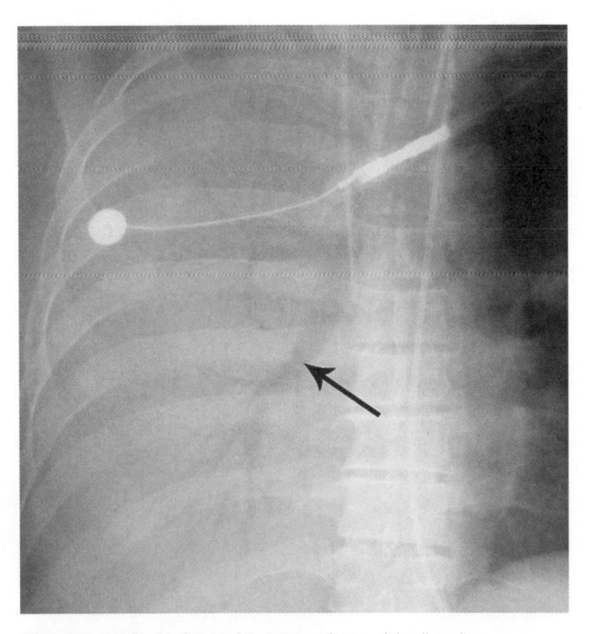

Figure 4.13 Air bronchograms (arrow) indicating extensive alveolar opacification. Air bronchograms are seen as a dark grey branching pattern due to air-filled bronchi outlined by opacified lung.

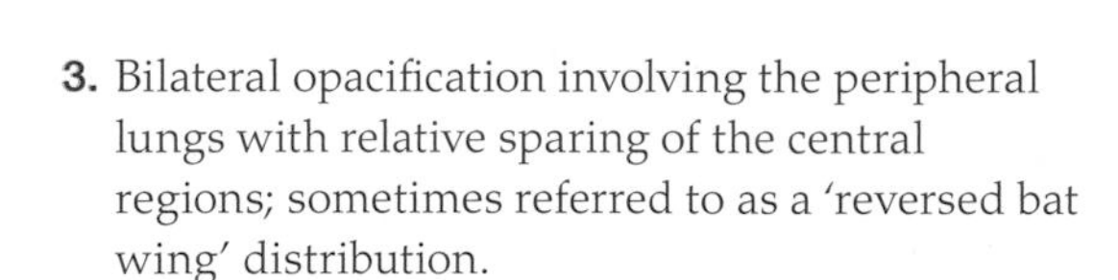

3. Bilateral opacification involving the peripheral lungs with relative sparing of the central regions; sometimes referred to as a 'reversed bat wing' distribution.

Alveolar opacification may be acute or chronic. Differential diagnosis lists based on the distribution of changes plus whether changes are acute or chronic may be developed.

CAUSES OF ALVEOLAR OPACIFICATION

Segmental/lobar alveolar pattern:

- Pneumonia (see below)
- Segmental/lobar collapse (see below)
- Pulmonary infarct
- Adenocarcinoma
- Contusion (associated with rib fractures, pneumothorax and other signs of trauma).

Acute bilateral central 'bat wing' pattern:

- Pulmonary oedema (Fig. 4.14):
  - Cardiac failure
  - Adult respiratory distress syndrome (ARDS)
  - Fluid overload
  - Drowning and other causes of aspiration
  - Head injury or other causes of raised intracranial pressure
  - Drugs and poisons (e.g. snake venom, heroin overdose)
  - Hypoproteinaemia (e.g. liver disease)
  - Blood transfusion reaction
- Pneumonia: *Pneumocystis jiroveci* pneumonia; TB; viral pneumonias; *Mycoplasma pneumoniae*
- Pulmonary haemorrhage: Goodpasture syndrome; anticoagulants; bleeding diathesis: haemophilia, disseminated intravascular coagulation (DIC).

Chronic bilateral central 'bat wing' pattern:

- Atypical pneumonia: TB, fungi
- Lymphoma and leukaemia
- Sarcoidosis: interstitial, nodular form much more common
- Pulmonary alveolar proteinosis.

Reversed 'bat wing' pattern:

- Chronic eosinophilic pneumonia
- Cryptogenic organizing pneumonia (COP)
- Granulomatosis with polyangiitis (formerly Wegener granulomatosis) (Fig. 4.15)

Figure 4.14 'Bat wing' pattern: pulmonary oedema. Extensive bilateral airspace opacification shows a parahilar distribution, known as the 'bat wing' pattern, with relative sparing of the lung periphery.

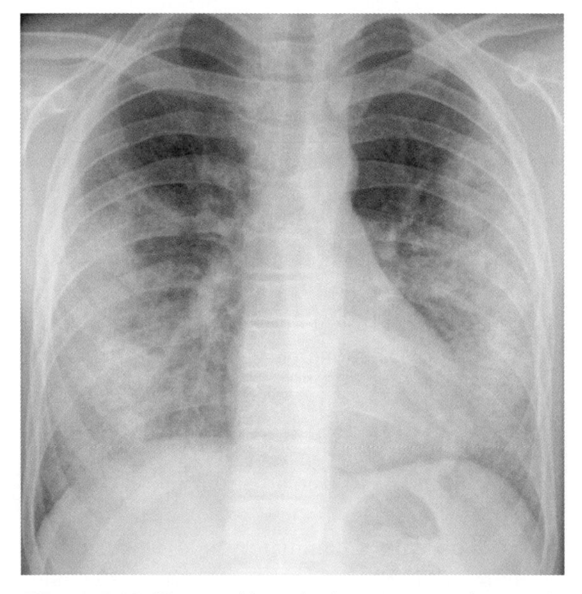

Figure 4.15 'Reversed bat wing' pattern: granulomatosis with polyangiitis. Note the presence of bilateral airspace opacity in a predominantly peripheral distribution with relative sparing of the central parahilar regions.

- Fat embolism: occurs 1–2 days after major trauma, particularly with fractures of the long bones of the lower limbs.

INTERSTITIAL OPACIFICATION

Three patterns of pulmonary opacification are seen in interstitial processes: linear, nodular and honeycomb pattern. These patterns may occur separately or together in the same patient, with considerable overlap in appearances often encountered.

Linear pattern:

- Network of fine lines running through the lungs due to thickened connective tissue septa
- Thickened interlobular septations (Kerley B or septal lines): short, thin lines predominantly in the lower zones extending 1–2 cm horizontally inwards from the lung surface (most reliable sign of interstitial oedema).

Nodular pattern:

- Nodules due to interstitial disease are small (1–5 mm), well defined and not associated with air bronchograms
- Nodules tend to be very numerous and are distributed evenly throughout the lungs.

Honeycomb pattern (Fig. 4.16):

- Honeycomb pattern represents the end stage of many of the interstitial processes listed below
- May also be seen with tuberous sclerosis, amyloidosis, neurofibromatosis and cystic fibrosis
- Honeycomb pattern implies extensive destruction of pulmonary tissue
- Thin-walled cysts that range in size from 3 to 10 mm replace the lung parenchyma
- Normal pulmonary vasculature is obscured
- Frequently complicated by pneumothorax.

CAUSES OF INTERSTITIAL OPACIFICATION

The list of interstitial disease processes is extensive. As with alveolar processes, CXR appearances are often non-specific. Short differential diagnosis lists of the more common disorders may be based on whether clinical presentation and CXR findings are acute, subacute or chronic. Chronic interstitial diseases may be categorized based on their distribution in the lungs, i.e. whether upper or lower zones are predominantly involved. These diseases are usually further characterized with CT.

Acute interstitial shadowing:

- Interstitial oedema: septal lines (Fig. 4.17); associated with cardiac enlargement and pleural effusions
- Acute interstitial pneumonia: usually viral.

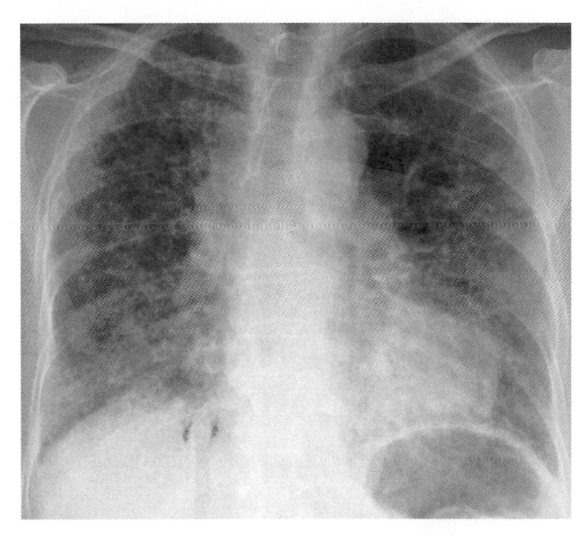

Figure 4.16 Honeycomb lung. Note the coarse interstitial opacity throughout both lungs with a 'shaggy' appearance of the cardiac borders and hemidiaphragms.

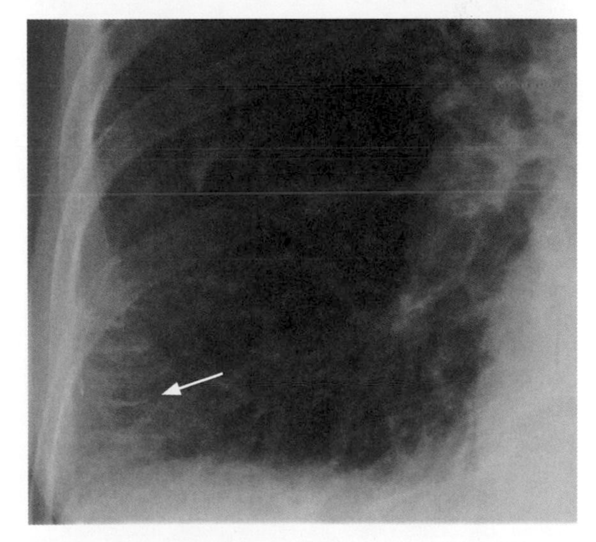

Figure 4.17 Septal (Kerley B) lines: interstitial oedema. Thickened septal lines are seen as short linear opacities extending into the lung from the pleural surface (arrow).

Subacute interstitial shadowing:

- Lymphangitis carcinomatosis: due to direct malignant infiltration and obstruction of the lymphatic pathways in the pulmonary interstitium (Fig. 4.18); may cause localized or diffuse interstitial shadowing
- Prominent linear and nodular shadowing with septal lines, often associated with mediastinal and/or hilar lymphadenopathy.

Chronic, upper zones:

- TB: upper lobe fibrosis; associated calcification in cavities (Fig. 4.19)
- Sarcoidosis: often associated with hilar lymphadenopathy, although pulmonary involvement alone occurs in 25% of cases
- Silicosis: associated with hilar lymph node calcification and enlargement; may also be associated with large confluent masses, i.e. progressive massive fibrosis (PMF)
- Extrinsic allergic alveolitis
- Bronchopulmonary aspergillosis
- Langerhans cell histiocytosis.

Chronic, lower zones:

- Idiopathic pulmonary fibrosis (IPF)

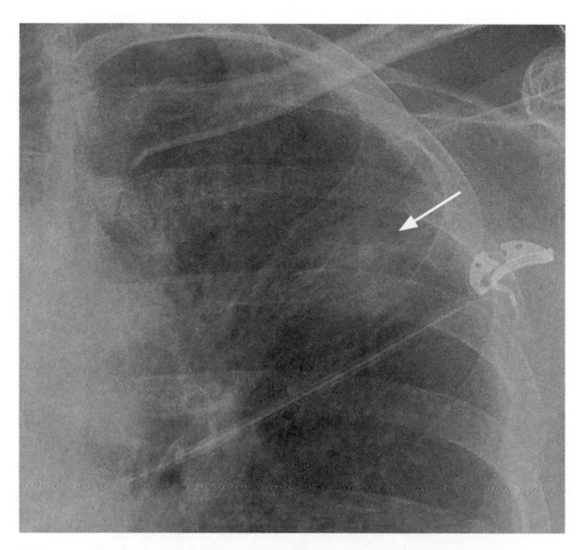

Figure 4.18 Lymphangitis carcinomatosis. A bronchogenic carcinoma is seen as a focal opacity (arrow). The coarse linear interstitial opacity throughout the left upper lobe indicates tumour invasion along the lymphatic channels in the lung, i.e. lymphangitis carcinomatosis.

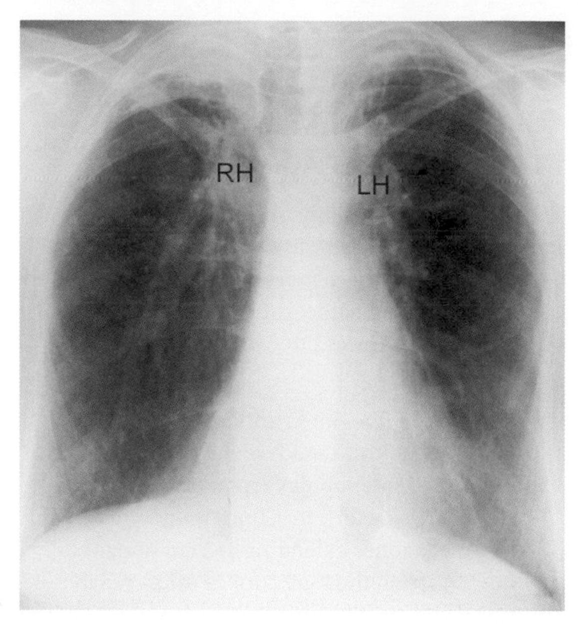

Figure 4.19 Upper lobe fibrosis. Note the ill-defined opacity at the lung apices. Elevation of the right and left hila (RH, LH) indicates volume loss in the upper lobes due to fibrosis.

- Asbestosis: may be associated with pleural plaques and calcification, particularly of the diaphragmatic pleura
- Connective tissue disorders: systematic lupus erythematosus (SLE); systemic sclerosis (scleroderma); dermatomyositis/polymyositis.

4.5.6 LOBAR PULMONARY CONSOLIDATION AND PNEUMONIA

Pulmonary consolidation occurs when air in the pulmonary alveoli is displaced by fluid (pus, blood and oedema), protein or cells. The radiographic signs of alveolar opacification are described above. Consolidation of a pulmonary lobe or segment is usually due to pneumonia, with other less common causes such as pulmonary infarct or contusion usually differentiated based on clinical history. Several radiographic signs may aid in localizing areas of pulmonary consolidation. These signs include consolidation adjacent to pulmonary fissures, the silhouette sign and increased density of the lower thoracic spine on a lateral view (Figs 4.20–4.28).

Table 4.4 Location of pulmonary consolidation or collapse according to fissure abutment.

Lobe of lung	Cause of straight margin
Right upper lobe (Fig. 4.20)	• Horizontal fissure inferiorly on PA film • Oblique fissure posteriorly on lateral film
Right middle lobe (Fig. 4.25)	• Horizontal fissure superiorly on PA film • Oblique fissure posteriorly on lateral film
Right lower lobe (Fig. 4.26)	• Oblique fissure anteriorly on lateral film • Collapse causes rotation and visualization of the oblique fissure on the PA film
Left upper lobe (Fig. 4.27)	• Oblique fissure posteriorly on lateral film
Left lower lobe (Fig. 4.28)	• Oblique fissure anteriorly on lateral film • Collapse causes rotation and visualization of the oblique fissure on the PA film

Abbreviation: PA, posteroanterior.

CONSOLIDATION ADJACENT TO FISSURES

Straight margins occur in the lungs at the pulmonary fissures. If an area of consolidation or collapse has a straight margin, that margin must abut a fissure (Fig. 4.20 and Table 4.4).

SILHOUETTE SIGN

The silhouette sign refers to loss of visualization of an anatomical structure or margin as a result of pathology, and is one of the most important principles in chest radiography. The key to understanding the silhouette sign is to remember the five principal densities that are recognized on plain radiographs (see Chapter 1 and Fig. 1.1): air/gas, fat, soft tissue/water, bone and contrast material/metal. The silhouette of an object will be seen with conventional radiography if its borders lie beside tissue of different density. This applies especially in the chest, where the hemidiaphragms, heart and mediastinal structures are well seen owing to their position adjacent to aerated lung. Should a part of lung lying against any of these structures become non-aerated owing to collapse, consolidation or a mass, the outline of that structure will no longer be seen (Fig. 4.21 and Table 4.5).

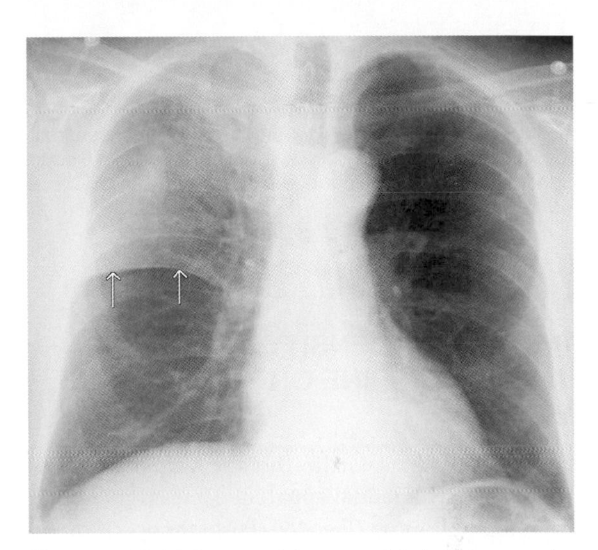

Figure 4.20 Right upper lobe consolidation: pneumonia. Note opacification of the right upper lobe bordered inferiorly by the horizontal fissure (arrows).

Table 4.5 Examples of the silhouette sign in the chest.

Part of lung that is non aerated	Border that is obscured
Right upper lobe (Fig. 4.20)	• Right border of ascending aorta • Right mediastinal margin
Right middle lobe (Fig. 4.21)	• Right heart border
Right lower lobe (Fig. 4.21)	• Right hemidiaphragm
Left upper lobe (Fig. 4.27)	• Aortic arch • Upper left cardiac border
Left lingula (Fig. 4.22)	• Left heart border
Left lower lobe (Fig. 4.23)	• Left hemidiaphragm • Descending aorta

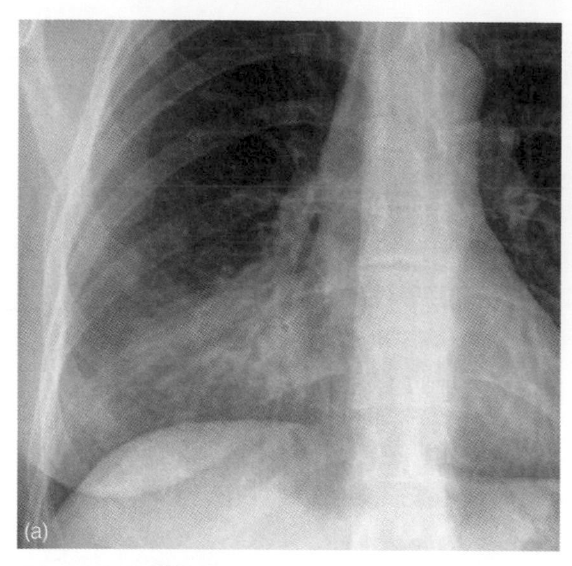

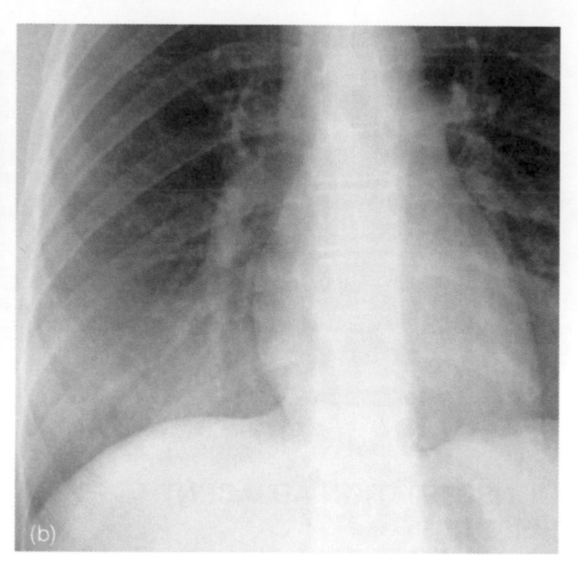

Figure 4.21 Silhouette sign: the presence or absence of visible radiographic borders can assist in the diagnosis and localization of pathology, as illustrated in these two examples. (a) Consolidation of the right middle lobe obscures the right heart border. The right hemidiaphragm can still be seen. (b) Consolidation of the right lower lobe. The right heart border can still be seen.

INCREASED DENSITY OF LOWER THORACIC SPINE ON THE LATERAL VIEW

On the lateral view, the thoracic vertebral bodies should show a gradual apparent decrease in density from top to bottom (Fig. 4.2). Posterior opacification in the right or left lower lobes may produce an apparent increase in density of the lower thoracic vertebral bodies. This may be the most obvious radiographic sign of lower lobe pneumonia (Fig. 4.23), particularly small areas of consolidation obscured by the heart on the PA view.

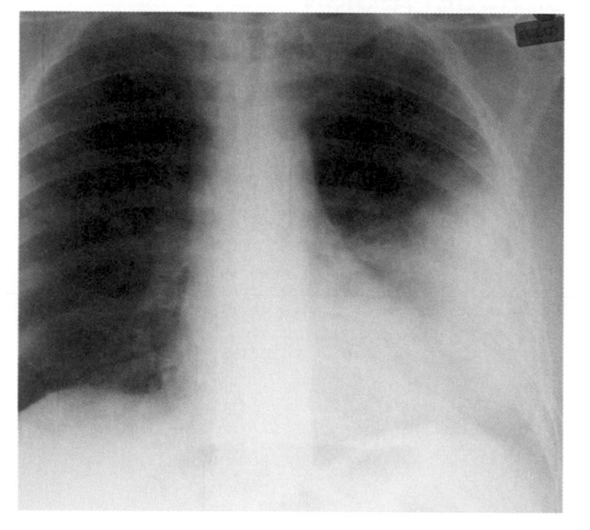

Figure 4.22 Lingula consolidation: pneumonia. Note that consolidation in the lingula obscures the left cardiac border.

4.5.7 PULMONARY COLLAPSE

Pulmonary collapse most commonly takes the form of linear or disc-like areas of focal collapse, referred to as linear or discoid atelectasis. Causes of linear atelectasis include:

- Postoperative hypoventilation
- Inflammatory or other painful pathology beneath the diaphragm, e.g. pancreatitis, acute cholecystitis
- Pulmonary embolus
- Following resolution of pneumonia (post inflammatory).

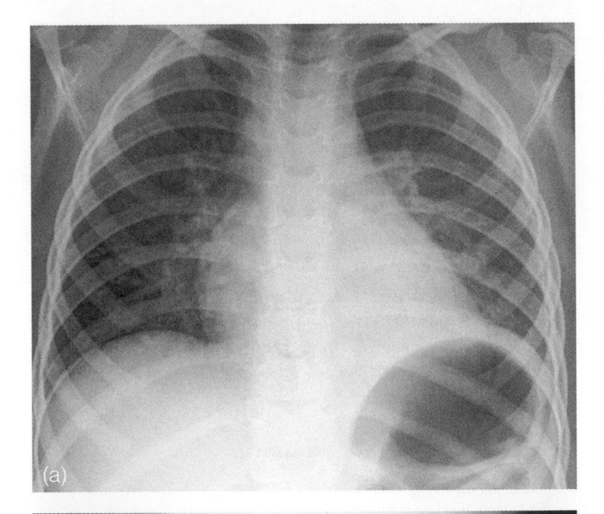

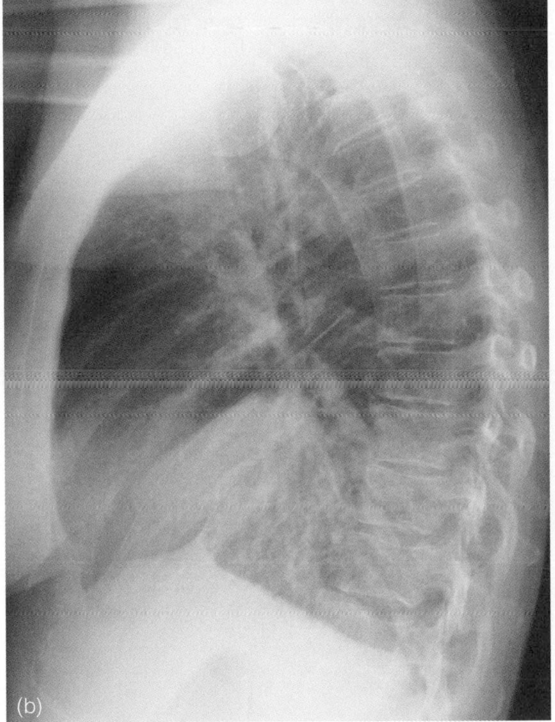

Figure 4.23 Left lower lobe consolidation: pneumonia. (a) On the posteroanterior view, consolidation of the left lower lobe produces opacity behind the left heart and loss of definition of the medial aspect of the left hemidiaphragm. (b) On the lateral view, consolidation in either lower lobe may produce an apparent increase in density of the lower thoracic vertebral bodies.

More extensive collapse may involve pulmonary segments or entire lobes. Causes of pulmonary lobar or segmental collapse include:

- Bronchial obstruction:
  - Tumour
  - Foreign body
  - Mucous plug, e.g. bronchiectasis, asthma, cystic fibrosis
- Passive collapse due to external pressure on the lung:
  - Pneumothorax
  - Pleural effusion or haemothorax
  - Diaphragmatic hernia (neonate)
- Scarring or fibrosis:
  - TB (upper lobes)
  - Radiation pneumonitis (post radiotherapy).

GENERAL SIGNS OF LOBAR COLLAPSE

The most important initial sign for differentiating lobar collapse from consolidation is decreased volume of the affected lung. Other signs of collapse include:

- Displacement of pulmonary fissures
- Local increase in density due to non-aerated lung
- Elevation of the ipsilateral hemidiaphragm
- Displacement of the hilum
- Displacement of the mediastinum towards the side of collapse
- Compensatory overinflation of adjacent lobes
- Loss of visualization of anatomical structures: silhouette sign.

SPECIFIC SIGNS OF LOBAR COLLAPSE

Each hilum may be thought of as a hinge, upon which the lung may rotate should there be upper or lower lobe collapse. The upper lobes tend to collapse upwards and anteriorly; the lower lobes collapse inferiorly and posteriorly. This leads to predictable radiographic appearances of the various types of lobar collapse, as summarized in Table 4.6 and illustrated in Figs 4.24–4.28.

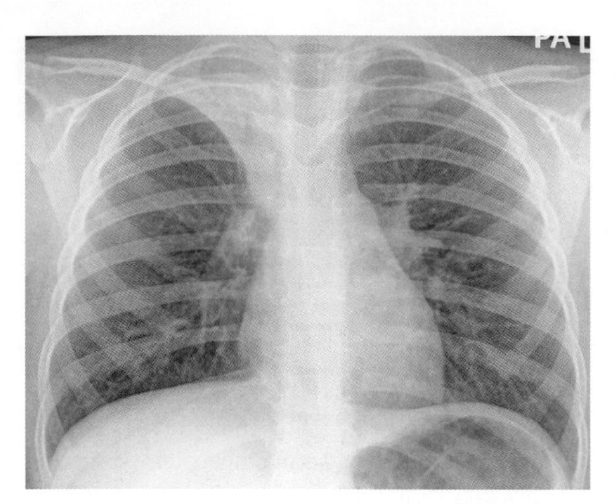

Figure 4.24 Right upper lobe collapse. Note the right upper zone opacity with a reduced volume of the right hemithorax and elevation of the horizontal fissure.

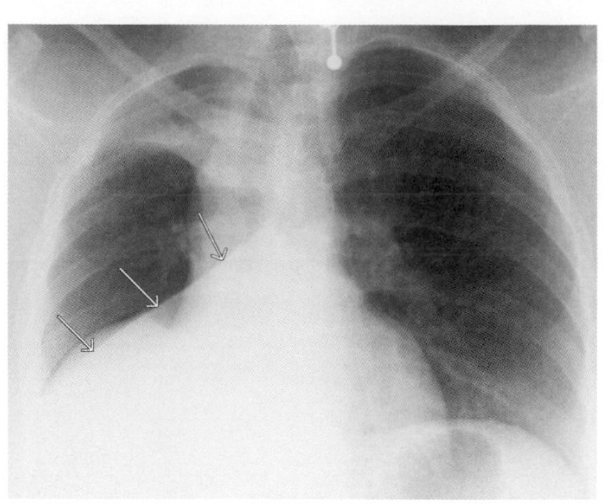

Figure 4.26 Right lower lobe collapse. A triangular opacity behind the right heart (arrows) with loss of definition of the right hemidiaphragm. The right heart border is still seen. Note that, in this case, the right upper lobe is also collapsed.

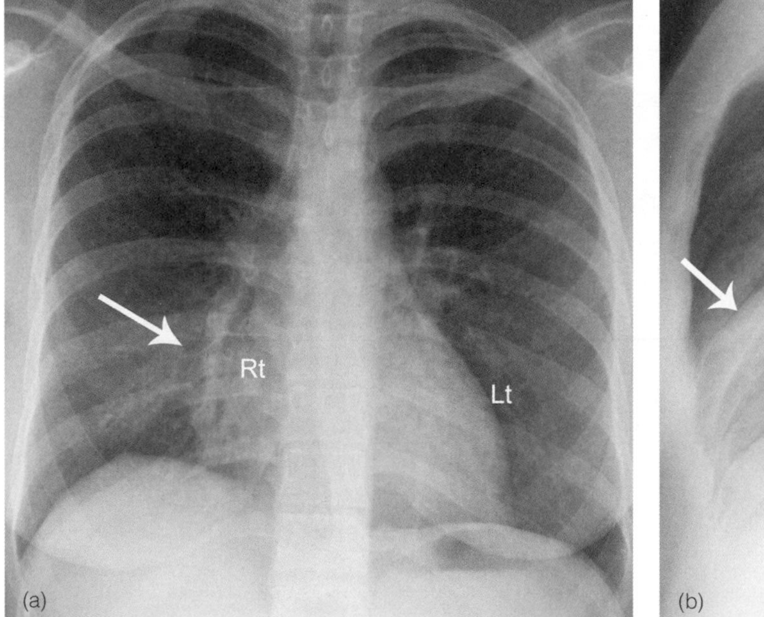

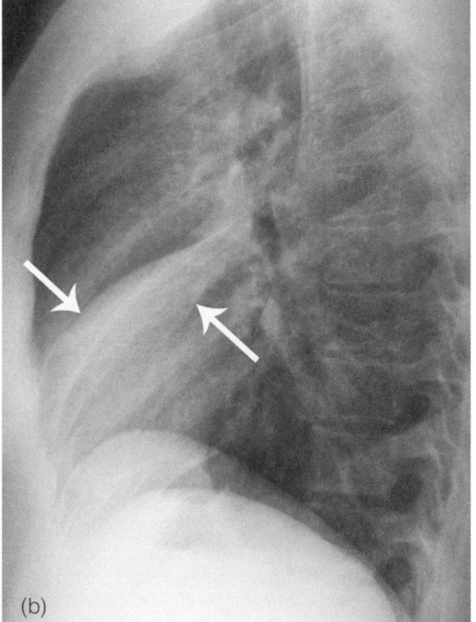

Figure 4.25 Right middle lobe collapse. (a) Posteroanterior view shows loss of volume on the right with opacity (arrow) obscuring the right heart border (Rt). Compare this with the left heart border (Lt), which is clearly seen. (b) Lateral view shows the typical triangular-shaped opacity produced by a collapsed right middle lobe (arrows).

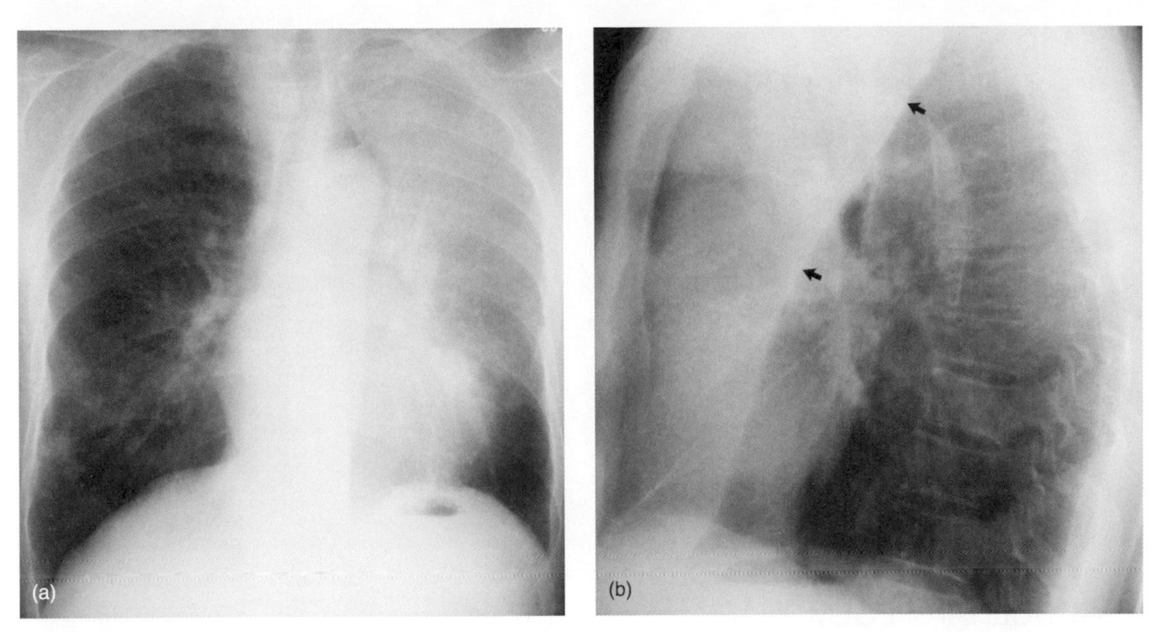

Figure 4.27 Left upper lobe collapse. (a) Posteroanterior view shows loss of volume on the left and opacity in the left upper zone. The aortic arch can be seen because of elevation of the aerated left lower lobe. (b) Lateral view shows the typical pattern of left upper lobe collapse with the oblique fissure pulled upwards and anteriorly (arrows).

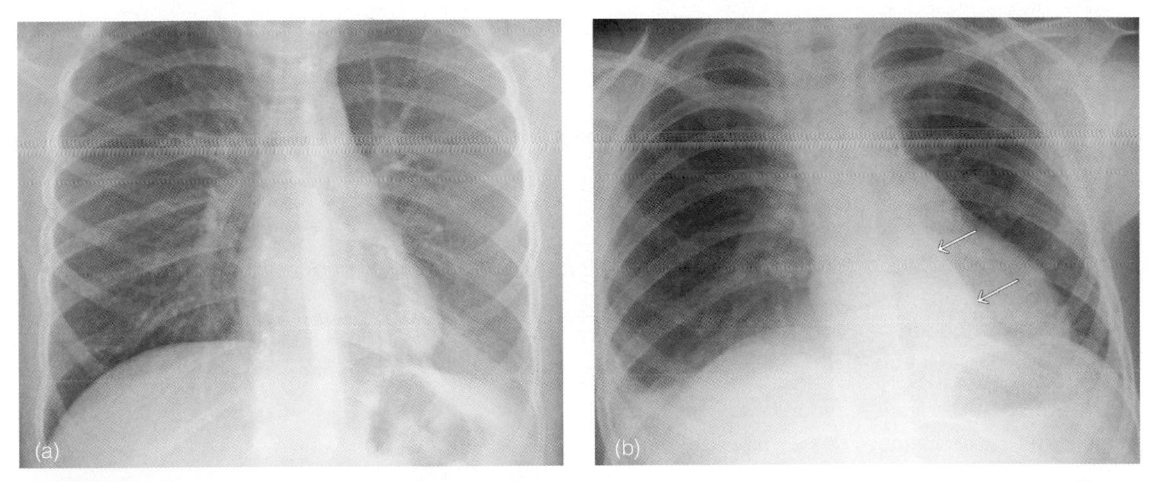

Figure 4.28 Left lower lobe collapse: two separate examples. (a) Note the loss of volume on the left, opacity behind the left heart and blurring of the left hemidiaphragm. (b) A more classical, though less commonly seen, pattern of left lower lobe collapse with a sharply defined triangular opacity behind the left heart (arrows).

Table 4.6 Specific features of lobar collapse.

Lobe	Direction of collapse	Hilum displacement	Increased density	Silhouette sign
Right upper	Upwards, anterior	Right, upwards	Right upper zone	Right mediastinum
Right middle	Anterior	None	PA: right midzone Lateral: triangular opacity overlying the heart	Right heart border
Right lower	Downwards, posterior	Right, downwards	Triangular opacity: right base	Right hemidiaphragm
Left upper	Upwards, anterior	Left, upwards	Left upper and midzone	Aortic arch[a] Upper left heart border
Left lower	Downwards, posterior	Left, downwards	Triangular opacity: left base, behind heart	Left hemidiaphragm, descending aorta

Abbreviation: PA, posteroanterior.
[a]Note that in complete collapse of the left upper lobe the aortic arch may be visible. This is because the apical segment of the left lower lobe may be pulled upwards and forwards enough such that aerated lung lies beside the aortic arch (luftsichel sign).

4.5.8 SOLITARY PULMONARY NODULE OR MASS

A solitary pulmonary nodule is a common incidental finding on CXR. It is defined as a spherical lung opacity seen on CXR or CT, measuring less than 3 cm in diameter and not associated with pulmonary collapse, pneumonia or lymphadenopathy. Opacities larger than 3 cm are referred to as masses and are more likely to be malignant.

Differential diagnosis of a solitary pulmonary nodule:

- Bronchogenic carcinoma (Fig. 4.29)
- Granuloma, including tuberculoma
- Solitary metastasis
- Carcinoid tumour
- Arteriovenous malformation.

The aim of investigation and follow-up of pulmonary nodules is to diagnose those that are malignant and to facilitate early resection.

Features associated with a higher likelihood of malignancy:

- Evidence of rapid growth on serial CXR examinations
- Ill-defined margin and spiculation
- Size greater than 3 cm
- No calcification.

Features associated with a lower likelihood of malignancy:

- Calcification
- Well-defined margin:
    - Small size: most granulomas measure 0.3–1.0 cm in diameter
- Unchanged on serial CXR examinations.

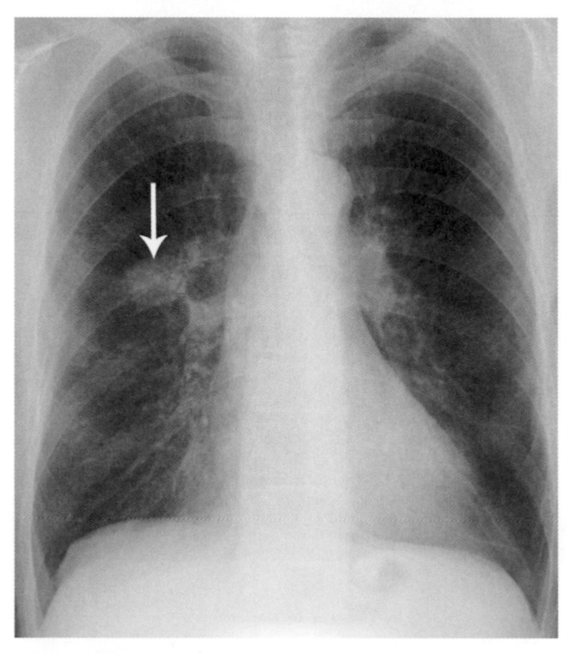

Figure 4.29 Solitary pulmonary nodule (arrow): bronchogenic carcinoma.

Findings on CXR that are sufficiently predictive of a benign aetiology to preclude further investigation are calcification and lack of growth over 2 years. Comparison with previous CXRs is therefore essential if these are available. These benign features are present in a minority of solitary pulmonary nodules and most require further imaging investigations, particularly when there are underlying risk factors for lung cancer. Major risk factors include cigarette smoking, exposure to asbestos and a history of lung cancer in a first-degree relative.

For notes on further investigation and classification of pulmonary nodules, see Chapter 5.

4.5.9 MULTIPLE PULMONARY NODULES

Whereas a solitary pulmonary nodule is commonly seen as an incidental finding, this is less often the case with multiple pulmonary nodules. More commonly, multiple pulmonary nodules are seen in symptomatic patients or in patients with underlying disease, such as immunosuppression or malignancy.

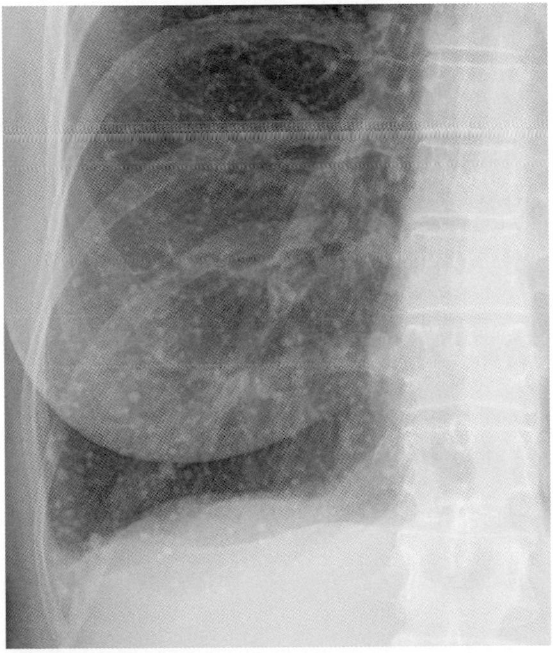

Figure 4.30 Multiple calcified granulomas due to previous varicella-zoster viral (chickenpox) pneumonia seen as innumerable small dense opacities scattered throughout the lung.

A common exception to this would be multiple small, calcified granulomas, which may indicate previous infection, including TB or varicella-zoster viral (chickenpox) pneumonia (Fig. 4.30).

Differential diagnosis of multiple pulmonary nodules:

- Granulomas
- Metastases (Fig. 4.31):
  - Usually well defined
  - Nodules of varying size
  - More common peripherally and in the lower lobes
  - Cavitation seen in squamous cell carcinomas, sarcomas and colorectal metastases
- Abscesses:
  - Cavitation: thick, irregular wall
  - Usually due to *Staphylococcus aureus*
- Fungal infection:
  - More common in immunocompromised patients, e.g. bone marrow transplant in children
- Hydatid cysts:
  - Often quite large, i.e. 10 cm or more

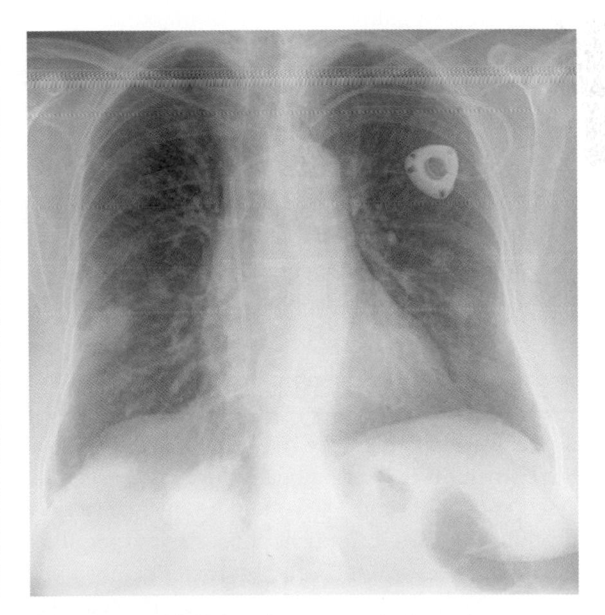

Figure 4.31 Multiple pulmonary metastases from colorectal carcinoma. Note the bilateral soft-tissue nodules of variable size and the left-sided portacath for chemotherapy.

- Granulomatosis with polyangiitis:
  - Cavitation of nodules common
  - Associated paranasal sinus disease
- Multiple arteriovenous malformations.

4.5.10 EMPHYSEMA

Emphysema refers to enlarged airspaces secondary to permanent destruction of the alveolar walls. Centrilobular emphysema is the most common form; it occurs in smokers and predominantly affects the upper lobes. Panlobular emphysema occurs in association with α_1-antitrypsin deficiency; it tends to predominantly affect the lower lobes.

CXR signs of emphysema (Fig. 4.32):

- Overexpanded lungs:
  - Flattening of the hemidiaphragms, best seen on lateral CXR
  - Hemidiaphragms lie below the anterior end of the sixth rib on a frontal view
  - Increased retrosternal airspace on a lateral film
  - Beware incorrect diagnosis of pulmonary overexpansion in a young, athletic patient capable of a large inspiration
- Decreased pulmonary vascular markings causing hyperlucent lungs
- Narrow mediastinum
- Increased AP diameter of the chest, with, in some cases, kyphosis and anterior bowing of the sternum
- Bulla formation: bullae are seen as thin-walled air-containing cavities
- Pulmonary arterial hypertension: prominent main pulmonary arteries.

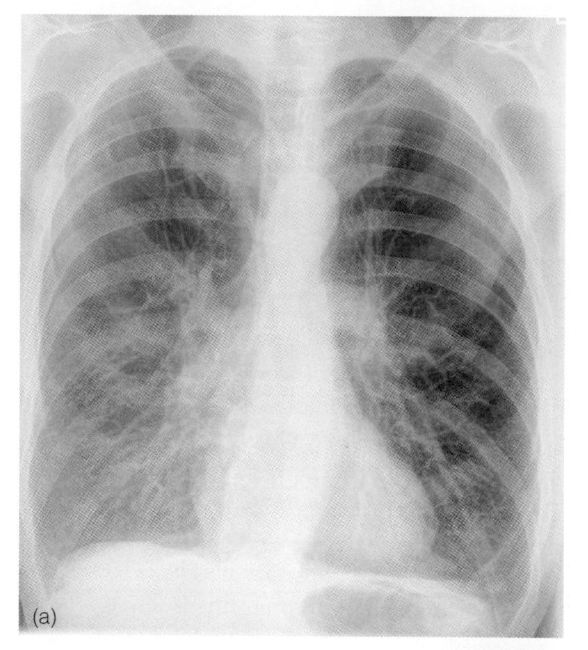

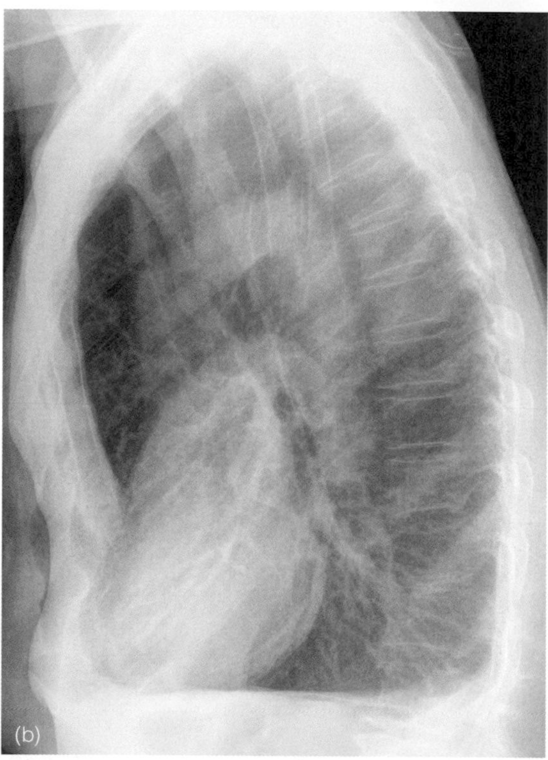

Figure 4.32 Emphysema. (a) Posteroanterior radiograph showing overexpansion of both lungs. (b) Lateral radiograph showing flattening of the hemidiaphragms and increased size of the retrosternal airspace posterior to the sternum.

4.5.11 BRONCHIECTASIS

Bronchiectasis refers to irreversible dilatation of the bronchi. It is often idiopathic or may be seen in association with multiple conditions, including cystic fibrosis, allergic bronchopulmonary aspergillosis, mycobacterial infection, post bacterial infection, chronic aspiration, severe asthma and congenital conditions such as Kartagener syndrome. The common factor is chronic inflammation and obstruction of airways, leading to dilatation.

CXR signs of bronchiectasis include:

- Parallel 'tram-track' opacity due to thickened bronchial walls
- Ring-like opacity in which dilated bronchi are seen end-on
- Air–fluid levels in severely dilated cyst-like bronchi.

CXR is relatively insensitive for the diagnosis of bronchiectasis; CT is usually required for definitive diagnosis and to accurately assess the extent of disease.

4.5.12 PLEURAL DISORDERS

Pleural disorders include accumulation of fluid in the pleural spaces (pleural effusion), air leaks (pneumothorax and pneumomediastinum) and pleural soft-tissue thickening and plaque formation.

PLEURAL EFFUSION

Pleural effusion is the accumulation of fluid in the pleural space between the visceral and parietal pleural layers. The radiographic appearances of pleural effusion are generally the same regardless of the nature of the fluid, which may include transudate, exudate, blood (haemothorax), pus (empyema) or lymph (chylothorax).

Signs of pleural effusion on erect CXR (Fig. 4.33):

- Homogeneous dense opacity at the base of the lung
- Concave upper surface higher laterally than medially, producing a meniscus
- Small pleural effusions produce blunting of the normal sharp angle between the lateral curve of the diaphragm and the inner chest wall, referred to as blunting of the costophrenic angle
- Large pleural effusions displace the mediastinum towards the contralateral side.

The lateral view is more sensitive to the presence of small pleural effusions than the PA view. It is estimated that about 300 mL of fluid is required to show costophrenic angle blunting on the PA, whereas only 100 mL is required to produce this sign (posteriorly) on the lateral view.

Variations to the 'normal' appearance of pleural effusion:

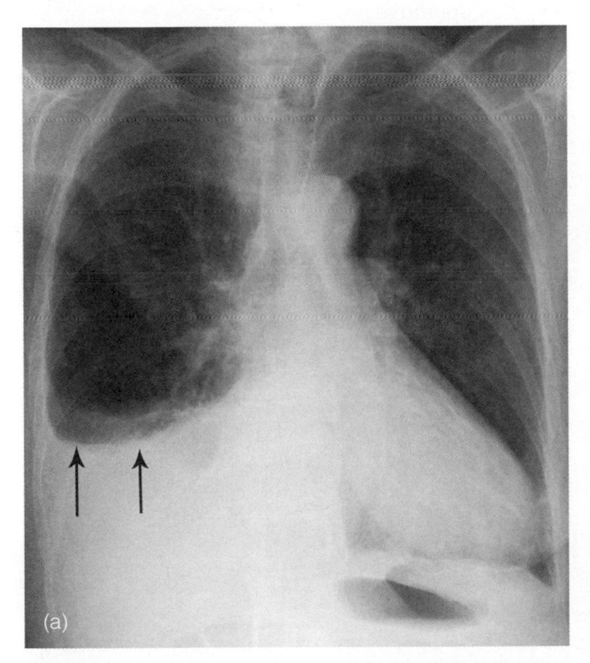

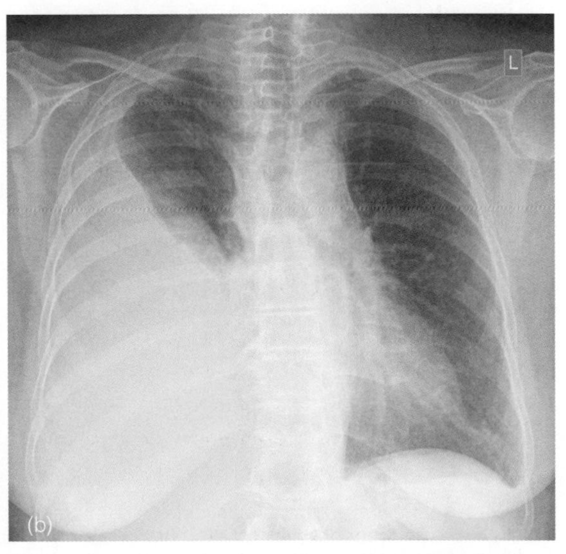

Figure 4.33 Pleural effusion. (a) Pleural effusion producing a fluid level at the right base (arrows). The outer edge of the fluid tracks a small distance up the chest wall, producing a typical meniscus shape. (b) Massive right pleural effusion.

- Loculations, i.e. failure of pleural fluid to layer out in a dependent fashion:
  - Pleural fluid may accumulate laterally or over the lung apices and may resemble pleural masses
- Causes of loculation of pleural fluid include:
  - Pleural scarring
  - Distortion of the lung due to collapse, fibrosis or surgery
  - Complex, thick fluid, e.g. empyema
- Fluid accumulating in a pulmonary fissure may mimic a pulmonary mass (pulmonary pseudotumour)
- Subpulmonic effusion: fluid trapped beneath the lung produces opacity parallel to the diaphragm with a convex upper margin.

Signs of pleural fluid on supine CXR include opacity over the lung apex (pleural cap) and increased opacity of the hemithorax, through which lung structures can still be seen (Fig. 4.34). There is often loss of definition of the hemidiaphragm and blunting of the costophrenic angle. The opacity caused by pleural effusion in a supine patient may be differentiated from pulmonary consolidation by the absence of air bronchograms.

Causes of pleural effusion:

- Cardiac failure:
  - Bilateral pleural effusions, right usually larger than left
- Malignancy:
  - Bronchogenic carcinoma
  - Metastatic
  - Mesothelioma
- Infection:
  - Bacterial pneumonia
  - TB
  - Mycoplasma
  - Empyema
  - Subphrenic abscess
- Pulmonary infarct from pulmonary embolism
- Pancreatitis: effusion is usually left-sided
- Trauma: associated with rib fractures
- Connective tissue disorders:
  - Rheumatoid arthritis
  - SLE
- Liver failure
- Renal failure
- Meigs syndrome: associated with ovarian tumour.
- Asbestos exposure
- Postoperative.

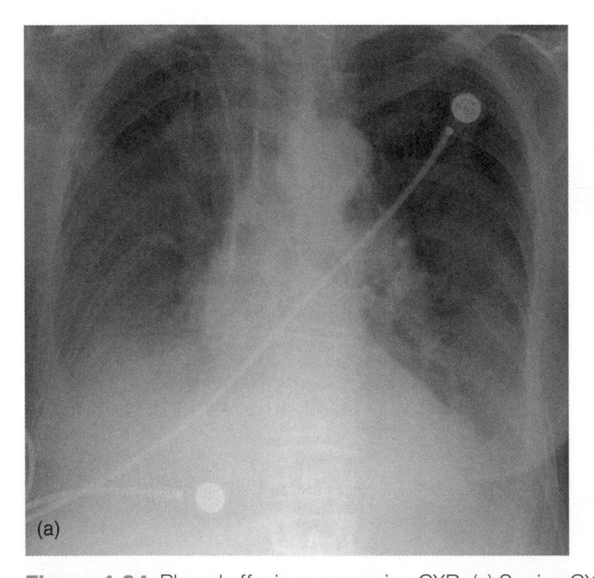

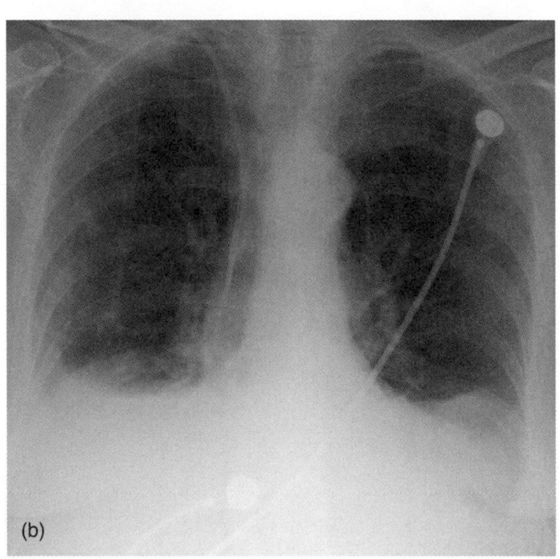

Figure 4.34 Pleural effusions on supine CXR. (a) Supine CXR: pleural effusions produce vague opacity over both lower zones with poor definition of each hemidiaphragm. Lack of air bronchograms and visualization of the pulmonary structures helps to differentiate pleural effusions from pulmonary consolidation. (b) Erect CXR confirms the diagnosis of bilateral pleural effusions.

PNEUMOTHORAX

Pneumothorax is the accumulation of air in the pleural space and is usually well seen on a normal inspiratory PA film. The diagnosis of small pneumothorax may be easier on an expiratory film. This is because of the reduced volume of the lung in expiration, which makes the pneumothorax look relatively larger. Whether the film is performed in inspiration or expiration, the sign to look for is the lung edge outlined by air in the pleural space (Fig. 4.35).

Tension pneumothorax occurs with continued air leak into the pleural space, producing increased intrapleural pressure; this expands the hemithorax and further compresses the lung, causing lung collapse. Venous return may be compromised, which can be life-threatening.

CXR signs of tension pneumothorax (Fig. 4.36):

- Marked collapse and distortion of the ipsilateral lung
- Increased volume of the ipsilateral hemithorax:
  - Contralateral displacement of the mediastinum
  - Depressed ipsilateral hemidiaphragm
  - Increased ipsilateral intercostal space.

Supine AP CXR may have to be performed in patients in an intensive care unit (ICU) or following severe trauma. Pleural air lies anteromedially and beneath the lung so that the usual appearance of a pneumothorax as described for an erect PA film is not seen.

Signs of pneumothorax on a supine CXR (Fig. 4.37):

- Mediastinal structures, including the heart border, inferior vena cava (IVC) and SVC, are sharply outlined by adjacent free pleural air
- Upper abdomen appears lucent because of overlying air
- Deep lateral costophrenic angle (deep sulcus sign).

Causes of pneumothorax:

- Spontaneous:
  - Tall, thin males
  - Smokers
- Iatrogenic:
  - Percutaneous lung biopsy
  - Complication of ventilation
  - Central venous line or cardiac pacemaker insertion
- Trauma: associated with rib fractures
- Emphysema

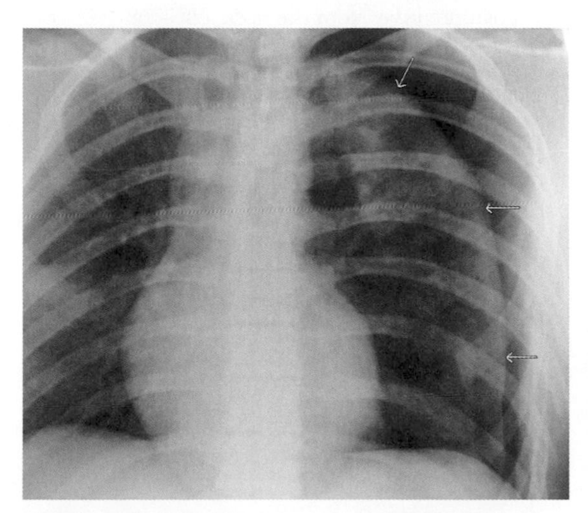

Figure 4.35 Pneumothorax. The pleural edge of the partly collapsed lung (arrows) is outlined by the pneumothorax.

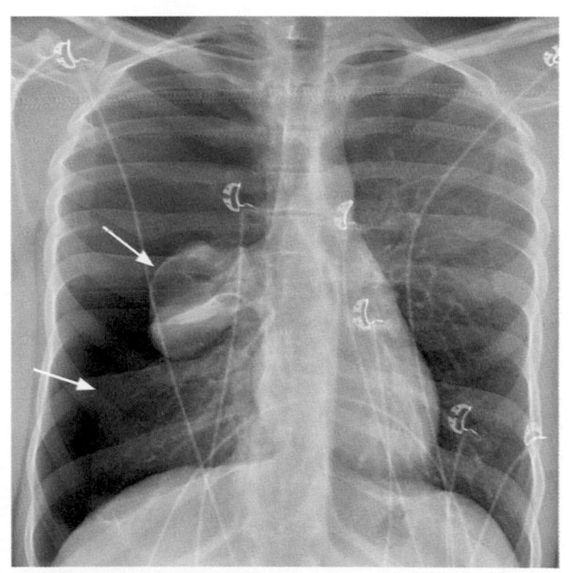

Figure 4.36 Tension pneumothorax. Massive pneumothorax and marked collapse of the right lung (arrows) and expansion of the right hemithorax characterized by increased space between the right ribs, a flattened right hemidiaphragm and mediastinal shift to the left.

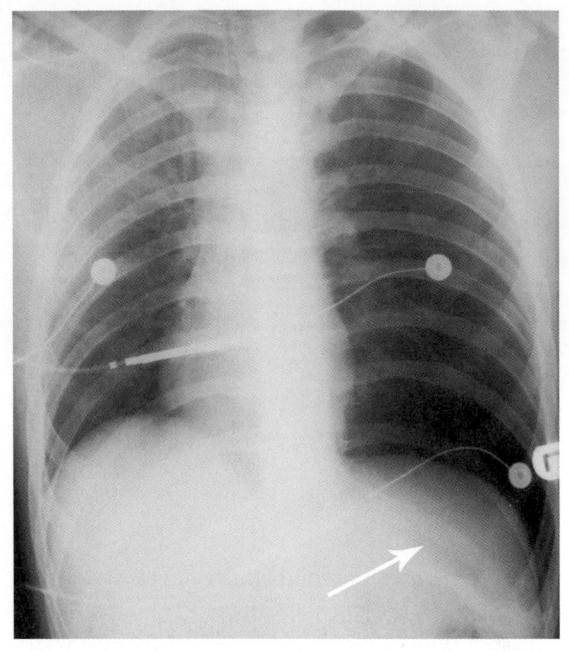

Figure 4.37 Supine pneumothorax. Pneumothorax in a supine patient shows as an area of lucency over the lower left hemithorax and upper left abdomen (arrow). Also note the increased volume on the left, indicating tension.

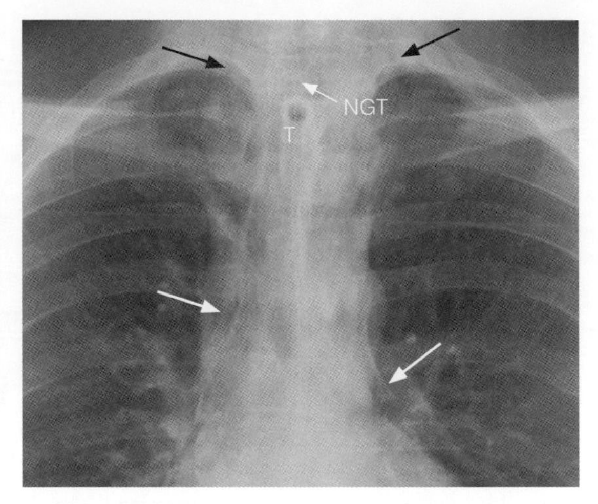

Figure 4.38 Pneumomediastinum. Streaky lucencies representing gas in both sides of the mediastinum (white arrows) extending into the neck (black arrows). Note the tracheostomy (T) and nasogastric tube (NGT).

- Malignancy: high incidence with osteosarcoma metastases
- Honeycomb lung
- Lymphangiomyomatosis: interstitial disease of young women; associated with tuberous sclerosis
- Cystic fibrosis.

PNEUMOMEDIASTINUM

Pneumomediastinum is an air leak into the connective tissues of the mediastinum.

Radiographic signs of pneumomediastinum are due to air outlining the normal mediastinal structures (Fig. 4.38):

- Strips of air outlining the left side of the mediastinum
- Air around the aorta, pulmonary arteries and pericardium
- Subcutaneous air extending upwards into the soft tissues of the neck.

Causes of pneumomediastinum:

- Spontaneous: following severe coughing or strenuous exercise
- Asthma
- Foreign body aspiration in neonates
- Chest trauma
- Oesophageal perforation: tumour, severe vomiting and endoscopy
- Barotrauma: ventilator or scuba diving
- Postoperative: from the neck, chest or retroperitoneum.

PLEURAL THICKENING/PLAQUE

Pleural thickening or plaque formation may show various radiographic appearances:

- Blunting of costophrenic angles, mimicking pleural effusion
- Soft-tissue thickening over the lungs, including the lung apices
- Calcification of the pleural surfaces due to previous pleural haemorrhage or infection
- Pleural plaques:
    - Convex, pleural-based opacities when seen in profile
    - Less well-defined opacities when not in profile

- May be calcified, especially with a history of asbestos exposure.

Causes of pleural thickening or pleural plaque formation:

- Secondary to trauma:
  - Associated with healed rib fractures
  - Dense layer of soft tissue, often calcified
- Following empyema:
  - More common over the lung bases
  - Often calcified
- TB
- Asbestos exposure:
  - Irregular pleural thickening and pleural plaques (Fig. 4.39)
  - Almost always bilateral
  - Calcification common, especially of diaphragmatic pleura
  - Note that pleural disease is not asbestosis; the term 'asbestosis' refers to the interstitial lung disease secondary to asbestos exposure (see Chapter 5)
- Mesothelioma:
  - Diffuse or localized pleural mass
  - Rib destruction uncommon
  - Large pleural effusions common
  - Pleural plaques elsewhere in 50%
- Pancoast tumour:
  - Primary apical lung neoplasm
  - Rib destruction with irregular pleural thickening
  - Causes Horner syndrome and lower brachial plexus radiculopathy and muscle wasting
- Pleural metastases:
  - Often obscured by associated pleural effusion.

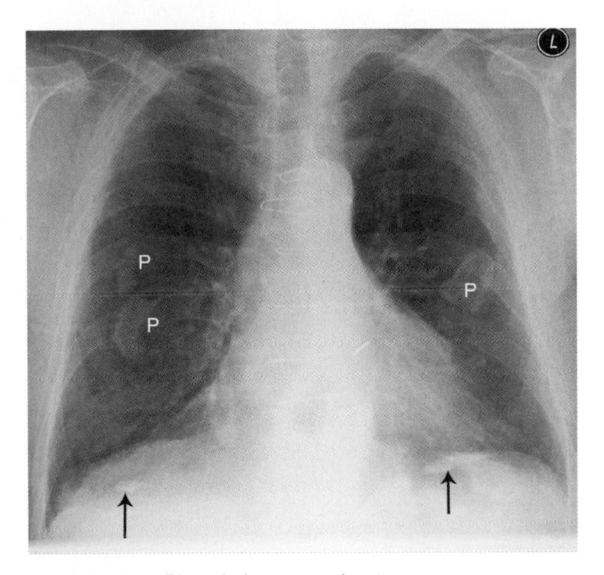

Figure 4.39 Pleural plaques: asbestos exposure. Multiple plaques (P) are seen as well-defined, though irregular opacities projected over the lungs. Also note the linear regions of pleural calcification (arrows).

5 Respiratory system and chest

This chapter is primarily concerned with the investigation of diseases of the lung. Imaging of the heart and aorta is discussed in Chapter 6, and imaging following chest trauma in Chapter 12.

5.1 IMAGING OF RESPIRATORY DISEASE

Common symptoms due to respiratory disease include cough, the production of sputum, haemoptysis, dyspnoea and chest pain. These symptoms may be accompanied by systemic manifestations, including fever, weight loss and night sweats. An accurate history plus findings on physical examination, in particular auscultation of the chest, are vital in directing further investigation and management. The history and examination may be supplemented by relatively simple tests such as white cell count, erythrocyte sedimentation rate (ESR) and sputum analysis for culture or cytology. A variety of pulmonary function tests may also be performed, including spirometry, measurements of gas exchange, such as CO diffusing capacity and arterial blood gas, and exercise testing. In some cases, more sophisticated and invasive tests such as flexible fibreoptic bronchoscopy, bronchoalveolar lavage and video-assisted thoracoscopic surgery (VATS) may be required.

A chest radiograph (chest X-ray, CXR) is requested for virtually all patients with respiratory symptoms. See Chapter 4 for an overview of CXR interpretation, including notes on common findings. Computed tomography (CT) is the next most performed investigation for diseases of the respiratory system and chest. Positron emission tomography (PET)-CT is also commonly used, particularly in the context of diagnosis and staging of bronchogenic carcinoma. Magnetic resonance imaging (MRI) may occasionally be used for specific indications, e.g. to confirm that a mediastinal lesion is a cyst. Furthermore, MRI is the imaging investigation of choice for disorders of the spine (see Chapter 10), including neurogenic tumours that may appear on CXR as a posterior mediastinal mass.

This chapter will provide an overview of the many and varied roles of CT in the investigation of chest disorders, followed by discussions of imaging of pulmonary infections and diffuse lung diseases, the approach to pulmonary nodules and the principles of staging of lung cancer.

5.2 COMPUTED TOMOGRAPHY IN THE INVESTIGATION OF CHEST DISORDERS

CT of the chest may be used in several ways, as outlined below.

5.2.1 FURTHER CHARACTERIZATION OF CHEST RADIOGRAPH FINDINGS

- Mediastinal mass (Fig. 5.1):
  - Accurate localization
  - Characterization of the internal contents of the mass: fat, air, fluid and calcification
  - Displacement or invasion of the adjacent structures, such as aorta, heart, trachea, oesophagus, vertebral column and chest wall
- Hilar mass:
  - Greater sensitivity than CXR for the presence of hilar lymphadenopathy
  - Greater specificity in differentiating lymphadenopathy or a hilar mass from enlarged pulmonary arteries

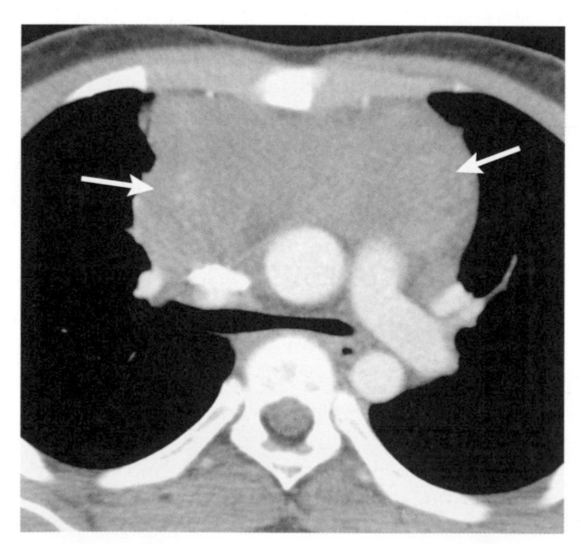

Figure 5.1 Hodgkin disease: CT. CT shows an anterior mediastinal mass (arrows) due to confluent lymphadenopathy.

- Characterization of a pulmonary nodule or mass seen on CXR:
  - More accurate than plain films for the presence of calcification or fat
  - Other factors that are also well assessed by CT include cavitation and the relation of a mass to the chest wall or mediastinum
  - Intravenous contrast material may help to identify aberrant vessels and arteriovenous malformations
- Suspected vascular anomaly as a cause for abnormality on CXR:
  - Azygos continuation of the inferior vena cava (IVC)
  - Partial anomalous pulmonary venous drainage
- Characterization of pleural disease:
  - CT provides excellent delineation of pleural abnormalities, which may produce confusing appearances on CXR
  - Pleural masses, fluid collections, calcifications and tumours such as mesothelioma are well shown, as are complications such as rib destruction, mediastinal invasion and lymphadenopathy.

5.2.2 COMPUTED TOMOGRAPHY AS THE PRIMARY INVESTIGATION OF CHOICE IN RESPIRATORY OR CARDIOVASCULAR DISEASE

- Staging of bronchogenic carcinoma (often with fluorodeoxyglucose (FDG)-PET):
  - Greater sensitivity than CXR for the presence of mediastinal or hilar lymphadenopathy, for ipsilateral or contralateral metastases and for complications such as chest wall or mediastinal invasion and cavitation
- Detection of pulmonary metastases (often with FDG-PET):
  - CT has greater sensitivity than CXR for the detection of pulmonary metastases in the staging of extrapulmonary malignancy
- Complicated infection and pleural effusion
- Chest trauma (see Chapter 12)

- Diseases of the thoracic aorta:
  - Thoracic aortic aneurysm
  - Aortic dissection.

5.2.3 HIGH-RESOLUTION COMPUTED TOMOGRAPHY

High-resolution CT (HRCT) is a modified chest CT technique whereby thin 1- to 2-mm sections provide highly detailed views of the lung parenchyma. With modern CT scanners, thin sections can be reconstructed from the acquired data. Alternately, HRCT may be performed by acquiring thin sections at 10- to 20-mm intervals through the lungs. HRCT occasionally may be augmented by acquisition with the patient prone to diagnose subtle posterior subpleural interstitial lung disease, and by an expiratory scan to highlight regions of 'air trapping' in patients with suspected inflammatory or obstructive bronchial disease. HRCT is performed for specific indications where diseases of the lung parenchyma are suspected:

- Bronchiectasis (Fig. 5.2):
  - As well as showing dilated bronchi, HRCT accurately shows the anatomical distribution of changes, in addition to complications such as scarring, collapse, consolidation and mucous plugging
- Interstitial lung disease:
  - HRCT is more sensitive and specific than CXR in the diagnosis of many interstitial lung diseases, e.g. sarcoidosis, pulmonary fibrosis, lymphangitis carcinomatosis and Langerhans cell histiocytosis
- Atypical infections:
  - HRCT provides a diagnosis of many atypical infections earlier and with greater specificity than plain CXR
  - Examples include infections that occur in immunocompromised patients such as pneumocystis pneumonia, aspergillosis and candidiasis
  - As well as assisting with diagnosis, HRCT may be useful for monitoring disease progress and response to therapy
- Chronic lung diseases in children:
  - HRCT is used to monitor changes associated with cystic fibrosis, such as mucous plugging and pulmonary collapse, acute infective episodes, and acute bronchopulmonary aspergillosis (ABPA)
  - Other examples of childhood lung disease where HRCT may be helpful include chronic lung disease of infancy and interstitial lung diseases, e.g. neuroendocrine hyperplasia of infancy (NEHI)
- Normal CXR in symptomatic patients:
  - HRCT has a definite role in the assessment of patients with an apparently normal CXR despite strong clinical indications of respiratory disease, including dyspnoea, chest pain, haemoptysis and abnormal pulmonary function tests
  - In such cases, the much greater sensitivity of HRCT may provide a diagnosis or direct further investigations such as lung biopsy.

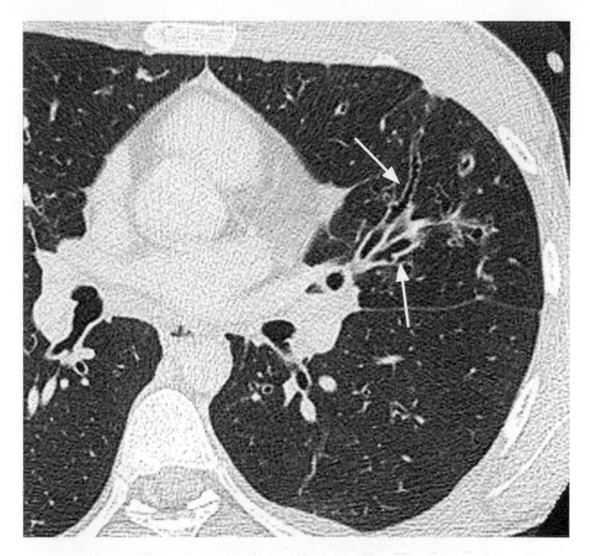

Figure 5.2 Bronchiectasis: high-resolution CT. Dilated bronchi in the left upper lobe are seen on CT as tubular thick-walled bronchi (arrows).

5.2.4 LOW (RADIATION) DOSE COMPUTED TOMOGRAPHY SCREENING FOR LUNG CANCER

Low-dose CT screening for lung cancer is currently recommended by the US Preventive Services Task Force for people aged between 50 and 80 who have

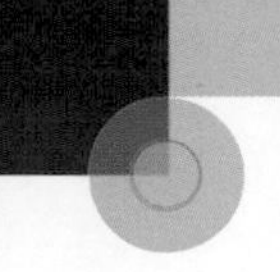

at least a 20-pack-year smoking history and who currently smoke or have ceased smoking within the past 15 years. A major problem with CT screening for lung cancer is the high incidence of benign nodules found on CT, with a large potential for false-positive studies. For this reason, a structured classification, the Lung Reporting and Data System (Lung-RADS), is used with low-dose screening to ascribe the risk of malignancy for various types and sizes of nodules. See section 5.5 for notes on lung nodules. Further details of Lung-RADS may be found on the companion website.

5.3 IMAGING FINDINGS IN PULMONARY INFECTIONS

Pulmonary infections are very common and occur in multiple different scenarios. Infections may be acquired in the community or may be seen in association with other comorbidities, such as recent surgery, malignancy and immune compromise. Imaging plays a major role in the diagnosis and management of pulmonary infection in multiple ways, including initial diagnosis, differentiation from other conditions that may present with acute respiratory symptoms and monitoring the response to therapy. Pulmonary infections are caused by a wide range of pathogens, including bacteria, viruses, fungi and parasites. Although imaging findings are often non-specific, it is often the case that imaging findings may assist in pinpointing specific aetiologies when correlated with appropriate clinical information. The following is a guide to the various appearances of infection on CXR and CT. This is followed by notes on a few specific infections and clinical scenarios. For further notes on respiratory infections in children, see Chapter 16.

5.3.1 SIGNS OF INFECTION ON CHEST RADIOGRAPH

CONSOLIDATION

Infective consolidation generally follows one of two patterns: bronchopneumonia and lobar consolidation. Bronchopneumonia produces small ill-defined opacities around bronchi that may become confluent. Consolidation filling an entire lobe is uncommon in an era of early initiation of antibiotic therapy, and lobar pneumonia is more commonly seen as a small segmental or subsegmental region of consolidation. Organisms that commonly cause pneumonia include *Streptococcus pneumoniae, Haemophilus influenzae, Klebsiella pneumoniae* and *Mycoplasma pneumoniae.* Expansion of a lobe with bulging pulmonary fissures may be seen with *Klebsiella*.

CAVITATION

Cavitation may occur within areas of consolidation and may progress to form an abscess. This is usually associated with more aggressive organisms such as *Staphylococcus aureus* and *Pseudomonas aeruginosa.* Cavities and abscesses are seen as air-filled spaces, with air–fluid levels on erect radiographs.

PLEURAL EFFUSION

Non-infected parapneumonic pleural effusions are commonly seen in association with consolidation. They are usually small and resolve with treatment of the underlying infection.

NODULES

Solitary lung nodules may be seen in certain infections, including *Mycobacterium tuberculosis* (tuberculosis [TB]) and hydatid disease. Multiple nodules may be seen in a variety of infections, including TB, angioinvasive aspergillosis and those caused by non-tuberculous mycobacteria, such as *Mycobacterium avium intracellulare* (MAC) and *Mycobacterium kansasii.*

MILIARY PATTERN

The miliary pattern refers to multiple small opacities measuring up to 3 mm spread throughout the lungs. The miliary pattern indicates haematogenous spread of infection. It is seen in primary and post-primary TB, and less commonly with other infections, including histoplasmosis.

5.3.2 SIGNS OF INFECTION ON COMPUTED TOMOGRAPHY

CT can detect all of the above-described CXR signs of infection; these signs are generally detected earlier and with greater accuracy on CT (Fig. 5.3). Other signs of infection that may only be detected accurately with CT are described below.

GROUND GLASS OPACITY

Ground glass opacity refers to diffuse opacity that is less dense than consolidation, and through which pulmonary bronchovascular structures can still be seen. It indicates cellular infiltration into the pulmonary interstitium with partial filling of alveoli and may be seen adjacent to areas of consolidation.

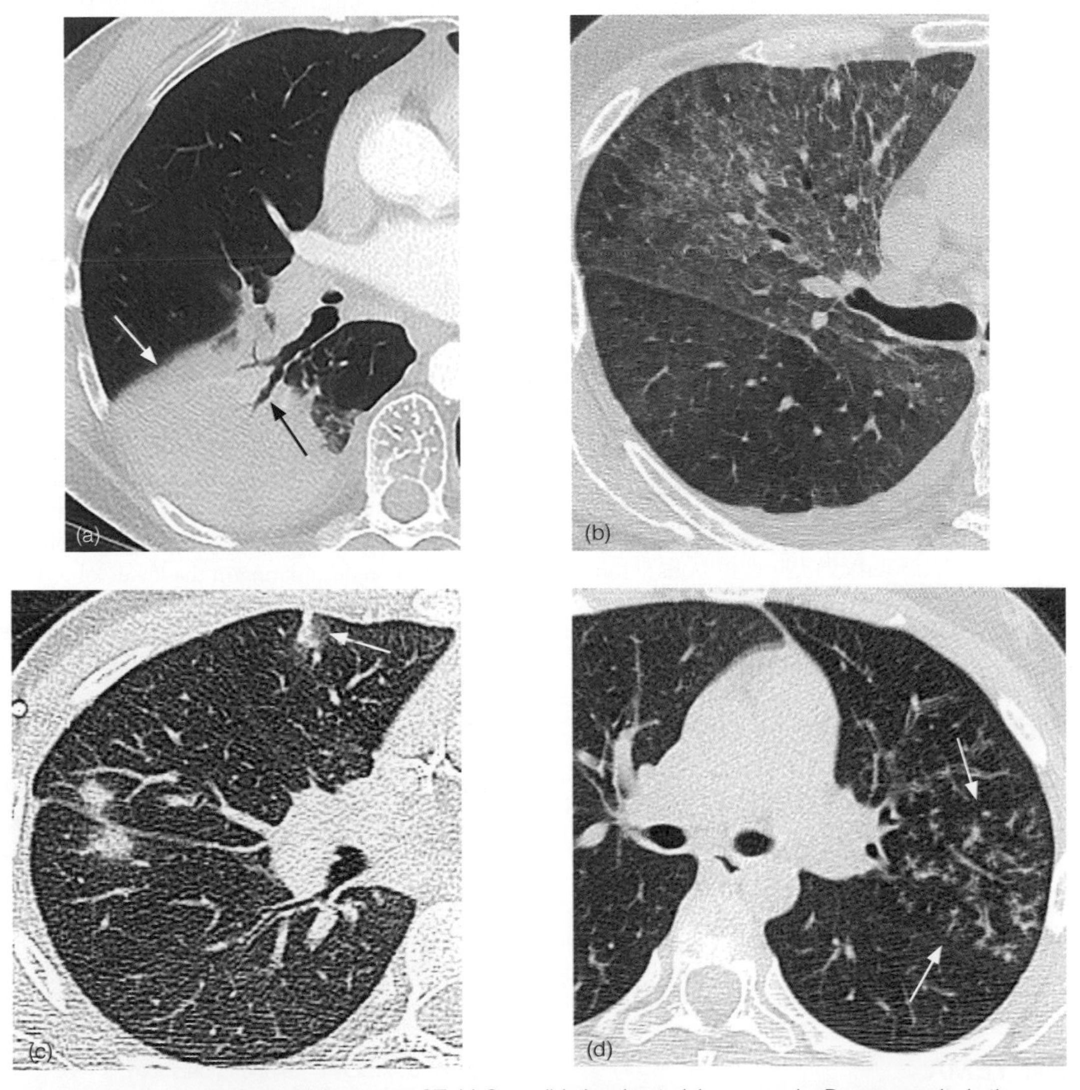

Figure 5.3 Examples of patterns of infection on CT. (a) Consolidation: bacterial pneumonia. Dense opacity in the right lower lobe, through which pulmonary structures cannot be seen (white arrow). Also note air bronchograms (black arrow). (b) Ground glass opacity: *Pneumocystis jiroveci* pneumonia. Diffuse opacity in the right upper lobe through which pulmonary structures can be seen. (c) Nodular opacity: invasive aspergillosis. Multiple irregularly shaped nodules, one of which shows a ground glass periphery or 'halo' (arrow). (d) Tree-in-bud sign: *Mycobacterium avium intracellulare.* Multiple small branching opacities in the left upper lobe representing opacification of small, distal bronchioles (arrows).

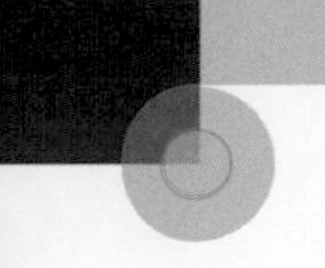

Ground glass opacity is a common feature of viral pneumonia, i.e. pneumonia caused by *M. pneumoniae,* and of opportunistic infections such as those caused by *Pneumocystis jiroveci*.

'CRAZY PAVING'

Crazy paving is a flooring method whereby irregularly shaped stones or tiles are laid to form a haphazard pattern. Crazy paving on CT is due to a combination of thickened interlobular septations and partial alveolar filling. This produces a random linear pattern on a background of ground glass opacity. First described as a sign of pulmonary alveolar proteinosis, crazy paving may also be seen in various infections, including influenza, other viral infections and *P. jiroveci*.

HALO SIGN

The halo sign refers to a peripheral zone of ground glass opacity surrounding a pulmonary nodule. It is encountered in infections that invade blood vessels and is produced by a rim of alveolar haemorrhage surrounding a pulmonary infarct. The halo sign is highly suggestive of angioinvasive aspergillosis in patients with febrile neutropenia. A variant of the halo sign, also seen with angioinvasive aspergillosis, is the reverse halo or atoll sign, which appears as a rim of consolidation surrounding a central zone of ground glass opacity.

TREE-IN-BUD SIGN

The tree-in-bud sign is produced by bronchiolitis, i.e. infection of terminal bronchioles (also referred to as 'small airways'). The tree-in-bud sign consists of multiple small nodular 'Y' or 'V' shaped branching opacities, often associated with adjacent underlying bronchiectasis. It may be caused by aspiration, and is also seen with a variety of infections, including those caused by fungi and MAC.

EMPYEMA

Empyema refers to infected pleural fluid. It presents on CXR as a localized pleural opacity, occasionally with an air–fluid level, but may be difficult to differentiate from a parapneumonic non-infected effusion. Empyema is commonly associated with the formation of an enclosing membrane and is best diagnosed on CT. CT may also be useful for guided aspiration and drainage of empyema.

5.3.3 VIRAL PNEUMONIA

Viral pneumonia may be caused by a variety of DNA and RNA viruses in immunocompetent and immunocompromised hosts. CXR findings are often subtle and non-specific, including consolidation, patchy ground glass opacities and nodules. CT findings relate to the biological behaviour of the virus. Influenza and adenoviruses invade the epithelium lining bronchi and bronchioles, producing a tree-in-bud pattern of bronchiolitis on CT followed by diffuse consolidation or a bronchopneumonia pattern. Respiratory syncytial virus (RSV) produces a variety of findings, including multifocal consolidation, nodules and bronchial wall thickening.

Coronavirus infection is of particular relevance at the time of writing, with the global pandemic caused by coronavirus disease 2019 (COVID-19) in its third year. As with other types of viral pneumonia, CXR findings in COVID-19 infection are often subtle early in symptomatic disease. More obvious findings are non-specific, such as diffuse bilateral peripheral consolidation predominating in the lower lobes (Fig. 5.4).

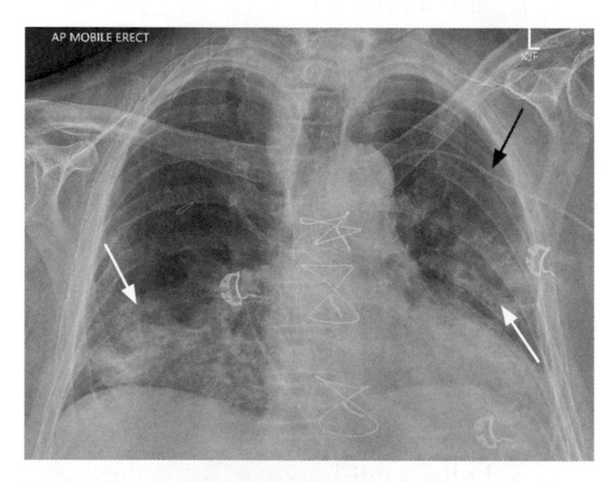

Figure 5.4 COVID-19 pneumonia. CXR shows bilateral regions of airspace opacification in keeping with severe viral pneumonia (white arrows). Also note a percutaneously inserted central venous catheter (PICC) via the left arm (black arrow), plus sternal wires and left mediastinal surgical clips indicating previous coronary artery bypass graft surgery.

CT is more sensitive for the early detection of COVID-19 pneumonia and for monitoring disease progression. CT findings include patchy ground glass opacities, which may progress to become more extensive. With disease progression a crazy paving pattern may be seen as well as regions of consolidation. It is also worth remembering that many patients with COVID-19 have comorbidities, and other causes of pulmonary disease may be encountered. CT findings, including mediastinal lymphadenopathy, pulmonary nodules and pleural effusions, would suggest alternative diagnoses.

5.3.4 TUBERCULOSIS

PRIMARY TUBERCULOSIS

Primary TB is usually asymptomatic. The healed pulmonary lesion of primary TB may be seen on CXR as a small calcified peripheral pulmonary nodule (Ghon focus), usually located in the upper lobes, with a calcified hilar lymph node (Ranke complex).

POST-PRIMARY PULMONARY TUBERCULOSIS (REACTIVATION TB)

Post-primary TB has a predilection for the apical and posterior segments of the upper lobes plus the apical segments of the lower lobes. Variable CXR appearances may include ill-defined areas of alveolar consolidation and thick-walled irregular cavities. Haemoptysis, aspergilloma ('fungus ball'), tuberculous empyema and a bronchopleural fistula may complicate cavitation. Subsequent fibrosis may cause volume loss in the upper lobes. Fibrosis and calcification usually indicate disease inactivity and healing, but one should never diagnose inactive TB on a single CXR; serial radiographs are essential to prove inactivity.

MILIARY TUBERCULOSIS

See Miliary pattern in section 5.3.1.

5.3.5 LUNG INFECTIONS IN IMMUNOCOMPROMISED HOSTS

Immunocompromise may be caused by diseases such as acquired immunodeficiency syndrome (AIDS), diabetes, malnutrition and malignancy, and by therapies such as chemotherapy for cancer, prolonged corticosteroids and organ transplants. Presenting symptoms including cough and dyspnoea may be mild and non-specific; early imaging with CT is often the key to timely diagnosis. A variety of opportunistic infections may be seen in immunocompromised hosts, including those listed below.

PNEUMOCYSTIS JIROVECI PNEUMONIA

Typical findings of *Pneumocystis jiroveci* pneumonia (PJP) are bilateral perihilar ground glass opacities, with sparing of the lung peripheries (Fig. 5.3b). A crazy paving pattern may also be seen.

ANGIOINVASIVE ASPERGILLOSIS

Usually caused by *Aspergillus fumigatus*, angioinvasive aspergillosis is the commonest fungal infection in immunocompromised patients with neutropenia, such as those with haematological malignancies and haematopoietic stem cell transplant. The typical CT finding in angioinvasive aspergillosis is multiple nodules with surrounding ground glass opacities, i.e. the halo sign (Fig. 5.3c).

NON-TUBERCULOUS MYCOBACTERIA

Non-tuberculous mycobacteria, most commonly MAC and *M. kansasii*, may produce a variety of patterns on CT. These include multiple nodules, tree-in-bud opacities (Fig. 5.3d), bronchiectasis and, in chronic cases, regions of atelectasis in the right middle lobe and lingula.

5.4 DIFFUSE LUNG DISEASES

Perhaps a more appropriate title for this section would be 'lung diseases that produce diffuse abnormalities on imaging'. Diffuse lung diseases represent a diverse group of disorders that produce varied appearances on CXR and are usually more accurately characterized on CT. The clinical presentation of these disorders is often non-specific, consisting of typical respiratory symptoms such as cough and shortness of breath. Appearances on CT are also often quite non-specific. The aim of this section is to provide a brief guide on how radiologists approach these disorders systematically to arrive at either a specific diagnosis or a short list of differential diagnoses.

When assessing diffuse lung pathology on CT, a systematic approach would be to assess the distribution (where is it?) and pattern (what does it look like?) of changes. This is followed by correlation with other associated imaging findings, and with clinical details, which may include specific blood tests, the results of spirometry and extrapulmonary manifestations. Finally, the chronicity of findings may be established by comparison with prior relevant images.

Although some disorders show a random distribution, others show a predilection for particular lung regions. The distribution of the abnormality is assessed by dividing the lungs into zones. First, the lung may be divided into central and peripheral zones, where the periphery consists of the outer 3–4 cm deep to the pleural surface and also along the fissures. The central zone consists of the remainder of the lung. Second, the lung is divided into upper, middle and lower zones in the craniocaudal direction.

In terms of pattern, diffuse lung diseases may produce a variety of appearances, including solid nodules, cavitating nodules, ground glass opacities and diffuse interstitial opacity. Of particular importance with respect to diffuse interstitial disease is the differentiation between two common patterns: usual interstitial pneumonia (UIP) and non-specific interstitial pneumonia (NSIP). Both of these entities show a peripheral lower zone distribution. UIP is characterized by decreased lung volume and the appearance of thick-walled, 3- to 10-mm, air-containing cystic spaces that replace normal lung parenchyma. This cystic change is referred to as 'honeycombing'; in UIP, it typically occurs with a subpleural and basal predominance (Fig. 5.5). NSIP is characterized by decreased lung volume and ground glass opacities, with minimal or no honeycombing.

UIP and NSIP are commonly idiopathic or may be associated with connective tissue disorders (systemic sclerosis, systemic lupus erythematosus (SLE), rheumatoid arthritis (RA), etc.), asbestos or other dust exposures and medication toxicity. When idiopathic,

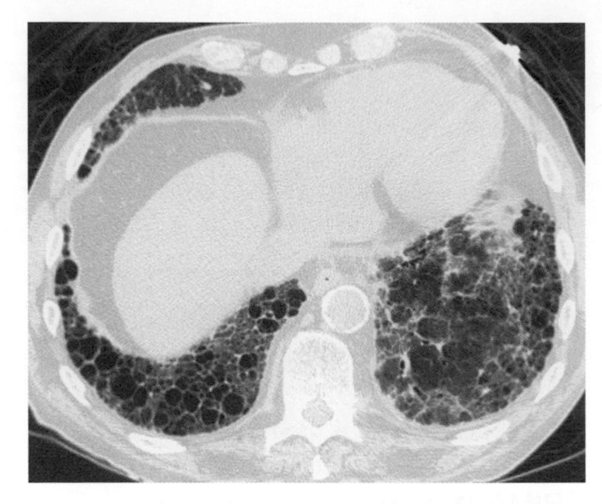

Figure 5.5 Honeycomb lung: high-resolution CT (HRCT). HRCT in a patient with end-stage idiopathic pulmonary fibrosis shows replacement of normal pulmonary parenchyma with air-filled cysts and coarse linear markings.

UIP is termed idiopathic pulmonary fibrosis (IPF). The importance of differentiation of these patterns is that NSIP may respond to steroid therapy and generally has a more favourable prognosis than UIP. Although a complete discussion of diffuse lung diseases is beyond the scope of this book, Table 5.1 provides a summary of some of the more commonly encountered conditions, emphasizing the approach to diagnosis on CT as outlined above.

5.5 LUNG NODULES

The two most used imaging investigations for a solitary pulmonary nodule are CT and FDG-PET, with CT the first investigation of choice in most instances. Lung nodules are common incidental findings on CXR and chest CT. They are also commonly found on CT examinations of other areas, including the abdomen, neck and spine, where parts of the lungs may be visualized. Some nodules may be classified as likely to be benign on CXR or CT by the presence of calcification or fat or by a lack of growth on comparison with previous studies. In most cases, however, these factors are not present and further assessment and classification are required. The assessment of lung nodules has become more complicated based on the recent realization that adenocarcinoma of the lung has multiple pathological subtypes that have protean

Table 5.1 Diffuse lung diseases on CT.

Disease	Distribution	Pattern	Other imaging findings	Specific clinical details
IPF	Lower, peripheral	UIP		Progressive dyspnoea
Connective tissue disorders	Lower, peripheral	UIP/NSIP	Dilated oesophagus in systemic sclerosis	• Known history of CTD • CRP and ESR • Autoantibodies
Asbestosis	Lower, peripheral	UIP/NSIP	Pleural plaques and calcifications	Asbestos exposure
Sarcoidosis	Upper/middle	Small nodules, predominantly along bronchovascular structures	Hilar and mediastinal lymphadenopathy	Extrapulmonary manifestations, e.g. uveitis
Granulomatosis with polyangiitis	Random	Nodules, often with cavitation		• Paranasal sinus and kidney disease • ANCA
Chronic eosinophilic pneumonia	Peripheral	Ground glass opacity and consolidation		Peripheral eosinophilia

Abbreviations: ANCA, anti-neutrophil cytoplasmic antibody; CRP, C-reactive protein; ESR, erythrocyte sedimentation rate; IPF, idiopathic pulmonary fibrosis; NSIP, non-specific interstitial pneumonia; UIP, usual interstitial pneumonia.

findings on CT, including scar-like lesions and focal regions of diffuse ground glass opacification.

Based on their appearances on CT (Fig. 5.6), lung nodules are classified into the following categories:

- Solid nodule (SN):
  - Homogeneous soft-tissue density
- Semisolid (or subsolid) nodule (SSN):
  - Composed of a mixture of solid and ground glass components
- Ground glass (non-solid) nodule (GGN):
  - Seen as a focal area of hazy opacification
  - Bronchial and vascular structures may be seen through this opacity
  - Differential for this appearance includes focal inflammatory change or adenocarcinoma
- Perifissural lung nodule (PFN):
  - Most common appearance is a soft-tissue density nodule with a flat surface in contact with a pulmonary fissure
  - May appear as oval or triangular on transverse images and flat on coronal or sagittal images
  - Virtually always benign.

The Fleischner Society has developed guidelines for the reporting and follow-up of pulmonary nodules in patients aged over 35; these guidelines are based on nodule classification and size, nodule multiplicity and patient risk factors (Table 5.2).

Factors that would indicate a high risk include patient factors such as smoking history and old age. Nodules that have spiculated or irregular outlines are also considered high risk.

For multiple nodules, the most suspicious-appearing nodule should guide further management based on the above guidelines. The Fleischner Society guidelines do not apply in patients aged under 35 or in patients with a known history of malignancy or immunocompromise. They also do not apply in low-dose CT screening for lung cancer, where Lung-RADS is used.

Lung nodules may be further assessed with FDG-PET and/or biopsy. FDG-PET may be useful to characterize solitary pulmonary nodules where other imaging is unhelpful, e.g. to differentiate mass-like scarring from malignancy. Neoplastic masses show an increased uptake of FDG. FDG-PET is unable to accurately characterize lesions less than 1 cm in diameter, and false-positive findings may occur in active inflammatory lesions.

Lesions that have positive findings for malignancy on CT or FDG-PET usually require biopsy. Biopsy may be performed percutaneously with CT guidance, via bronchoscopy, with VATS or by open surgical biopsy and resection. The main risk of CT-guided lung biopsy is pneumothorax. These are usually small and settle spontaneously; however, they may occasionally require management with a chest tube. Haemoptysis may also occur; this is usually minimal and self-limiting.

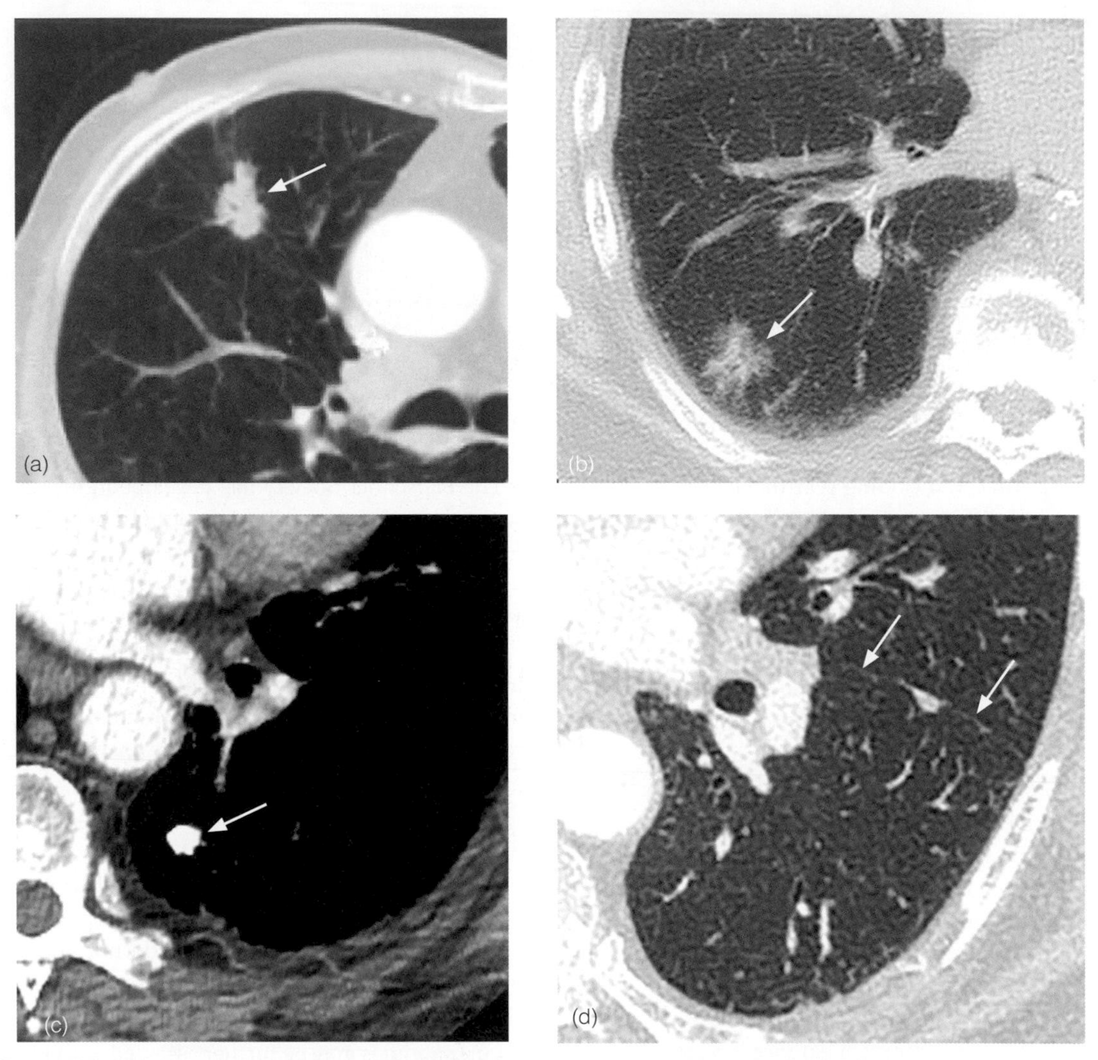

Figure 5.6 Examples of lung nodules seen on CT. (a) Solid: non-small cell lung cancer (NSCLC). Irregularly shaped, spiculated nodule of uniform soft-tissue density (arrow). (b) Subsolid: adenocarcinoma. Irregularly shaped nodule with a mixture of solid and ground glass components (arrow). (c) Calcified: granuloma. Calcified nodule seen as a dense opacity (arrow). (d) Perifissural: benign intrapulmonary lymph node. Soft-tissue nodule with a flat margin where it abuts the oblique fissure, which is seen as a thin straight line traversing the lung (arrows).

Table 5.2 The Fleischner Society guidelines for follow-up of a single pulmonary nodule.

Nodule type	Nodule size (mm)	Low-risk patient	High-risk patient
Solid	<6	No follow-up	Optional CT at 12 months
	6–8	• CT at 6–12 months • Consider CT at 18–24 months	• CT at 6–12 months • CT at 8–24 months
	>8	• Consider CT at 3 months • FDG-PET or biopsy	• Consider CT at 3 months • FDG-PET or biopsy
Semisolid	<6	No follow-up	
	≥6	• CT at 6–12 months to confirm persistence; if unchanged and solid component remains <6 mm, annual CT for 5 years • Consider CT at 18–24 months	
Ground glass	<6	No follow-up	
	≥6	CT at 6–12 months to confirm persistence; then CT every 2 years for 5 years	

5.6 BRONCHOGENIC CARCINOMA

Bronchogenic carcinoma is classified into small cell lung cancer (SCLC) and non-small cell lung cancer (NSCLC). SCLS accounts for about 15% of new cases of bronchogenic carcinoma and is more aggressive than NSCLC.

5.6.1 DIAGNOSIS

Most bronchogenic carcinomas are initially diagnosed on CXR. CXR may be performed for investigation of a specific symptom such as haemoptysis or weight loss in a smoker. Alternatively, bronchogenic carcinoma may be an incidental finding on a CXR performed for other reasons, such as before an anaesthetic or as part of a routine medical check-up. The usual appearance of a bronchogenic carcinoma on CXR is a pulmonary nodule or mass (Fig. 5.7). Also, as discussed above, adenocarcinoma of the lung may have a variety of appearances, including scar-like lesions and focal ground glass opacities. Complications of bronchogenic carcinoma that may produce a more complex appearance on CXR include:

- Segmental/lobar collapse
- Persistent areas of consolidation
- Hilar lymphadenopathy
- Mediastinal lymphadenopathy
- Pleural effusion

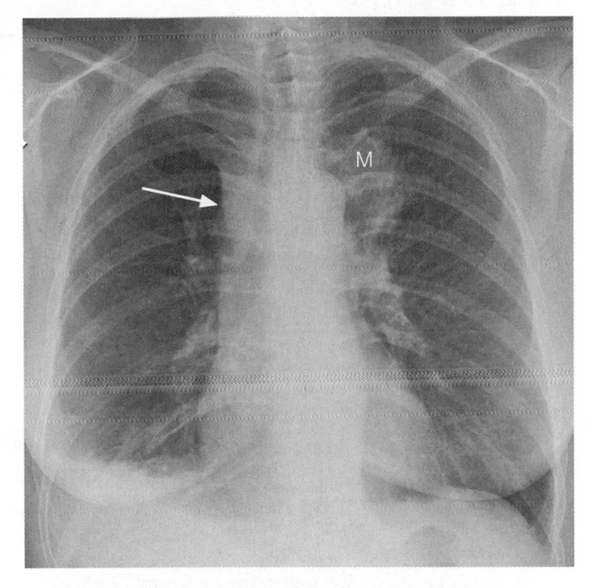

Figure 5.7 Lung cancer: CXR. Large medial left upper zone mass (M). Also note the widened right mediastinum indicating paratracheal lymphadenopathy (arrow) and right pleural effusion.

- Invasion of adjacent structures: mediastinum, chest wall
- Metastases: lungs, bones.

CT is more accurate than CXR for the diagnosis of mediastinal lymphadenopathy, hilar lymphadenopathy, mediastinal invasion and chest wall invasion. CT may also be used for primary diagnosis when the CXR is negative and the presence of a tumour is suspected on clinical grounds, e.g. haemoptysis, positive sputum cytology or paraneoplastic syndrome.

The diagnosis of cell type is important: first, to confirm the diagnosis of bronchogenic carcinoma; second, to classify the tumour. Tumour cells may be obtained from sputum cytology or from aspiration of pleural fluid. More commonly, some form of invasive biopsy will be required as follows:

- Centrally located tumours: bronchoscopy and biopsy
- Peripheral tumours: CT-guided biopsy
- Very small masses or tumours in difficult locations such as deep to the scapula: open biopsy or VATS.

5.6.2 STAGING

FDG-PET-CT is the imaging modality of choice for the staging of bronchogenic carcinoma (Fig. 5.8). The tumour–node–metastasis (TNM) system is used to stage bronchogenic carcinoma:

- 'T' includes features such as tumour size and evidence of chest wall or mediastinal invasion
- 'N' refers to regional hilar or mediastinal lymph node involvement
- 'M' refers to distant metastasis.

SCLC is often staged using a two-stage system, in which patients are classified as having limited or extensive disease. Limited disease is tumour confined to one hemithorax and to regional lymph nodes, which usually implies that the tumour is confined to a region small enough to be treated with radiotherapy. Extensive disease describes SCLC that has spread to the contralateral lung or lymph nodes or to distant organs. Further details of bronchogenic cancer staging may be found on the companion website.

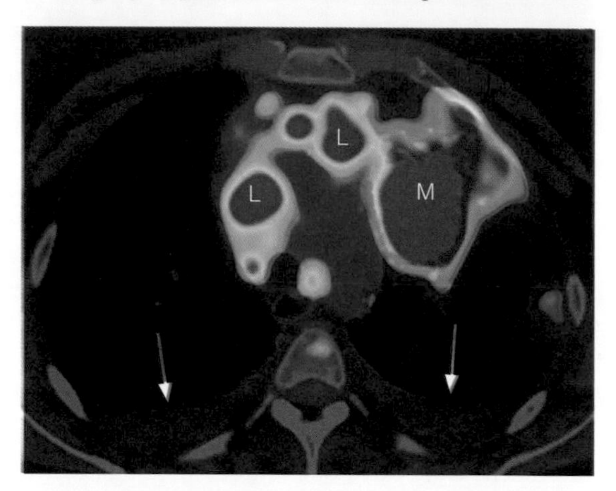

Figure 5.8 Lung cancer: FDG-PET-CT. Intensely avid left upper lobe mass (M) and mediastinal lymphadenopathy (L). Also note the bilateral pleural effusions (arrows).

SUMMARY

Clinical presentation	Investigation of choice	Comment
Respiratory symptoms, including cough, shortness of breath, pleuritic chest pain, haemoptysis	CXR	CT as specifically indicated
Pulmonary infection	CXR	CT for specific scenarios, e.g. immunocompromised hosts, monitoring viral pneumonia such as that caused by COVID-19
Diffuse lung disease	HRCT	See Table 5.1 for a summary of common diffuse lung diseases
Solitary pulmonary nodule	• CT • FDG-PET-CT • Biopsy	See Table 5.2 for guidelines on the follow-up of pulmonary nodules
Staging of bronchogenic carcinoma	FDG-PET-CT	CT if PET-CT is not available

Abbreviation: HRCT, high-resolution CT.

6 Cardiovascular system

The epidemiology of atherosclerotic cardiovascular disease has evolved over the past few decades. Effective therapies for lipid disorders and hypertension plus reduced cigarette smoking have seen a reduction in the classical risk factors in the industrialized world. Vaccination programmes, effective treatment of acute infections and improved sanitation have improved life expectancy in the developing world, such that individuals survive longer with increased prevalence of non-communicable chronic diseases such as atherosclerosis. At the same time, there is currently a worldwide epidemic of obesity, and high-level tobacco use continues in many populations in Asia and Central and South America. For these and other reasons, atherosclerotic cardiovascular disease is a growing global health problem.

Imaging of cardiovascular disease encompasses the heart and coronary arteries, peripheral arteries, venous thromboembolism, venous insufficiency and hypertension. The last decade has seen significant advances in cardiac imaging with computed tomography (CT) and magnetic resonance imaging (MRI). These modalities complement, and in many cases replace, longer established techniques of radiography, ultrasound (US) and scintigraphy.

6.1 IMAGING OF THE HEART

6.1.1 RADIOGRAPHY

The most common uses of X-rays in cardiac disease are in the assessment of cardiac failure and its treatment and to exclude other causes of chest pain in suspected myocardial ischaemia. See Chapter 4 for an overview of the assessment of the heart and pulmonary vessels, plus other relevant findings such as pulmonary oedema and pleural effusion on chest radiograph (chest X-ray, CXR).

6.1.2 ECHOCARDIOGRAPHY

Echocardiography combines the direct visualization of cardiac anatomy, Doppler analysis of flow rates through valves and septal defects and colour Doppler. Colour Doppler helps in the identification of septal defects and quantification of gradients across stenotic valves.

Indications for echocardiography include:

- Quantification of cardiac function:
  - Systolic function: measurement of the ejection fraction (Fig. 6.1)

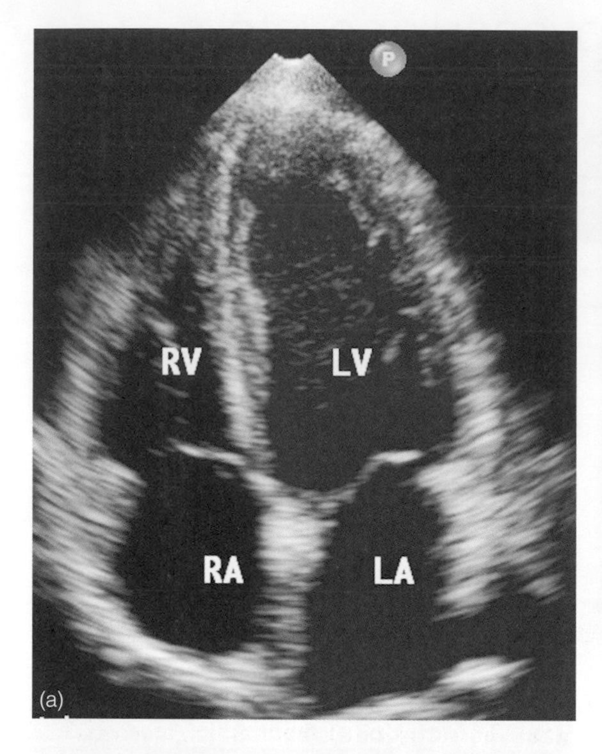

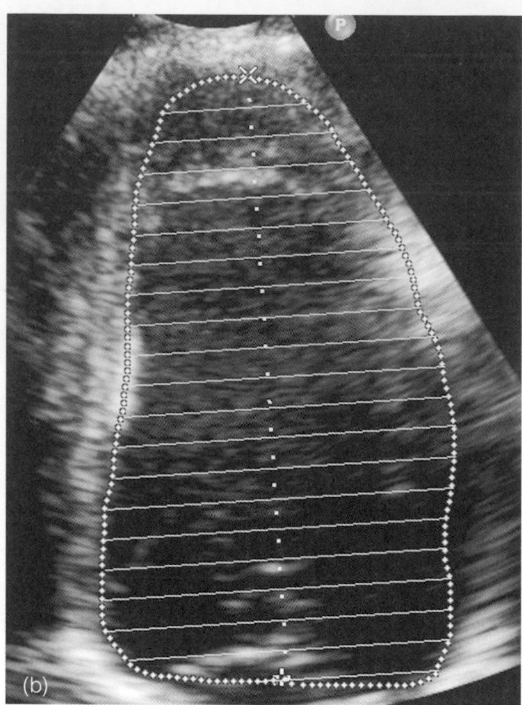

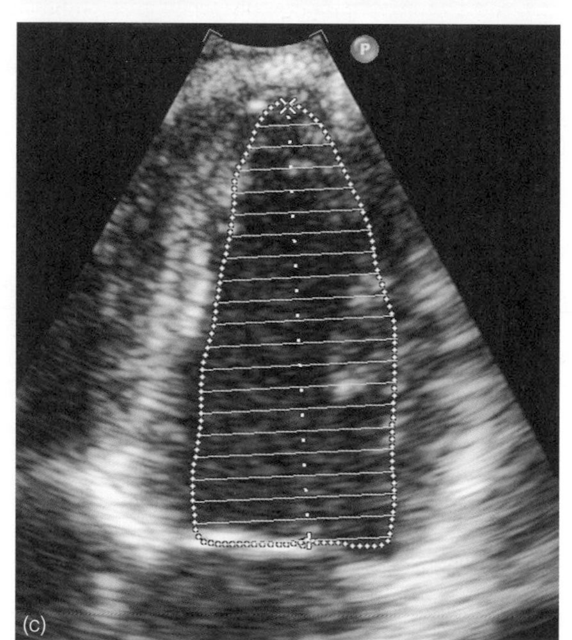

Figure 6.1 Calculation of ejection fraction: echocardiography. (a) Apical four-chamber view of the heart: left atrium (LA), left ventricle (LV), right atrium (RA), right ventricle (RV). (b) Measurement of left ventricular volume at end diastole. (c) Measurement of left ventricular volume in systole.

- Quantification of stroke volume and cardiac output
- Measurement of chamber volumes and wall thicknesses
- Diastolic function: measurement of left ventricular 'relaxation'

- Congenital heart disease
- Diagnosis and quantification of valvular dysfunction
- Stress echocardiography: diagnosis of regional wall motion abnormalities induced by exercise or medication as a sign of coronary artery disease (CAD)
- Miscellaneous: cardiac masses, pericardial effusion, aortic dissection.

The accuracy of echocardiography may be further enhanced by the injection of microbubble contrast agents. Indications for contrast enhanced echocardiography include:

- Cardiac chamber visualization and measurement in technically challenging cases
- Diagnosis of intracardiac shunts such as a patent foramen ovale.

Transoesophageal echocardiography (TOE) is a specialized echocardiographic technique that uses a transoesophageal probe. TOE overcomes the difficulty of imaging through the anterior chest wall, especially in patients with emphysema, in whom the heart may be obscured anteriorly by overexpanded lung. TOE also provides improved imaging of the thoracic aorta and may be used to diagnose aortic diseases such as acute aortic dissection.

6.1.3 COMPUTED TOMOGRAPHY

Modern multidetector and dual-source CT scanners can image the heart and coronary arteries during the diastolic (resting) phase of a single heartbeat (Fig. 6.2).

Current roles of cardiac CT include:

- Quantification of coronary artery calcium expressed as a coronary artery calcium score
- CT coronary angiography (CTCA) in patients at risk for CAD
- CT myocardial perfusion imaging: single-phase or dynamic perfusion imaging during stress with the vasodilator agents adenosine and dipyridamole

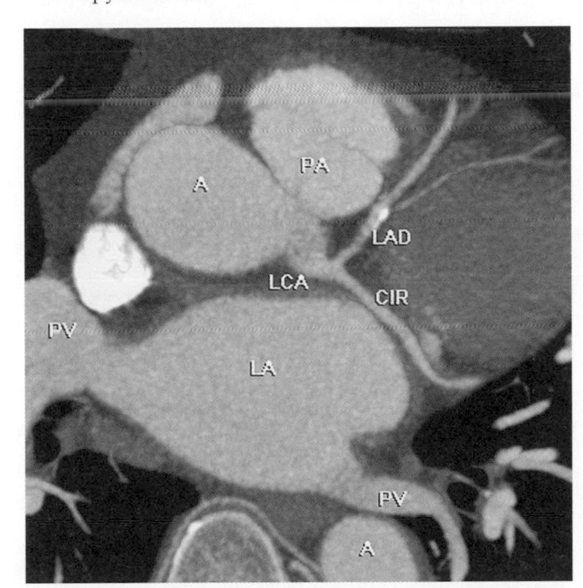

Figure 6.2 CT angiogram of the coronary arteries: normal anatomy. Note the following structures: ascending aorta (A), circumflex artery (CIR), left atrium (LA), left anterior descending artery (LAD), left coronary artery (LCA), pulmonary artery (PA), pulmonary veins (PV).

- Anatomical assessment prior to various procedures, e.g. mapping of the left atrium and pulmonary veins prior to radiofrequency catheter ablation for atrial fibrillation; planning of transcatheter aortic valve implantation (TAVI) with measurement of the aortic valve annulus and mapping of the coronary artery origins
- Postprocedure imaging, e.g. post TAVI to confirm appropriate positioning and to assess for valve leaflet thickening; CTCA for assessment of the patency of coronary artery bypass grafts (CABG) and stents
- Infective endocarditis: perivalvular abscess and fistula.

6.1.4 CORONARY ANGIOGRAPHY

Coronary angiography is performed by placement of preshaped catheters into the origins of the coronary arteries and injection of contrast material. Vascular access is via the groin (femoral artery) or wrist (radial artery). Coronary angiography may be combined with therapeutic interventions, including coronary artery angioplasty and stent deployment.

6.1.5 MAGNETIC RESONANCE IMAGING

Cardiac MRI (CMR) is an established modality in the investigation of cardiac disease.

Current applications of CMR include:

- Quantification of cardiac function: calculation of ejection fraction, myocardial thickness and regional wall motion where echocardiography is difficult or equivocal
- Congenital heart disease: complementary to echocardiography
- Cardiomyopathy, e.g. hypertrophic obstructive cardiomyopathy (HOCM), arrhythmogenic right ventricular cardiomyopathy (ARVC)
- Cardiac anatomy where echocardiography is difficult or equivocal, e.g. left ventricular aneurysm (Fig. 6.3)
- Myocardial perfusion imaging: dynamic perfusion imaging during stress with

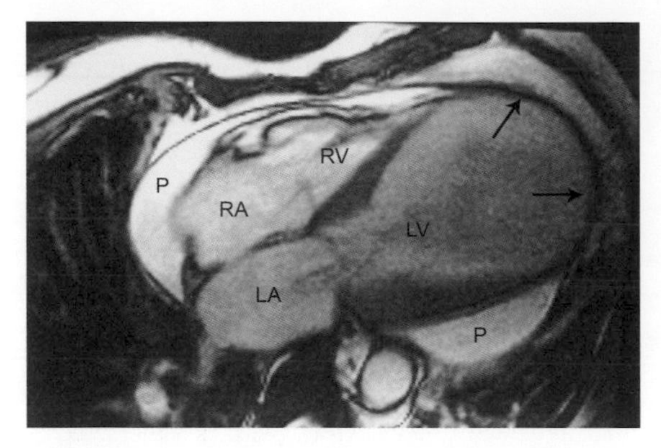

Figure 6.3 Left ventricular aneurysm: MRI. Transverse MRI scan showing a 'four-chamber' view of the heart. Note the left atrium (LA), left ventricle (LV), right atrium (RA), right ventricle (RV), pericardial effusion (P). The apex of the left ventricle has a markedly thinned wall and is dilated (arrows).

vasodilator agents, e.g. regadenoson, or inotropic agents, e.g. dobutamine
- Infarct scan: gadolinium accumulates in infarcted myocardium on delayed scans, differentiating infarction from non-ischaemic infiltrative disease and cardiomyopathy
- Aortic disease: aneurysm, dissection, coarctation
- Myocarditis, e.g. coronavirus disease 2019 (COVID-19)
- Miscellaneous: cardiac masses; pericardial disease.

6.1.6 SCINTIGRAPHY: GATED MYOCARDIAL PERFUSION IMAGING

Myocardial perfusion scintigraphy is performed with ^{99m}Tc-sestamibi, ^{99m}Tc-tetrofosmin or fluorodeoxyglucose–positron emission tomography (FDG-PET). Indications for myocardial perfusion imaging, which may also be performed with CT or MRI, include:

- Acute chest pain with normal or inconclusive electrocardiogram (ECG)
- Abnormal stress ECG in patients at low or intermediate risk of CAD (high-risk patients should have coronary angiography)
- Determine haemodynamic significance of CAD
- Assess cardiac risk prior to major surgery.

6.2 CONGESTIVE CARDIAC FAILURE

Dyspnoea may have a variety of causes, including cardiac and respiratory diseases, anaemia and anxiety states. Certain features in the clinical history may be helpful in diagnosis, such as whether dyspnoea is acute or chronic, worse at night or accentuated by lying down (orthopnoea). Initial tests include a full blood count, ECG and CXR, followed by pulmonary function tests when a respiratory cause such as emphysema or asthma is suspected. Congestive cardiac failure (CCF) is the commonest cardiac cause of dyspnoea and is the result of systolic or diastolic dysfunction or a combination of the two. Systolic dysfunction refers to a reduction in the amount of blood pumped as a result of failure of ventricular contraction. Diastolic dysfunction refers to failure of ventricular relaxation between contractions, leading to reduced filling of the ventricular chambers.

The commonest underlying cause of CCF is ischaemic heart disease. Other causes include valvular heart disease, hypertension, hypertrophic cardiomyopathy, infiltrative disorders such as amyloidosis, pericardial effusion or thickening, or congenital heart disease. Imaging is performed to confirm that CCF is the cause of dyspnoea, to quantify and classify cardiac dysfunction and to identify an underlying cause. CXR and echocardiography are the usual imaging tests employed for the initial assessment of CCF. Coronary artery imaging with CT or angiography is indicated where an ischaemic cause for CCF is suspected.

6.2.1 CHEST RADIOGRAPH SIGNS OF CONGESTIVE CARDIAC FAILURE

(Also see Chapter 4.)

- Cardiac enlargement (cardiomegaly):
  - Cardiothoracic ratio is unreliable as a one-off measurement
  - Of more significance is an increase in heart size on serial CXRs
- Pulmonary vascular redistribution:
  - Upper lobe blood vessels larger than those in the lower lobes

- Interstitial oedema:
  - Reticular (linear) pattern with thickened septal (Kerley B) lines
- Alveolar oedema:
  - Fluffy, ill-defined areas of alveolar opacity in a bilateral central or 'bat wing' distribution
- Pleural effusions
  - Pleural effusions associated with CCF tend to be larger on the right.

6.2.2 ECHOCARDIOGRAPHY

Echocardiography may be used to calculate cardiac chamber size and wall thickness and to diagnose the presence of valvular dysfunction and pericardial effusion. Systolic dysfunction may be diagnosed and quantified by calculation of the left ventricular ejection fraction. The ejection fraction is a measurement of the amount of blood ejected from the left ventricle with systolic contraction. To calculate the ejection fraction, the volume of the left ventricle is calculated at the end of diastole (D) and then at the end of systole (S). The left ventricular volume may be calculated by various methods. Figure 6.1 illustrates the modified Simpson's biplane method. The ejection fraction, expressed as a percentage, is calculated by the following formula: $(D - S)/D \times 100$. Normal values for ejection fraction are $70 \pm 7\%$ for males and $65 \pm 10\%$ for females.

Other measurements such as stroke volume and cardiac output may be calculated with echocardiography. Measurements of left ventricular relaxation may also be done to assess diastolic dysfunction.

6.3 ISCHAEMIC HEART DISEASE

6.3.1 OVERVIEW OF CORONARY ARTERY DISEASE

CAD is the leading cause of death worldwide. Mortality and disability rates due to CAD are increasing in industrialized and developing countries. CAD is a diffuse disease of the coronary arteries characterized by atheromatous plaques. Plaques may cause stenosis of coronary arteries, limiting blood flow to the myocardium. During the development of atheromatous plaques, the external membranes of the coronary arteries may expand outwards. As a result of this arterial remodelling phenomenon, significant coronary atherosclerosis may be present without narrowing of the vessel lumen (non-stenosing plaque). Rupture of atherosclerotic plaques with subsequent arterial thrombosis leads to acute cardiac events (acute cardiac syndrome) such as unstable angina, myocardial infarction and sudden death. Instability and rupture of atherosclerotic plaques is mediated by inflammatory factors and may occur with stenosing or non-stenosing plaques.

CAD with multiple arterial stenoses may present clinically with chronic cardiac disease, most commonly cardiac failure. CCF in this context is caused by pump failure as a result of ischaemic myocardium. CCF due to CAD is commonly associated with chronic stable angina.

The roles of imaging in CAD include:

- Screening for CAD
- Diagnosis and quantification of CAD in acute cardiac syndrome
- Planning of revascularization procedures, including CABG, and interventional procedures, such as angioplasty and coronary artery stent placement
- Assessment of myocardial viability
- Assessment of cardiac function.

6.3.2 SCREENING FOR CORONARY ARTERY DISEASE

The Framingham risk score is a well-recognized tool used to provide a global risk assessment for future 'hard' cardiac events, including myocardial infarction and sudden death. Based on gender and age, cholesterol and high-density lipoprotein (HDL) levels, systolic blood pressure and tobacco use, individuals are categorized as low, intermediate or high risk. This approach has limited accuracy in predicting the presence of CAD and the occurrence of acute cardiac syndrome, which may occur in the absence of known risk factors. Multiple imaging modalities are available for improved assignment of risk level and for direct visualization of CAD.

COMPUTED TOMOGRAPHY CALCIUM SCORING

CT is highly sensitive to the presence of coronary artery calcification (Fig. 6.4). The amount of coronary artery calcification increases with the overall burden of coronary atherosclerotic disease. Software programs quantify coronary artery calcium detected by CT and provide a coronary calcium score. Calcium scores adjusted for age and gender, in combination with other known risk factors, can provide a more accurate assignment of risk category in individual patients. A calcium score of zero is a strong indicator of a very low risk of subsequent cardiac events, though it does not exclude non-calcified plaque. Calcium scoring may also be useful for monitoring CAD in patients undergoing medical treatments for risk factor reduction.

COMPUTED TOMOGRAPHY CORONARY ANGIOGRAPHY

CTCA is an established ECG-gated technique for the diagnosis of CAD (Fig. 6.5). CTCA requires a relatively low heart rate (ideally ≤60 beats per minute); patients are usually administered beta-blocker medication prior to scanning and vasodilatory sublingual nitrates at the time of scanning. Advantages of CTCA include:

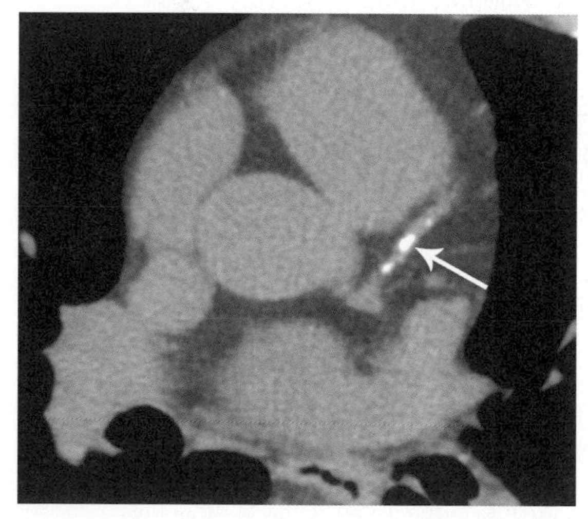

Figure 6.4 CT coronary calcium scoring. Note calcification in the left anterior descending artery (arrow) in a middle-aged man with atherosclerosis of the coronary arteries.

- Non-invasiveness
- Ability to image non-stenotic plaques in the vessel wall
- Very high negative predictive value, i.e. a normal CTCA examination is an excellent indicator of the absence of clinically significant CAD.

Indications for CTCA include:

- Investigation of choice for the diagnosis of CAD in low- to intermediate-risk patients
- Diagnosis of indeterminate chest pain, specifically exclusion of a cardiac cause
- Planning of catheter-directed interventions, angioplasty and stent deployment
- Assess grafts in patients following CABG.

The Coronary Artery Disease Reporting and Data System (CAD-RADS) is a standardized reporting method relevant to CTCA. CAD-RADS is used for patients with two different clinical presentations:

- Stable chest pain
- Acute chest pain, negative first troponin, negative or non-diagnostic ECG and low to intermediate risk (thrombolysis in myocardial infarction (TIMI) risk score <4).

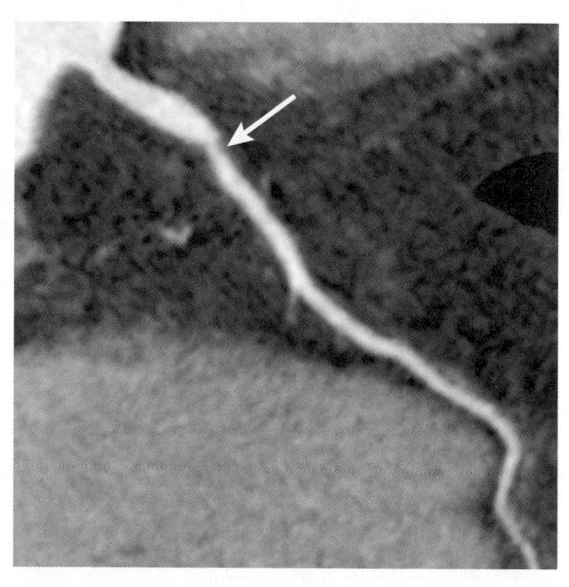

Figure 6.5 Coronary artery stenosis: CT coronary angiography (CTCA). Stenosis is seen as a focal narrowing of the contrast-filled arterial lumen (arrow).

Based on the most severe coronary artery lesion, a CAD-RADS score is applied under whichever of these categories is applicable, along with an accompanying clinical recommendation. Further details on CAD-RADS may be found on the companion website.

CATHETER CORONARY ANGIOGRAPHY

In the past, catheter coronary angiography has been the standard method for the diagnosis of CAD. Coronary angiography remains the investigation of choice in acute cardiac syndrome and in patients at high risk for the presence of CAD. The major limitation of coronary angiography is that it only provides an image of the vessel lumen. Only atherosclerotic plaques that cause significant narrowing of the lumen of the coronary artery are diagnosed with coronary angiography. Non-stenosing plaques, which may be at risk of rupture, are not diagnosed with coronary angiography.

EXERCISE STRESS TESTING

Screening tests may be performed to identify clinically silent CAD, to calculate the risk of future acute cardiac events and to identify those patients who may benefit from revascularization procedures. These screening tests are designed to detect abnormalities such as ECG changes or regional ventricular wall motion abnormalities in response to exercise or pharmacologically induced myocardial stress. An abnormal exercise test has a high predictive value for the presence of obstructive CAD.

Methods of exercise stress testing include:

- Stress ECG: ST segment depression induced by exercise
- Stress echocardiogram: segmental wall motion abnormalities induced by exercise
- Myocardial perfusion scintigraphy (Fig. 6.6).

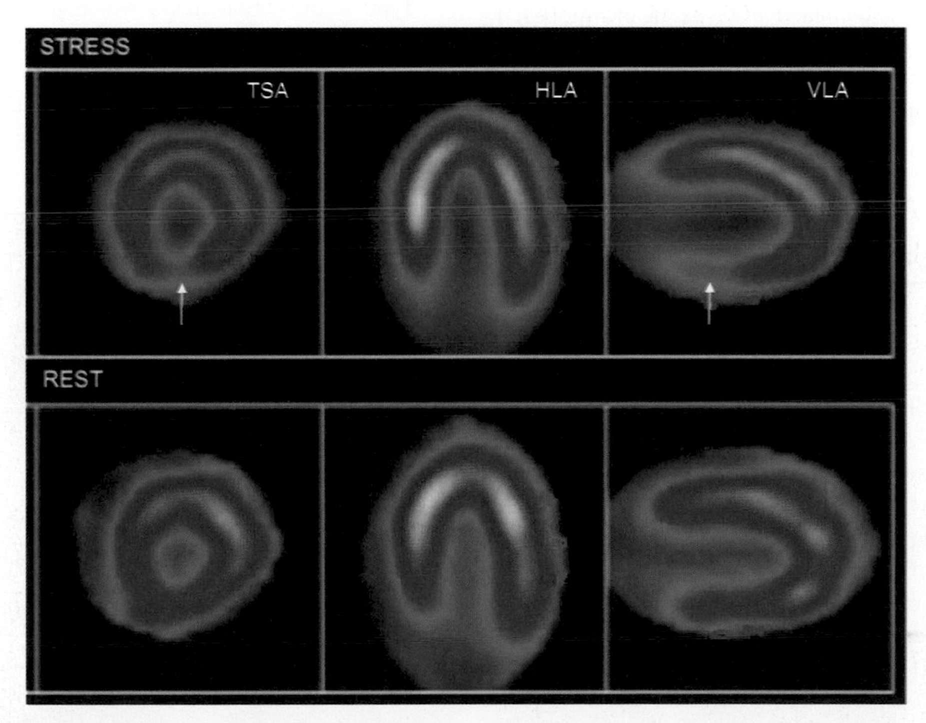

Figure 6.6 Myocardial ischaemia: ^{99m}Tc myocardial perfusion single photon emission CT (SPECT). Images are displayed in three planes. From left to right, these are transverse short axis (TSA), horizontal long axis (HLA) and vertical long axis (VLA). The top three images are with myocardial stress; the lower three are at rest. The TSA and VLA stress images show a region of reduced perfusion in the inferior wall of the left ventricle (arrows). This region shows improved perfusion at rest, indicating a reversible ischaemic defect.

6.3.3 ACUTE CHEST PAIN

As outlined in section 6.3.1, sudden rupture of an atherosclerotic plaque with subsequent arterial thrombosis and occlusion may lead to acute cardiac events such as sudden death, myocardial infarction and acute unstable angina. The classical symptoms of acute angina are chest pain and tightness radiating to the jaw and left arm. Other causes of acute chest pain include aortic dissection, pulmonary embolism (PE), gastro-oesophageal reflux, muscle spasm and a variety of respiratory causes. Initial work-up for a cardiac cause includes ECG and serum markers such as CK-MB and cardiac troponins. Initial imaging assessment in the acute situation consists of a CXR to look for evidence of cardiac failure and to diagnose a non-cardiac cause of chest pain such as pneumonia or pneumothorax. Coronary angiography is indicated in patients with ECG changes or elevated serum markers. Interventional procedures aimed at restoring coronary blood flow, including coronary artery angioplasty and stent deployment, may also be performed acutely. CTCA may also be used in the acute situation, including as part of a 'triple rule out' protocol to diagnose or exclude CAD, aortic dissection and PE.

6.3.4 MYOCARDIAL VIABILITY AND CARDIAC FUNCTION

Further imaging in the setting of CAD and ischaemic heart disease consists of tests of myocardial viability. Myocardial perfusion scintigraphy assesses the amount of viable versus non-viable myocardium, and echocardiography quantifies cardiac function and can diagnose complications of myocardial infarction such as papillary muscle rupture, ventricular septal defect, left ventricular aneurysm and pericardial effusion.

Cardiac CT and MRI may also be used to assess myocardial viability and cardiac function in patients with CAD. Both provide a quantitative assessment of ventricular wall motion and can assess myocardial perfusion at rest and with pharmacologically induced stress. CT myocardial perfusion imaging can be combined with CTCA to assess the functional significance of any identified coronary arterial stenosis.

6.4 AORTIC DISSECTION

Aortic dissection occurs when a tear in the surface of the intima allows blood to flow into the aortic wall. This creates a false lumen, with re-entry of blood into the true lumen occurring more distally. Dissection may involve the aorta alone or may cause occlusion of major arterial branches.

Aortic dissection usually presents with acute chest pain, which is often described as a 'tearing' sensation. Chest pain may be anterior, or posterior between the scapulae, and may radiate more distally as the dissection progresses. Aortic dissections are classified by the Stanford system into types A and B:

- Type A: any dissections involving the ascending aorta or aortic arch proximal to the origin of the left subclavian artery, regardless of distal extent
- Type B: dissection confined to the aorta distal to the origin of the left subclavian artery.

Type A dissection has a worse prognosis than type B because of an increased risk of coronary artery occlusion, rupture into the pericardium and aortic valve regurgitation. In general, type A is treated surgically and type B with medical therapy and endovascular repair.

CXR is performed in the initial assessment of the patient with chest pain. In the context of suspected aortic dissection, CXR is mainly to exclude other causes of chest pain prior to more definitive investigation. Most of the CXR signs that may be seen with aortic dissection, such as pleural effusion, are non-specific and may be seen in a range of other conditions. Alterations to the contour of the aortic arch and displacement of intimal calcification may be more specific but are only occasionally seen (Fig. 6.7).

Contrast CT angiography (CTA) of the chest is the investigation of choice for suspected aortic dissection (Fig. 6.8). CT is used in the evaluation of suspected aortic dissection to:

- Confirm the diagnosis by demonstration of the dissection flap
- Classify the dissection as type A or B
- Define the true and false lumens
- Identify involvement or occlusion of arterial branches, including the coronary arteries

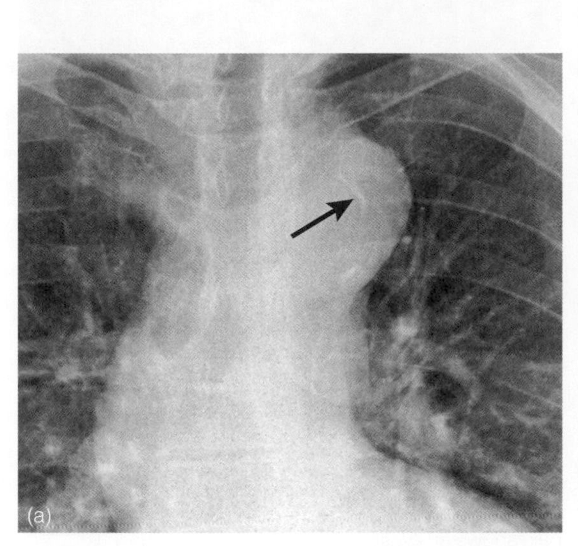

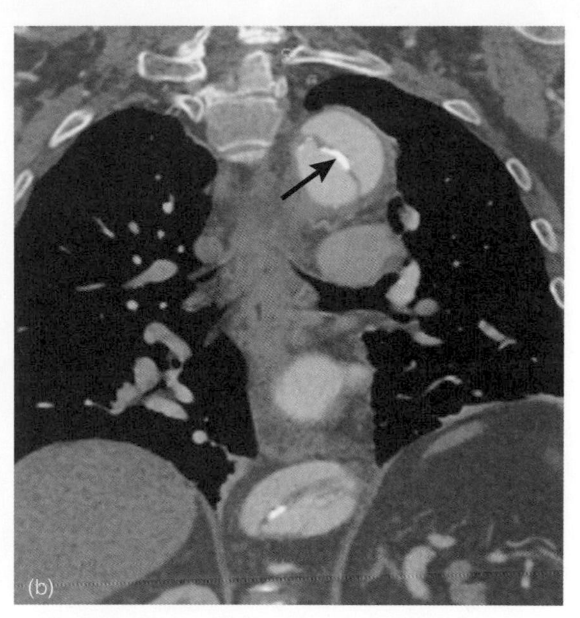

Figure 6.7 Aortic dissection: CXR and CT. (a) CXR shows intimal calcification (arrow) displaced centrally by blood in the false lumen. (b) Coronal contrast-enhanced CT in the same patient shows a true lumen and a false lumen separated by an intimal flap. The intimal flap contains calcification (arrow), which is displaced on CXR.

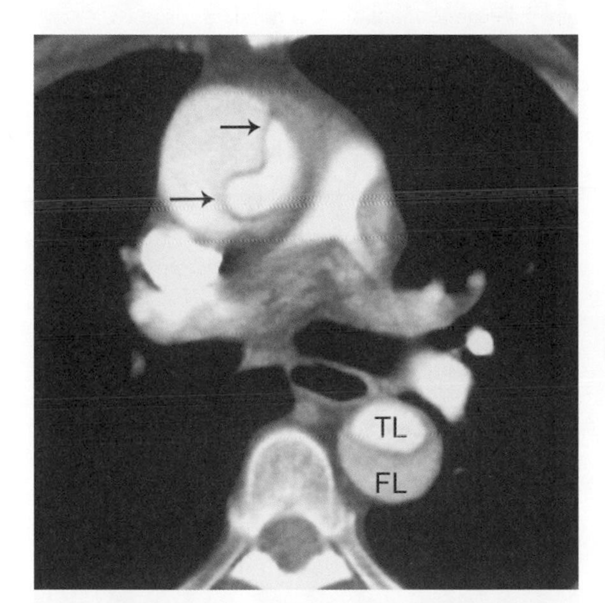

Figure 6.8 Aortic dissection: CT. Note the thin intimal flap in the ascending aorta (arrows). In the descending aorta the flap is seen separating the true lumen (TL) from the false lumen (FL).

- Demonstrate bleeding: mediastinal haematoma, haemothroax or pericardial effusion.

Depending on local availability and expertise, TOE or MRI may be used to confirm the diagnosis in difficult or equivocal cases. TOE may also be performed at the bedside in critically ill patients.

6.5 ABDOMINAL AORTIC ANEURYSM

Abdominal aortic aneurysm (AAA) is generally defined as an abdominal aortic diameter of greater than 4 cm. AAA is usually caused by weakening of the aortic wall as a result of atherosclerosis. This weakening leads to dilatation of the aorta, which is usually progressive. AAA may present clinically as a pulsatile abdominal mass or occasionally with acute abdominal pain due to leakage. More commonly, AAA is an incidental finding on imaging performed for other reasons, including US or CT of the abdomen or radiograph of the lumbar spine. Radiographic signs of AAA may include a soft-tissue mass with curvilinear calcification.

6.5.1 ULTRASOUND

Most small aneurysms less than 5 cm in diameter may be managed conservatively with regular clinical and imaging surveillance.

Indications for surgical or endoluminal repair include:

- Diameter greater than 5.4 cm in males; 4.9 cm in females
- Diameter expansion greater than 1 cm in 1 year
- Symptoms attributable to AAA.

US is the investigation of choice for initial measurement and definition of AAA in some countries, but is being replaced by CT.

Based on diameter measurement, further surveillance or management may be recommended as follows:

- 3.0–3.9 cm: repeat US in 5 years
- 4.0–4.9 cm: repeat US in 6 months
- greater than 4.9 cm: refer to a vascular surgeon.

6.5.2 COMPUTED TOMOGRAPHY

Except for emergency situations, imaging is usually required for preoperative planning prior to surgical or endoluminal repair of AAA. CTA is the investigation of choice for measurement, definition of anatomy and diagnosis of complications such as leakage (Fig. 6.9). Treatment planning prior to percutaneous stent placement (see section 6.11.2) requires precise CT measurements of aneurysm diameter and length, distance from renal arteries and diameter and length of common iliac arteries (Fig. 6.10). CT may also be performed after stent deployment or surgical repair for diagnosis of complications such as infection, occlusion and endoleak, or less common complications such as aortoduodenal fistula and retroperitoneal fibrosis.

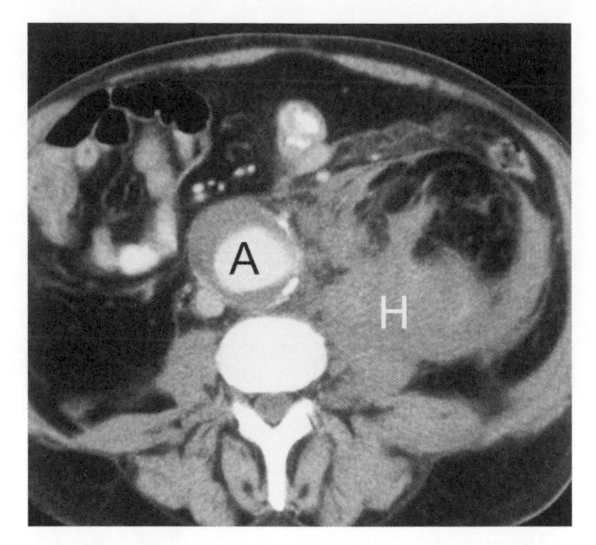

Figure 6.9 Leaking abdominal aortic aneurysm: CT. CT obtained in a patient with acute onset of abdominal pain shows an aortic aneurysm (A) and a large left retroperitoneal haematoma (H).

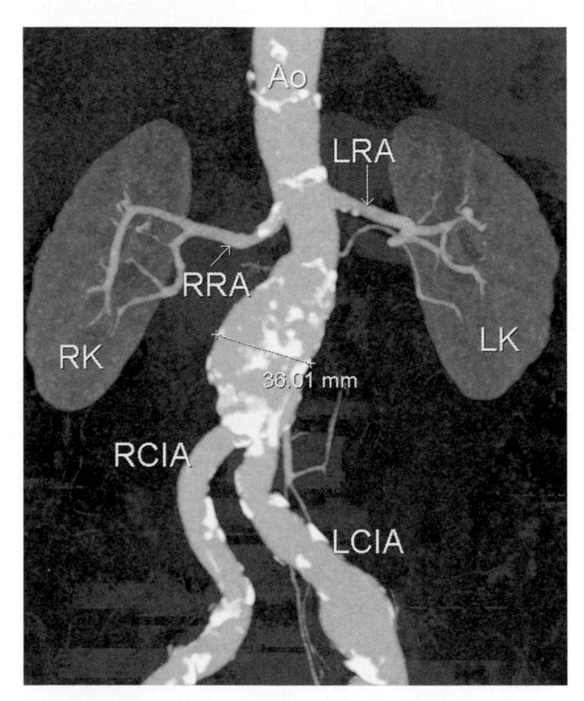

Figure 6.10 Abdominal aortic aneurysm: CT. A reconstructed image from a CT angiogram shows the following structures: aorta (Ao), left and right common iliac arteries (LCIA, RCIA), left and right kidneys (LK, RK), left and right renal arteries (LRA, RRA).

6.6 PERIPHERAL VASCULAR DISEASE

The commonest clinical presentation of the patient with peripheral vascular disease (PVD) is claudication, which is characterized by muscle pain and weakness and is reproducibly produced by a set amount of exercise and relieved by rest. Patients with severe arterial disease may have pain at rest or soft-tissue changes such as ischaemic ulcers and gangrene. Non-arterial causes of claudication such as spinal stenosis and chronic venous occlusion may be seen in 25% of cases.

6.6.1 PHYSIOLOGICAL TESTING AND DOPPLER ULTRASOUND

The diagnosis of PVD in patients with claudication may be confirmed with non-invasive physiological tests:

- Ankle–brachial index (ABI)
- Pulse volume recordings
- Segmental pressures, including measurements performed at rest and following exercise.

A normal ABI at rest and following exercise usually excludes significant peripheral arterial disease; in such cases, no further arterial imaging is required. The non-invasive vascular laboratory combines physiological tests with Doppler US imaging to define those patients requiring angiography and possible further treatment – either surgery or interventional radiology. Signs of arterial stenosis on Doppler US include visible narrowing of the artery seen on two-dimensional and colour images associated with a focal zone of increased flow velocity and an altered arterial wave pattern distally. Doppler US is particularly useful for differentiating focal stenosis from diffuse disease and occlusion. Other arterial abnormalities, such as aneurysm, pseudoaneurysm and arteriovenous malformation (AVM), are well seen, and Doppler US is also useful for postoperative graft surveillance.

Therapy is required if physiological testing with or without Doppler US demonstrates significant peripheral arterial disease in a patient with claudication. In these cases, a complete accurate assessment of the arterial system from the aorta to the arteries in the foot is required. The choice of modality often depends on local expertise and availability and includes CTA, MR angiography (MRA) or catheter angiography.

6.6.2 COMPUTED TOMOGRAPHY ANGIOGRAPHY AND MAGNETIC RESONANCE ANGIOGRAPHY

CTA and MRA are used for planning of therapy for PVD. CTA and MRA can display highly accurate images of the peripheral vascular system without arterial puncture. Problems with MRA include long examination times, inability to image patients with cardiac pacemakers and artefacts from surgical clips and metallic stents. CTA has very short examination times, uses less radiation than catheter angiography and is usually not significantly degraded by stents and surgical clips. CTA has fewer technical problems than MRA and is more widely used for assessment of PVD (Fig. 6.11).

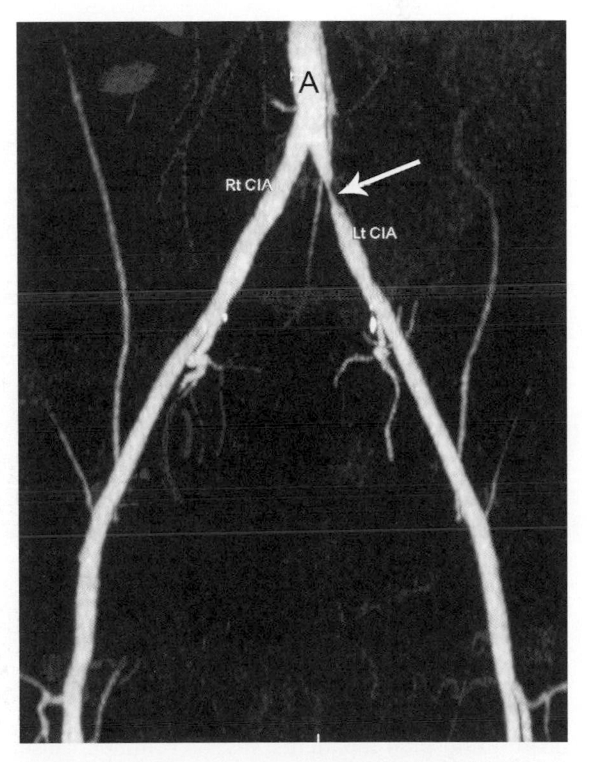

Figure 6.11 Stenosis of the left common iliac artery (Lt CIA): CT angiogram. Compare the focal narrowing due to the stenosis (arrow) with the normal smooth outline of the right common iliac artery (Rt CIA) and aorta (A).

6.6.3 CATHETER ANGIOGRAPHY

Catheter angiography refers to the placement of selective arterial catheters and injection of contrast material to outline arterial anatomy. Most catheters are placed via femoral artery puncture and less commonly via the brachial, axillary or radial artery. Catheter insertion is performed by the Seldinger technique as follows:

1. Artery punctured with a needle
2. Wire threaded through the needle into the artery
3. Needle removed, leaving the wire in the artery
4. Sheath inserted over the wire into the artery
5. Catheter inserted into the sheath.

A wide array of preshaped catheters is available that allow selective catheterization of most major arteries in the body. Postprocedure care following catheter angiography consists of bed rest for a few hours with observation of the puncture site for bleeding and swelling. The complication rate of modern angiography is very low and is most commonly related to the arterial puncture:

- Haematoma at the puncture site
- False aneurysm (pseudoaneurysm) formation
- Arterial dissection
- Embolism due to dislodgement of atheromatous plaques.

Other possible complications of catheter angiography relate to the use of iodinated contrast material (allergy and contrast-induced nephropathy; see Chapter 2). With the widespread use of less invasive diagnostic methods such as Doppler US, CTA and MRA, catheter angiography is more usually performed in association with interventional techniques such as angioplasty, arterial stent placement and thrombolysis (see section 6.11).

6.7 PULMONARY EMBOLISM

PE is one of the commonest preventable causes of death in hospital inpatients. PE is a common cause of morbidity and mortality in postoperative patients, as well as in patients with other risk factors such as prolonged bed rest, malignancy and cardiac failure. Symptoms of PE may include pleuritic chest pain, shortness of breath, cough and haemoptysis; a large number of PEs are clinically silent. Clinical signs such as hypotension, tachycardia, reduced oxygen saturation and ECG changes (S1 Q3 T3) are non-specific and often absent. As such, the clinical diagnosis of PE is problematical and usually requires confirmation with imaging studies including CXR, CT pulmonary angiography (CTPA) and ventilation/perfusion nuclear lung scan (V/Q scan).

The rate of negative imaging studies can be reduced by assignment of a pretest probability of PE in a patient presenting with a suggestive history and clinical findings using a logical clinical assessment system and a D-dimer assay. The most widely used clinical model is the Simplified Wells Scoring System, in which points are assigned:

	Score
• Leg pain, swelling and tenderness suggestive of deep venous thrombosis (DVT):	3.0
• Heart rate greater than 100 beats/minute:	1.5
• Immobilization for three or more consecutive days:	1.5
• Surgery in the previous 4 weeks:	1.5
• Previous confirmed DVT or PE:	1.5
• Haemoptysis:	1.0
• Malignancy:	1.0
• Alternative diagnosis less likely than PE:	3.0

The pretest probability is assigned depending on the points score:

- Less than 2: low
- 2–6: moderate
- More than 6: high

D-dimer is a plasma constituent present when fibrin is released from active thrombus. A positive D-dimer assay is non-specific; a negative D-dimer has a very high negative predictive value. The diagnosis of PE is reliably excluded if the clinical pretest probability is low and the D-dimer assay is negative. In such patients, imaging with CTPA or scintigraphy is not indicated. Imaging is indicated when the clinical pretest probability is moderate or high or when the D-dimer assay is positive.

6.7.1 CHEST RADIOGRAPH

CXRs are often normal in patients with suspected PE. Signs of PE on CXR include pleural effusion, a localized area of consolidation contacting a pleural surface (Hampton hump) or a localized area of collapse. These signs are non-specific and often absent. The main role of CXR in this context is to diagnose other causes for the patient's symptoms, such as pneumonia. CXR may also assist in the interpretation of a V/Q scan.

6.7.2 COMPUTED TOMOGRAPHY PULMONARY ANGIOGRAPHY

In most circumstances, CTPA is the investigation of choice for confirming the diagnosis of PE. PEs are seen on CTPA as filling defects within contrast-filled pulmonary arteries (Fig. 6.12). Right ventricular dysfunction ('right heart strain') may occur with large occlusive emboli and may be indicated on CTPA by dilatation of the right ventricle, enlargement of the pulmonary trunk and flattening or bowing of the interventricular septum. CTPA is highly sensitive and specific with a very low incidence of intermediate or equivocal results. It may also establish alternative diagnoses such as pneumonia or aortic dissection. The main disadvantage of CTPA is radiation dose, which is a particular issue in young women because of the absorbed radiation dose to the breasts. In some centres scintigraphy may be offered to young women, particularly if pregnant. However, modern CT scanners have lower radiation doses, narrowing the difference in radiation exposure between CTPA and scintigraphy.

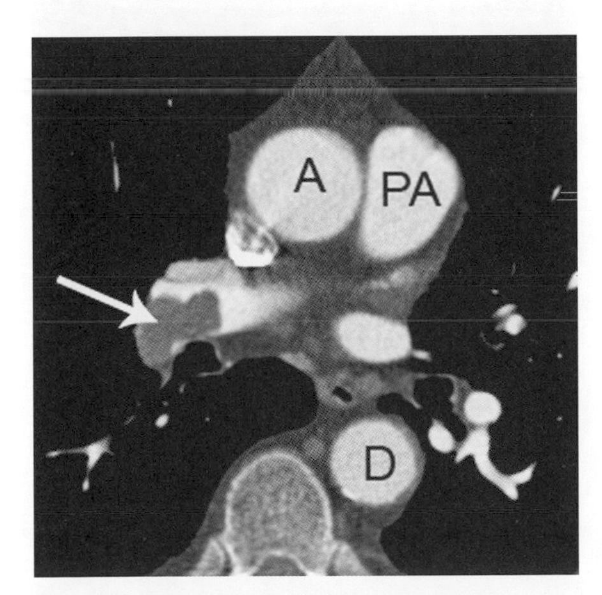

Figure 6.12 Pulmonary embolism: CT pulmonary angiography (CTPA). Pulmonary embolus seen as a low-density filling defect in the right pulmonary artery (arrow). Also note the ascending aorta (A), descending aorta (D), main pulmonary artery (PA).

Spectral CT using various techniques as described in Chapter 1, including low mono-energetic reconstructions (low monoE) for 'iodine boosting' of the pulmonary arteries, as well as Z-effective and iodine maps for lung perfusion assessment, may enhance the diagnostic performance of CTPA.

6.7.3 SCINTIGRAPHY: VENTILATION/PERFUSION NUCLEAR LUNG SCAN

Scintigraphy is indicated in certain circumstances, including in patients with a history of previous allergic reaction to intravenous contrast material and in young or pregnant women because the absorbed radiation dose to the breasts is much lower than with CTPA.

V/Q scan consists of the following:

- Ventilation (V) phase: ventilation with ^{99m}Tc-Technegas (30- to 60-nm carbon particles)
- Perfusion (Q) phase: intravenous injection of ^{99m}Tc-macroaggregated albumen (MAA); aggregates have a mean diameter of 30–60 μm and are trapped in the pulmonary microvasculature on first pass through the lungs
- Perfusion phase is then compared with the ventilation phase.

The diagnostic hallmark of PE is one or more regions of V/Q mismatch, i.e. a region of lung where perfusion is reduced or absent and ventilation is preserved. Currently, single photon emission CT (SPECT) offers excellent anatomical detail of pulmonary perfusion and improves sensitivity for small PEs. SPECT criteria for the diagnosis of PE are at least one large (segmental or larger) mismatched defect or two or more small (subsegmental) mismatched defects. Historically, V/Q scans were graded as low, intermediate or high probability of PE based on the Prospective Investigation of Pulmonary Embolism Diagnosis

(PIOPED) trials. V/Q scans performed without Technegas or based on planar imaging alone may be reported according to PIOPED probability criteria.

6.8 DEEP VENOUS THROMBOSIS

DVT of the leg presents clinically with local pain and tenderness accompanied by swelling. Risk factors for the development of DVT include:

- Hospitalization and immobilization
- Trauma
- Surgery, particularly surgery to the lower limb or major abdominal surgery
- Malignancy
- Obesity
- History of previous DVT
- Factor V Leiden.

Sequelae of DVT include:

- PE
- Recurrent DVT
- Post-thrombotic syndrome, in which venous incompetence and stasis cause chronic leg pain, swelling and venous ulcers.

Doppler US is the investigation of choice for suspected DVT. US is highly accurate in the diagnosis of DVT and may detect conditions that can mimic DVT, such as a ruptured Baker cyst.

Signs of DVT on US examination (Fig. 6.13) include:

- Visible thrombus within the vein
- Non-compressibility of the vein
- Failure of venous distension with Valsalva's manoeuvre
- Lack of normal venous Doppler signal
- Loss of flow on colour images.

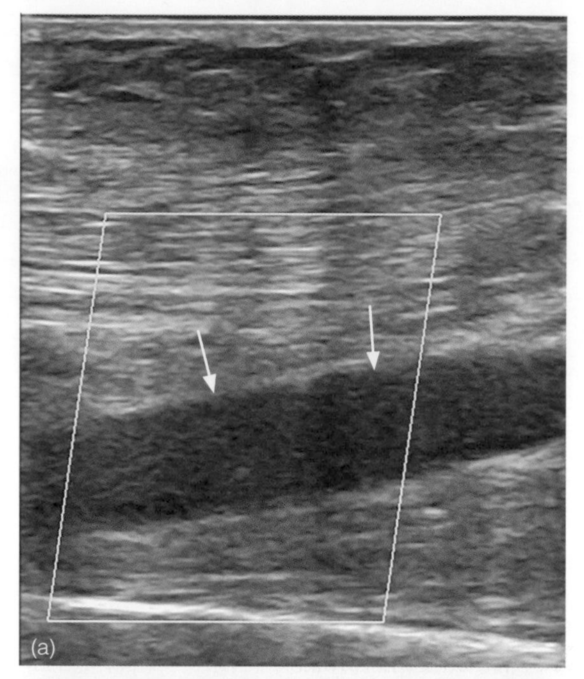

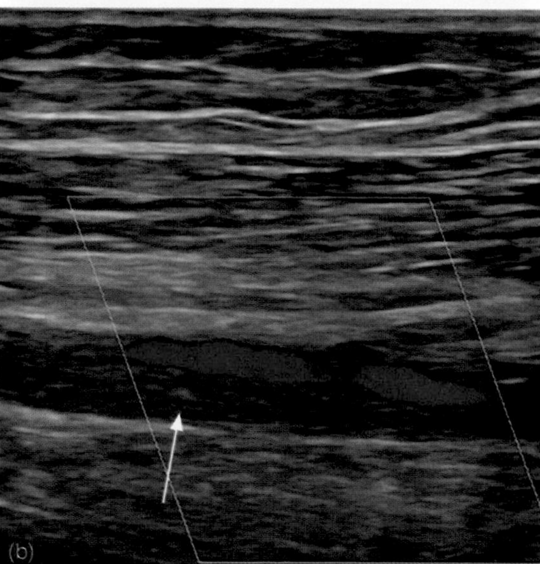

Figure 6.13 Deep venous thrombosis (DVT): duplex US. (a) Occlusive thrombus: hypoechoic soft tissue seen filling the femoral vein with no blood flow identified (arrows). (b) Non-occlusive thrombus: seen as hypoechoic soft tissue in the femoral vein (arrow), with residual blood flow seen on colour Doppler as blue colour.

6.8.1 UPPER LIMB DEEP VENOUS THROMBOSIS

Upper limb DVT usually presents clinically with acute onset of upper limb swelling. Risk factors for upper limb DVT include:

- Central venous catheters, including percutaneously inserted central venous catheters (PICCs)

- Trauma
- In young adult patients, especially bodybuilders, upper limb DVT may occur secondary to compression of the subclavian vein between the first rib and clavicle (Paget–Schroetter syndrome)
- Superior vena cava (SVC) compression by mediastinal tumour or lymphadenopathy.

Doppler US is the first investigation of choice for suspected upper limb DVT. If Doppler US is negative, contrast-enhanced CT is indicated to provide further assessment of the large central veins, including the SVC. Venography and thrombolysis may be indicated for acute thrombosis of the axillary or subclavian veins. In cases of SVC compression by tumour or lymph node mass, stent deployment may provide palliation.

6.9 VENOUS INSUFFICIENCY

For the patient with varicose veins for whom surgery is contemplated, US with Doppler is the imaging investigation of choice for assessment. The competence of a leg vein, deep or superficial, is determined with Doppler US using calf compression and release. A competent vein will show no or minor reflux (reversal of flow) on release of calf compression. Incompetence is defined as reflux of greater than 0.5 seconds in duration. The following information may be obtained with Doppler US:

- Patency and competence of the deep venous system from the common femoral vein to the lower calf
- Competence and diameter of the saphenofemoral junction and long saphenous vein
- Identification of duplications, tributaries and varices arising from the long saphenous vein
- Competence and diameter of the saphenopopliteal junction
- Document location and variants of the saphenopopliteal junction
- Course and connections of superficial varicose veins
- Identification of incompetent perforator veins connecting the deep and superficial systems and their position in relation to anatomical landmarks such as the groin crease, knee crease and medial malleolus.

To assist with surgical planning marks may be placed on the skin over incompetent perforating veins preoperatively. For clarity, a diagram of the venous system based on the US examination is usually provided.

6.10 HYPERTENSION

Most patients with hypertension have primary (essential) hypertension. The clinical challenge is to identify the small percentage of patients with secondary hypertension and to delineate any treatable cause. All patients with hypertension should have a CXR for the diagnosis of cardiovascular complications (cardiomegaly, aortic valve calcification, cardiac failure) and to establish a baseline for monitoring of future changes or complications such as aortic dissection. Further imaging investigation of hypertension is indicated in the following:

- Children and young adults less than 40 years old
- Hypertension that is severe or malignant in nature
- Failure of antihypertensive medication
- Renal dysfunction
- Certain clinical signs such as a bruit heard over the renal arteries
- Clinical evidence of endocrine disorders.

The more common causes of secondary hypertension include:

- Renal artery stenosis
- Chronic renal failure
- Endocrine disorders such as phaeochromocytoma, primary hyperaldosteronism and Cushing syndrome; for notes on imaging of these disorders, see Chapter 8.

6.10.1 RENAL ARTERY STENOSIS

Initial screening for renal artery stenosis may be performed with Doppler US or scintigraphy.

Doppler US is non-invasive, does not use radiation and should be the initial investigation of choice where local expertise is available. A major limitation of US is obscuration of renal arteries by overlying bowel gas and obesity. Scintigraphy with ^{99m}Tc-DTPA (see Table 1.1) may be used where US is technically inadequate. The use of an angiotensin-converting enzyme (ACE) inhibitor such as intravenous enalapril maleate increases the accuracy of the study. CTA or MRA may be used for further relatively non-invasive imaging when the above screening tests are equivocal.

When the screening tests are positive, renal angiography and interventional radiology are indicated. Most patients with renal artery stenosis are treated with interventional radiology, i.e. percutaneous transluminal angioplasty (PTA) and stent insertion. The goals of treatment with interventional radiology are normal blood pressure or hypertension that can be controlled medically plus improved renal function.

6.11 INTERVENTIONAL RADIOLOGY OF THE PERIPHERAL VASCULAR SYSTEM

6.11.1 CENTRAL VENOUS ACCESS

Interventional radiologists use a combination of US and fluoroscopic guidance in acquiring long-term access to the central venous system. US is used to obtain initial venous access. US can localize the vein, confirm its patency and diagnose relevant anatomical variants. Fluoroscopic guidance is used to confirm the final position of the catheter. In general, a central venous catheter should be positioned with its tip at the junction of the SVC and right atrium.

Indications for central venous access include:

- Chemotherapy
- Antibiotic therapy
- Hyperalimentation
- Haemodialysis.

The type of device depends largely on the period for which venous access is required. The most used devices are:

- PICCs:
  - Short- to intermediate-term central venous access
  - Inserted with US guidance via a peripheral arm vein above the elbow (basilic vein most commonly); patients generally prefer this over cubital fossa placement as they are able to use their arm
- Tunnelled catheters (Fig. 6.14):
  - Intermediate-term access
  - Internal jugular vein is usually the preferred route for insertion
  - A subcutaneous tunnel is made with blunt dissection from a skin incision in the upper chest wall to the venous access site
  - The venous catheter is pulled through this subcutaneous tunnel with a tunnelling device and inserted into the internal jugular vein

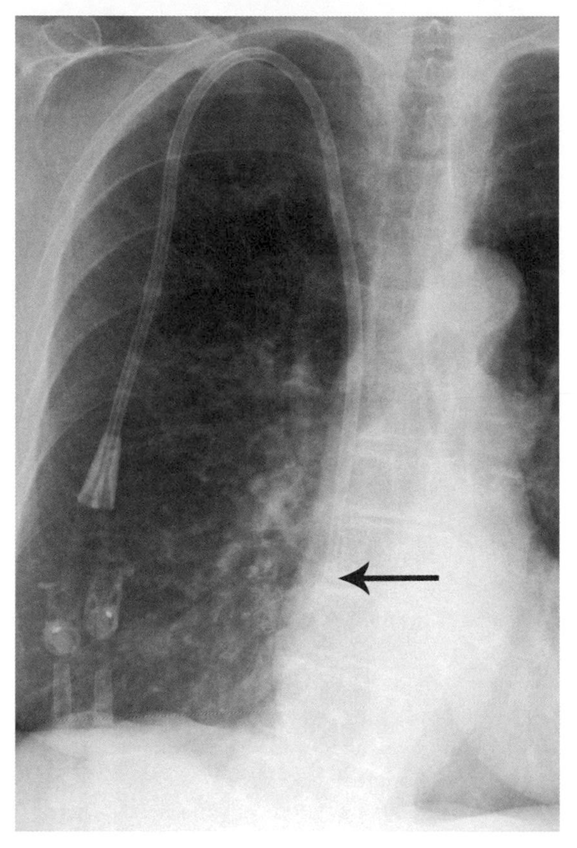

Figure 6.14 Tunnelled central venous port. The tip of the catheter is well positioned at the junction of the superior vena cava and right atrium (arrow).

  - The catheter is held at the skin insertion site with a purse-string suture
- Implanted ports:
  - Longer term (3 months or more) intermittent access
  - Particularly suitable for cyclical chemotherapy
  - Access ports are made of steel, titanium or plastic
  - A subcutaneous pocket is fashioned in the chest wall for the port
  - Venous access is via the internal jugular or subclavian vein
  - After placement, the skin is sutured over the port.

PICC insertion requires only local anaesthetic; the other methods usually require sedation or, in some cases including children, general anaesthetic. All venous access techniques are performed under conditions of strict sterility. Complications of venous access may include the following:

- Infection: the rate of infection is expressed as the number of infections per 10,000 catheter-days
  - PICCs: 4–11
  - Tunnelled catheters: 14
  - Implantation ports: 6
- Catheter blockage due to thrombosis and fibrin sheath formation: 3–10%
- Venous thrombosis (upper limb DVT): 1–2%
- Other complications such as catheter malposition and kinking are rare with careful placement.

6.11.2 AORTIC STENTS

Endoluminal devices combining metallic stents with Dacron graft material may be used to treat aneurysms of the abdominal aorta. These devices are inserted percutaneously via femoral artery puncture, removing the need for open surgery. Covered stents consist of a tube of Dacron graft material that is held open by a series of self-expanding metal stents and are the most commonly used endoluminal device for endovascular aneurysm repair (EVAR). EVAR usually has three components: an inverted 'Y' shaped graft that sits in the aorta with the lower limbs of the 'Y' projecting into the common iliac arteries, and two shorter grafts for the common iliac arteries.

The aims of EVAR are to reconstitute a normal lumen in the centre of the aneurysm and to prevent aneurysm rupture by excluding the aneurysm sac from blood flow and arterial pressure. Complications of EVAR include graft migration, kinking and distortion, and endoleak. Endoleak refers to blood flow in the aneurysm sac outside the graft. Endoleak is an important complication to recognize as it implies that the aneurysm sac is exposed to arterial pressure, increasing the risk of further dilatation and rupture. Postprocedural imaging consists of radiographs to confirm graft position and structural integrity plus US or contrast-enhanced CT to exclude endoleak (Fig. 6.15).

Covered stents may also be deployed in the aortic arch and thoracic aorta for the treatment of type B aortic dissection and thoracic aortic aneurysm. Various designs and configurations are deployed, depending on the site and extent of thoracic aortic pathology, plus the need to protect the origins of aortic arch branches.

6.11.3 PERCUTANEOUS TRANSLUMINAL ANGIOPLASTY

The usual indication for PTA is a short-segment arterial stenosis in a patient with clinical evidence of limb ischaemia. PTA consists of positioning a balloon catheter in the stenosed arterial segment then balloon inflation to expand the stenosis. Pressure readings proximal and distal to the stenosis before and after dilatation may be performed, plus a postdilatation angiogram to assess the result (Fig. 6.16). Postprocedure care following PTA consists of haemostasis at the arterial puncture site and bed rest. Patients may be maintained on low-dose aspirin or heparin following a complicated procedure. Complications are uncommon and include arterial occlusion, arterial rupture, haemorrhage and distal embolization.

6.11.4 ARTERIAL STENT PLACEMENT

Arterial stents are commonly used by interventional radiologists in the management of stenotic

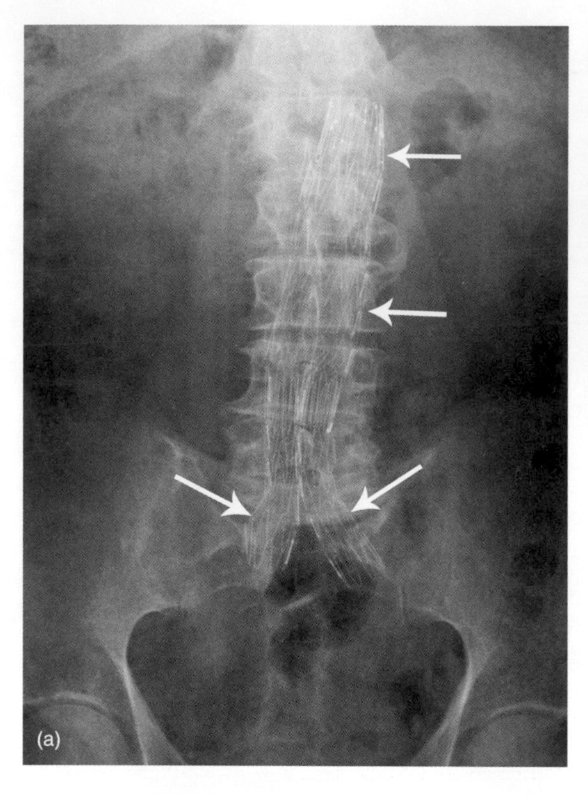

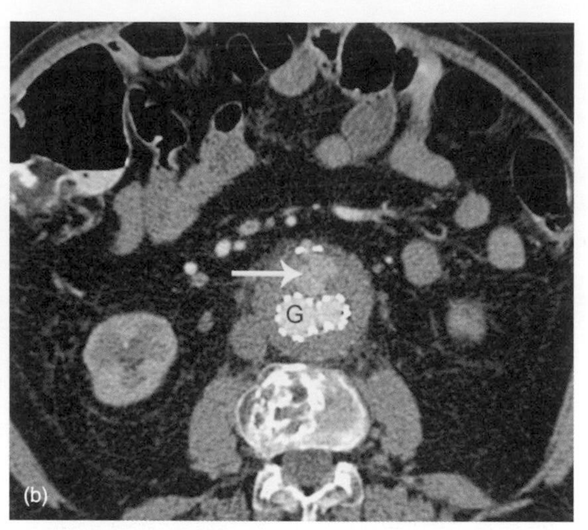

Figure 6.15 Covered stent (arrows) for aortic aneurysm. (a) Abdomen radiograph (AXR) shows the position of the stent graft (arrows). (b) CT with intravenous contrast injection shows the stent graft (G) within the aortic aneurysm. Note the presence of contrast enhancement in the aneurysm sac anterior to the graft, indicating an endoleak (arrow).

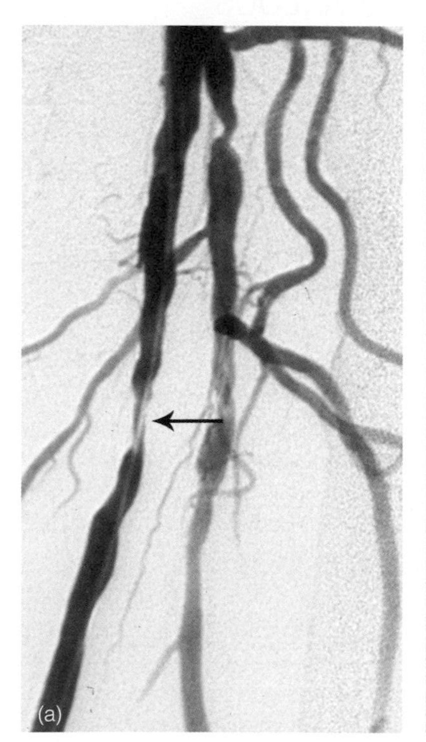

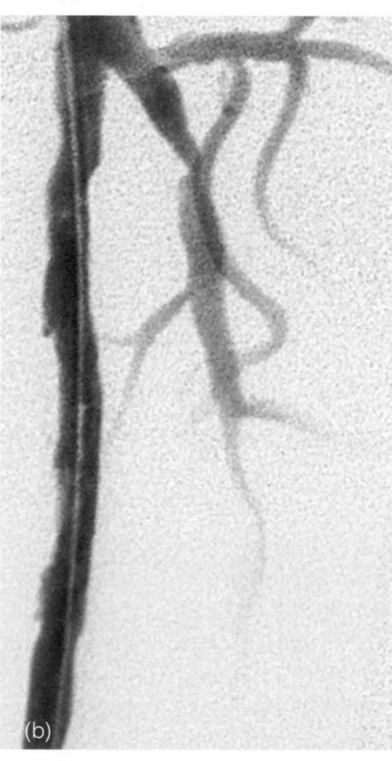

Figure 6.16 Percutaneous transluminal angioplasty (PTA). (a) Catheter angiography shows a stenosis of the superficial femoral artery in the upper thigh (arrow). (b) Following PTA, the stenosis is no longer seen.

and occlusive arterial disease. Indications for stent deployment include:

- Severe or heavily calcified iliac artery stenosis/occlusion
- Acute failure of PTA due to recoil of the vessel wall
- PTA complicated by arterial dissection
- Late failure of PTA due to recurrent stenosis.

Arterial stents are of two types: balloon-expandable and self-expanding. Self-expanding stents consist of stainless-steel spring filaments woven into a flexible self-expanding band.

6.11.5 ARTERIAL THROMBOLYSIS

Indications for thrombolysis in the peripheral vascular system include:

- Acute or acute-on-chronic arterial ischaemia
- Arterial thrombosis complicating PTA
- Surgical graft thrombosis
- Acute upper limb DVT.

Thrombolysis is performed via arterial puncture or venous puncture for upper limb DVT. A catheter is positioned in or just proximal to the thrombosis followed by infusion of a thrombolytic agent such as urokinase or tissue plasminogen activator (tPA) Regular follow-up angiograms or venograms are performed to ensure dissolution of the thrombus with repositioning of the catheter as required. PTA or arterial stent deployment may be performed for any underlying stenosis. The patient is maintained on anticoagulation therapy following successful thrombolysis.

Contraindications of thrombolysis include:

- Bleeding diathesis
- Active or recent bleeding from any source
- Recent surgery, pregnancy or significant trauma.

Complications of thrombolysis may include:

- Haematoma formation at the arterial puncture site
- Distal embolization of partly lysed thrombus
- Systemic bleeding, including cerebral haemorrhage, haematuria and epistaxis.

6.11.6 VASCULAR EMBOLIZATION

Vascular embolization refers to selective delivery of a variety of embolic materials.

Uses of vascular embolization include:

- Control of bleeding:
  - Trauma: penetrating injuries, hepatic or renal injury, pelvic trauma
  - AVMs and aneurysms
  - Severe epistaxis
- Management of tumour:
  - Palliative: embolic materials labelled with cytotoxic agents, radioactive isotopes or monoclonal antibodies
  - Definitive treatment for tumours of vascular origin, e.g. aneurysmal bone cyst
  - Preoperative to decrease vascularity or deliver chemotherapy
- Systemic AVM: definitive treatment, preoperative, palliative.

For vascular embolization the embolic material is delivered through an arterial catheter, either a standard diagnostic angiographic catheter or one of several specialized superselective catheters. These include microcatheters, which can be coaxially placed through a larger guiding catheter to gain distal access in small arteries. Embolic materials include:

- Metal coils with or without thrombogenic fibres attached
- Particles such as polyvinyl alcohol particles
- Glue: superglue acrylates
- Detachable balloons: latex or silicon
- Gelfoam pledgets
- Absolute alcohol
- Chemotherapeutic agents
- Resin microspheres loaded with yttrium-90.

The type of material used depends on the site, blood flow characteristics, whether a permanent or temporary occlusion is required, the type of catheter in use and the personal preference of the operator. Vascular embolization requires high-quality digital subtraction angiography (DSA) imaging facilities to monitor the progress of embolization and to diagnose complications.

Complications of vascular embolization may include:

- Inadvertent embolization of normal structures
- Pain
- Postembolization syndrome: fever, malaise and leukocytosis 3–5 days after embolization.

6.11.7 INFERIOR VENA CAVA FILTER INSERTION

In certain situations, self-expanding metallic filters may be deployed in the IVC to prevent PE. IVC filters may be deployed via the groin (common femoral vein) or neck (internal jugular vein). Most are positioned in the infrarenal segment of the IVC. Indications for IVC filtration include:

- PE or DVT, where anticoagulation therapy is contraindicated
- Recurrent PE despite anticoagulation
- High-risk surgical or trauma patients.

Permanent or removable filters may be used (Fig. 6.17). Complications of IVC filtration are rare and may include femoral vein or IVC thrombosis, perforation of the IVC and filter migration.

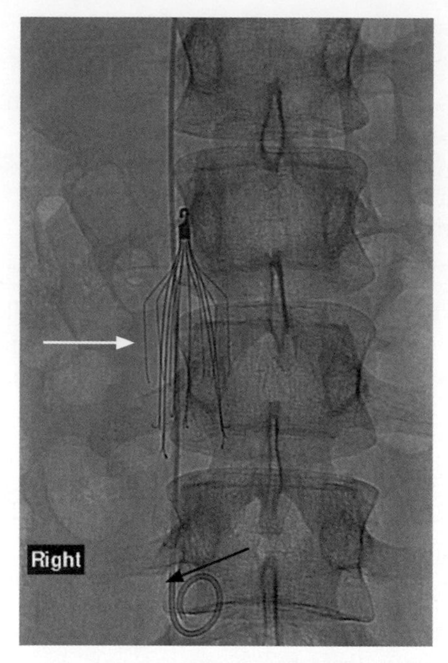

Figure 6.17 Removable inferior vena cava (IVC) filter in the IVC seen on venography as an umbrella-shaped metal opacity to the right of the spine (white arrow). This image is taken just prior to removal of the filter. A contrast study is required to exclude IVC thrombus prior to filter removal, for which a pigtail catheter has been inserted via the internal jugular vein (black arrow). The filter is removed by grasping the small hook at its upper end.

SUMMARY

Clinical presentation	Investigation of choice	Comment
Congestive cardiac failure	• CXR • Echocardiography	

Screening for coronary artery disease	• Exercise stress testing
	  • ECG
	  • Echocardiography
	  • Perfusion scintigraphy
	• CT calcium score
	• CT coronary angiography
		Choice of modality depends on:
		• Clinical presentation
		• Cardiac risk factors
		• Local expertise and availability

Myocardial viability	• Myocardial perfusion scintigraphy • Echocardiography • CT/MR myocardial perfusion	
Aortic dissection	CT	
Abdominal aortic aneurysm	• US for surveillance • CT for preoperative planning • US/CT for EVAR follow-up	
Claudication: PVD	• Physiological testing and Doppler US • CTA/MRA	Catheter angiography largely replaced by CTA and MRA for diagnosis of PVD
Pulmonary embolism	CTPA (spectral CT)	V/Q scintigraphy in selected cases
Deep venous thrombosis	Duplex US	
Venous incompetence	Duplex US	
Hypertension: suspected renal artery stenosis	• Duplex US/scintigraphy • CTA/MRA	

Abbreviations: CTA, CT angiography; CTPA, CT pulmonary angiography; ECG, electrocardiogram; EVAR, endovascular aneurysm repair; MR, magnetic resonance; MRA, MR angiography; PVD, peripheral vascular disease; V/Q, ventilation/perfusion.

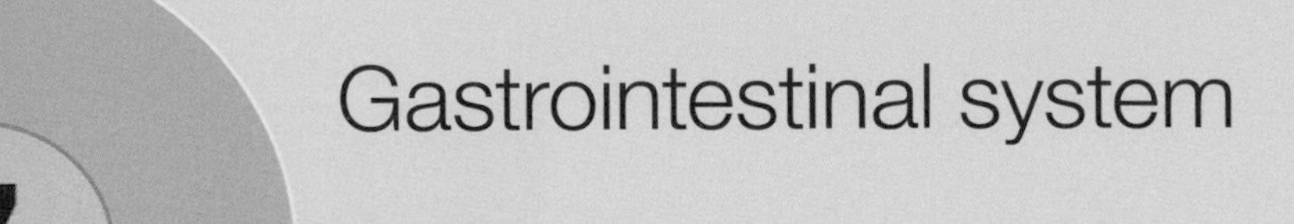

7 Gastrointestinal system

7.1 HOW TO READ AN ABDOMEN RADIOGRAPH

With the widespread use of ultrasound (US) and computed tomography (CT) in the imaging of abdominal disorders, the abdomen radiograph (abdomen X-ray, AXR) is less commonly performed in modern practice. Indications for AXR include:

- Suspected intestinal obstruction
- Perforation of the gastrointestinal tract (GIT)
- Follow-up of urinary tract calculi
- Foreign bodies due to penetrating injuries, ingestion or insertion (see Fig. 4.4).

The standard abdominal series consists of three radiographs as follows:

- Supine anteroposterior (AP) abdomen: standard projection used in all cases
- Erect chest radiograph (chest X-ray, CXR) to look for the following:
  - Free gas beneath the diaphragm
  - Chest complications of abdominal conditions, e.g. pleural effusion in pancreatitis
  - Chest conditions presenting with abdominal pain, e.g. lower lobe pneumonia
- Erect AP abdomen: used to look for fluid levels and free gas in cases of suspected intestinal obstruction or perforation.

Owing to several variable factors, including body habitus, distribution of bowel gas and the size of individual organs, such as the liver, the 'normal' AXR may show a wide range of appearances. For this reason, a methodical approach is important and the following checklist of 'things to look for' should be used (Fig. 7.1):

- Hollow organs:
  - Stomach
  - Small bowel: usually contains no visible gas, although a few non-dilated gas-filled loops may be seen in elderly patients as a normal finding
  - Large bowel
  - Bladder: seen as a round, soft-tissue 'mass' arising in the midline from the pelvic floor
- Solid organs: liver, spleen, kidneys, uterus
- Margins: diaphragm; psoas muscle outline; flank stripe, otherwise known as the properitoneal fat line

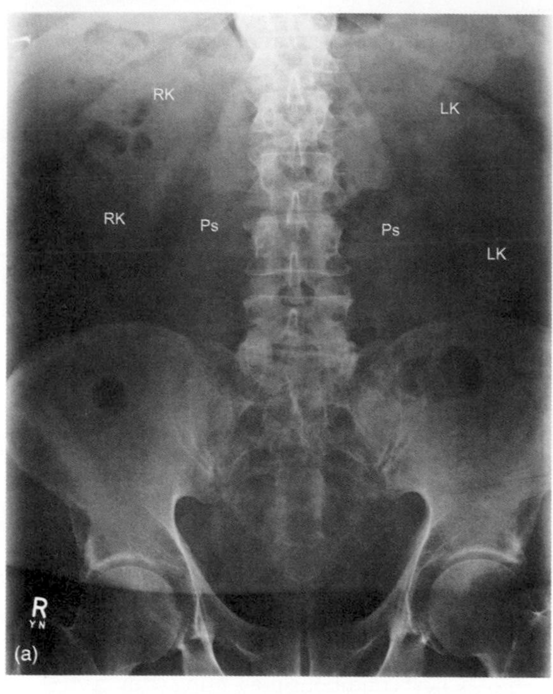

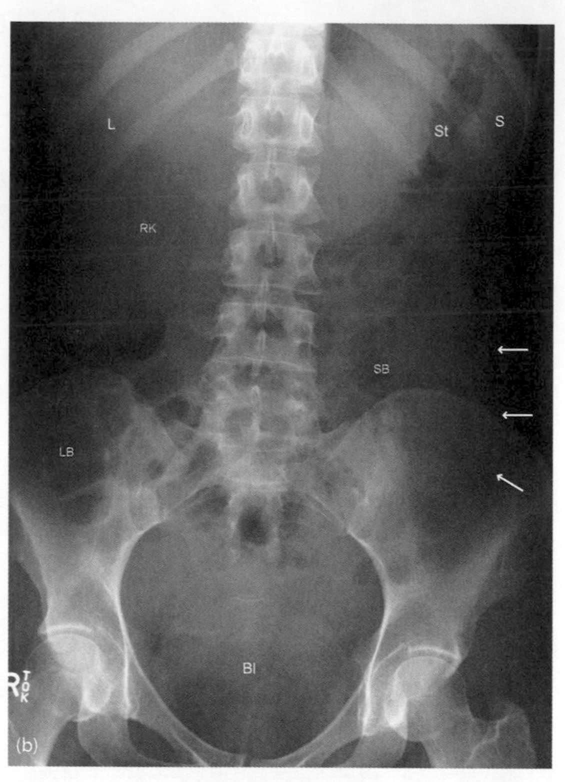

Figure 7.1 Normal AXR. (a) Note the following: left kidney (LK), psoas muscles (Ps), right kidney (RK). According to the principles explained in Chapter 1 the margins of the kidneys and psoas muscles are outlined by retroperitoneal fat. (b) Note the following structures: bladder (Bl), liver (L), large bowel (LB), right kidney (RK), spleen (S), small bowel (SB), stomach (St) and the properitoneal fat stripe (arrows).

- Bones: lower ribs, spine, pelvis, hips and sacroiliac joints
- Calcifications:
  - Aorta
  - Other arteries: the splenic artery is often calcified in the elderly and is seen as tortuous calcification in the left upper abdomen
  - Phleboliths: small, round calcifications with central lucency within pelvic veins; very common even in young patients and should not be confused with ureteric calculi
  - Lymph nodes: often due to previous infection and is common in the right iliac fossa and pelvis
  - Costal cartilages commonly calcify in older patients.

7.2 CONTRAST STUDIES OF THE GASTROINTESTINAL TRACT

Many contrast studies of the GIT, such as barium meal, barium enema and small bowel follow-through, have been replaced by more accurate studies, including endoscopy, colonoscopy, CT colonography, magnetic resonance (MR) enterography, wireless capsule enteroscopy, push enteroscopy, and double- and single-balloon enteroscopy.

Contrast studies are now performed for specific indications, such as:

- Limited contrast enema to assess surgical anastomoses
- Contrast swallow following bariatric surgery (gastric banding, sleeve gastrectomy and Roux-en-Y gastric bypass)

- GIT contrast studies are still used in children (see Chapter 16):
  - Upper GIT studies for malrotation
  - Enema with dilute barium for the diagnosis of large bowel pathology such as Hirschsprung disease.

7.2.1 CONTRAST SWALLOW

Contrast swallow is a relatively simple and non-invasive investigation in which the patient is asked to swallow liquid contrast material and images are obtained as it passes through the oesophagus. Barium is usually used, although for checking the integrity of surgical anastomoses a water-soluble material such as Gastrografin or other iodinated contrast material is preferable. Gastrografin should not be used if pulmonary aspiration is suspected as it may induce pulmonary oedema as a result of its high osmolarity if it enters the lungs.

Indications for contrast swallow include:

- Dysphagia
- Swallowing disorders in the elderly following stroke or central nervous system (CNS) trauma
- Suspected gastro-oesophageal reflux
- Following oesophageal surgery.

Detailed assessment of swallowing function and oesophageal motility may be obtained with a 'modified contrast swallow'. This involves ingestion of liquids and solids of varying consistencies under the supervision of a speech pathologist and radiologist with video recording of swallowing.

7.3 DYSPHAGIA

Dysphagia refers to the subjective feeling of swallowing difficulty caused by a variety of structural or functional disorders of the oral cavity, pharynx, oesophagus or stomach. Endoscopy is the first investigation of choice when oesophageal malignancy is suspected on clinical grounds. Advantages of endoscopy include direct visualization of the mucosal surface of the oesophagus, performance of biopsies as well as other interventions such as dilatation and stent placement. In most other instances, or where endoscopy has limited availability, barium swallow is the simplest and cheapest screening test for the investigation of dysphagia. For many conditions, barium swallow is sufficient for diagnosis; for others it will guide further investigations. Some of the more common findings in patients with dysphagia are:

- Stricture of the oesophagus, i.e. a localized region of constant narrowing
  - Intrinsic stricture due to a disease process of the wall of the oesophagus can usually be differentiated from extrinsic compression on barium swallow
  - Intrinsic stricture of the oesophagus may be due to oesophageal carcinoma, peptic stricture secondary to gastro-oesophageal reflux, corrosive ingestion or systemic sclerosis
  - All strictures seen on barium swallow should undergo endoscopic assessment and biopsy, as should areas of ulceration and mucosal irregularity
  - Stricture due to external compression (extrinsic stricture) may be caused by aberrant blood vessels, mediastinal tumours or lymphadenopathy
  - Extrinsic stricture seen on barium swallow should be investigated further with CT
- Carcinoma of the oesophagus:
  - Appearances of oesophageal carcinoma depend on the pattern of tumour growth
  - Early lesions: mucosal irregularity and ulceration
  - More advanced lesions: irregular strictures with elevated margins
  - Further staging: fluorodeoxyglucose–positron emission tomography–CT (FDG-PET-CT) to assess local invasion and mediastinal lymphadenopathy, as well as to exclude hepatic and pulmonary metastases
- Sliding hiatus hernia:
  - Range in size from a small clinically insignificant hernia to the entire stomach lying in the thorax (i.e. thoracic stomach), which is at risk of volvulus
  - CXR sign: apparent round mass containing a fluid level lying behind the heart
- Pharyngeal pouch (Zenker diverticulum):

  - Weakness of the posterior wall of the lower pharynx may lead to the formation of a pharyngeal pouch
  - Contrast-filled pouch projects posteriorly and to the left above the cricopharyngeus muscle (Fig. 7.2)
  - CXR sign: if large there may be an air–fluid level
- Achalasia:
  - Dilated oesophagus that may also be elongated and tortuous with a smoothly tapered lower end
  - CXR signs: an air–fluid level in the mediastinum, an absent gastric air bubble and evidence of aspiration pneumonia
- Motility disorders of the oesophagus:
  - Dysphagia due to abnormal oesophageal motility is common in elderly patients and may also be seen in association with reflux oesophagitis, early achalasia and various causes of neuropathy, including diabetes
- Patients with swallowing disorders due to CNS problems, such as stroke or Parkinson disease, or following laryngectomy may be assessed with modified barium swallow
- Dysphagia in immunocompromised patients:
  - Usually due to infectious oesophagitis
  - Commonest causative organism in human immunodeficiency virus (HIV)-positive patients is *Candida albicans*; dysphagia in these patients is often treated empirically with antifungal therapy
  - Other causes include herpes simplex and cytomegalovirus
  - Endoscopy is indicated to obtain specimens for laboratory analysis if dysphagia in an immunocompromised patient fails to settle on antifungal therapy.

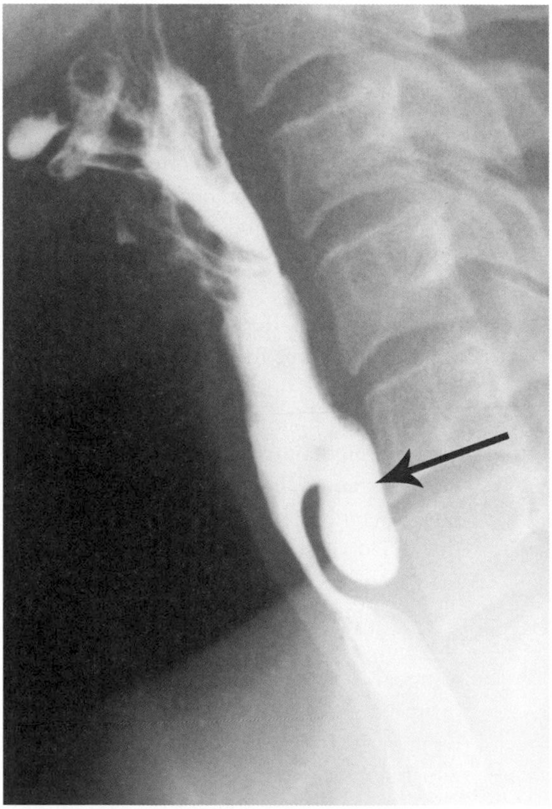

Figure 7.2 Pharyngeal pouch: barium swallow. A pharyngeal pouch (arrow) is seen on a lateral view projecting posteriorly from the lower pharynx.

7.4 ACUTE ABDOMEN

Acute abdominal pain is a common clinical problem that encompasses a wide range of pathologies. Key diagnostic points may be obtained from the initial history and examination, including:

- Location of the pain
- Associated fever
- History of previous or recent surgery
- Prior history of similar pain
- Signs that may indicate intestinal obstruction, such as abdominal distension, vomiting and altered bowel habit
- Features of peritonism.

The clinical history and examination may be accompanied by laboratory investigations such as white cell count and pancreatic enzymes. Imaging may be used to complement – not replace – clinical assessment. Where the diagnosis is obvious on clinical grounds and/or AXR, more sophisticated imaging is not required. Indications for AXR in a setting of acute abdomen are suspected bowel obstruction or perforation of the GIT. AXR may be negative or misleading in many of the other common causes of acute abdomen.

CT and US are commonly used where clinically indicated. US is useful for assessment of the solid organs and for the diagnosis of gallstones. CT is commonly used in the assessment of acute abdominal pain. One of the most important reasons for this is the ability of CT to display inflammation or oedema in fat. Inflammatory change is very well shown on CT as streaky soft-tissue density or infiltration within the darker fat (Fig. 7.3), commonly referred to as fat stranding. This is an extremely useful sign on CT that often helps to localize pathology that may otherwise be overlooked. CT is less sensitive in the assessment of very thin or cachectic patients in whom abdominal fat planes may be absent.

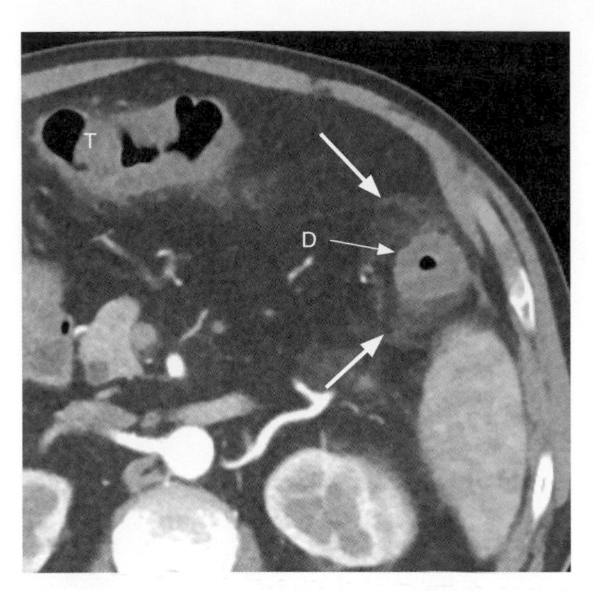

Figure 7.3 Infectious colitis: CT. Note the thickening of the wall of the transverse (T) and descending (D) colon, with fat stranding seen as wispy soft-tissue density in the pericolic fat (arrows).

7.4.1 PERFORATION OF THE GASTROINTESTINAL TRACT

Perforation of the GIT may be due to peptic ulceration, inflammation, including acute diverticulitis and appendicitis, or blunt or penetrating injury, including iatrogenic trauma. Perforation of the stomach, small intestine and most of the colon produces free gas in the peritoneal cavity (pneumoperitoneum). Perforation of the duodenum and posterior rectum results in free retroperitoneal gas (pneumoretroperitoneum).

Radiographic signs of free gas:

- Erect CXR: gas beneath the diaphragm (Fig. 7.4)
- Supine abdomen: gas outlines anatomical structures such as the liver, falciform ligament and spleen; bowel walls are seen as white lines outlined by gas on both sides, i.e. inside and outside the bowel lumen (Rigler sign) (Fig. 7.5)
- Free gas is also identified on an erect abdomen film
- If the patient is too ill to stand then either decubitus or shoot-through lateral films can be performed.

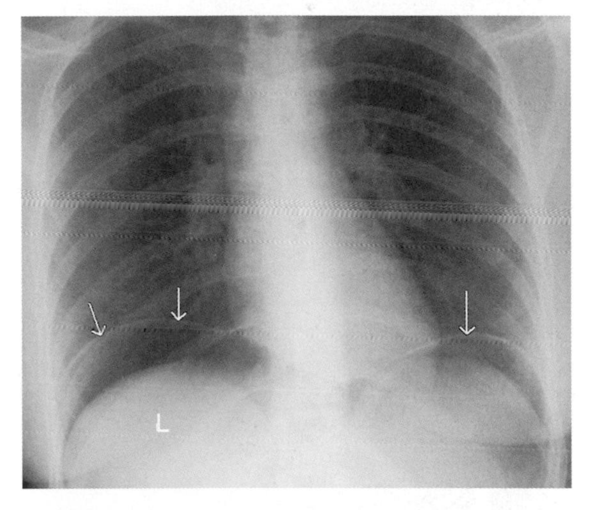

Figure 7.4 Free gas: erect CXR. Free gas is seen beneath the diaphragm (arrows). Free gas on the right separates the liver (L) from the right diaphragm.

7.4.2 SUSPECTED SMALL BOWEL OBSTRUCTION

The clinical presentation of small bowel obstruction (SBO) is abdominal pain and vomiting, progressing to acute abdomen with abdominal distension and tenderness. Causes of SBO in adults include:

- Adhesions due to previous surgery, trauma or infection
- Strangulated hernia
- Small bowel neoplasm
- Gallstone ileus.

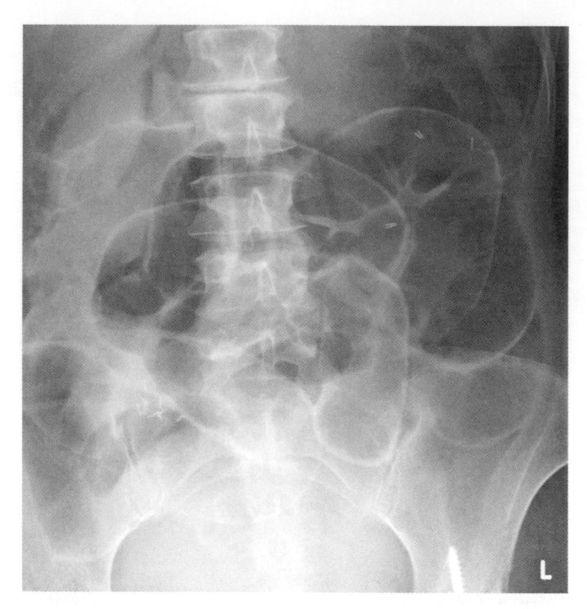

Figure 7.5 Free gas: AXR. Free gas in the peritoneal cavity causes clear delineation of both sides of the bowel wall. Compare the appearances of these bowel lops with those visualized in Figure 7.1. Multiple small metal clips are also present, indicating previous surgery.

In children, causes of SBO include strangulated hernia, congenital malformation, intussusception and malrotation (see Chapter 16).

AXR is the primary investigation of choice in suspected SBO. Situations in which AXR may be less accurate include partial or early obstruction and closed-loop obstruction. Although most SBOs may be diagnosed with clinical assessment and AXR, in modern practice CT is commonly used as it is more accurate and more likely to provide a specific diagnosis and offer surgical planning.

Signs of SBO on AXR (Fig. 7.6):

- Dilated small bowel loops, which have the following features:
  - Central location
  - Numerous
  - Greater than 3.0 cm in diameter
  - Small radius of curvature
  - Valvulae conniventes, seen as thin white lines that are thin, numerous, close together and extend right across the bowel
  - Do not contain solid faeces
- Multiple fluid levels on the erect AXR
- 'String of beads' sign on the erect AXR owing to small gas pockets trapped between valvulae conniventes
- Absent or little air in the large bowel.

The differential diagnosis of dilated small bowel loops on AXR is paralytic ileus. Paralytic ileus may

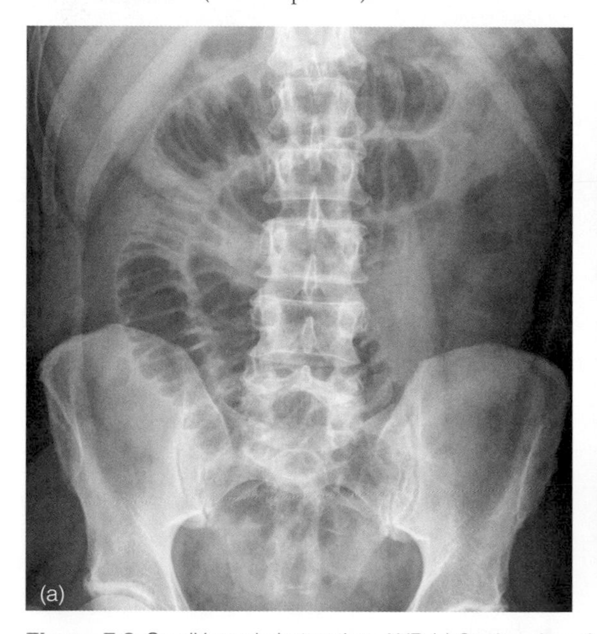

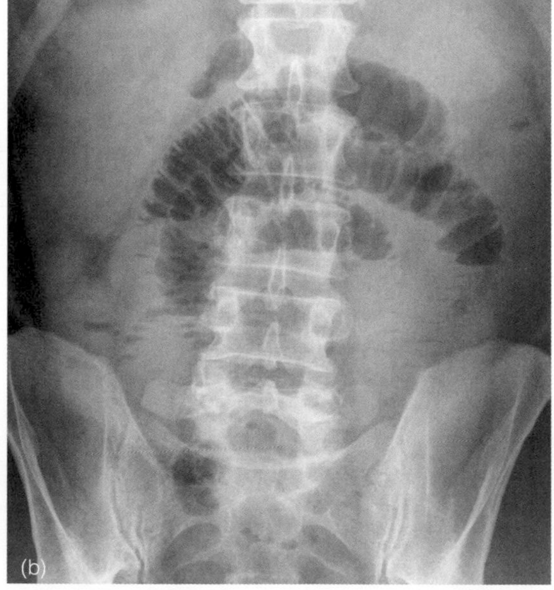

Figure 7.6 Small bowel obstruction: AXR (a) Supine view showing multiple loops of small bowel. Note the features of small bowel loops as described in the text. (b) Erect view showing multiple relatively short gas–fluid levels.

be generalized or localized. Localized ileus refers to dilated loops of bowel ('sentinel loops'), usually small bowel, overlying a local inflammation:

- Right upper quadrant (RUQ): acute cholecystitis
- Left upper quadrant: acute pancreatitis
- Lower right abdomen: acute appendicitis.

Generalized ileus refers to non-specific dilatation of small and large bowel, which may occur postoperatively or with peritonitis. Scattered irregular fluid levels are seen on the erect radiograph (Fig. 7.7).

CT is highly accurate for establishing the diagnosis of SBO, defining the location and cause of obstruction and diagnosing associated strangulation. CT signs of SBO include:

- Dilated small bowel loops measuring greater than 3.0 cm in diameter
- Small bowel transition point
  - The point where dilated bowel becomes non-dilated or collapsed (Fig. 7.8)
  - Presence of faecalized small bowel contents (small bowel faeces sign).

In patients with SBO, a definable transition point on CT and no visible cause of obstruction, a presumptive diagnosis of obstruction as a result of adhesions can be made, particularly if there is a history of prior abdominal surgery. Specific causes of SBO that may occasionally be diagnosed on CT include strangulated hernia and gallstone ileus.

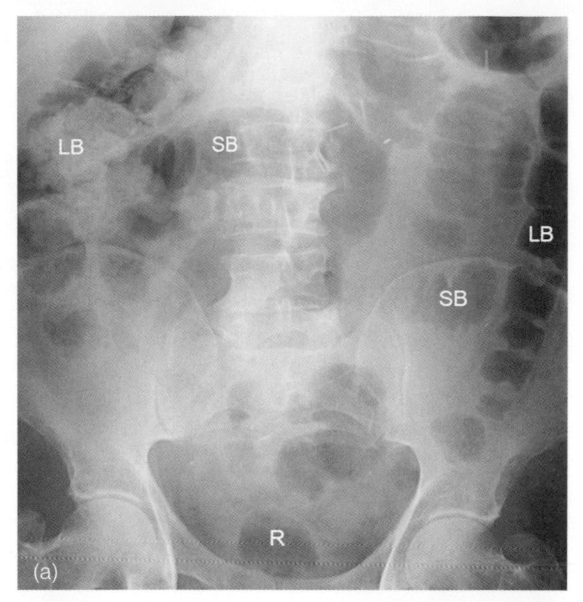

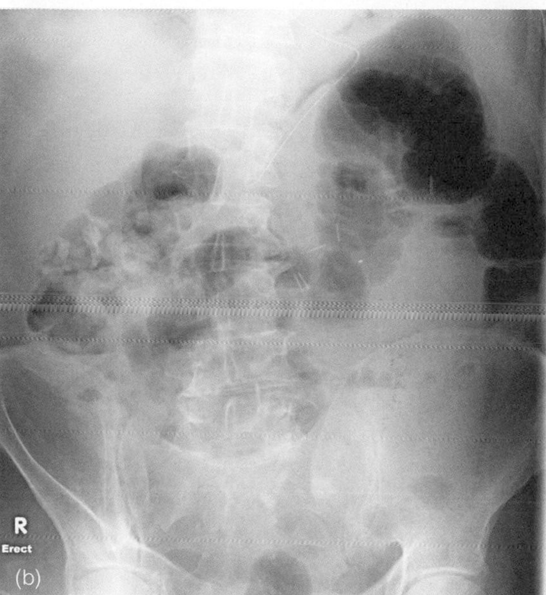

Figure 7.7 Generalized ileus: AXR (a) Supine view shows dilated loops of both large (LB) and small bowel (SB). Gas is seen distally in the rectum (R), making a mechanical obstruction unlikely. (b) Erect view showing only scattered gas–fluid levels.

STRANGULATED HERNIA

The term 'hernia' refers to abnormal protrusion of intra-abdominal contents, usually peritoneal fat and bowel loops. Inguinal hernia accounts for about 80% of abdominal wall hernias. Femoral hernia is more common in elderly women. Other types of external hernia include umbilical hernia and hernia related to previous surgery, either incisional or parastomal. Most hernias present with an inguinal or abdominal wall mass that increases in size when the patient stands or strains. Occasionally, hernias may become strangulated and present with localized pain and intestinal obstruction.

Strangulated hernia is seen on CT as dilated small bowel loops entering a gas-containing soft-tissue mass in the inguinal or femoral canal or in the abdominal wall. Non-dilated, collapsed loops can be followed distally. Gas in the bowel wall within the hernia indicates incarceration and bowel wall infarction.

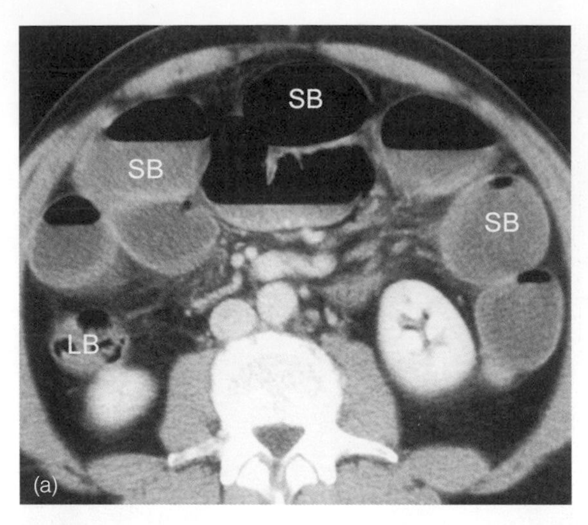

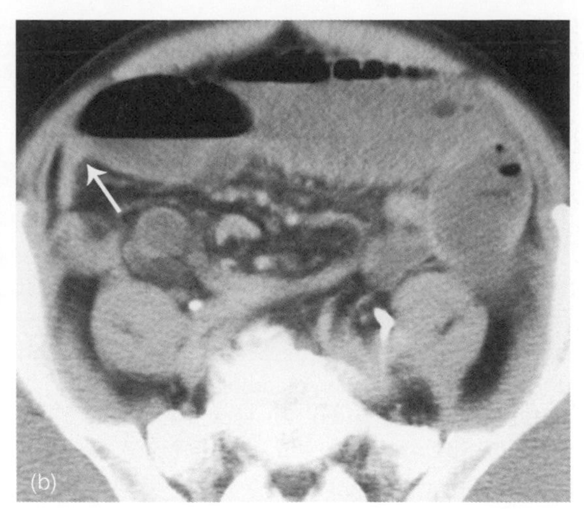

Figure 7.8 Small bowel obstruction: CT. (a) Note the dilated loops of small bowel (SB) containing gas–fluid levels and non-dilated large bowel (LB). (b) Abrupt transition from dilated to non-dilated small bowel (arrow), indicating mechanical SBO.

GALLSTONE ILEUS

Gallstone ileus refers to SBO secondary to gallstone impaction and usually occurs in the setting of chronic cholecystitis. A large gallstone erodes through the inflamed gallbladder wall to enter the duodenum and becomes impacted in the distal small bowel, causing SBO.

Signs of gallstone ileus on CT and AXR (Rigler triad):

- SBO
- Gas in the biliary tree (pneumobilia), seen as a branching pattern of gas density in the RUQ
- Calcified gallstone lying in an abnormal position, usually in the right iliac fossa.

7.4.3 SUSPECTED LARGE BOWEL OBSTRUCTION

Large bowel obstruction (LBO) may have a subacute to chronic presentation with abdominal pain, distension and constipation. The commonest cause for such a presentation is colorectal carcinoma (CRC). More acute presentations of LBO may be seen with sigmoid volvulus, caecal volvulus and diverticulitis. Most cases of LBO are diagnosed with clinical assessment and AXR.

Signs of LBO on AXR (Fig. 7.9):

- Dilated large bowel loops, which have the following features:
  - Peripheral location
  - Few in number
  - Large: greater than 6.0 cm diameter (>9.0 cm for the caecum)
  - Wide radius of curvature
  - Haustra, seen as thick white lines that are widely separated and may or may not extend right across the bowel (compare these features with those of the small bowel valvulae conniventes described in section 7.4.2)
  - Contain solid faeces
- Small bowel may also be dilated if the ileocaecal valve is 'incompetent'.

Depending on which large bowel lops are dilated, an approximate level of obstruction may be suggested on AXR. With respect to the cause of LBO, AXR appearances are generally non-specific and non-diagnostic. Cases where a specific diagnosis may be made with AXR include caecal volvulus and sigmoid volvulus.

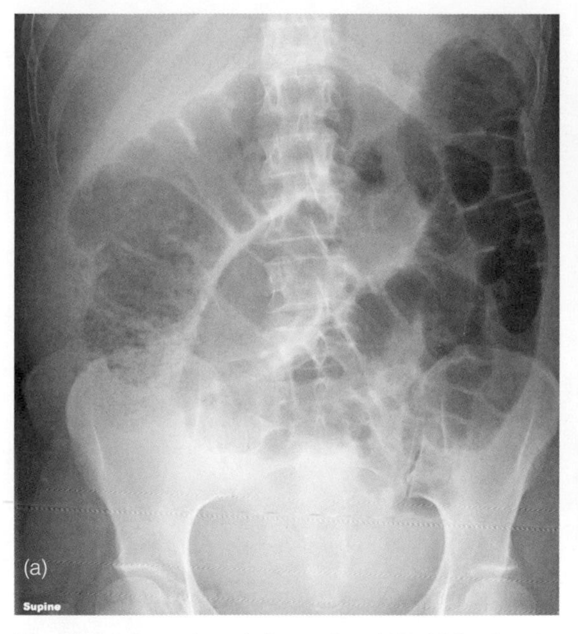

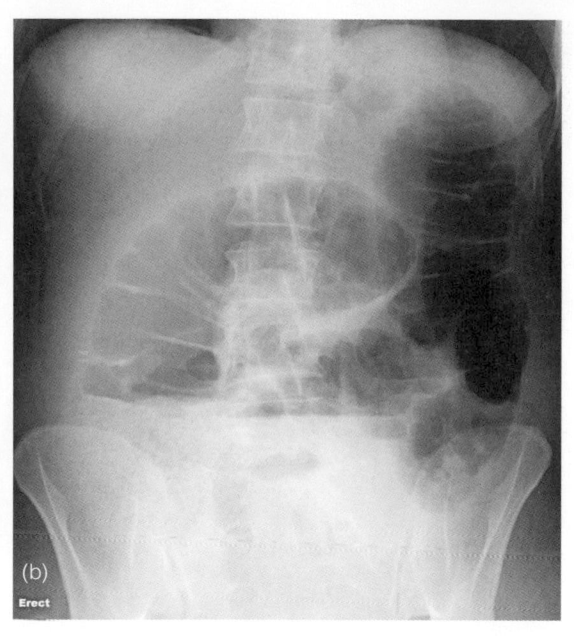

Figure 7.9 Large bowel obstruction: AXR. (a) Supine view showing multiple dilated loops of large bowel. Note the thick haustral folds and compare with the small bowel valvulae conniventes shown in Figure 7.6. (b) Erect view showing fluid levels.

CAECAL VOLVULUS

Caecal volvulus refers to twisting and obstruction of the caecum. Caecal volvulus occurs most commonly in patients aged 20–40 and is associated with an abnormally long mesentery and malrotation.

Radiographic signs of caecal volvulus (Fig. 7.10):

- Markedly dilated caecum containing one or two haustral markings
- The dilated caecum may lie in the right iliac fossa or left upper quadrant
- Attached gas-filled appendix
- Small bowel dilatation
- Collapse of the left half of the colon.

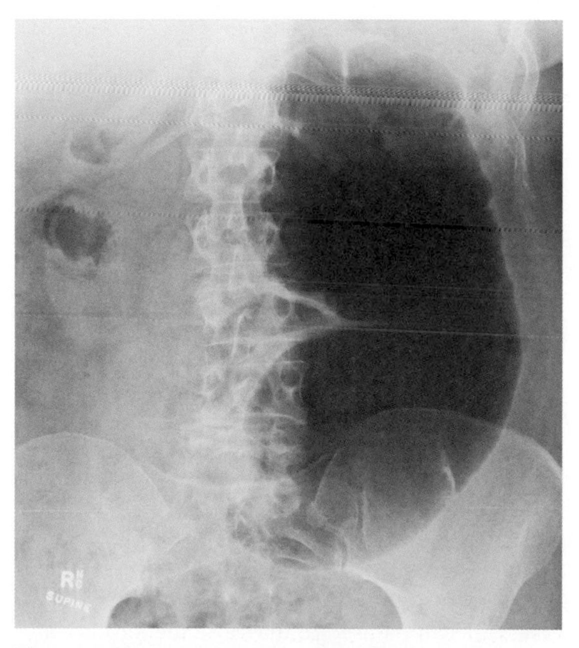

Figure 7.10 Caecal volvulus: AXR. Massively distended caecum passing across to the left. This is differentiated from sigmoid volvulus by its shape plus the absence of large bowel dilatation.

SIGMOID VOLVULUS

Sigmoid volvulus refers to twisting of the sigmoid colon around its mesenteric axis with obstruction and marked dilatation. Sigmoid volvulus occurs in elderly and chronic psychiatric patients.

Radiographic signs of sigmoid volvulus (Fig. 7.11):

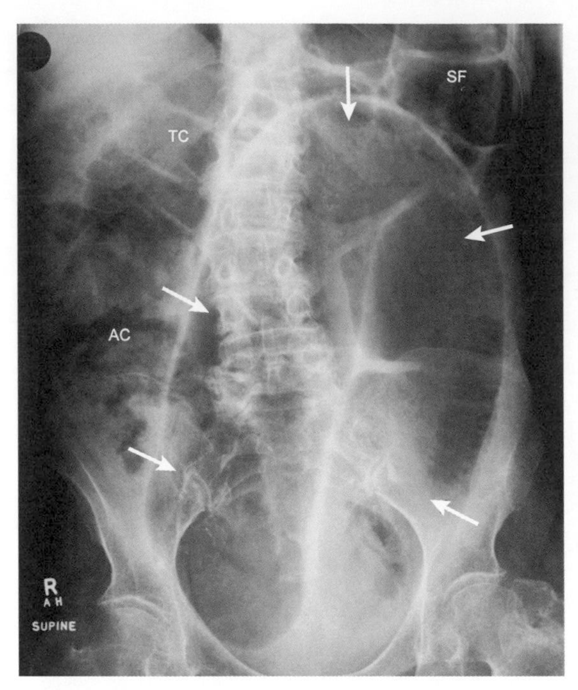

Figure 7.11 Sigmoid volvulus: AXR. Note the typical inverted 'U' appearance of sigmoid volvulus (arrows). Also note dilatation of the ascending colon (AC), splenic flexure (SF), transverse colon (TC). Note the characteristic overlap of dilated left colon and sigmoid loop below the splenic flexure.

- Massively distended sigmoid loop in the shape of an inverted 'U', which can extend above T10 and overlap the lower border of the liver
- Usually has no haustral markings
- The outer walls and adjacent inner walls of the 'U' form three white lines that converge towards the left side of the pelvis (coffee bean sign)
- Overlap of the dilated descending colon: 'left flank overlap' sign (good differentiating feature from caecal volvulus in which the remainder of the large bowel is not dilated).

COMPUTED TOMOGRAPHY

CT may be used for the assessment of difficult or equivocal cases of LBO (Fig. 7.12). In the majority of cases, CT can be used to diagnose the location and cause of obstruction. CT may also be used to diagnose other relevant findings, such as liver metastases in the case of an obstructing tumour.

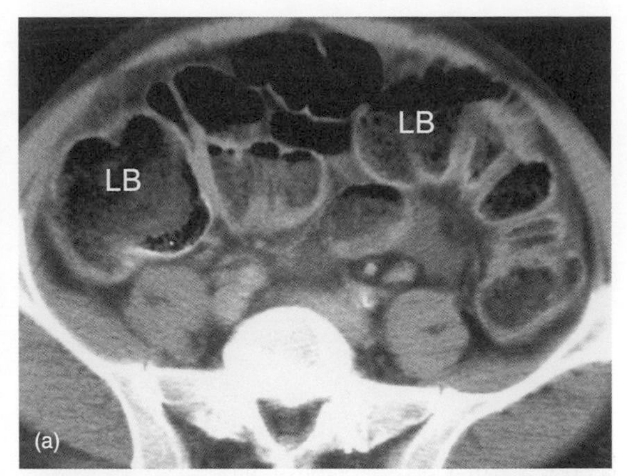

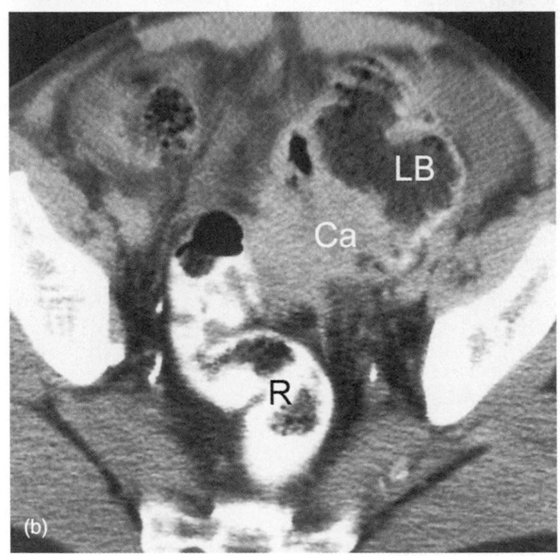

Figure 7.12 Large bowel obstruction due to carcinoma: CT. (a) Dilated loops of large bowel (LB). (b) Carcinoma (Ca) seen as a soft-tissue mass in the sigmoid colon proximal to the rectum (R).

7.4.4 RIGHT UPPER QUADRANT PAIN

The primary diagnostic consideration in adult patients with acute RUQ pain is acute cholecystitis.

ULTRASOUND

US is the most sensitive investigation for the presence of gallstones and is therefore the investigation of choice for suspected acute cholecystitis. The diagnosis of acute cholecystitis is usually made by confirming the presence of gallstones in a patient with RUQ pain and fever (Fig. 7.13). Other signs of acute cholecystitis that may be seen with US include thickening of the gallbladder wall, fluid surrounding the gallbladder and localized tenderness to direct probe pressure (Fig. 7.14).

SCINTIGRAPHY

Scintigraphy with ^{99m}Tc-labelled iminodiacetic acid (IDA) compounds has a limited role in difficult cases where clinical assessment and US are doubtful.

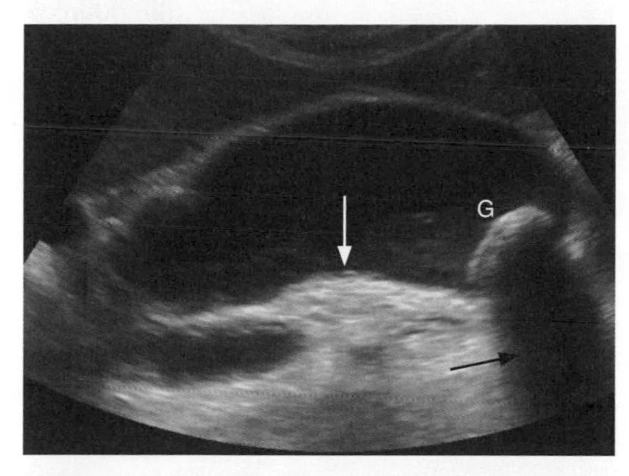

Figure 7.13 Gallstone and sludge: US. Large gallstone (G) in the fundus of the gallbladder seen as a round hyperechoic focus with acoustic shadowing (black arrow). There is also a layer of dependent echogenic material indicating sludge (white arrow).

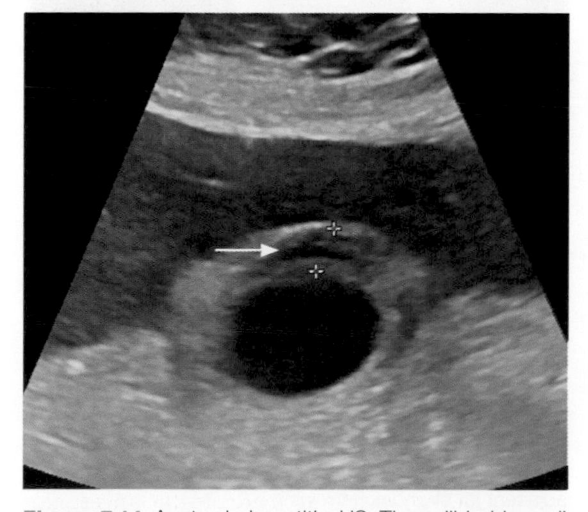

Figure 7.14 Acute cholecystitis: US. The gallbladder wall is thickened (+), with a thin hypoechoic layer indicating oedema (arrow).

Acute cholecystitis is diagnosed on IDA scan by non-visualization of the gallbladder with good visualization of the common bile duct and duodenum 1 hour after injection.

COMPUTED TOMOGRAPHY

CT may be used where US is negative and/or where alternate diagnoses are being considered. Because the density of gallstones often approximates that of bile, CT is much less sensitive than US for the detection of gallstones unless they contain calcification or gas. The use of spectral CT can improve the detection of cholesterol gallstones. CT signs of gallbladder inflammation include thickening of the gallbladder wall with infiltrative streaking in adjacent fat.

7.4.5 RIGHT LOWER QUADRANT PAIN

The commonest cause of acute right lower quadrant (RLQ) pain is acute appendicitis. The differential diagnosis includes inflammatory bowel disease (IBD), mesenteric adenitis and gynaecological pathology in female patients. Although most cases of acute appendicitis are confidently diagnosed on clinical grounds, imaging may significantly lower the number of negative appendicectomies. Imaging is particularly useful in patients with atypical features on history and/or in young females where gynaecological pathologies such as ectopic pregnancy or pelvic inflammatory disease are suspected.

ULTRASOUND

When imaging is required, US is the initial investigation of choice in children, thin patients and women of childbearing age. An inflamed appendix appears on US as a blind-ending, thick-walled tubular structure with hypervascularity on colour Doppler imaging (Fig. 7.15). Approximately one-third of appendixes are retrocaecal in location, which limits identification. In such cases, the identification rate can be increased by rolling the patient left side down. If still unidentifiable, the absence of secondary signs such as hyperechoic fat or free fluid may be sufficient to adopt a conservative management approach.

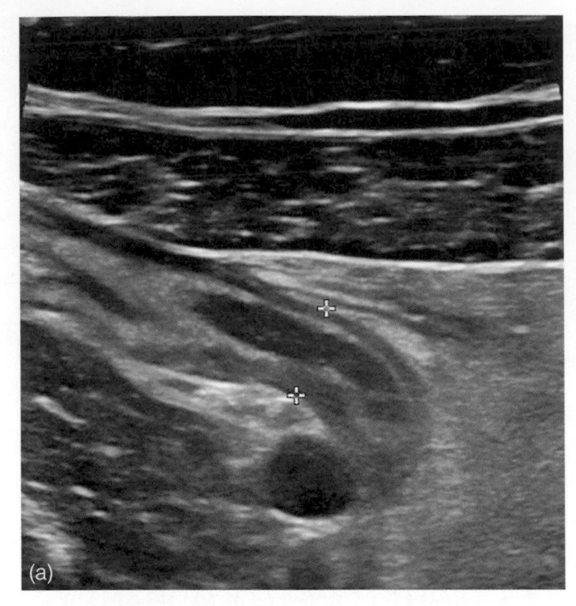

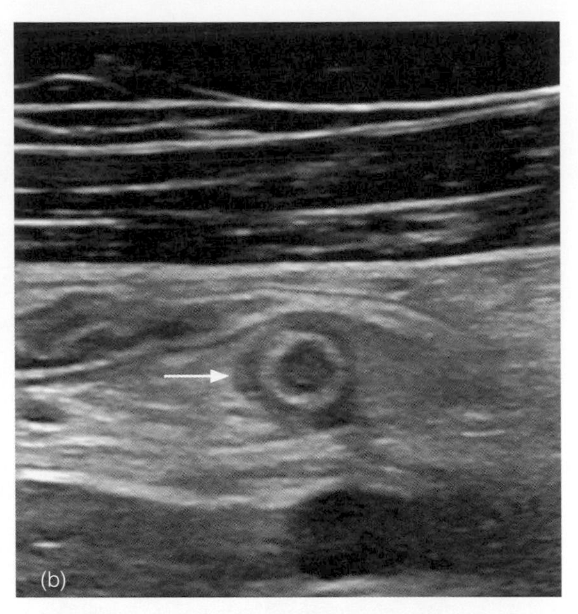

Figure 7.15 Acute appendicitis: US. (a) Acutely inflamed appendix seen as a non-compressible blind-ending tubular structure (+) in the right iliac fossa. (b) Cross-sectional view of the inflamed appendix showing a target-like appearance (arrow).

COMPUTED TOMOGRAPHY

For most adult patients, excluding women of childbearing age, CT is the imaging investigation of choice in the assessment of RLQ pain (Fig. 7.16). Advantages of CT include its proven accuracy in the diagnosis of appendicitis and related complications and its use to diagnose alternative causes of RLQ pain. The ability of CT to identify a normal appendix in most patients, plus its high level of sensitivity to inflammatory change, mean that a negative CT has a very high negative predictive value.

7.4.6 LEFT LOWER QUADRANT PAIN

The primary diagnostic consideration for patients with acute left lower quadrant (LLQ) pain is acute diverticulitis. The term 'acute diverticulitis' encompasses a range of inflammatory pathologies that occur secondary to diverticulosis, including bowel wall and pericolonic inflammation, perforation, abscess and sinus or fistula tracts. US should be used in women of childbearing age in whom gynaecological pathology such as ectopic pregnancy or pelvic

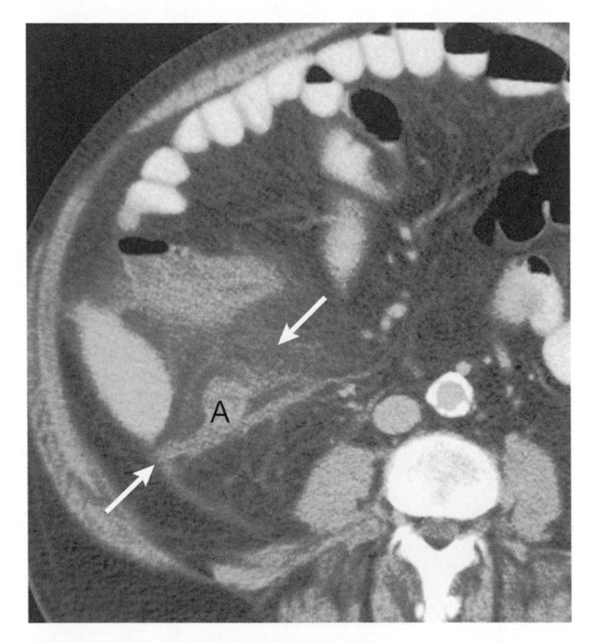

Figure 7.16 Acute appendicitis: CT. Transverse CT shows a swollen appendix (A) as a round opacity with adjacent fat stranding (arrows).

inflammatory disease would be more likely than acute diverticulitis.

CT is otherwise the investigation of choice for assessment of acute LLQ pain. CT is highly accurate for the diagnosis of acute diverticulitis; where diverticulitis is not present, it may suggest alternative diagnoses such as SBO, pelvic inflammatory disease and renal colic. CT signs of acute diverticulitis include localized bowel wall thickening and soft-tissue stranding or haziness in pericolonic fat. Often, an inflamed diverticulum is seen in the epicentre of the fat stranding (Fig. 7.17). Gas in the bladder may indicate the formation of a colovesical fistula (Fig. 7.18). Epiploic appendagitis is focal inflammation centred on the fat-containing epiploic appendages anterior to the distal descending and sigmoid colon that may mimic acute diverticulitis.

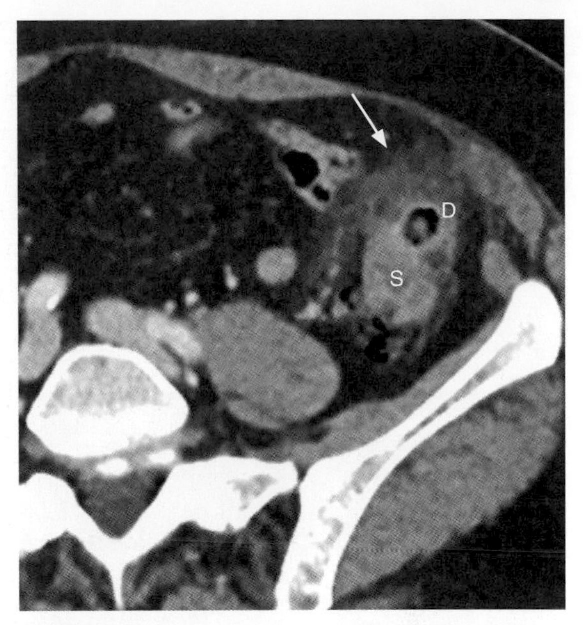

Figure 7.17 Sigmoid diverticulitis: CT. Acute sigmoid wall thickening (S) and pericolic fat stranding (arrow) centred on a large diverticulum (D).

7.4.7 RENAL COLIC AND ACUTE FLANK PAIN

Acute flank pain describes pain of the posterolateral abdomen from the lower thorax to the pelvis. The most common cause of acute flank pain is ureteral obstruction caused by an impacted renal calculus. For this reason, the terms acute flank pain and renal colic are often used interchangeably.

The term 'acute flank pain' more accurately reflects the fact that non-renal causes may produce similar symptoms to genuine renal colic. Non-renal causes of acute flank pain include appendicitis, ovarian cyst torsion or haemorrhage, diverticulitis, IBD and pancreatitis.

Other renal causes of acute flank pain include acute pyelonephritis, urothelial cell carcinoma of the ureter causing obstruction and 'clot colic', i.e. ureteric colic due to a blood clot complicating haematuria. In the patient with acute flank pain, initial assessment is directed towards confirming or excluding urinary tract obstruction secondary to a ureteric calculus.

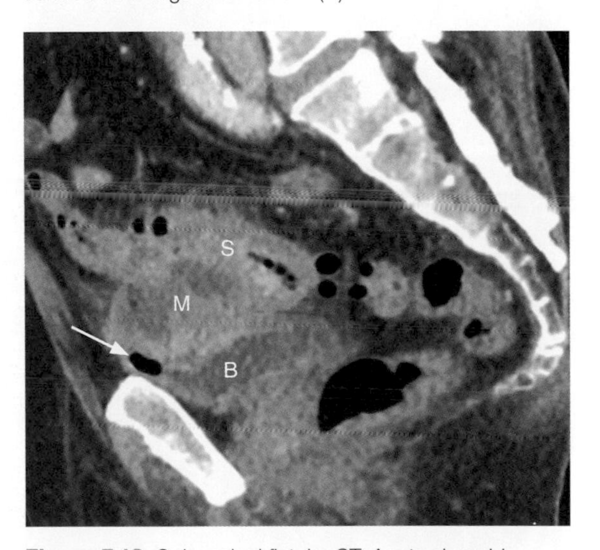

Figure 7.18 Colovesical fistula: CT. Acute sigmoid diverticulitis (S) with an inflammatory mass (M) communicating inferiorly into the bladder (B). Note gas in the bladder lumen anteriorly (arrow), indicating fistulous connection with the bowel.

COMPUTED TOMOGRAPHY

CT without contrast enhancement is the imaging test of choice for acute flank pain. Virtually all renal stones are identified on CT, including cystine, urate, xanthine and matrix stones, which are generally not seen on AXR. The only exceptions are stones due to crystal precipitation in patients with HIV taking indinavir. The likelihood of a ureteric calculus passing spontaneously is largely related to size. A calculus of 5 mm or less will usually pass, whereas a calculus of 10 mm or more is likely to become lodged. Stone position and size are accurately assessed on CT.

CT signs of urinary tract obstruction:

- Dilatation of the ureter above the calculus
- Dilatation of the renal pelvis and collecting system
- Soft-tissue stranding in the perinephric fat due to distended lymphatic channels (Fig. 7.19).

CT of the kidneys, ureters and bladder (KUB) is performed as a non-contrast scan. The patient is prone, which allows differentiation between calculi impacted at the vesicoureteric junction (VUJ) and those that have already passed into the bladder. A major advantage of CT is that non-renal causes of acute flank pain may also be diagnosed. Spectral CT can characterize uric acid renal calculi that can be treated with dissolution therapy (Fig. 7.20).

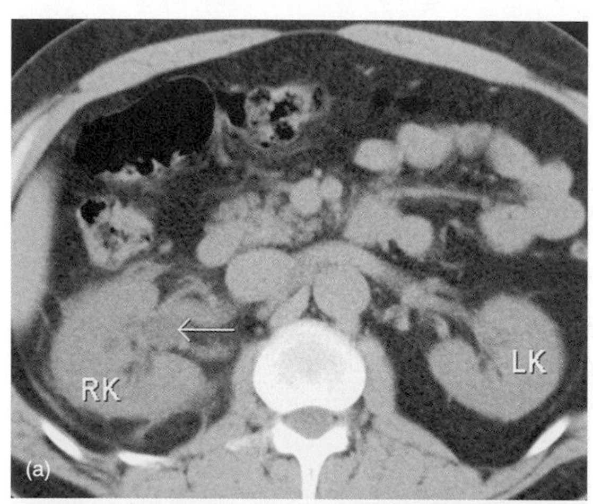

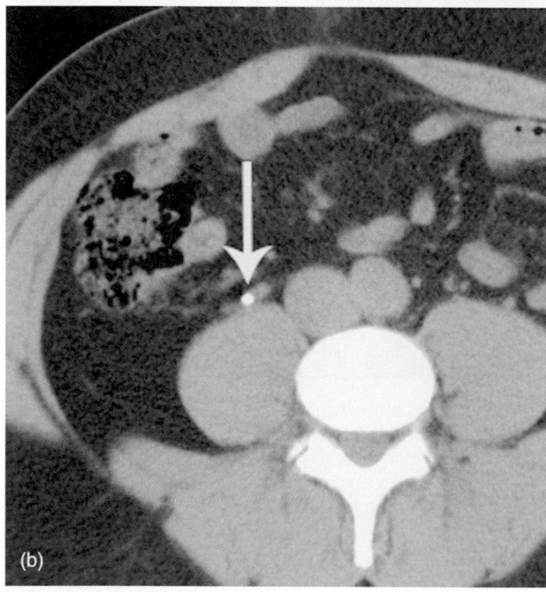

Figure 7.19 Ureteric calculus: CT. Non-enhanced CT performed in a patient with right renal colic. (a) Right kidney (RK), dilated right renal pelvis (arrow), left kidney (LK). (b) Ureteric calculus (arrow).

RADIOGRAPH OF THE KIDNEYS, URETERS AND BLADDER

A KUB radiograph refers to a supine AXR used to diagnose and follow up renal or ureteric calculi. Where possible, follow-up of ureteric or renal calculi should be with a KUB radiograph, as this will result in less radiation exposure than a repeat CT. KUB radiographs can be performed when an obstructing urinary tract calculus is diagnosed on CT to confirm that the calculus is visible and therefore amenable to follow-up with radiographs. KUB radiographs may then be used to confirm spontaneous passage of a calculus or to direct further management. KUB radiographs may also be performed after external shock wave lithotripsy or percutaneous calculus extraction to check for residual fragments in the urinary tract.

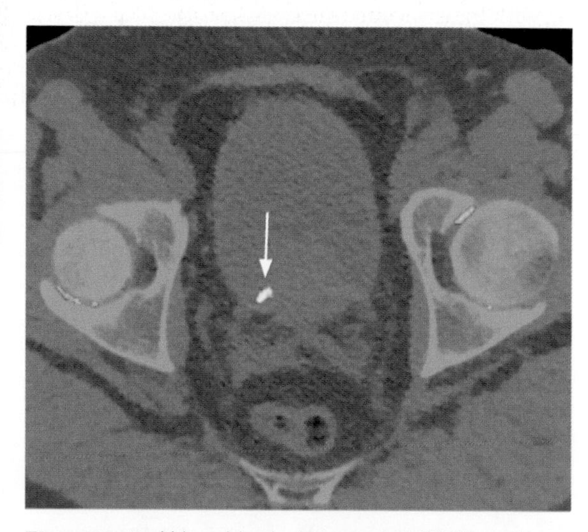

Figure 7.20 Uric acid calculus: spectral CT. The uric acid colour map is overlaid on the conventional non-contrast CT of the kidneys, ureters and bladder (KUB). This shows a uric acid calculus at the right vesicoureteric junction (arrow). Note the scan was performed with the patient prone and the image has been flipped vertically.

Ninety per cent of renal calculi contain sufficient calcium to be visible on KUB radiographs. Cystine stones (3%) are faintly opaque and may be visualized on KUB radiographs with difficulty. Uric acid stones (5%) are not visible on KUB radiographs. Rare xanthine and matrix stones are also lucent. Note that opacities seen on KUB radiographs/AXR thought to be renal or ureteric calculi need to be differentiated from other causes of calcification, such as arterial calcification, calcified lymph nodes and pelvic phleboliths. Phleboliths are small round calcifications in pelvic veins, often with a lucent centre. Phleboliths are extremely common and are visible on AXR in most adults.

7.4.8 ACUTE PANCREATITIS

Acute pancreatitis usually presents with severe acute epigastric pain. Risk factors for the development of acute pancreatitis include heavy alcohol intake and the presence of gallstones. The initial evaluation for suspected pancreatitis consists of biochemical tests, including amylase and lipase levels. CT is the imaging investigation of choice for the diagnosis of acute pancreatitis. CT signs in early pancreatitis may precede elevation of serum enzymes. CT signs of acute pancreatitis include diffuse or focal pancreatic swelling with indistinct margins, thickening of surrounding fascial planes and peripancreatic fat stranding (Fig. 7.21). CT performed during infusion of contrast material can differentiate necrotic non-enhancing tissue from viable enhancing tissue; the presence of pancreatic necrosis is associated with a significantly increased mortality.

Complications of pancreatitis such as phlegmon, abscess and pseudocyst are well shown on CT (Fig. 7.22). CT can also be used to guide percutaneous aspiration and drainage procedures. Indications for percutaneous drainage of a fluid collection associated with acute pancreatitis include:

- Suspected abscess
- Enlarging cyst on follow-up imaging
- Symptoms due to mass effect on adjacent structures.

US is usually indicated in patients with acute pancreatitis, primarily to search for gallstones and to assess the biliary tree.

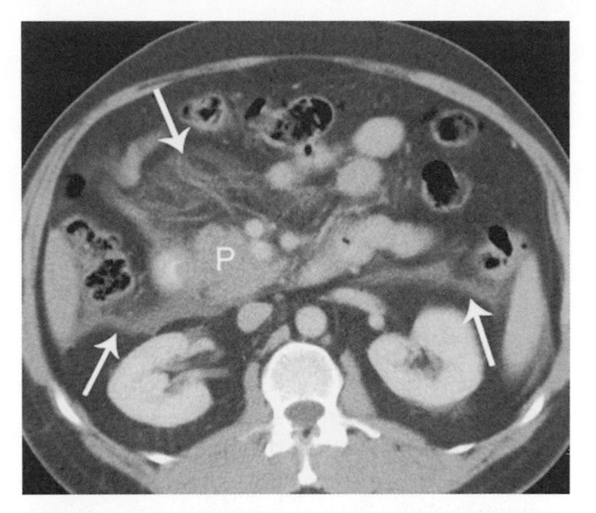

7.21 Acute pancreatitis: CT. Pancreas (P) is swollen with adjacent fat stranding and thickening of fascial planes (arrows).

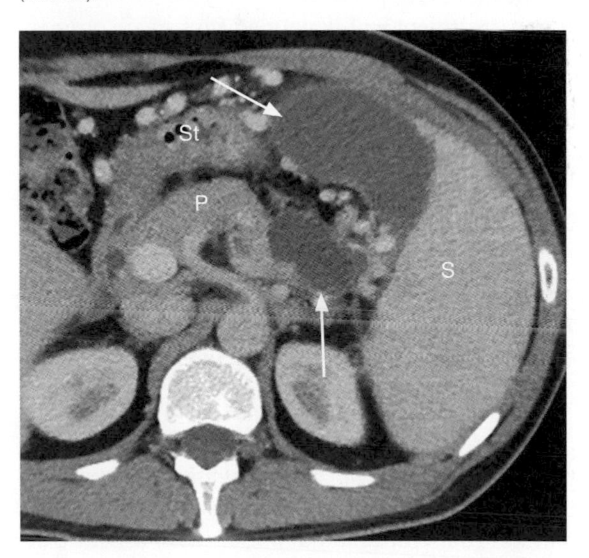

Figure 7.22 Pancreatic pseudocysts: CT. Fluid density collections (arrows) associated with the pancreatic tail and spleen (S) representing pseudocysts from recent acute pancreatitis. Also note stomach (St), body of pancreas (P).

7.4.9 ACUTE MESENTERIC ISCHAEMIA

Acute mesenteric ischaemia (AMI) is caused by abrupt disruption of blood flow to or from the bowel. Arterial occlusion is far more common than venous occlusive disease. AMI usually presents with a sudden onset of severe abdominal pain and bloody diarrhoea. The goal of diagnosis and therapy in AMI is the prevention or limitation of bowel infarction. Prompt diagnosis requires a high index of suspicion and early referral for angiography in patients with clinical evidence of AMI. The most common causes of arterial AMI are superior mesenteric artery (SMA) embolus, SMA thrombosis and non-occlusive SMA vasospasm. SMA embolism occurs in patients with a history of cardiac disease, a previous embolic event or simultaneous peripheral artery embolus. SMA thrombosis is usually associated with an underlying stenotic atherosclerotic lesion in the SMA. Portal vein thrombosis is seen in patients with hypercoagulable states, such as malignancy, portal hypertension or sepsis.

Depending on the cause and clinical situation, particularly the presence or absence of peritoneal signs, treatment will be immediate surgery or interventional radiology. Interventional radiology consists of thrombolysis via a selective catheter, which may be followed by angioplasty of any underlying stenosis or vasodilator (e.g. papaverine) infusion for SMA vasospasm.

7.5 INFLAMMATORY BOWEL DISEASE

The two forms of IBD are Crohn disease (CD) and ulcerative colitis (UC). Patients with IBD present with abdominal pain and diarrhoea. Extraintestinal manifestations may occur, including rashes, arthritis, ocular problems and sclerosing cholangitis. The clinical course after initial presentation usually consists of intermittent episodes of diarrhoea or intestinal obstruction, as well as complications such as infected sinus tracts, fistulae and abscesses. The main roles of imaging at initial presentation are to confirm the diagnosis and assess the distribution of disease. Follow-up examinations are frequently required to assess the efficacy of therapy and to diagnose complications.

AXR is relatively insensitive and non-specific for the definitive diagnosis of IBD. AXR is useful in patients with severe symptoms for the diagnosis of toxic megacolon, perforation or obstruction. Colonoscopy is contraindicated by these findings.

7.5.1 CROHN DISEASE

CD is characterized by transmural granulomatous inflammation with deep ulceration, sinuses and fistula tracts. The disease may involve any part of the GIT from mouth to anus with small bowel involvement alone in 30%, large bowel in 30% and both small and large bowel in 40%. Involvement is discontinuous with normal bowel between diseased segments ('skip lesions').

Cross-sectional imaging techniques – MR enterography and CT enterography – are used for diagnosis and follow-up of CD. Scintigraphy with ^{99m}Tc-HMPAO (see Table 1.1) and ^{99m}Tc-labelled sucralfate may be used in some centres to define the anatomical location of disease and to diagnose relapse in patients with known IBD.

MR enterography refers to MR of the abdomen following ingestion of fluid to distend the small bowel. Hyoscine or glucagon is often injected intravenously to temporarily halt peristalsis. Intravenous gadolinium is also included to show abnormal enhancement of inflamed bowel wall (Fig. 7.23). MR enterography is highly accurate for the diagnosis of bowel wall inflammation and for the demonstration of complications such as sinus tracts, fistulae, abscesses and strictures. The lack of ionizing radiation makes MR enterography particularly useful for the diagnosis

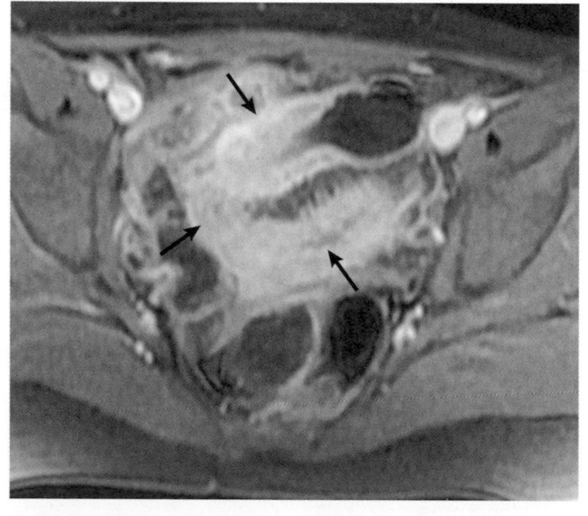

Figure 7.23 Crohn disease: magnetic resonance enterography. Transverse T1-weighted contrast-enhanced MRI of the lower abdomen shows an inflamed segment of small bowel. The inflamed segment shows irregular thickening and marked enhancement (arrows).

and follow-up of young patients with CD and other patients with chronic conditions of the small bowel that may require repeated follow-up examinations.

CT enterography may be used where MR studies are unavailable. The major limitation of CT enterography is the radiation dose; this is particularly relevant in young patients requiring repeated follow-up examinations.

7.5.2 ULCERATIVE COLITIS

UC is a disease of the large bowel characterized by mucosal ulceration and inflammation.

The rectum is involved in virtually all cases with disease extending proximally in the colon. The distribution of disease is continuous with no 'skip lesions'. The initial diagnosis of UC involving the colon is usually by endoscopy, either sigmoidoscopy or colonoscopy, including biopsy. Where colonoscopy is unavailable or contraindicated CT may be performed to show bowel wall thickening and adjacent inflammatory changes in pericolic fat.

7.6 GASTROINTESTINAL BLEEDING

The goals of the diagnosis and treatment of patients with acute GIT bleeding are:

- Haemodynamic resuscitation
- Localization and diagnosis of the source of bleeding
- Control of blood loss either by endoscopic haemostatic therapy, by interventional radiology or by surgery.

7.6.1 UPPER GASTROINTESTINAL TRACT BLEEDING

Upper GIT bleeding is defined as bleeding from the oesophagus to the duodenojejunal flexure (ligament of Treitz). Acute upper GIT bleeding usually presents with haematemesis and/or melaena. It can usually be distinguished clinically from acute lower GIT bleeding, which presents with red blood loss per rectum. The causes of acute upper GIT bleeding include peptic ulcer disease, erosive gastritis, varices, Mallory–Weiss tear and carcinoma. An upper GIT source for GIT bleeding is diagnosed by emergency upper GIT endoscopy in most cases. Endoscopic haemostatic therapies include injection of sclerosants, injection of vasoconstrictors, thermal coagulation and mechanical methods.

7.6.2 LOWER GASTROINTESTINAL TRACT BLEEDING

Common causes of acute lower GIT bleeding are angiodysplasia and diverticular disease. Although colonic diverticula are more prevalent in the sigmoid colon, up to 50% of bleeding from diverticular disease occurs in the ascending colon. Less common causes of lower GIT bleeding include IBD, colonic carcinoma, solitary rectal ulcer and following polypectomy. Lower GIT bleeding is first investigated by sigmoidoscopy. If sigmoidoscopy is negative, CT angiography and scintigraphy are used to diagnose and localize bleeding. This may be followed by catheter angiography and interventional radiology.

COMPUTED TOMOGRAPHY ANGIOGRAPHY

In many centres, CT angiography has replaced red blood cell (RBC) scintigraphy as the initial investigation of choice for investigation of acute lower GIT bleeding. A multiphase contrast-enhanced study shows a bleeding point as a localized 'blush' of contrast, which persists and becomes more diffuse on the later venous phase. Identification of a bleeding source on CT angiography usually leads to treatment with surgery or interventional radiology (Fig. 7.24).

RED BLOOD CELL SCINTIGRAPHY

RBC scintigraphy with ^{99m}Tc-labelled RBCs shows a GIT bleeding point as an area of increased activity. Scintigraphy is less anatomically specific than CT angiography; for this reason, surgery based on RBC scintigraphy alone is not recommended. RBC scintigraphy should be seen as a screening test used to direct further investigation:

- Positive scintigraphy will increase the accuracy of subsequent angiography

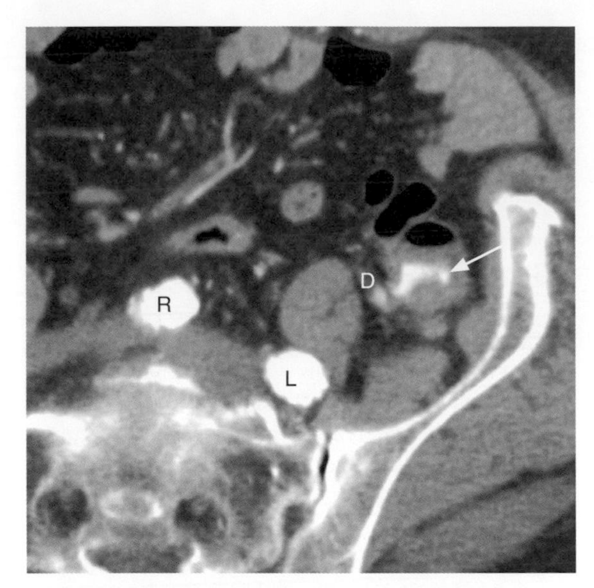

Figure 7.24 Lower gastrointestinal tract bleeding: CT. CT performed during the arterial phase of contrast enhancement with dense enhancement of the right (R) and left (L) common iliac arteries. Diverticular haemorrhage is seen as leakage of contrast material from a bleeding diverticulum (D) into the colonic lumen (arrow).

- Negative scintigraphy implies that subsequent angiography is unlikely to identify a bleeding point; elective colonoscopy would be the next investigation in such cases.

ANGIOGRAPHY AND INTERVENTIONAL RADIOLOGY

Catheter angiography is performed in acute GIT bleeding to achieve haemostasis by superselective catheterization and embolization of bleeding vessels or infusion of vasoconstrictors (e.g., vasopressin). This may be a definitive treatment or may provide stabilization of bleeding prior to surgery.

7.7 COLORECTAL CARCINOMA

7.7.1 SCREENING FOR COLORECTAL CARCINOMA

CRC is the second leading cause of cancer death in Western society. CRC may present clinically with LBO, GIT bleeding or less specifically with weight loss or anaemia. A large percentage of CRCs show locally invasive disease or distant metastases at the time of presentation.

The concept of the adenoma–carcinoma sequence describes the well-demonstrated fact that the vast majority of CRCs develop from small adenomatous polyps through a series of genetic mutations. The adenoma–carcinoma sequence is a slow process: 5.5 years, on average, is required for large adenomas greater than 10 mm diameter to develop into CRC, with 10–15 years for small adenomas (<5 mm). Colonic polyps are very common; not all are adenomas and not all will develop cancer. Most polyps less than 5 mm in diameter are hyperplastic polyps or mucosal tags, which are not cancer precursors. Less than 1% of adenomas up to 1 cm in diameter contain cancer, with cancer in small polyps (<5 mm) being extremely rare.

Given the above concepts, it would seem logical that screening for CRC should be targeted at detecting larger, more advanced adenomas with a high malignant potential rather than trying to identify every single polyp regardless of size, the majority of which will never develop cancer. The risk for the development of CRC may be stratified into three categories:

- Average risk: age older than 50
- Moderate risk: a past personal history of a large adenoma or CRC or first-degree relative with a large adenoma or CRC
- High risk: IBD; hereditary non-polyposis CRC syndromes; familial polyposis syndromes.

Various screening strategies are available and include faecal occult blood testing, colonoscopy and CT colonography. All have limitations, including accuracy, patient reluctance and a lack of community awareness. Faecal occult blood testing is non-specific with a high false-positive rate and will not detect adenomas or cancers that do not bleed. Colonoscopy provides the most complete and thorough examination and is the reference standard for evaluation of the colon.

Advantages of colonoscopy:

- Detection of polyps and cancers with a high degree of accuracy

- Direct visualization of the mucosal surface
- Able to diagnose flat adenomas as well as inflammatory mucosal disease
- Biopsy and polypectomy.

Limitations of colonoscopy:

- Relative expense and variable availability
- Need for sedation and bowel preparation
- Incompletion rate of 5–10% owing to colonic tortuosity or obstruction
- Complications such as perforation, bleeding and splenic injury can rarely occur.

CT colonography is a multidetector CT technique with the potential to play a role in screening for CRC. CT colonography consists of the following:

- Patient's colon is thoroughly 'cleansed' prior to the procedure with commercially available preparation kits
- Faecal tagging: ingestion of contrast material prior to CT will cause any retained faecal material to be of high density and therefore easily distinguished from polyps
- Patient is placed on the CT table and a rectal tube inserted
- Colon is distended with room air or CO_2
- Two CT scans – first supine and then prone using a low radiation dose CT technique
- Images are reviewed on a computer workstation with software applications that allow instant multiplanar and three-dimensional reconstructions, as well as specialized algorithms for viewing of the mucosal surface (Fig. 7.25).

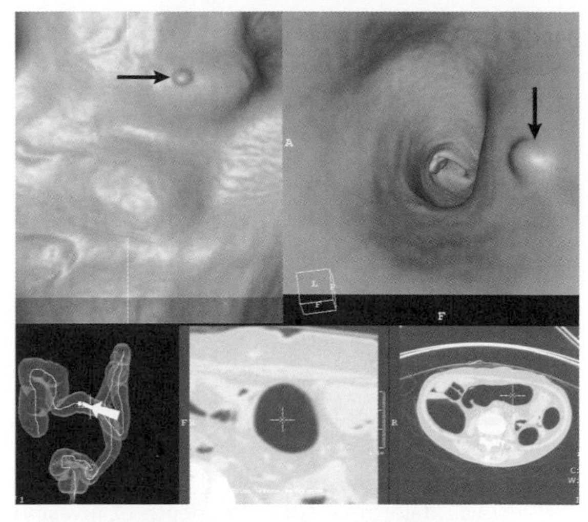

Figure 7.25 CT colonography: image showing the type of software used for reporting of CT colonography. Simultaneous display of cross-sectional and three-dimensional images allows accurate appraisal of the mucosal surface of the colon. In this example, there is a 5-mm polyp in the mid-transverse colon (arrows).

CT colonography has a sensitivity of over 90% for the detection of polyps measuring 10 mm or more (Fig. 7.26). The limitations of CT colonography are:

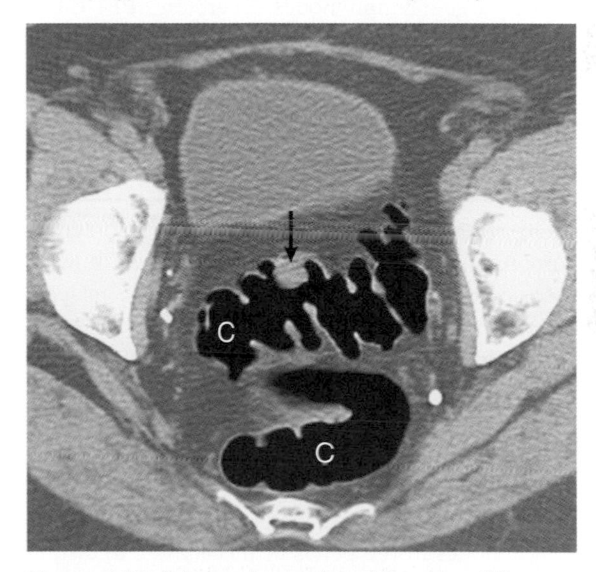

Figure 7.26 Adenomatous polyp of the colon: CT colonography. The colon (C) is distended with air. This transverse view shows a round polyp (arrow) arising in the sigmoid colon.

- Inability to reliably identify flat adenomas or mucosal inflammation
- Low reported sensitivities for the detection of small polyps (<5 mm)
- Biopsy and polypectomy cannot be performed.

Because of these limitations, CT colonography cannot replace colonoscopy.

Indications for CT colonography include:

- Failed colonoscopy
- Evaluation of the colon proximal to an obstruction
- Where colonoscopy or sedation are contraindicated.

7.7.2 STAGING OF COLORECTAL CARCINOMA

Key factors in the tumour–node–metastasis (TNM) staging of CRC are the presence and depth of invasion of the bowel wall, invasion through the bowel wall, invasion of adjacent structures, involvement of regional lymph nodes and metastasis to distant sites such as liver, non-regional lymph nodes, skeleton and lung.

FDG-PET-CT is the imaging investigation of choice for the detection of locally invasive disease, lymphadenopathy and distant metastases in patients with CRC. CT may be used where PET scanning is unavailable. The two most critical factors influencing survival data in CRC are the depth of invasion of the bowel wall and the presence or absence of lymph node metastases. Unfortunately, two limitations of PET-CT are the assessment of depth of wall invasion and detection of microscopic metastases in non-enlarged lymph nodes. Therefore, PET-CT is accurate for advanced disease though less so for earlier non-invasive disease.

7.7.3 STAGING OF RECTAL CARCINOMA

Most rectal carcinomas are annular or polypoid tumours that invade the wall of the rectum. Tumour invasion occurs through the layers of the rectal wall, i.e. mucosal layer, submucosa and muscularis propria. Tumours that have invaded through the full thickness of the rectal wall may then extend into the surrounding mesorectal fat. Tumour may then invade adjacent structures, such as the bladder or seminal vesicles, or may perforate into the peritoneal cavity. Rectal carcinoma may also spread to regional lymph nodes in the pelvis or metastasize to distant sites such as the abdominal lymph nodes or liver.

Management options for rectal carcinoma include surgery, chemotherapy and radiotherapy. Surgery for rectal carcinoma is potentially curative and consists of complete removal of the rectum and surrounding mesorectal fat and lymphatics, i.e. total mesorectal excision (TME). Less invasive techniques such as transanal endoscopic microsurgery (TEMS) may be used for early-stage low rectal tumours. For higher stage tumours neoadjuvant chemotherapy or a combination of neoadjuvant chemotherapy and radiotherapy may be used prior to surgery. For advanced invasive disease or metastatic disease, non-curative surgery such as local excision and stoma may be used to palliate obstruction. Furthermore, locally advanced tumours that respond well to neoadjuvant chemoradiotherapy may be amenable to a 'watch and wait' approach, whereby serial imaging is performed to exclude recurrent or progressive disease that may require surgery.

From the above, it can be seen that accurate TNM staging of rectal carcinoma is essential for directing management. Because the rectum is surrounded by a layer of mesorectal fat with a fixed position in the pelvis, it is amenable to high-resolution imaging with magnetic resonance imaging (MRI). MRI can differentiate the layers of the rectal wall and is therefore able to accurately assess the depth of invasion of rectal tumour (Fig. 7.27). It is also accurate for the assessment of small regional mesorectal lymph nodes, as well as other relevant prognostic features such as invasion of veins. Furthermore, MRI is used for surveillance imaging post adjuvant or neoadjuvant therapy. MRI is the investigation of choice for local staging of rectal cancer. PET-CT or CT is used for the exclusion or detection of distant metastases.

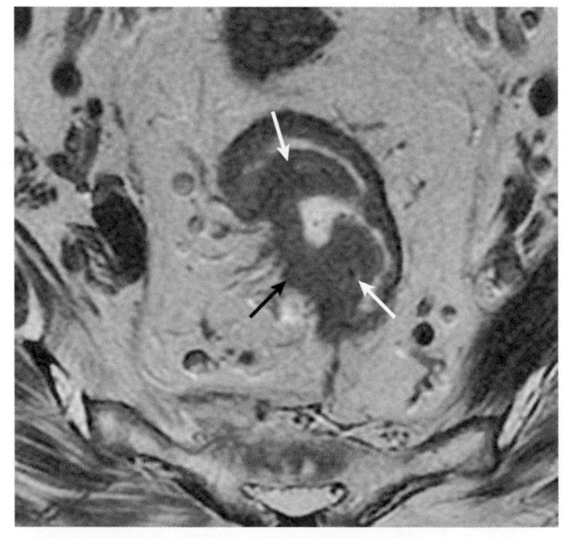

Figure 7.27 Carcinoma of the rectum: MRI. Transverse T2-weighted MRI of the rectum shows an annular (ring-shaped) tumour (white arrows). Note the nodular irregularity at the junction of the tumour and mesorectal fat, indicating tumour extension through the full thickness of the rectal wall (black arrow).

Further details of TNM staging of colorectal cancer may be found on the companion website.

7.8 DIFFUSE LIVER DISEASE: STEATOSIS, FIBROSIS AND CIRRHOSIS

Deranged liver function tests (LFTs) is a common indication for imaging of the liver. Raised liver enzymes are found in multiple scenarios, including incidentally in patients having screening blood tests. Among the many causes of liver disease, non-alcoholic fatty liver disease (NAFLD) is increasing in incidence. Like other forms of chronic liver disease, it may lead to the development of hepatic cirrhosis and hepatocellular carcinoma (HCC).

7.8.1 HEPATIC STEATOSIS

Also known as 'fatty liver', hepatic steatosis is the abnormal accumulation of intracellular fat in hepatocytes. Hepatic steatosis has multiple causes, including:

- NAFLD
- Alcohol abuse
- Chemotherapy
- Steroid use
- Chronic hepatitis.

US provides excellent assessment of the hepatic parenchyma. In NAFLD, and other causes of hepatic steatosis, the liver shows increased parenchymal echogenicity. In severe cases, the US beam becomes attenuated, such that deep portions of the liver are poorly visualized. An associated phenomenon that is commonly seen on US is focal fatty sparing. As the name suggests, this refers to regions of normal-appearing hepatic parenchyma. On US fatty sparing appears as relatively hypoechoic regions that tend to occur in typical locations adjacent to the gallbladder and falciform ligament and deep to the hepatic capsule.

Hepatic steatosis shows on CT as reduced parenchymal attenuation (Fig. 7.28). This is manifest on non-contrast CT as an absolute liver density measurement of less than 40 HU or hepatic parenchymal attenuation less than that of the spleen. Hepatic

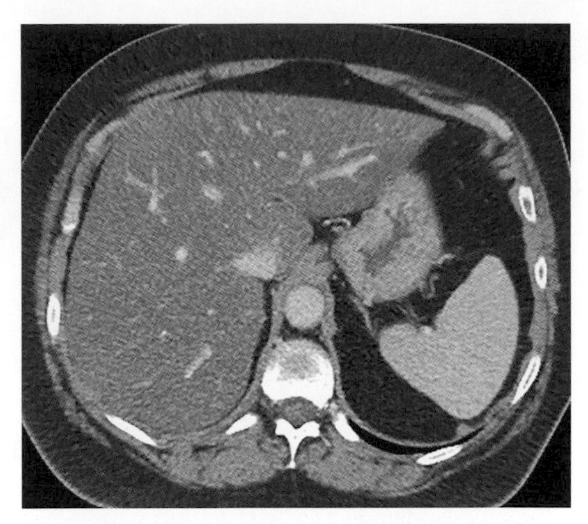

Figure 7.28 Hepatic steatosis: CT. Note that the hepatic parenchyma is of low attenuation, indicating markedly increased fat content. Compare this with the normal-appearing parenchyma in Figure 7.30.

steatosis is a common incidental finding on CT performed for other reasons.

Most MRI liver imaging protocols include chemical shift imaging to assess the hepatic parenchyma. Chemical shift imaging exploits the slightly different precession frequency of hydrogen atoms in water from those in fat. At certain time intervals, the hydrogen atoms in water and fat will be perfectly in phase; at other times, they will be out of phase. A good analogy is to think of two children on swings in a playground, one swinging slightly faster than the other. At certain times, both children will be at the top of their arcs at the same time; at other intervals, the swings will be at opposite ends of their arcs. Where fat and water molecules are in close contact, such as in fat-rich hepatocytes, scans timed to detect the molecules in phase will show high signal, while scans timed to be out of phase (opposed phase) will show reduced signal. With chemical shift MRI, hepatic steatosis shows reduced hepatic parenchymal signal on out-of-phase scans.

7.8.2 FIBROSIS AND CIRRHOSIS

Cirrhosis is an irreversible process that is a common pathological end point resulting from various liver diseases. These include alcoholic liver disease, chronic viral hepatitis (hepatitis B and C) and NAFLD. It is characterized by loss of the normal hepatic architecture with nodules interspersed with bands of fibrosis. Cirrhosis may be complicated by portal hypertension and is also associated with an increased risk of HCC. Cirrhosis that is asymptomatic is referred to as compensated and is often found incidentally on imaging performed for other reasons. Decompensated cirrhosis is associated with clinical manifestations, including jaundice, encephalopathy, ascites and variceal haemorrhage.

ULTRASOUND

Features of cirrhosis on US include:

- Coarse, heterogeneous hepatic parenchymal echotexture
- Nodular hepatic outline
- Relatively reduced size of the right lobe hepatic segments (V, VI, VII and VIII)
- Relatively enlarged caudate lobe (segment I).

Features of portal hypertension on US include:

- Splenomegaly
- Ascites
- Varices
- Doppler US abnormalities
  - Slow or reversed portal venous flow
  - Portal vein thrombosis.

In a patient with cirrhosis, US is used as a screening tool to assess for signs of portal hypertension and for the development of HCC. Focal lesions in cirrhosis may be due to causes other than HCC, such as regenerative or dysplastic nodules. New or growing lesions found on serial US are further characterized with MRI (or CT) and reported using the Liver Imaging Reporting and Data System (LI-RADS) (see section 7.9.5).

COMPUTED TOMOGRAPHY AND MAGNETIC RESONANCE IMAGING

Signs of hepatic cirrhosis and portal hypertension on CT and MRI are equivalent to those described for US, i.e. nodular liver that may be associated with splenomegaly, ascites and varices. A lack of enhancement of the portal vein indicates thrombosis. Portosystemic shunts and venous varices are easily identified.

SHEAR WAVE ELASTOGRAPHY

In the development of cirrhosis, the diseased liver passes through increasingly severe and extensive changes of fibrosis over several years. Various staging systems may be used, such as the five-stage Metavir (an acronym of 'meta-analysis of histological data in viral hepatitis') classification from 0 (normal) through increasingly severe stages 1–3 to stage 4 (cirrhosis). The diagnosis of early-stage fibrosis is important as changes may be reversible or at least stoppable with lifestyle changes and other interventions. Biopsy is the gold standard for the diagnosis but is invasive and carries a level of risk.

As described in Chapter 1, shear wave elastography (SWE) is a non-invasive method for measuring tissue stiffness. Applied to the liver, SWE is gaining acceptance as a useful tool in the imaging of liver disease. SWE is performed in conjunction with real-time US examination. This allows appropriate positioning of a region of interest in the parenchyma of the right lobe of the liver, avoiding structures that would interfere with shear wave velocity such as large blood vessels (Fig. 7.29). Multiple (usually about 10) measurements of shear wave velocity are made.

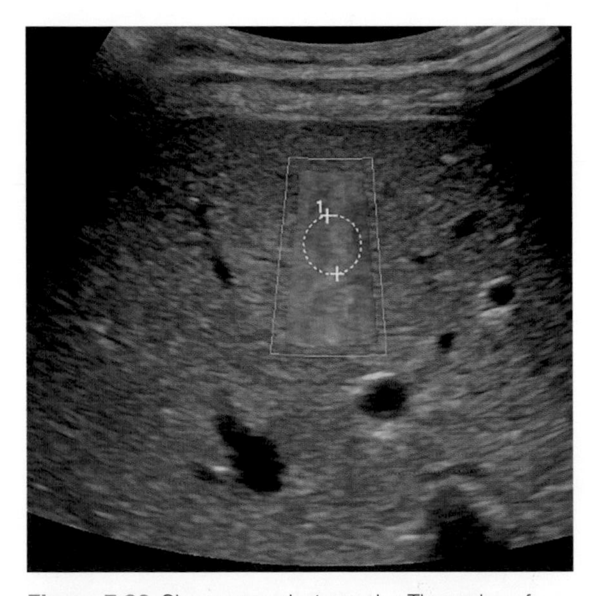

Figure 7.29 Shear wave elastography. The region of interest (ROI) is shown as a circle within a colour-filled box superimposed on an US image of the liver. The ROI is positioned within the hepatic parenchyma, away from the liver capsule and separate from hepatic blood vessels.

Tissue stiffness is reported as the median shear wave velocity expressed as m/s or as kilopascals (kPa). SWE is particularly accurate and reproducible in viral liver disease and NAFLD.

7.9 DETECTION AND CHARACTERIZATION OF LIVER MASSES

Liver masses may present clinically in several ways:

- Upper abdominal pain, often described as 'dragging' in nature
- Acute abdominal pain that may be caused by sudden haemorrhage
- Sudden deterioration in liver function owing to HCC occurring in a cirrhotic liver.

Many liver masses are discovered as incidental findings during imaging investigation of unrelated symptoms. Liver masses may also be detected during imaging screening of the liver for metastases in a patient with a known primary malignancy. The characterization of liver masses, whether in the setting of a known malignancy or underlying cirrhosis, is an important goal of diagnostic imaging. The choice of imaging technique may vary depending on the clinical context, as well as local availability and expertise. Liver masses, listed in Table 7.1, usually have characteristic appearances on US, CT and MRI.

Table 7.1 Commonly encountered liver masses.

Benign	Malignant
• Simple cyst • Haemangioma • Focal nodular hyperplasia • Adenoma	• Metastases • Hepatocellular carcinoma • Cholangiocarcinoma

7.9.1 DYNAMIC IMAGING STUDIES

Dynamic imaging of the liver is possible because the liver receives a dual blood supply. The hepatic artery supplies 25% of hepatic blood flow whereas the portal vein supplies the remaining 75%.

Three phases of contrast enhancement occur following intravenous injection of a bolus of contrast material:

- Arterial phase: begins at around 25 seconds after commencement of injection
- Portal venous phase: begins at around 70 seconds, after blood has circulated through the mesentery, intestine and spleen
  - o 75% of the liver's blood supply is from the portal vein; therefore, maximum enhancement of liver tissue occurs in the portal venous phase
- Equilibrium or transition phase: several minutes after injection there is redistribution of contrast material to the extracellular space.

Most liver tumours derive their blood supply from the hepatic artery and receive less blood supply than surrounding liver, i.e. they are hypovascular. It follows then that maximum lesion conspicuity for most liver tumours, including metastases, will occur in the portal venous phase of contrast enhancement. Note that this is due to background liver enhancement, not enhancement of the tumour. Hypovascular tumours are seen as low-attenuation masses visualized against high-attenuation enhancing liver (Fig. 7.30).

Some liver tumours are hypervascular in that they receive more blood supply than surrounding liver. For these tumours maximum lesion conspicuity occurs in the arterial phase of contrast enhancement (Fig. 7.31). Examples of hypervascular lesions best seen in the arterial phase are HCC, focal nodular hyperplasia (FNH) and hypervascular metastases. Hypervascular metastases are less common than hypovascular metastases and may be seen with carcinoid tumour, renal cell carcinoma and melanoma.

Three methods are available for dynamic imaging of the liver: contrast-enhanced US (CEUS), multiphase CT with iodinated contrast material and MRI with gadolinium.

7.9.2 ULTRASOUND

US is often the first investigation performed for a suspected liver mass as it is non-invasive and relatively inexpensive. Characterization of a lesion as a simple cyst on US usually means that further investigation

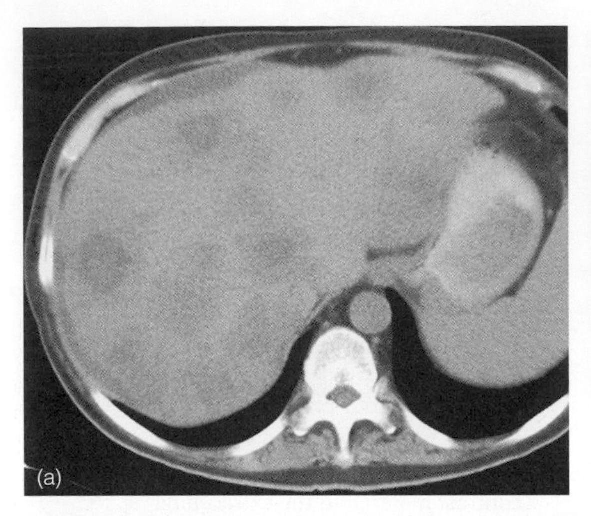

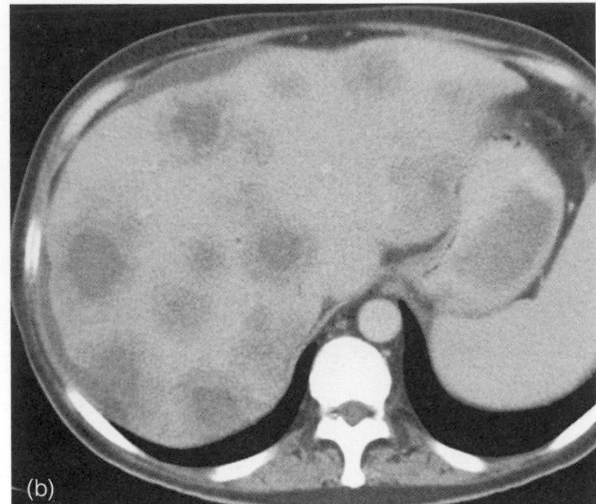

Figure 7.30 Hepatic metastases: CT. (a) Non-contrast CT of the liver shows multiple low-attenuation lesions throughout the liver. (b) CT during the portal venous phase of contrast enhancement shows multiple low-attenuation metastases, more obvious than on the non-contrast scan.

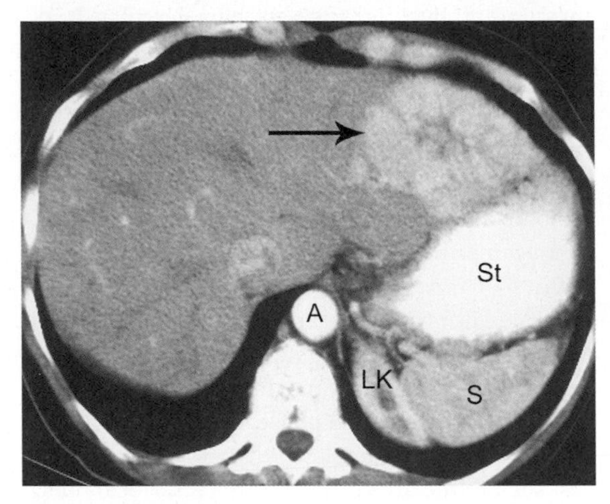

Figure 7.31 Focal nodular hyperplasia (FNH): CT. CT of the liver during the arterial phase of contrast enhancement shows the typical pattern of FNH with an intensely enhancing mass (arrow) containing a central non-enhancing scar. Also note aorta (A), left kidney (LK), spleen (S), stomach (St).

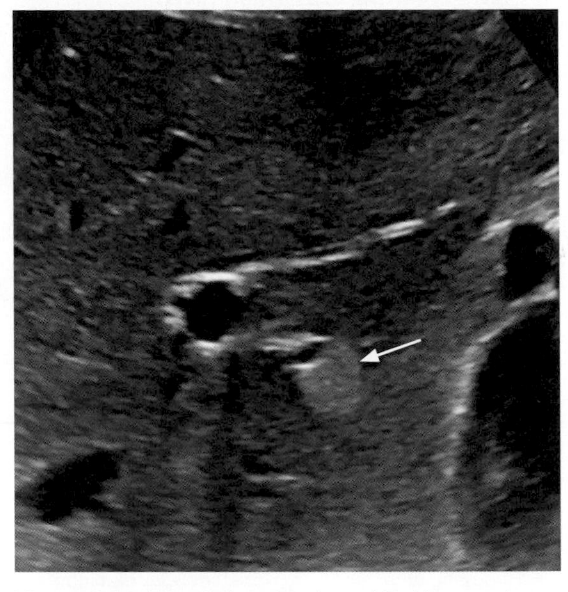

Figure 7.32 Hepatic haemangioma: US. Haemangioma shows as a well-defined hyperechoic lesion (arrow).

is not required. A solid mass detected on US will in most circumstances require further characterization with dynamic imaging, i.e. CEUS, CT or MRI.

Other roles for US in hepatic masses:

- Follow-up of a known mass, e.g. suspected haemangioma where US is used to confirm lack of growth (Fig. 7.32)
- US-guided biopsy
- Intraoperative US: a high-frequency US probe is directly applied to the surface of the liver during surgery to detect metastases.

Limitations of US in the detection of liver lesions:

- Less accurate for the detection of lesions high in the liver near the diaphragmatic surface,

particularly where the liver lies high up under the rib cage
- Hepatic steatosis (fatty liver): fatty infiltration produces an increasingly echogenic (bright) liver with deeper parts poorly seen on US.

7.9.3 COMPUTED TOMOGRAPHY

CT provides accurate anatomical localization and characterization of mass contents such as fluid, fat or calcification. Complications of HCC such as invasion of the portal vein and arteriovenous shunting are well demonstrated with CT. As well as lesion detection, multiphase liver CT is often useful for liver mass characterization based on the contrast enhancement pattern. Common examples of this include differentiation of common benign masses such as haemangioma and FNH from more sinister lesions. Haemangioma and FNH are usually asymptomatic, though large lesions may produce pain. Characterization of these lesions is particularly important in patients with known primary malignancy in whom metastatic disease is suspected. Most haemangiomas show a typical peripheral nodular enhancement pattern in the arterial phase, and this is usually adequate for diagnosis. FNH is usually isointense to liver on non-enhanced and portal venous phases, with intense enhancement on the arterial phase plus a non-enhancing central scar.

7.9.4 MAGNETIC RESONANCE IMAGING

MRI is used commonly for liver lesion detection and characterization, and in many centres has replaced CT as the primary investigation of choice. Fast imaging sequences allow imaging of the liver during a single breath-hold. As with CT, MRI may be performed during the arterial, portal venous and equilibrium phases of contrast enhancement following intravenous injection of gadolinium (Fig. 7.33). The role of MRI for liver lesion detection and characterization has been expanded with the use of the gadolinium-based hepatobiliary contrast agents gadoxetic acid (Gd-EOB-DTPA) and gadobenate dimeglumine (Gd-BOPTA). Hepatobiliary contrast agents are taken up by functioning hepatocytes and

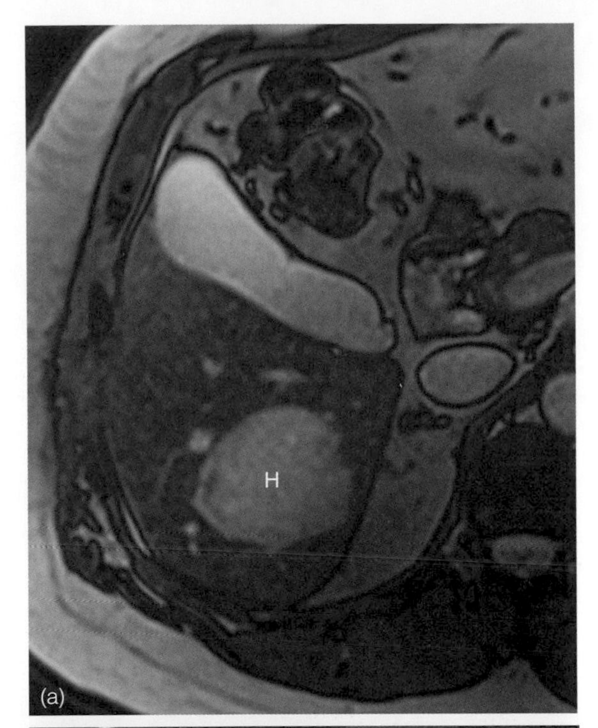

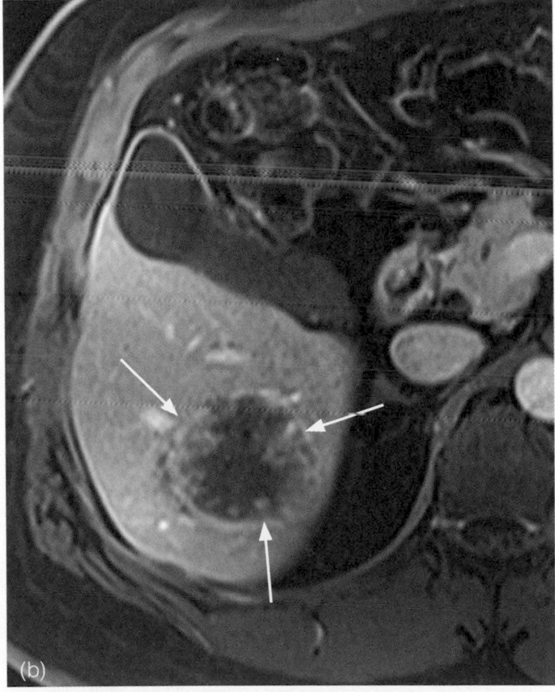

Figure 7.33 Hepatic haemangioma: MRI. (a) T2-weighted image. Haemangioma (H) shows as a mass with intensely high signal. (b) Arterial phase contrast-enhanced T1-weighted image. Haemangioma shows peripheral nodular enhancement (arrows).

excreted in bile. On delayed imaging – known as the hepatobiliary phase (10–20 minutes post injection for Gd-EOB-DTPA) – these agents produce increased signal of the liver and biliary tree. Certain liver masses such as FNH and cirrhotic dysplastic nodules take up the hepatobiliary agents and therefore show increased signal on the hepatobiliary phase (Fig. 7.34). Other lesions, including metastases, haemangioma and most HCCs, show as filling defects outlined by the high-signal hepatic parenchyma.

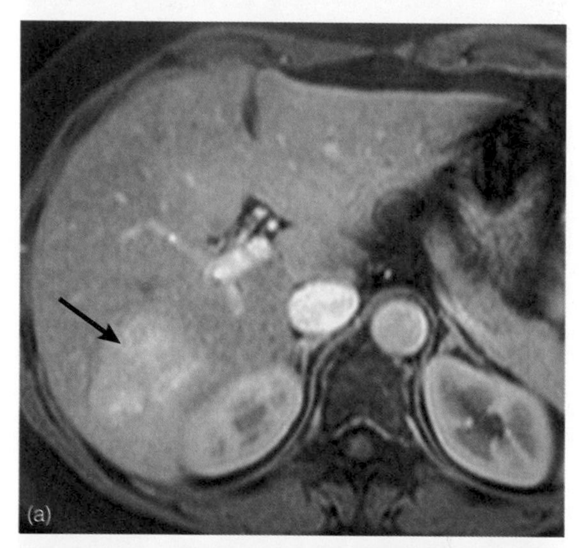

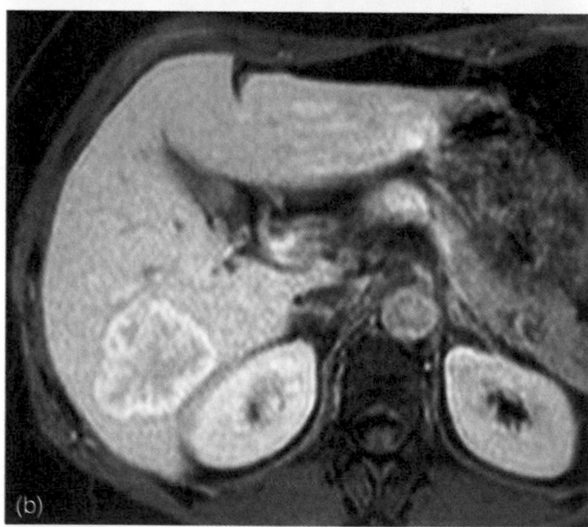

Figure 7.34 Focal nodular hyperplasia (FNH): MRI with hepatobiliary contrast agent. (a) Transverse T1-weighted MRI during the arterial phase of contrast enhancement shows an enhancing hypervascular mass (arrow). (b) Hepatobiliary phase scan shows continued enhancement of the lesion, strongly favouring a diagnosis of FNH.

7.9.5 LIVER IMAGING REPORTING AND DATA SYSTEM

LI-RADS provides a standardized framework for reporting liver imaging in patients at risk of developing HCC. LI-RADS is used in patients aged over 18 with hepatic cirrhosis, with chronic hepatitis B or with a prior or current history of HCC, including liver transplant candidates and recipients. It may be applied with multiphase contrast-enhanced imaging with MRI, CT and US. LI-RADS has gained wide acceptance owing to several factors:

- Increasing incidence of cirrhosis, and therefore risk of HCC, owing to alcoholic and viral liver disease, plus the rapidly increasing incidence of NAFLD
- Risks associated with liver biopsy
- Well-established evidence that LI-RADS criteria closely parallel tumour biology, and therefore provide an accurate method of diagnosing HCC without resort to biopsy
- Availability of treatments for HCC, including percutaneous ablation, selective delivery of chemotherapy and radiotherapy and liver transplant.

LI-RADS categorizes lesions (termed 'observations') by size and then assesses for various imaging signs (Fig. 7.35):

- Arterial phase hyperenhancement
- Venous or transition phase hypoenhancement ('washout')
- Enhancing border around the lesion on the venous or transition phase ('capsule')
- Growth on serial scans.

Based on these findings, plus other ancillary features, a LI-RADS category is assigned. Each category has a corresponding conclusion that can guide further management, e.g. LI-RADS 5: 'definitely HCC'. Further details of LI-RADS may be found on the companion website.

7.10 IMAGING INVESTIGATION OF JAUNDICE

Causes of jaundice may be divided into two broad categories:

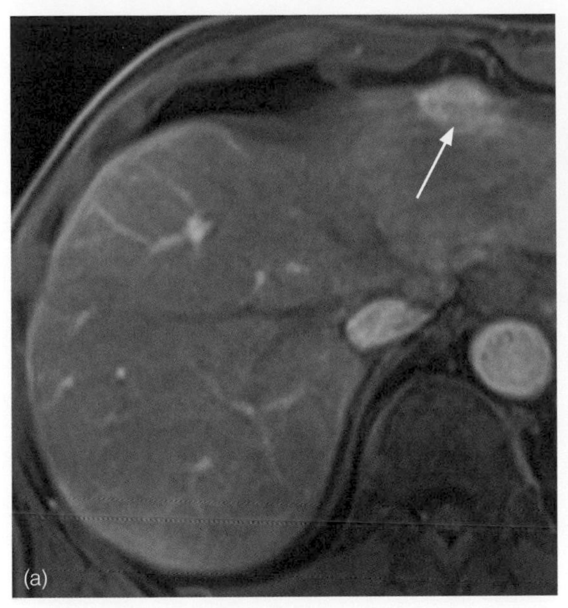

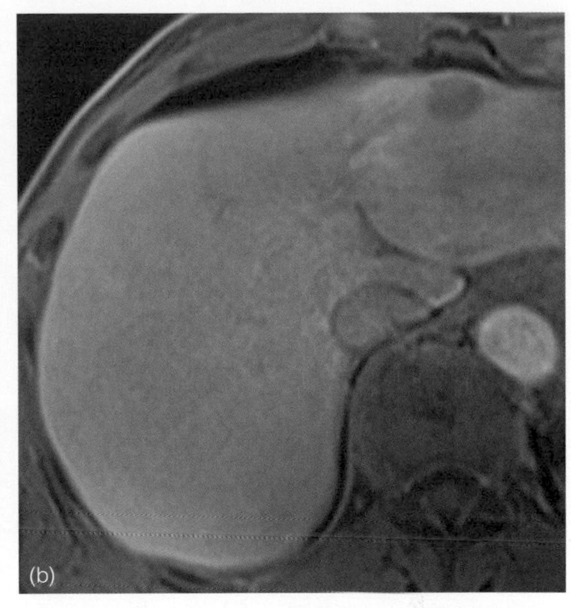

Figure 7.35 Hepatocellular carcinoma: multiphase contrast-enhanced MRI. (a) Arterial phase: lesion is higher signal than liver parenchyma, indicating arterial phase enhancement (arrow). (b) Venous phase: the lesion is lower signal than liver parenchyma, indicating venous phase washout.

- Mechanical biliary obstruction
- Intrahepatic biliary stasis, also known as hepatocellular or non-obstructive jaundice.

Based on clinical findings such as pain and stigmata of liver disease, plus biochemical tests of liver function, the distinction between these categories can be made in most patients. Imaging has no significant role in hepatocellular jaundice, other than US guidance of liver biopsy. Mechanical biliary obstruction may occur at any level from the liver to the duodenum. Causes include gallstones in the bile ducts, pancreatic carcinoma (see section 7.10.7), cholangiocarcinoma, carcinoma of the ampulla of Vater or duodenum, iatrogenic biliary stricture, chronic pancreatitis, liver masses and sclerosing cholangitis. The roles of imaging are to determine the presence, level and cause of biliary obstruction.

7.10.1 ULTRASOUND

US is the first imaging investigation of choice for the jaundiced patient. As well as imaging the hepatic parenchyma (see section 7.8), US provides excellent visualization of the biliary tree. Common bile duct diameter measurements are graded as follows: normal, less than 6 mm; equivocal, 6–8 mm; dilated, more than 8 mm (Fig. 7.36). The site and cause of obstruction are defined on US in only 25% of cases as overlying duodenal gas often obscures the lower end of the common bile duct (Fig. 7.37). Associated dilatation of the main pancreatic duct suggests obstruction at the level of the pancreatic head or ampulla of

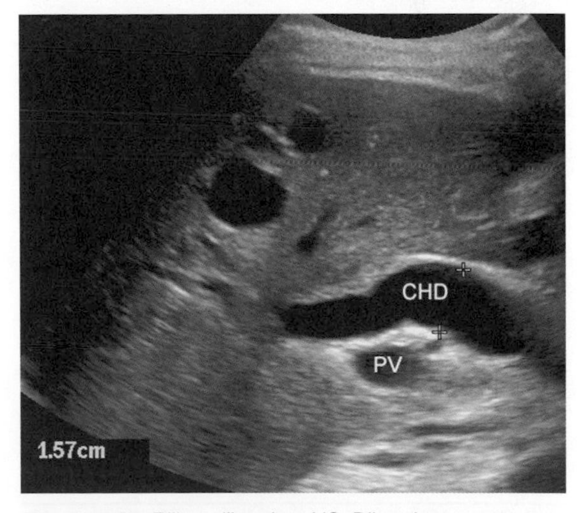

Figure 7.36 Biliary dilatation: US. Dilated common hepatic duct (CHD) seen as an anechoic tubular structure anterior to the portal vein (PV).

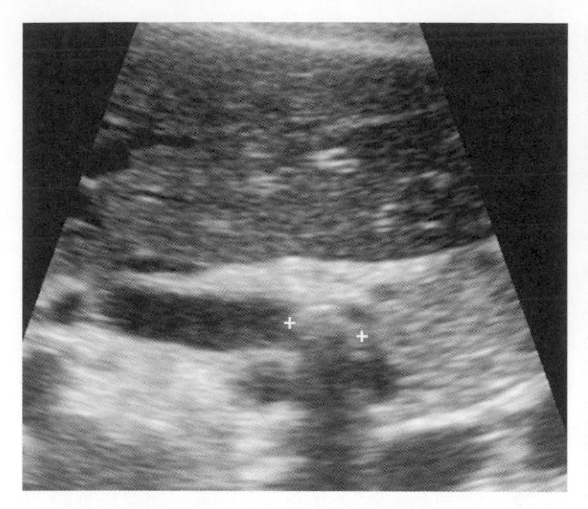

Figure 7.37 Choledocholithiasis: US. Biliary calculus seen as a hyperechoic focus (+) in the common bile duct.

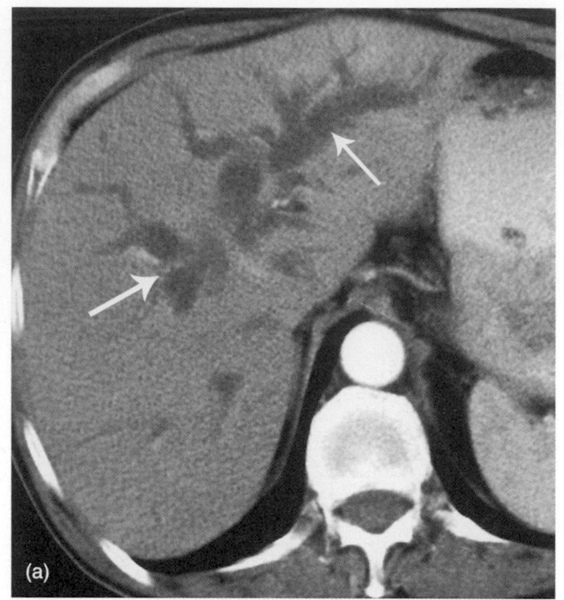

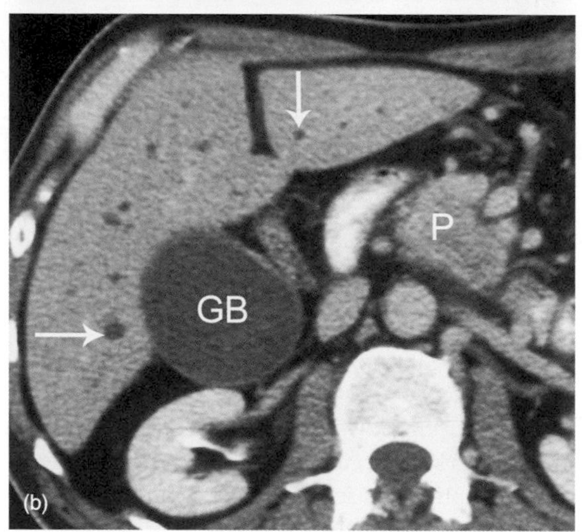

Figure 7.38 Biliary obstruction due to carcinoma of the head of the pancreas: CT. (a) Dilated bile ducts seen on CT as a low-attenuation branching pattern (arrows) in the liver. (b) Note enlargement of the head of the pancreas (P) due to tumour and the distended gallbladder (GB).

Vater (double-duct sign). Depending on the results of US, further investigation may be directed as follows:

- Bile ducts not dilated: hepatocellular jaundice is considered and liver biopsy may be indicated
- Bile ducts dilated as a result of biliary calculus: endoscopic retrograde cholangiopancreatography (ERCP) and sphincterotomy or surgery
- Bile ducts dilated as a result of a soft-tissue mass: multiphase CT for further characterization
- Bile ducts dilated without an obvious cause: CT may be performed as this has a higher rate of diagnosis of the cause of biliary obstruction than US (Fig. 7.38).

Depending on the findings, US and CT may be followed by more definitive imaging of the biliary system with magnetic resonance cholangiopancreatography (MRCP), CT cholangiography, endoscopic US (EUS), ERCP or percutaneous transhepatic cholangiography (PTC).

7.10.2 MAGNETIC RESONANCE CHOLANGIO-PANCREATOGRAPHY

MRCP is non-invasive, does not involve ionizing radiation and does not require intravenous contrast material. MRCP uses heavily T2-weighted images that show stationary fluids such as bile as high signal, with moving fluids and solid tissues as low signal. The bile ducts and gallbladder are therefore seen as bright structures on a dark background (Fig. 7.39). MRCP is unaffected by bilirubin levels and may be

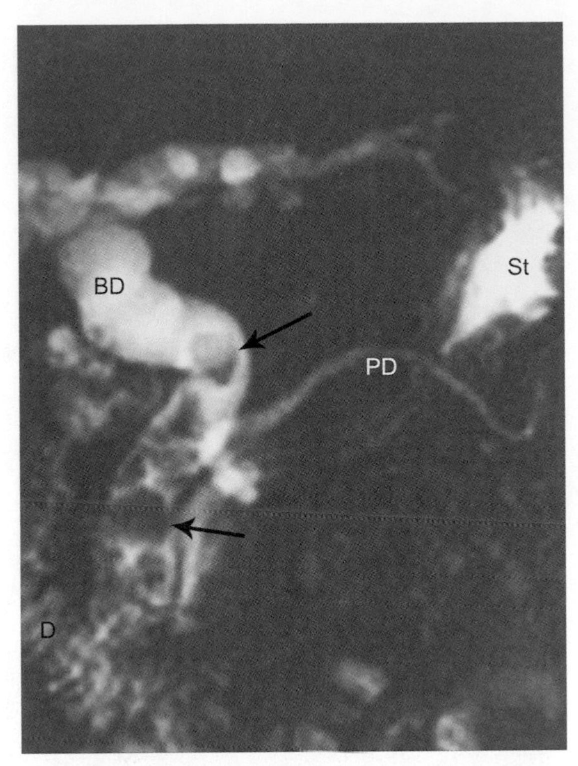

Figure 7.39 Choledocholithiasis: magnetic resonance cholangiopancreatography (MRCP). Biliary calculi are seen as filling defects (arrows) within the dilated bile ducts (BD). Also note duodenum (D), pancreatic duct (PD), stomach (St).

combined with other sequences to provide more comprehensive imaging of the liver and pancreas.

MRCP has largely replaced diagnostic ERCP as the investigation of choice for imaging of the biliary system, including assessment of jaundiced patients with dilated bile ducts on US. MRCP is commonly used prior to laparoscopic cholecystectomy to diagnose bile duct calculi and bile duct variants, and to avoid intraoperative exploration of the common bile duct.

7.10.3 COMPUTED TOMOGRAPHY CHOLANGIOGRAPHY

CT cholangiography involves a slow intravenous infusion of an iodine-containing cholangiographic agent (meglumine iotroxate) to opacify the bile ducts, followed by CT. CT cholangiography is a reasonably reliable method of imaging the biliary system. It may be used when MRCP and the other more invasive methods listed below are contraindicated or not available. The disadvantages of CT cholangiography include radiation exposure, allergy to contrast material and non-visualization of the bile ducts in patients with hyperbilirubinaemia.

7.10.4 ENDOSCOPIC ULTRASOUND

As the name suggest, EUS combines a small US probe with an endoscope. EUS is highly sensitive in the detection of small biliary and pancreatic tumours. EUS may be used to guide biopsy of small masses or cyst aspiration. The limitations of EUS include limited availability, difficulty of interpretation following biliary stent placement or sphincterotomy and technical difficulties following gastric surgery.

7.10.5 ENDOSCOPIC RETROGRADE CHOLANGIO-PANCREATOGRAPHY

For ERCP, the ampulla of Vater is identified endoscopically and a small cannula passed into it under direct endoscopic visualization. Contrast material is then injected into the biliary and pancreatic ducts and images acquired (Fig. 7.40). When MRCP is not available, ERCP is used to assess biliary obstruction diagnosed on US or CT. ERCP is the investigation of choice for suspected distal biliary obstruction that may require interventions such as sphincterotomy, basket retrieval of stones, biliary biopsy or biliary stent placement. The disadvantages of ERCP include:

- Complications, including pancreatitis (relatively uncommon though may be devastating when they do occur)
- Technical failure in up to 10%.

7.10.6 PERCUTANEOUS TRANSHEPATIC CHOLANGIOGRAPHY

PTC is indicated for the assessment of high biliary obstruction at the level of the porta and where biliary obstruction cannot be outlined by ERCP owing to previous biliary diversion surgery. PTC is performed under fluoroscopy with a fine needle passed into a

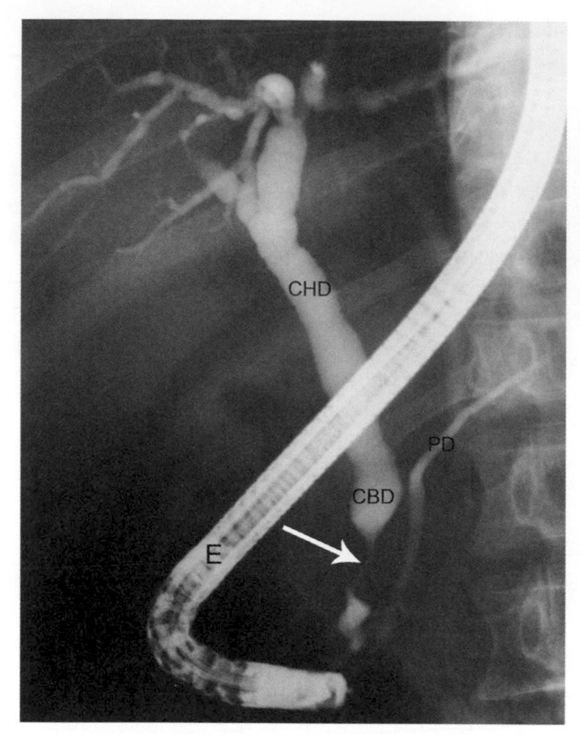

Figure 7.40 Cholangiocarcinoma: endoscopic retrograde cholangiopancreatography (ERCP). Stricture (arrow) of the distal common bile duct (CBD) due to cholangiocarcinoma. Also note endoscope (E), common hepatic duct (CHD), pancreatic duct (PD).

peripheral bile duct in the liver and contrast material injected to outline the biliary system. PTC is often accompanied by biliary stent placement for the relief of biliary obstruction. Patient preparation for PTC should include clotting studies and antibiotic cover to prevent septicaemia due to release of infected bile.

7.10.7 PANCREATIC CARCINOMA

Over 90% of pancreatic malignancies are ductal adenocarcinomas. Although they may present with obstructive jaundice, the most common clinical presentation is abdominal pain. Carcinoma in the head of the pancreas may be seen on US as a hypoechoic mass with associated biliary and pancreatic duct dilatation. CT is the investigation of choice for staging. The key feature that governs resectability is involvement of local blood vessels, specifically the coeliac axis and SMA. Contact and encirclement of 180° or more of a blood vessel's circumference by tumour tissue as seen on CT is a highly accurate predictor of unresectability (Fig. 7.41). Further details of staging of pancreatic ductal adenocarcinoma may be found on the companion website.

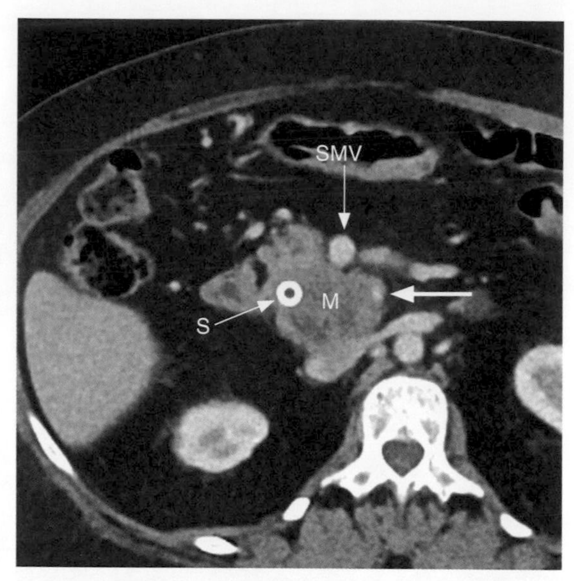

Figure 7.41 Pancreatic ductal adenocarcinoma: CT. A heterogeneous mass (M) can be seen expanding the pancreatic head. This is encasing and compressing the superior mesenteric artery (arrow), indicating unresectability. Note that the superior mesenteric vein (SMV) is not encased. Also note a biliary stent (S).

7.11 INTERVENTIONAL RADIOLOGY OF THE LIVER AND BILIARY TRACT

7.11.1 LIVER BIOPSY

The two broad indications for image-guided liver biopsy are liver mass and diffuse liver disease. Liver biopsy may be performed under CT or US guidance. Core biopsy is usually required, as fine-needle aspiration may not provide sufficient material for diagnosis. Not all liver masses should undergo biopsy:

- Bleeding may complicate biopsy of haemangioma
- Seeding of tumour cells may occur along the needle track following biopsy of HCC

- Most liver masses are characterized with imaging as above and managed surgically or non-surgically without biopsy.

Biopsy of liver masses is restricted to a few specific indications:

- Liver metastases and an unknown primary tumour
- Known extrahepatic primary tumour and a liver mass that cannot be characterized with imaging.

Use of a coaxial needle technique with placement of a Gelfoam plug in the biopsy track may reduce the risk of haemorrhage.

7.11.2 PERCUTANEOUS LIVER TUMOUR ABLATION

Percutaneous tumour ablation may be used to treat HCC or hepatic metastases. US or CT may be used for procedure guidance. A variety of ablation techniques are available under three broad categories:

- Injection of substances that cause cell death, such as ethanol or heated saline
- Thermal:
  - Radiofrequency ablation (RFA)
  - Microwave ablation
  - Cryotherapy
- Non-thermal ablation: irreversible electroporation (IRE).

Post-procedure follow-up imaging with multiphase contrast-enhanced MRI or CT is performed to assess the response to treatment.

7.11.3 TRANSARTERIAL CHEMOEMBOLIZATION

Transarterial chemoembolization (TACE) is used for the treatment of HCC and involves the following:

- Catheter angiography of the liver to outline the arterial anatomy and tumour blood supply
- Superselective microcatheter placement into hepatic artery branches supplying the tumour
- Injection of a chemotherapeutic agent in an emulsion with iodized oil
- Injection of an arterial embolizing agent.

A modification of TACE uses drug-eluting beads (DEB-TACE), which are microspheres of polyvinyl alcohol and a hydrophilic monomer loaded with doxorubicin, a chemotherapeutic agent. The microspheres lodge in the tumour and gradually release the doxorubicin. Regardless of precise technique, TACE induces tumour necrosis through a combination of blockage of the blood supply and localized delivery of a chemotherapeutic agent.

7.11.4 SELECTIVE INTERNAL RADIATION THERAPY

Selective internal radiation therapy (SIRT) is used for the treatment of HCC and inoperable hepatic metastases from colorectal carcinoma. SIRT involves the following:

- Catheter angiography of the liver to outline the arterial anatomy and tumour blood supply
- Superselective microcatheter placement into hepatic artery branches supplying the tumour
- Injection of resin (or glass) microspheres loaded with the β-particle-emitting radioisotope yttrium-90.

SIRT induces tumour necrosis through a combination of blockage of the blood supply and local delivery of radiotherapy (brachytherapy).

7.11.5 NON-SURGICAL MANAGEMENT OF BILE DUCT STONES

Non-surgical management of bile duct stones is normally done via ERCP, with widening of the lower end of the common bile duct (sphincterotomy) and removal of stones via a small wire basket. Occasionally, bile duct stones may be removed via a T-tube tract. This may be done via basket removal or flexible choledochoscope. The T-tube should be *in situ* for at least 4 weeks post surgery to ensure a 'mature' tract that is able to accept wires and catheters. Complications are rare and may include pancreatitis, cholangitis and bile leak.

7.11.6 NON-SURGICAL MANAGEMENT OF MALIGNANT BILIARY OBSTRUCTION

A range of palliative procedures may be used to assist in the management of biliary obstruction caused by malignancies arising from the liver, bile ducts, pancreas and gallbladder. Indications are as follows:

- Symptomatic relief: relief of pruritus, pain or cholangitis
- Non-resectable tumour of the bile ducts, head of pancreas or liver
- Medical risk factors that make surgery unsafe or impossible.

Methods vary with the type of tumour and its location, plus local expertise and preferences:

- Endoscopic: 'from below' for mid- to low biliary obstruction
- Percutaneous: 'from above' for high biliary obstruction or where the second part of the duodenum is inaccessible to endoscopy owing to tumour or prior surgery
- Combined percutaneous–endoscopic.

Internal biliary stents are made of plastic or self-expanding metal and are better accepted by patients as they avoid the potential problems of external biliary drains, such as skin irritation, pain, bile leaks and risk of dislodgement.

7.11.7 PERCUTANEOUS CHOLECYSTOSTOMY

Percutaneous cholecystostomy (drainage of the gallbladder) may be useful in the management of acute cholecystitis when the surgical risks are unacceptable. Using US guidance, the gallbladder is punctured, a wire passed through the needle and a drainage catheter placed in the gallbladder over the wire. Non-resolution of pyrexia within 48 hours may indicate gangrene of the gallbladder, requiring surgery. A cholecystogram is performed once the acute illness has settled, with contrast material injected through the drainage catheter. Stones causing cystic duct obstruction may require surgery; otherwise, the catheter is removed.

7.11.8 TRANSJUGULAR INTRAHEPATIC PORTOSYSTEMIC STENT SHUNT

A major cause of mortality and morbidity in patients with hepatic cirrhosis is haemorrhage from oesophageal varices. The transjugular intrahepatic portosystemic stent shunt (TIPSS) procedure is performed in the setting of portal hypertension for chronic, recurrent variceal haemorrhage not amenable to sclerotherapy. TIPSS is an interventional technique used to form a shunt from the portal system to the systemic venous circulation, thus reducing portal venous pressure. The liver is imaged with Doppler US prior to the procedure to exclude malignancy and confirm the patency of the portal vein.

Complications of TIPSS:

- Procedural complications: intraperitoneal haemorrhage, portal vein thrombosis, shunt occlusion
- Hepatic encephalopathy
- Renal failure
- Pulmonary oedema.

SUMMARY

Clinical presentation	Investigation of choice	Comment
Dysphagia	• Endoscopy where malignancy suspected • Barium swallow for other indications	
Perforation of GIT	AXR	
Small bowel obstruction	• AXR • CT	
Large bowel obstruction	AXR	
Right upper quadrant pain	US	
Right lower quadrant pain	CT	US in children and women of childbearing age
Left lower quadrant pain	CT	US in children and women of childbearing age
Renal colic/flank pain	CT	AXR/KUB if ureteric calculus seen on CT
Acute pancreatitis	CT	US to search for gallstones
Acute mesenteric ischaemia	• CT angiogram • Interventional radiology	
Crohn disease	• Colonoscopy • MR enterography	AXR in acute presentation
Ulcerative colitis	Colonoscopy	AXR in acute presentation
Upper GIT bleeding	Endoscopy	
Lower GIT bleeding	• CT angiogram • Interventional radiology	Treat bleeding with interventional radiology or surgery
Hepatic steatosis	US	
Hepatic cirrhosis	US	Includes US for HCC screening
Hepatic fibrosis	Shear wave elastography	
Liver mass: detection	US	CT or MRI following US
Liver mass: characterization	Multiphase contrast-enhanced imaging: MRI, CT, US	
Jaundice	• US • MRCP	Other imaging/intervention as indicated: ERCP, PTC

Abbreviations: ERCP, endoscopic retrograde cholangiopancreatography; GIT, gastrointestinal tract; HCC, hepatocellular carcinoma; KUB, kidneys, ureters and bladder radiograph; MR, magnetic resonance; MRCP, magnetic resonance cholangiopancreatography; PTC, percutaneous transhepatic cholangiography.

8 Urogenital tract

8.1 IMAGING INVESTIGATION OF THE UROGENITAL TRACT

Ultrasound (US) and computed tomography (CT) are the principal imaging investigations used for assessment of the urinary tract in both males and females. Magnetic resonance imaging (MRI) is used as a problem-solving modality in the characterization of renal and adrenal masses and in the diagnosis and staging of prostatic carcinoma. US, CT and MRI will be discussed extensively throughout this chapter. Other imaging modalities and techniques used in the investigation of urinary tract disease are outlined below. Imaging of gynaecological disease is discussed in Chapter 15.

8.1.1 SCINTIGRAPHY

RENOGRAM (RENAL SCINTIGRAPHY)

Renal scintigraphy with ^{99m}Tc-DTPA or ^{99m}Tc-MAG3 (see Table 1.1) is used to assess renal function and urodynamics, including calculation of the percentage of total renal function contributed by each kidney. Renal scintigraphy is used in renal transplant to assess transplant perfusion and function, diagnose rejection or acute tubular necrosis and detect urinary leak or outflow obstruction.

For other specific indications, modifications to renal scintigraphy may be used as follows:

- Diuresis renogram:
  - Renal scintigraphy with injection of furosemide
  - Indication: differentiation of mechanical urinary tract obstruction from non-obstructive hydronephrosis (Fig. 8.1)
- Angiotensin-converting enzyme (ACE) inhibitor renogram:
  - Renal scintigraphy with injection of captopril
  - Indication: screening test for renal artery stenosis in suspected renovascular hypertension.

RENAL CORTICAL SCINTIGRAPHY

Indications for renal cortical scintigraphy with ^{99m}Tc-DMSA (see Table 1.1):

- Acute pyelonephritis in infants and young children
- Renal scars complicating urinary tract infection in children (see Chapter 16).

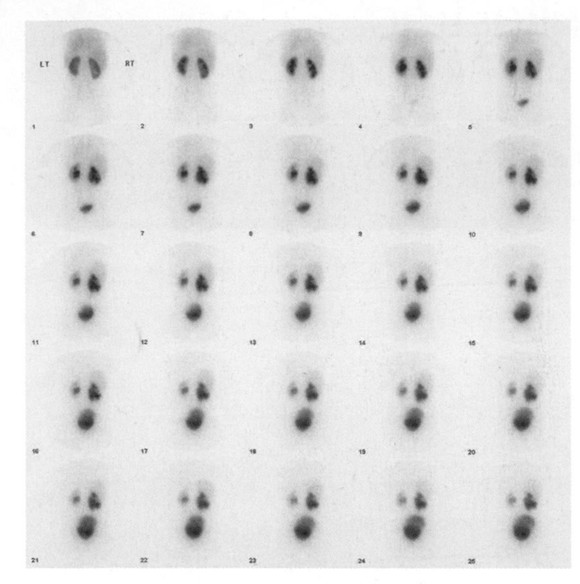

Figure 8.1 Right pelviureteric junction obstruction and hydronephrosis: MAG3 furosemide scan. Sequential series of images taken from 1 to 25 minutes after injection of ^{99m}Tc-MAG3. Normal uptake and excretion of MAG3 by the left kidney. Increased accumulation of MAG3 in the dilated right renal collecting system, indicating mechanical obstruction. Note that the images are acquired posteriorly, so the left kidney is shown on the left of the image unlike most other cross-sectional imaging.

8.1.2 RETROGRADE PYELOGRAM

Retrograde pyelogram (RPG) is usually performed in the operating theatre, in conjunction with formal cystoscopy. At cystoscopy, the ureteric orifice is identified and a catheter passed into the ureter. Contrast material is then injected via this catheter to outline the collecting system and ureter. Indications for RPG:

- Further definition of upper renal tract lesions identified by other imaging studies such as CT
- Haematuria where other imaging studies are normal or equivocal
- Guide for various interventional procedures, including removal of ureteric calculus and ureteric stent placement.

8.1.3 ASCENDING URETHROGRAM

For an ascending urethrogram, a small catheter is passed into the distal urethra and contrast material injected. Radiographs are obtained in the oblique projection to show the urethra in profile. Indications for an ascending urethrogram:

- In the setting of trauma prior to urethral catheterization in a male patient with an anterior pelvic fracture or dislocation, or with blood at the urethral meatus (see Chapter 12)
- Suspected urethral stricture, which may be the result of previous trauma or inflammation.

8.1.4 MICTURATING CYSTOURETHROGRAM

A micturating cystourethrogram (MCU) is also known as a voiding cystourethrogram (VCU). For MCU, the bladder is filled with contrast material via a urethral catheter. Images of the contrast-filled bladder are obtained. The catheter is then removed and radiographs are taken during micturition. Indications for MCU:

- Assessment of urinary tract infection in children (see Chapter 16)
- Following radical prostatectomy to check the surgical anastomosis and the integrity of the bladder base
- Assess posterior urethral problems in male adults
- Stress incontinence in female adults.

8.2 PAINLESS HAEMATURIA

Painless haematuria may be classified clinically as macroscopic or microscopic. Initial clinical tests in patients with haematuria consist of urine culture to exclude infection, examination of urine for protein and red cell casts and measurement of blood pressure.

Over 70% of cases of haematuria have no demonstrable cause. Demonstrable causes of haematuria include:

- Urinary tract infection
- Urinary calculi
- Tumour of the urinary tract
- Trauma
- Glomerulonephritis
- Bleeding diathesis.

Other clinical symptoms and signs such as acute flank pain and fever usually accompany haematuria caused by urinary tract infection and ureteric calculi. Glomerulonephritis is suspected when haematuria is accompanied by heavy proteinuria and red cell casts. Glomerulonephritis is confirmed with renal biopsy, which is best performed with imaging guidance, usually US. Patients with glomerulonephritis should have a chest radiograph (chest X-ray, CXR) to exclude cardiomegaly and pulmonary oedema, plus a renal US to screen for underlying renal morphological abnormalities.

In the absence of compelling evidence of urinary tract infection or glomerulonephritis, painless haematuria should be assumed to be due to urinary tract tumour until proved otherwise. The imaging work-up of patients with painless haematuria is therefore directed at excluding or diagnosing renal cell carcinoma (RCC) and urothelial carcinoma (transitional cell carcinoma [TCC]). Urothelial carcinoma may occasionally produce a central renal mass, although most tumours occur in the bladder. Less commonly, a small tumour arises in the renal collecting system or ureter. Multifocal tumours are common. Large or advanced bladder tumours may invade beyond the bladder wall and cause hydronephrosis owing to obstruction of the distal ureters (Fig. 8.2). It follows from the above that the imaging evaluation of painless haematuria requires assessment of the renal parenchyma to exclude a renal mass plus visualization of the urothelium. This includes imaging of the collecting system, renal pelvis, ureters and bladder.

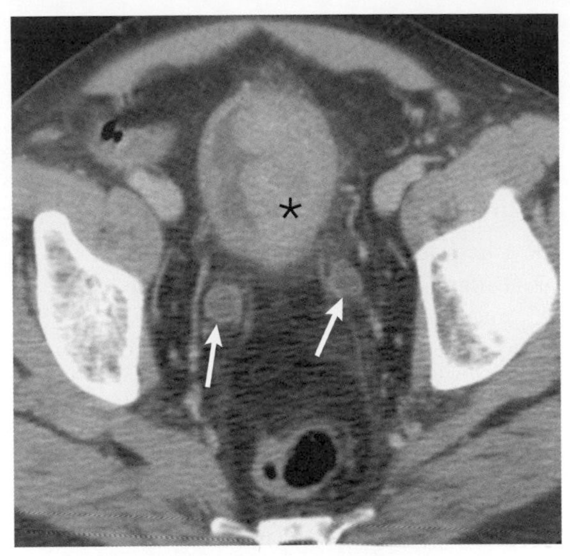

Figure 8.2 Urothelial tumour of the bladder: CT. Non-contrast-enhanced CT shows a large soft-tissue mass arising from the bladder (*). The tumour is obstructing the vesicoureteric junctions and causing obstruction and dilatation of the distal ureters (arrows).

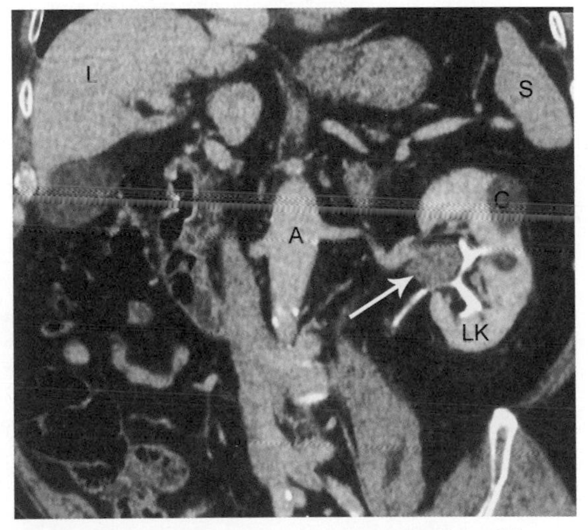

Figure 8.3 Urothelial tumour of the renal pelvis: CT urography. Urothelial tumour of the left kidney (LK) seen as a central mass (arrow) in the renal pelvis on a coronal CT image. Also note the aorta (A), left renal cyst (C), liver (L), spleen (S).

8.2.1 COMPUTED TOMOGRAPHY UROGRAPHY

CT urography is the investigation of choice for painless haematuria. CT urography is a term used to describe a contrast-enhanced CT technique designed to provide excellent delineation of the renal collecting systems, ureters and bladder, as well as cross-sectional images of the kidneys and adjacent structures. Although the precise method may vary, CT urography usually consists of a multiphase examination, including scans performed with sufficient delay after contrast material injection to allow opacification of the collecting systems and ureters (Fig. 8.3).

8.2.2 CYSTOSCOPY

Cystoscopy accompanied by ureteroscopy is the gold standard investigation for tumours of the lower urinary tract. Retrograde pyelography may also be performed at the time of cystoscopy when an upper urinary tract tumour is suspected.

8.2.3 ULTRASOUND

US of the urinary tract may supplement CT urography in selected cases. Indications for US include:

- Characterization of complex cysts
- Differentiation of complex cysts from solid masses.

Limitations of US in this context include:

- Incomplete visualization of the kidneys because of obesity or intestinal gas
- Non-visualization of non-dilated ureters
- Inability to visualize small urothelial tumours.

8.3 RENAL MASS

The goals of imaging a suspected renal mass include:

- Confirmation of the presence and site of a mass
- Classification into simple cyst, complicated cyst or solid mass
- Assessment of lesion contents, such as the presence of fat or calcification
- Differentiation of benign from malignant lesions
- Diagnosis of complications such as local invasion, venous invasion, lymphadenopathy and metastases.

Renal masses in children, including hydronephrosis, multicystic dysplastic kidney and nephroblastoma (Wilms tumour), are discussed in Chapter 16.

8.3.1 CLASSIFICATION OF RENAL MASSES

Renal masses may be classified with imaging into simple cysts, complex cysts and solid masses. Simple renal cysts are extremely common in adults. They are usually small and asymptomatic and are discovered incidentally on CT or US examinations of the abdomen. Occasionally, very large cysts may present with abdominal pain or a palpable abdominal mass. Simple cysts have thin walls and clear fluid contents.

A small percentage of benign cysts have more complex features and are classified as complex cysts. The causes of a complex cyst include a simple cyst complicated by haemorrhage or infection, a benign cyst containing septations or calcifications or a cystic tumour (Table 8.1).

Table 8.1 Bosniak classification of renal cysts.

Bosniak classification	CT features	Diagnosis	Malignant potential (%)	Management
I	• Thin wall • Low density • Non-enhancing	Simple cyst	0	No follow-up
II	• <3 cm • High density • Thin septations • Fine calcification	Benign, minimally complex cyst	0	No follow-up
IIF	• >3 cm with the same features as type 2 • Nodular calcification	Minimally complex cyst	5	Follow-up CT/MRI
III	• Thickened wall • Thickened smooth or irregular septations	Indeterminate cystic mass	55	Partial nephrectomy or RF ablation
IV	As for Bosniak III plus enhancing soft-tissue component	Malignant	100	• Staging • Partial or total nephrectomy

Abbreviation: RF, radiofrequency.

Most solid renal masses are malignant and RCC is the most common type. RCC may present clinically with haematuria or flank pain, and less commonly with pathological fracture or bone pain as a result of a skeletal metastasis. In many cases, RCC and other renal masses or cysts are found incidentally on US and CT examinations performed for other reasons. Over 60% of RCCs are diagnosed incidentally. Uncommonly, urothelial carcinoma may produce a mass centred in the collecting system and extending into the renal parenchyma. Other types of renal malignancy that may produce solid renal masses are lymphoma and metastases.

Angiomyolipoma (AML) is the commonest cause of a benign solid renal mass in adults. Eighty per cent of AMLs occur sporadically and are usually small and asymptomatic. Twenty per cent of AMLs occur in association with tuberous sclerosis. Rarely, large AMLs may present as a palpable abdominal mass or may be complicated by haemorrhage, causing acute abdomen and haematuria. AMLs contain fat, giving them a characteristic appearance on US and CT. Visible fat in a renal mass usually, but not always, implies a benign aetiology.

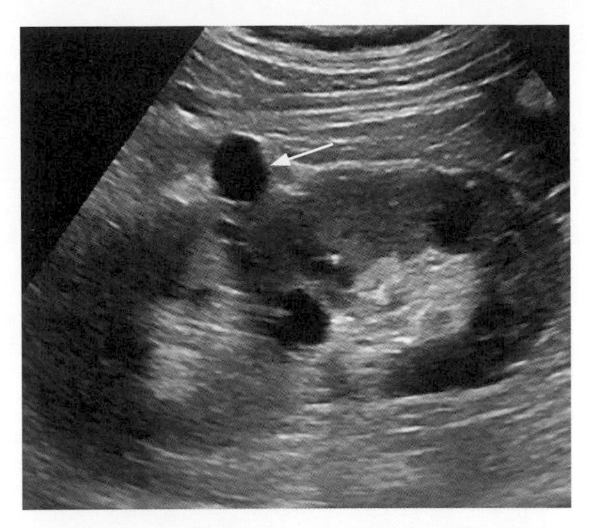

Figure 8.4 Simple renal cyst: US. Note the US features of a simple cyst (arrow): anechoic contents, smooth thin wall and no soft-tissue components.

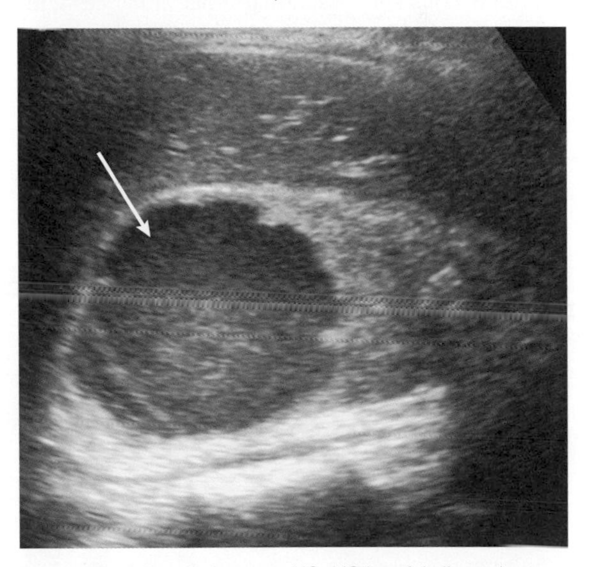

Figure 8.5 Renal abscess: US. US in a febrile patient with severe right flank pain shows a fluid collection in the upper pole of the right kidney (arrow). Note the echogenic fluid contents and the irregular wall, indicating a complex cystic lesion. US-guided aspiration confirmed the diagnosis of an abscess.

8.3.2 IMAGING OF RENAL MASSES

ULTRASOUND

US is the initial investigation of choice for the diagnosis of a suspected renal mass, followed by CT. US will accurately characterize a renal mass as a simple cyst, complex cyst or a solid mass. A simple cyst appears on US as a round anechoic (black) structure with a thin or invisible wall (Fig. 8.4). No further imaging is required for simple renal cysts diagnosed with US.

The term 'complex cyst' refers to a cyst with internal echoes that may be due to haemorrhage or infection, soft-tissue septations, calcifications or an associated soft-tissue mass (Fig. 8.5). A solid mass on US may show areas of increased echogenicity owing to calcification or fat or areas of decreased echogenicity owing to necrosis. Where RCC is suspected, US is also used to look for specific findings, such as invasion of the renal vein and inferior vena cava (IVC), lymphadenopathy and metastases in the liver and contralateral kidney. Complex cysts or solid renal masses found with US usually require further assessment with CT or MRI.

US may also be used as a guide for various procedures, including:

- Biopsy of solid lesions or complicated cysts

- Cyst aspiration for diagnostic and therapeutic purposes
- Cyst ablation by injection of ethanol
- Radiofrequency (RF) ablation of small tumours.

COMPUTED TOMOGRAPHY

Contrast-enhanced CT is used for further characterization of a solid lesion or complex cyst found on US. CT is more accurate than US for the characterization of the internal contents of a mass, particularly to show areas of fat to confirm the diagnosis of AML (Fig. 8.6). Based on CT appearances, cystic renal lesions may be classified according to the Bosniak system, last revised in 2019 (Table 8.1) (Figs 8.7 and 8.8).

The most common CT appearance of RCC is a heterogeneous soft-tissue mass that enhances with intravenous contrast material (Fig. 8.9). CT is also used for staging of RCC. Factors relevant to staging of RCC include the size of the tumour, invasion of local structures such as the adrenal gland, vascular invasion of the renal vein or IVC, lymphadenopathy and metastases in the liver and skeleton.

Further details of the tumour–node–metastasis (TNM) staging of RCC may be found on the companion website.

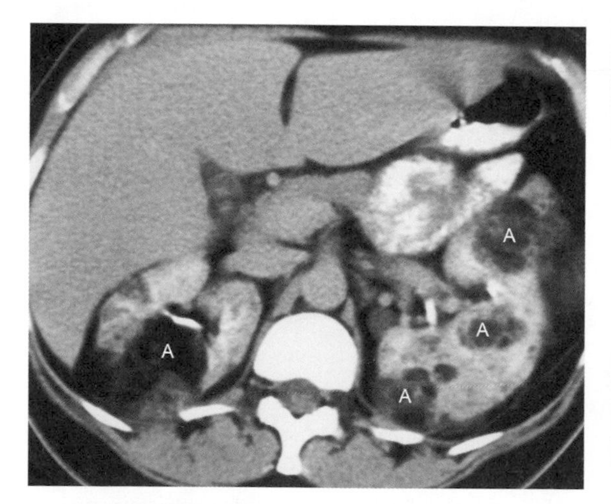

Figure 8.6 Angiomyolipoma: CT. Multiple angiomyolipomas (A) arising on both kidneys in a woman with tuberous sclerosis. Note the typical low-attenuation fat content well shown on CT.

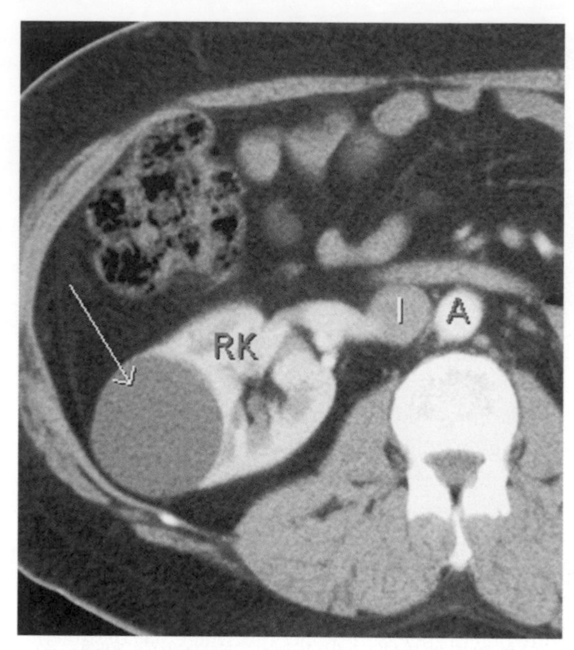

Figure 8.7 Simple renal cyst: CT. Note the CT features of a simple cyst (arrow) arising on the right kidney (RK): homogeneous low-attenuation contents, thin wall and sharp demarcation from the adjacent renal parenchyma. Also note inferior vena cava (I), aorta (A).

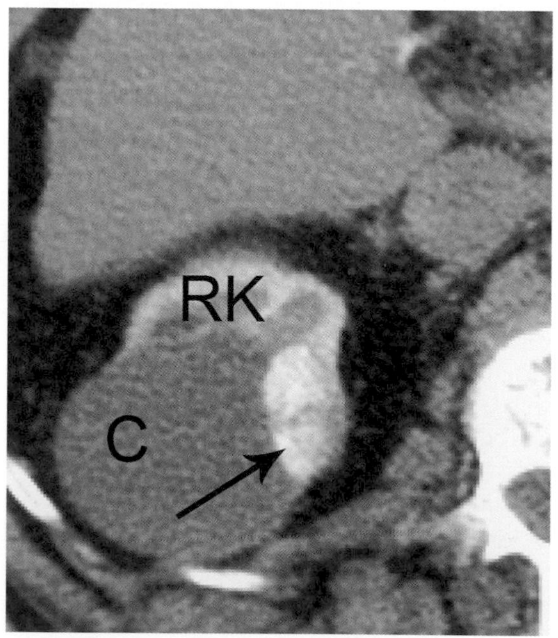

Figure 8.8 Renal cell carcinoma (RCC) arising in a cyst: CT. A cyst (C) arising on the right kidney (RK) contains a soft-tissue mural mass that enhances with intravenous contrast (arrow). This is the typical appearance of a Bosniak type IV cyst and indicates malignancy.

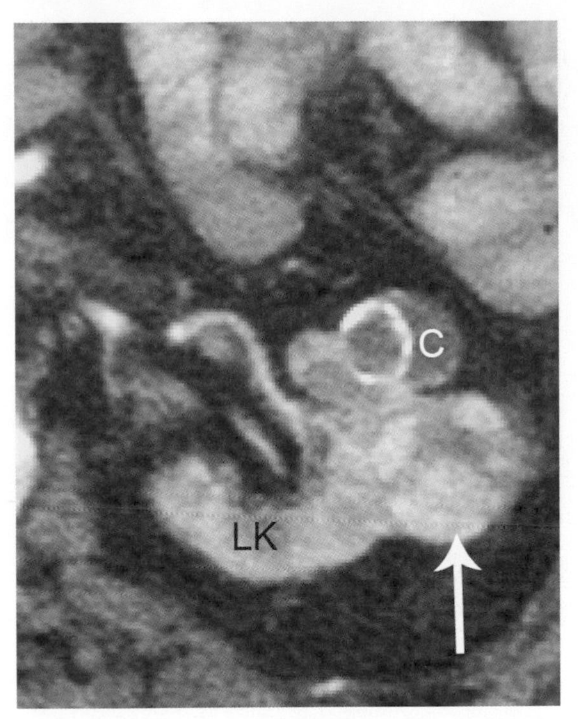

Figure 8.9 Renal cell carcinoma (RCC): CT. RCC seen as a small mass (arrow) arising on the left kidney (LK). Also note the presence of an adjacent partly calcified cyst (C).

MAGNETIC RESONANCE IMAGING

In many centres, MRI is used in preference to CT for the investigation and characterization of renal masses. MRI generally provides similar information to CT in the detection of specific features such as fat contents, septations and soft-tissue masses, as well as staging of renal cysts and tumours.

BIOPSY

Biopsy of renal masses is not commonly performed, as tumour seeding may occur and histological interpretation is often difficult. The most common indication for renal mass biopsy is for management of a small mass (<3 cm), where a positive biopsy result would indicate a non-operative approach.

Other indications for biopsy of a renal mass include:

- High suspicion for lymphoma
- Known or previous primary carcinoma elsewhere, especially lung, breast or stomach.

8.4 IMAGING IN PROSTATISM

The prostate gland consists of three zones. The peripheral zone (PZ) occupies the posterior prostate from apex to base. It is replaced anteriorly by the fibromuscular stroma (AFMS). Most prostatic cancer occurs in the PZ. The central zone is a small region posterior to the prostatic urethra and contains the ejaculatory ducts. The transition zone lies anterolateral to the prostatic urethra. It is small in young males but is the site of benign prostatic hyperplasia (BPH) in older men. The term 'central gland', used by some urologists, refers to the combined central and transition zones.

8.4.1 BENIGN PROSTATIC HYPERPLASIA

Prostatism refers to obstructive voiding symptoms due to prostatic enlargement. BPH with enlargement of the transition zone of the prostate is the commonest cause of symptomatic prostatic enlargement. Symptoms of prostatism include frequency, nocturia, poor stream, hesitancy and post-void fullness. The primary imaging investigation in the assessment of prostatism is urinary tract US (US of the kidneys, ureters and bladder [KUB]), which provides accurate assessment of the prostate, bladder and upper urinary tracts. Prostate dimensions are measured, and the approximate prostate volume is calculated by a simple formula: height × width × length × 0.5 (Fig. 8.10). The bladder is assessed for morphological changes indicating bladder obstruction, including bladder wall thickening and trabeculation, bladder wall diverticulum and bladder calculi. Bladder volume is measured before and after micturition. The kidneys are examined for hydronephrosis, asymptomatic congenital anomalies and tumours and renal calculi.

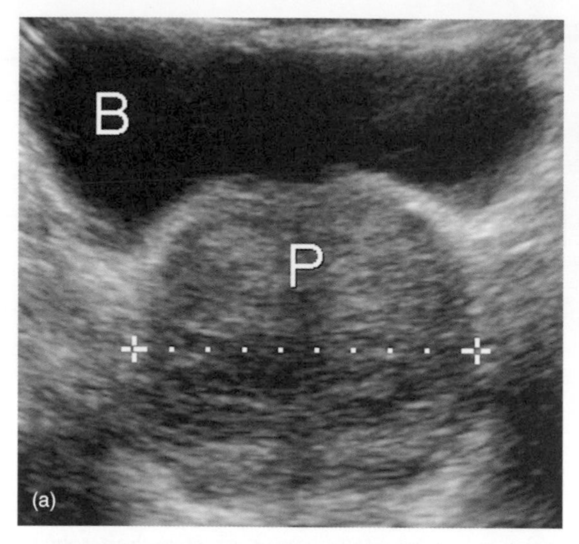

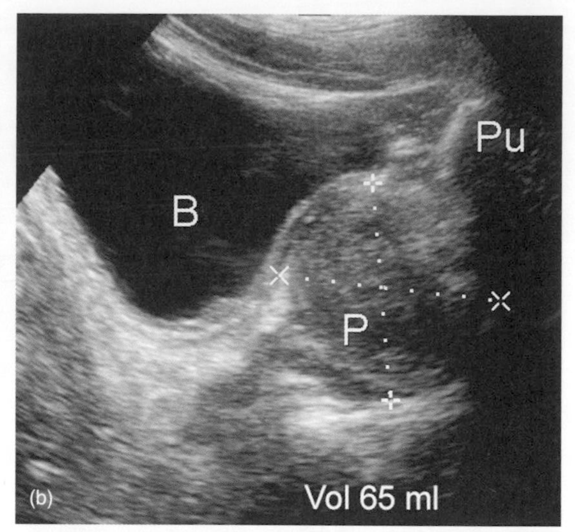

Figure 8.10 Prostate volume measurement: US. (a) Transverse plane. (b) Longitudinal plane. Note prostate (P), bladder (B), pubic bone (Pu).

8.5 ADENOCARCINOMA OF THE PROSTATE

8.5.1 DIAGNOSIS AND STAGING OF ADENOCARCINOMA OF THE PROSTATE

Prostate adenocarcinoma is the second most common cancer in males, its incidence increasing steadily with age. Outside screening, it may be diagnosed in several ways:

- Urinary tract symptoms, e.g. haematuria, obstructive voiding symptoms
- Histological examination of tissue 'chips' obtained by transurethral resection of the prostate (TURP) for presumed BPH
- Bone metastases may be the initial finding owing to a specific presentation such as bone pain or spinal cord compression
- Multiple sclerotic metastases are occasionally picked up as an incidental finding on a radiograph or CT performed for unrelated reasons, e.g. pre-anaesthetic CXR or CT for abdominal pain.

Most prostate carcinomas are diagnosed through screening. Screening methods include digital rectal examination (DRE) and prostate-specific antigen (PSA) blood assay. The issues with PSA screening include:

- PSA is non-specific and may be elevated in BPH and chronic prostatitis, as well as in prostatic carcinoma
- PSA is unable to differentiate low-risk tumours that may remain small and confined to the prostate from those that may cause local invasion and metastases.

An increasing PSA level in an individual patient is considered more significant than a single reading. If either DRE or PSA is abnormal, further assessment is recommended. In the past, this consisted of systematic transrectal or transperineal US-guided biopsies, targeting the PZ of the prostate. The problems with this approach include:

- Significant false-negative rate
- Overdiagnosis of clinically insignificant low-risk cancers
- Complications, most notably septicaemia, with a high incidence of antibiotic-resistant strains of *Escherichia coli*.

The staging of established prostate cancer incorporates TNM and other factors:

- T: local disease including extension beyond the prostate and invasion of seminal vesicles and other local structures
- N: regional lymph nodes (internal iliac and obturator)
- M: metastatic spread, most commonly to the skeleton and distant lymph nodes in the pelvis and abdomen
- PSA level
- Gleason score.

The Gleason score is a histology-based grading system. Neoplastic changes are graded from 1 to 5. Two grades are given: one for the most prevalent and one for the second most prevalent pattern in a biopsy sample. These grades are added to provide a Gleason score from 6 (3 + 3) to 10. Clinically significant disease is defined as a Gleason score greater than 6 and either a tumour size of 0.5 mL or higher or extraprostatic extension. TNM staging may be achieved by conventional imaging with single photon emission CT (SPECT)-CT, providing a combination of CT of the chest and abdomen and scintigraphic bone scan. Further details of staging of prostate adenocarcinoma may be found on the companion website.

Depending on staging, including the Gleason score, therapy may be curative (surgery or radiotherapy), palliative (antiandrogen therapy, chemotherapy) or consist of active surveillance in low-risk disease. Recurrence may occur following curative therapy. PSA levels should drop to zero following surgery and to a low-level nadir after radiotherapy. A PSA level of more than 0.2 ng/mL following surgery or more than 2 ng/mL above the nadir following radiotherapy with negative imaging is termed biochemical recurrence. This may be treated with androgen deprivation therapy. Cancer refractory to this treatment is termed castration-resistant prostate cancer (CRPC). Differentiation of localized or non-metastatic (nmCRPC) from distant or metastatic (mCRPC) disease may direct further therapy and determine the prognosis.

Currently, two imaging techniques – multiparametric MRI and prostate-specific membrane antigen (PSMA)–positron emission tomography (PET) – are radically changing the approach to diagnosis, staging and management of prostate cancer.

8.5.2 MULTIPARAMETRIC MAGNETIC RESONANCE IMAGING

Multiparametric MRI of the prostate consists of three sequences: (i) T2-weighted imaging, (ii) diffusion-weighted imaging (DWI) with apparent diffusion coefficient (ADC), and (iii) dynamic contrast-enhanced (DCE) imaging. Adenocarcinoma shows as a low-signal lesion on T2-weighted images, with diffusion restriction and a low ADC (Fig. 8.11). On DCE, owing to tumour neovascularity, there is rapid early enhancement with subsequent washout. Multiparametric MRI is reported using the Prostate Imaging Reporting and Data System, version 2.1 (PI-RADS v.2.1), which was last modified in 2019. Based on appearances on T2, DWI and ADC images, PI-RADS assigns a numerical scale from 1 to 5:

- PI-RADS 1: clinically significant cancer is highly unlikely to be present
- PI-RADS 2: clinically significant cancer is unlikely to be present
- PI-RADS 3: the presence of clinically significant cancer is equivocal
- PI-RADS 4: clinically significant cancer is likely to be present
- PI-RADS 5: clinically significant cancer is highly likely to be present.

Positive DCE imaging increases the equivocal score of PI-RADS 3 to PI-RADS 4. For further details on PI-RADS, see the companion website.

Multiparametric MRI has multiple established and evolving roles in prostate cancer imaging:

- Further assessment following negative biopsy when disease is clinically suspected
- Exclusion of clinically significant disease, thereby reducing the number of unnecessary biopsies
- Diagnosis and localization of clinically significant disease
- Targeted biopsy guidance
  - Cognitive guidance: operator targets US-guided biopsy based on a review of the magnetic resonance (MR) images

- Fusion biopsy in which software overlays MR images on real-time US
- Biopsy while in the MR machine using a specifically designed needle guidance system
- Staging: accurate visualization of the prostatic zonal anatomy as well as adjacent structures, including the neurovascular bundle and seminal vesicles
- Active surveillance for low-risk disease
- Follow-up post therapy
  - Exclude recurrent disease
  - Assess extent of biochemical recurrence.

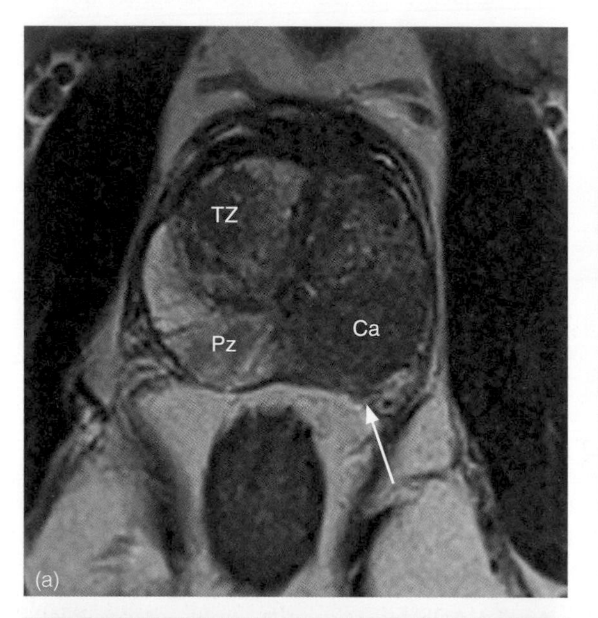

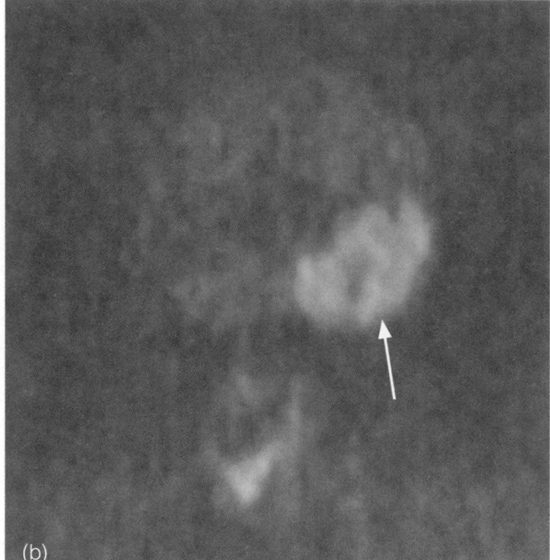

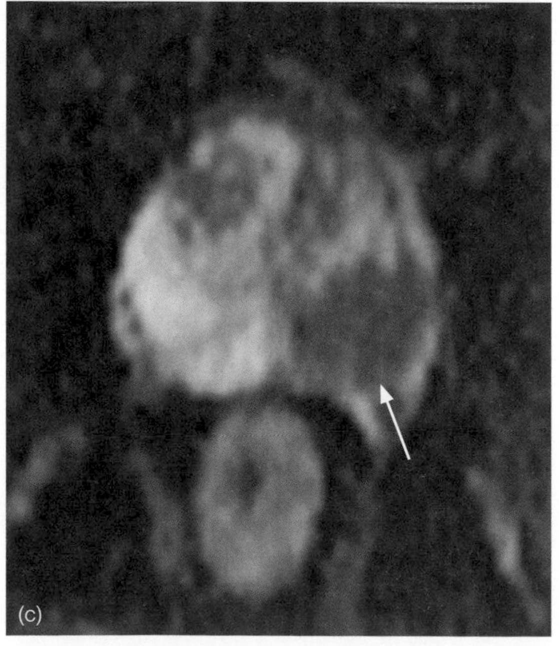

Figure 8.11 Prostate cancer (PI-RADS 5): multiparametric MRI. (a) Transverse T2-weighted image shows the typical appearance of a prostate adenocarcinoma with a large discrete region of low signal in the left peripheral zone (Ca). This shows a small extension through the prostatic capsule (arrow). Also note the normal high-signal within the right peripheral zone (PZ) and the slightly heterogeneous appearance of the transitional zones (TZ), in keeping with mild benign prostatic hyperplasia (BPH). (b) Diffusion-weighted imaging (DWI) shows high signal, indicating diffusion restriction corresponding to the lesion seen on T2 (arrow). (c) Apparent diffusion coefficient (ADC) map shows reduced signal, indicating low ADC values in the left peripheral zone lesion (arrow).

8.5.3 PROSTATE-SPECIFIC MEMBRANE ANTIGEN–POSITRON EMISSION TOMOGRAPHY

PSMA is a membrane glycoprotein expressed by normal prostate tissue, with levels up to 1000 times higher in prostate cancer. PET imaging can be performed with PSMA-targeted radiopharmaceuticals. ^{68}Ga-PSMA-PET has been found to have a high detection rate for prostate tumours and to be highly sensitive for nodal and distant metastases (Fig. 8.12).

Established and evolving roles for PSMA-PET in prostate cancer imaging include:

- Localization of tumour within the prostate, which may be complementary to multiparametric MRI
- Staging
- Localization of biochemical recurrence not visible on other imaging
- Differentiation of nmCRPC from mCRPC.

As an example of the emerging field of theranostics, PSMA molecules can be linked to a therapeutic radionuclide such as β-emitting lutetium-177 (^{177}Lu) or α-emitting actinium-225 (^{225}Ac). These combined imaging and therapeutic radiopharmaceuticals may have a role in the therapy of metastatic CRPC.

8.6 INVESTIGATION OF A SCROTAL MASS

US with colour Doppler is the first investigation of choice for a scrotal mass. The primary role of US is to differentiate intratesticular from extratesticular masses; in most cases, this is sufficient to distinguish malignant and benign lesions.

8.6.1 INTRATESTICULAR MASSES

Most (over 90%) intratesticular masses are malignant. The exceptions include testicular abscess, tuberculosis (TB), sarcoidosis and benign tumours such as Sertoli–Leydig tumours. Most intratesticular tumours are hypoechoic on US. Seminoma is seen as a localized hypoechoic mass outlined by surrounding hyperechoic testicular tissue (Fig. 8.13).

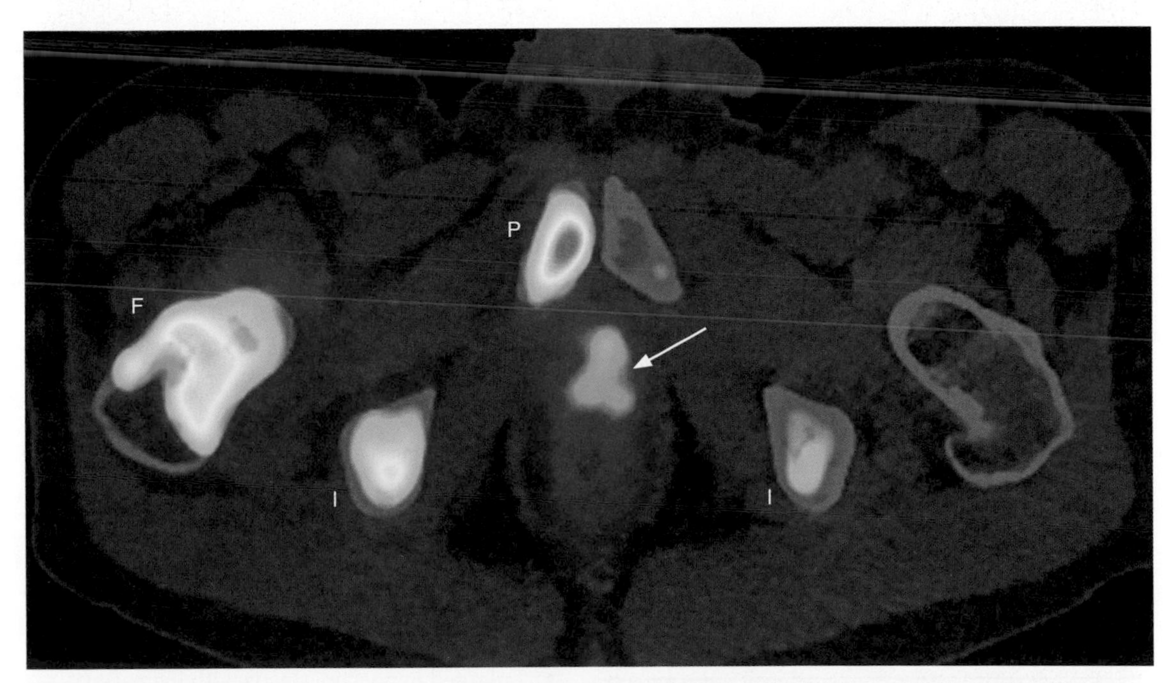

Figure 8.12 Prostate cancer: prostate-specific membrane antigen (PSMA) PET-CT. Intense PSMA avidity in the prostate gland consistent with a primary prostatic malignancy (arrow). Several intensely PSMA-avid bone metastases in the right pubic bone (P), bilateral ischial tuberosities (I) and right proximal femur (F).

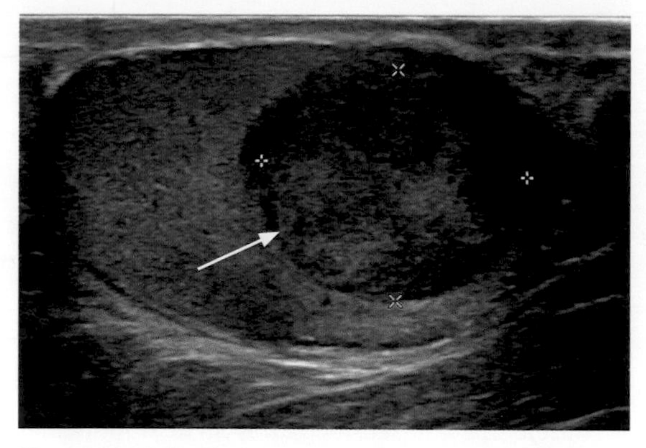

Figure 8.13 Testicular cancer: US. Round hypoechoic mass representing a seminoma in the lower pole of the testicle (arrow).

Occasionally, with a large seminoma the entire testicle is replaced by abnormal hypoechoic tissue. Other tumour types such as choriocarcinoma, embryonal cell carcinoma, teratoma and mixed tumours usually show a heterogeneous echotexture. Lymphoma of the testis is hypoechoic and homogeneous and may be focal or diffuse.

Staging of testicular tumour incorporates four factors:

1. T: local growth within the testes and invasion of adjacent structures, including spermatic cord and scrotal skin
2. N: spread to regional lymph nodes, including abdominal retroperitoneum
3. M: metastasis to distant lymph nodes or other organs, e.g. lung and brain
4. S: serum tumour marker levels:
   - Lactate dehydrogenase (LDH)
   - Human chorionic gonadotropin (HCG)
   - Alpha-fetoprotein (AFP).

Imaging for the staging of testicular tumours consists of scrotal US, abdomen CT for retroperitoneal lymphadenopathy and chest CT for mediastinal lymphadenopathy and pulmonary metastases. Further details of TNMS staging of testicular cancer may be found on the companion website.

8.6.2 EXTRATESTICULAR MASSES

Most (90%) extratesticular lesions are benign. The most encountered extratesticular masses are hydrocele, varicocele and epididymal cyst. Hydrocele is seen on US as anechoic fluid surrounding the testicle. Hydrocele may be congenital, idiopathic or secondary to inflammation, torsion, trauma or tumour. An epididymal cyst is a common incidental finding on scrotal US or may occasionally be large enough to present as a palpable mass. An epididymal cyst appears on US as a well-defined anechoic simple cyst in the head of the epididymis, i.e. posterolaterally at the superior pole of the testis.

Varicocele consists of dilated veins of the pampiniform plexus, producing a tortuous nest of veins seen well on US. The vascular nature of the mass is confirmed with colour Doppler. Most varicoceles occur on the left and present with a clinically obvious mass or with infertility. Small asymptomatic varicoceles are common incidental findings on scrotal US. Primary varicoceles are caused by venous incompetence and are the most common form. Secondary varicoceles are due to testicular vein compression such as by retroperitoneal lymphadenopathy. Large varicoceles associated with infertility or discomfort may be amenable to therapeutic embolization of the testicular vein.

8.7 ACUTE SCROTUM

An acute scrotum is usually unilateral and is defined as sudden, painful scrotal swelling. The main differential diagnosis in this situation is torsion versus acute epididymo-orchitis. Common causes of acute epididymo-orchitis are bacterial infection and mumps. Conditions other than testicular torsion that may mimic acute epididymo-orchitis include:

- Scrotal haematoma, which is usually related to trauma
- Torsion of testicular appendages
- Strangulated hernia
- Haemorrhage into a testicular tumour.

US signs of acute epididymo-orchitis:

- Enlarged hypoechoic epididymis with increased blood flow
- Enlarged hypoechoic testis with increased blood flow
- Surrounding fluid/hydrocele.

The need for early surgical exploration in suspected torsion gives imaging a role only in doubtful cases and where it is quickly available. When imaging is required, US with colour Doppler is the investigation of choice. US is quick, non-invasive and highly accurate at differentiating torsion from inflammation.

US signs of testicular torsion:

- Decreased spermatic cord Doppler signal and lack of blood flow in the testis
- Twisting of the spermatic cord (whirlpool sign)
- Testis may be normal in appearance or enlarged and hypoechoic.

Torsion may be an intermittent phenomenon and is therefore not excluded by a normal scrotal US.

8.8 ADRENAL IMAGING

The adrenal gland is essentially made up of two separate organs: the adrenal cortex and the adrenal medulla:

- Adrenal cortex: endocrine gland composed of fat-rich cells
  - Secretes cortisol, aldosterone and androgenic steroids
- Adrenal medulla: develops from the neural crest
  - Secretes adrenaline and noradrenaline.

Indications for imaging of the adrenal glands include:

- Endocrine syndromes
  - Cushing syndrome
  - Hyperaldosteronism
- Suspected phaeochromocytoma
- Incidentally discovered adrenal mass.

CT and MRI are both excellent modalities for imaging of the adrenal glands. Scintigraphy may occasionally be useful for specific indications. More specialized techniques, such as adrenal vein sampling and percutaneous biopsy, rarely may be required.

8.8.1 ADRENAL ENDOCRINE SYNDROMES

CUSHING SYNDROME

A common cause of Cushing syndrome is exogenous steroid therapy for chronic inflammatory conditions, such as polymyalgia rheumatica.

Non-iatrogenic causes of Cushing syndrome:

- Excessive adrenocorticotropic hormone (ACTH) production (70%) (Cushing disease)
  - Usually due to pituitary adenoma
- Ectopic ACTH production by tumours (10%)
  - Bronchial carcinoid, thymoma, islet cell tumour
- Adrenal disease (20%).

Adrenal causes of Cushing syndrome may be further classified as follows:

- Bilateral adrenal hyperplasia (70%)
- Unilateral adrenocortical adenoma (20%)
- Adrenal carcinoma (10%).

Biochemical assessment of the patient with Cushing syndrome includes measurement of serum ACTH and 24-hour cortisol levels. Elevated ACTH indicates excessive pituitary or ectopic production; low or undetectable levels of ACTH indicate adrenal disease. Imaging investigation of Cushing syndrome guided by biochemical testing is therefore as follows:

- Suspected pituitary source of ACTH: MRI of the pituitary gland
- Suspected ectopic source of ACTH: CT of the chest and abdomen
- Suspected adrenal disease: CT/MRI of the adrenal glands.

PRIMARY HYPERALDOSTERONISM (CONN SYNDROME)

Primary hyperaldosteronism is thought to be responsible for up to 10% of cases of hypertension. The diagnosis of primary hyperaldosteronism is established biochemically with measurement of the plasma aldosterone concentration to plasma renin activity ratio (PAC/PRA). The causes of primary hyperaldosteronism (Conn syndrome) include:

- Solitary unilateral adrenal adenoma (70%)
- Multiple adrenal adenomas (20%)
- Bilateral adrenal hyperplasia (10%)
- Adrenal carcinoma (rare).

CT or MRI of the adrenal glands is the initial investigation of choice. When bilateral adrenal disease is seen, or when CT/MRI is normal, bilateral selective adrenal vein sampling for aldosterone levels may be helpful to localize a small abnormality and therefore guide management.

PRIMARY ADRENAL INSUFFICIENCY (ADDISON DISEASE)

The causes of primary adrenal insufficiency (Addison disease) include:

- Idiopathic adrenal atrophy
  - Most common cause
  - Probable autoimmune aetiology
- Granulomatous disease
  - TB
  - Sarcoidosis
- Bilateral adrenal haemorrhage:
  - Birth trauma, hypoxia or sepsis in neonates
  - Anticoagulation therapy or sepsis in adults.

CT or MRI of the adrenal glands is the investigation of choice.

8.8.2 PHAEOCHROMOCYTOMA

Phaeochromocytoma is a tumour arising from chromaffin cells of the adrenal medulla; 90% occur in the adrenal gland and 10% in ectopic extra-adrenal locations. Most ectopic locations are within the abdomen along the sympathetic chain. Phaeochromocytoma usually presents with symptomatology related to excess catecholamine production:

- Paroxysmal or sustained hypertension
- Headaches, sweating, flushing
- Nausea and vomiting
- Abdominal pain.

Urine analysis reveals elevated levels of vanillylmandelic acid (VMA).

Phaeochromocytoma may also be discovered as a result of a hypertensive crisis brought on by surgery or some other stress; 10% arise as part of a syndrome, e.g. multiple endocrine neoplasia (MEN) IIa and IIb, familial phaeochromocytoma, tuberous sclerosis, von Hippel–Lindau disease and neurofibromatosis; 10% are malignant. Phaeochromocytomas are usually large tumours, measuring up to 12 cm in diameter with an average of around 5 cm.

CT of the abdomen, with particular attention to the adrenal glands, is the initial imaging investigation of choice in the diagnosis of phaeochromocytoma. When the adrenal glands are normal on CT and no obvious mass is seen elsewhere, PET-CT with a somatostatin analogue (tetraazacyclododecane–tetraacetic acid and tyrosine-3-octreotate [^{68}Ga-DOTATATE]) or whole-body scintigraphy with iodine-labelled metaiodobenzylguanidine (^{131}I-/^{123}I-MIBG) (see Table 1.1) may be useful.

8.8.3 THE INCIDENTALLY DISCOVERED ADRENAL MASS

Benign adrenal adenomas occur in 1–2% of the population. Incidental adrenal masses are a common finding on CT of the abdomen and may be informally termed adrenal 'incidentalomas'. Patients with an incidentally discovered adrenal mass should be assessed for clinical evidence of Cushing syndrome and hypertension; depending on the clinical findings, biochemical screening for Cushing syndrome, hyperaldosteronism or phaeochromocytoma may be indicated.

Adrenal mass is a particularly significant finding when there is a history of malignancy. Tumours with a high incidence of metastasis to the adrenal glands include melanoma, lung, breast, renal, gastrointestinal tract and lymphoma. Fifty per cent of adrenal masses seen in patients with primary carcinoma elsewhere are benign adenomas, not metastases. It is important to differentiate benign from malignant masses, specifically adrenal adenoma from adrenal metastasis or carcinoma.

CT features of a benign adrenal adenoma (Fig. 8.14) include:

- Small size (<3 cm)
- Smooth contour
- Low density on unenhanced scans because of the high fat content of normal adrenal cells.

CT features of adrenal carcinoma include:

- Relatively large size (>5 cm)
- Higher density on unenhanced scans with low density centrally due to necrosis
- Other evidence of malignancy, such as liver metastases, lymphadenopathy, venous invasion.

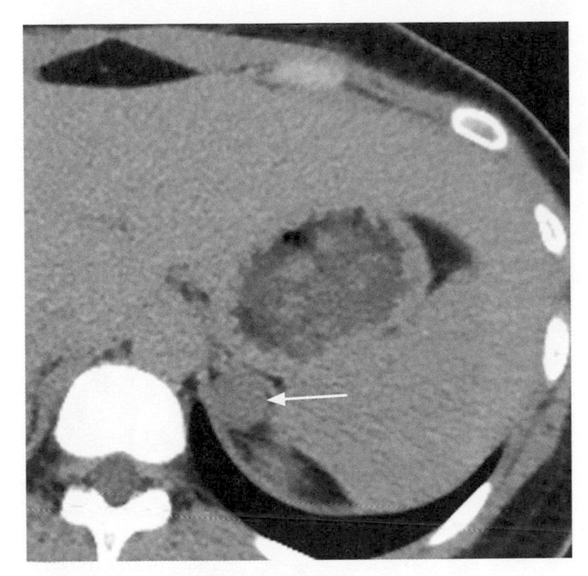

Figure 8.14 Adrenal adenoma: CT. Low-density left adrenal nodule (arrow).

Adrenal metastases also tend to be larger in size (>3 cm) and of higher density on unenhanced scans.

Equivocal lesions may be further assessed with multiphase contrast-enhanced CT. Attenuation values of the adrenal mass are measured before contrast injection and then at 60 seconds and 15 minutes after injection. Adrenal adenomas rapidly enhance and rapidly wash out; hence, they demonstrate low attenuation before contrast injection, high attenuation at 60 seconds and significantly reduced attenuation at 15 minutes. Adrenal metastases demonstrate slower washout.

MRI, including chemical shift imaging, may also be useful in differentiating adrenal adenoma from malignancy. Chemical shift imaging exploits the slightly different precession frequency of hydrogen atoms in water from those in fat. With chemical shift MRI, normal adrenal tissue and adrenal adenomas show reduced signal on out-of-phase scans (Fig. 8.15). Adrenal metastases show relatively increased signal on the out-of-phase scans, allowing differentiation from benign adrenal adenoma.

Rarely, when imaging cannot be used to confidently classify an adrenal mass as either benign or malignant, and when that adrenal mass is the only evidence of metastasis in a patient with a primary tumour, percutaneous biopsy under CT guidance may be required for definitive diagnosis.

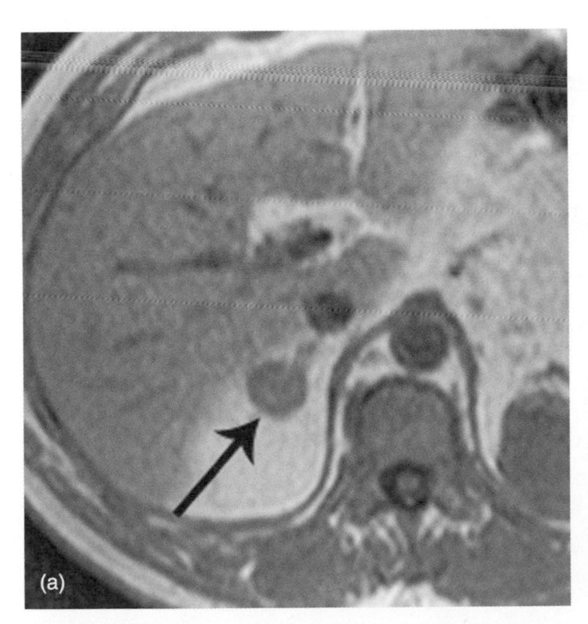

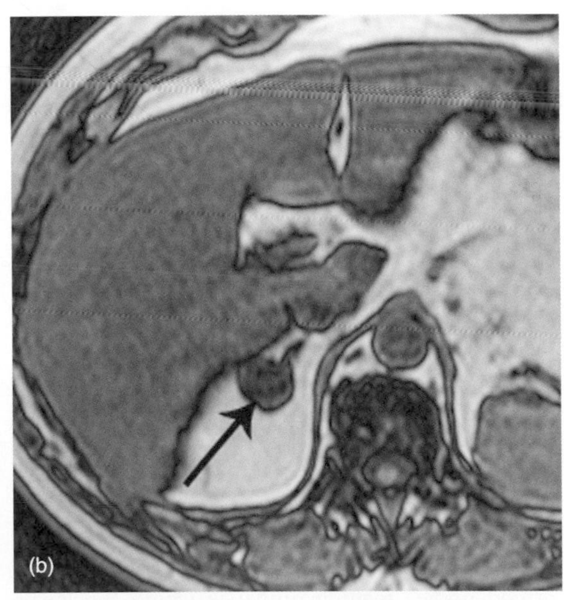

Figure 8.15 Adrenal adenoma: chemical shift MRI. (a) In-phase gradient echo scan shows a small round mass on the right adrenal gland (arrow). (b) Out-of-phase gradient echo scan shows reduced signal intensity in the mass (arrow) typical of an adrenal adenoma.

8.9 INTERVENTIONAL RADIOLOGY IN UROLOGY

8.9.1 PERCUTANEOUS NEPHROSTOMY

Percutaneous nephrostomy is percutaneous insertion of a drainage catheter into the renal collecting system. Indications for percutaneous nephrostomy include:

- Relief of urinary tract obstruction, which may be caused by ureteric calculus, carcinoma of the bladder, ureteric TCC or carcinoma of the prostate
- Pyonephrosis
- Leakage of urine from the upper urinary tract secondary to trauma or after surgery.

Percutaneous nephrostomy is performed with imaging guidance, either US and fluoroscopy or CT. Complications may include haematuria, which is usually mild and transitory, and vascular trauma, which is very rare with imaging guidance.

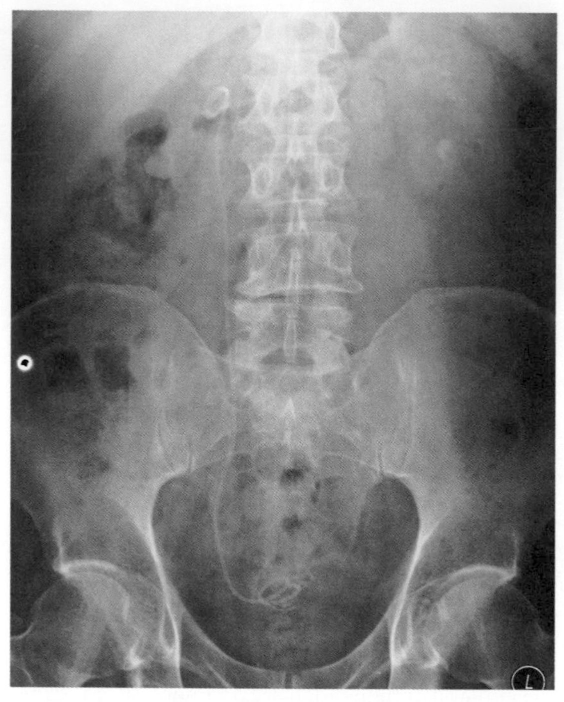

Figure 8.16 Ureteric stent well positioned with its upper end in the right renal pelvis and its lower end in the bladder. Also note the left renal calculi.

8.9.2 URETERIC STENT

Indications for ureteric stent insertion include:

- Malignant obstruction of the urinary tract caused by carcinoma of the bladder, prostate or cervix
- Pelviureteric junction obstruction
- Other benign obstructions of the urinary tract, e.g. retroperitoneal fibrosis, radiotherapy
- Following ureteric surgery
- Management of ureteric calculi, including after extracorporeal shock wave lithotripsy (ESWL) of large renal calculi (Fig. 8.16).

Ureteric stent insertion may be either retrograde or antegrade. Retrograde insertion is done via cystoscopy. Antegrade insertion is occasionally performed under imaging guidance where the lower ureter is occluded, making retrograde insertion impossible, or if percutaneous nephrostomy is performed concomitantly.

8.9.3 SHOCK WAVE LITHOTRIPSY

Shock wave lithotripsy uses highly focused sound waves to fragment renal or ureteric stones. When the shock waves are generated outside the body, the process is referred to as ESWL. Intracorporeal shock wave lithotripsy refers to shock waves generated inside the body through a ureteroscope. Shock wave lithotripsy is the technique of choice for the management of most renal stones.

8.9.4 PERCUTANEOUS NEPHROLITHOTOMY

Indications for percutaneous nephrolithotomy (PCNL):

- Failed ESWL
- Staghorn calculus
- Cystine or matrix calculus.

PCNL is usually performed under general anaesthetic. A retrograde ureteric catheter is inserted via cystoscopy to opacify the renal collecting system with contrast material and to prevent calculus fragments passing down the ureter. The renal collecting system is then punctured with a needle, followed by passage of a guidewire. A tract into the collecting system is made with a series of dilators and the renal stone is extracted.

8.9.5 RENAL ARTERY EMBOLIZATION

For general notes on vascular embolization, see section 6.11 in Chapter 6.

Indications for renal artery embolization include:

- Control of renal bleeding due to trauma, surgery or biopsy
- Treatment of arteriovenous malformation (AVM) and arteriovenous fistula, which are most often seen as a complication of nephrostomy or biopsy
- Palliation or preoperative reduction of vascular renal tumour, either RCC or large AML.

8.9.6 PERCUTANEOUS TUMOUR ABLATION

As stated above, over 60% of RCCs are diagnosed incidentally. Most of these are small, early-stage tumours (<4 cm) that are amenable to minimally invasive nephron-sparing treatment options. Such treatment options include open or laparoscopic partial nephrectomy and percutaneous tumour ablation. Percutaneous tumour ablation techniques are becoming widely available and include RF ablation and cryoablation. Both techniques involve precise intratumoral placement of probes under imaging guidance. Ablation procedures may be performed with local anaesthesia and conscious sedation or general anaesthesia. The choice of imaging guidance technique (US or CT) depends on multiple factors, including the size and position of the tumour, body habitus of the patient and local expertise and availability. Postprocedure follow-up includes:

- Observation for immediate complications such as pain
- Imaging with contrast-enhanced CT or MRI to ensure ablation of the tumour and exclude complications such as haemorrhage.

SUMMARY

Clinical presentation	Investigation of choice	Comment
Painless haematuria	CT urography and cystoscopy	US for further definition in selected cases
Renal mass	• US • CT/MRI	Biopsy in selected cases
Prostatism	US	
Diagnosis of prostate cancer	• Multiparametric MRI • US-guided biopsy	
Staging of adenocarcinoma of the prostate	• SPECT-CT bone scan • Multiparametric MRI	Evolving role for PSMA-PET
Scrotal mass	US	
Acute scrotum	US	
Phaeochromocytoma	CT/MRI abdomen	DOTATATE-PET or MIBG scintigraphy if CT/MRI negative
Incidental adrenal mass	• Multiphase contrast CT • Chemical shift MRI	

Abbreviations: DOTATATE, tetraazacyclododecane–tetraacetic acid and tyrosine-3-octreotate; MIBG, see Table 1.1; PSMA, prostate-specific membrane antigen; SPECT, single photon emission CT.

9 Central nervous system: brain

Computed tomography (CT) and magnetic resonance imaging (MRI) are the most common imaging investigations performed for assessment of brain disorders. MRI is the investigation of choice for most indications. The three most common exceptions are acute head trauma (see Chapter 12), suspected acute subarachnoid haemorrhage (SAH) and stroke, where CT is the initial imaging investigation. A skull radiograph (X-ray) may occasionally be performed for a few uncommon skull vault disorders, such as craniosynostosis (premature fusion of cranial sutures in infants), or as part of a skeletal survey, e.g. multiple myeloma (see Fig. 13.67) or suspected non-accidental injury in children. Cranial ultrasound (US) is a useful investigation in infants in whom the anterior fontanelle is open. Cranial US is used in the diagnosis and monitoring of intracranial haemorrhage in premature infants and is also a useful screening test in older infants for assessment of increasing head circumference. For discussion of traumatic brain injury, see Chapter 12.

9.1 SUBARACHNOID HAEMORRHAGE

Patients with non-traumatic spontaneous SAH present with sudden onset of severe headache, often accompanied by neck pain and stiffness, diminished consciousness and focal neurological signs. The most common causes of spontaneous SAH are a ruptured intracranial artery aneurysm in 80–90% and cranial arteriovenous malformation (AVM) in 5%. Less common causes include spinal AVM, coagulopathy, tumour and venous or capillary bleeding.

Most cerebral artery aneurysms are congenital 'berry' aneurysms. Berry aneurysms occur in 2% of the population and are multiple in 10% of cases. An increased incidence of berry aneurysms occurs in association with coarctation of the aorta and autosomal dominant polycystic kidney disease and connective tissue diseases. Some patients with sporadic aneurysms will have a family history of aneurysm or SAH. Most berry aneurysms occur around the circle of Willis, the most common sites being:

- Anterior communicating artery (AComA)
- Posterior communicating artery (PComA)
- Middle cerebral artery (MCA)
- Bifurcation of the internal carotid artery (ICA)
- Tip of the basilar artery.

The risk of aneurysm rupture is dependent on aneurysmal factors, such as size, morphology and location, and patient factors, such as hypertension, family history, bleeding diathesis and underlying predisposing conditions.

CT is the primary imaging investigation of choice in suspected SAH. Acute SAH shows on non-contrast CT as high-attenuation material (fresh blood) in the basal cisterns, Sylvian fissures, ventricles and cerebral sulci (Fig. 9.1). The possible aneurysmal cause of SAH is suggested by the location of the haemorrhage, e.g. blood concentrated in a Sylvian fissure indicates bleeding from the ipsilateral MCA. Complications of SAH visible on CT include hydrocephalus and ischaemia due to vasospasm. Hydrocephalus may occur within hours of haemorrhage owing to obstruction of the cerebrospinal fluid (CSF) pathways with blood.

CT that is positive for SAH is usually followed immediately by CT angiography (CTA) to diagnose and define the cause (Fig. 9.2). CTA can show the bleeding aneurysm, demonstrate the relationship of the neck of the aneurysm to the vessel of origin and diagnose multiple aneurysms, if present (10% of cases). The sensitivity of CTA in the detection of intracerebral aneurysms is very good, but catheter angiography is the most sensitive imaging modality, especially for aneurysms smaller than 2 mm.

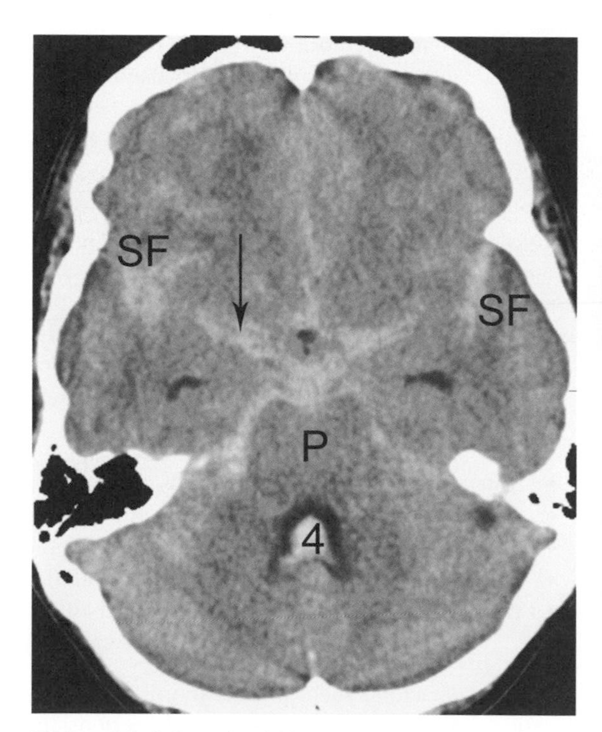

Figure 9.1 Subarachnoid haemorrhage. Acute blood is seen as high-density material in the basal cisterns (arrow), anterior to the pons (P), in the Sylvian fissures (SF) and in the fourth ventricle (4).

Interventional neuroradiologists play a major role in the management of SAH. The basic tool of interventional neuroradiology (INR) is the microcatheter. Microcatheters can be advanced coaxially through larger catheters to access vascular pathology deep in the brain. Vascular access is gained through the groin (common femoral artery) or wrist (radial artery). In the management of SAH, INR fulfils the following roles:

- Secure the aneurysm: coil embolization as an alternative to neurosurgical aneurysm clipping (Fig. 9.3)
- Diagnose and treat vasospasm: intra-arterial infusion of vasodilator drugs and balloon angioplasty
- Occlusion of inflow and outflow of AVMs.

Up to 5% of patients with a proven SAH have a normal CT at initial presentation. The sensitivity of CT for SAH is greatest in the first 6 hours after symptom onset. After this time, with sensitivity for SAH declining, patients with a negative CT for SAH may undergo diagnostic lumbar puncture to identify blood in the CSF or xanthochromia. Potential problems with lumbar puncture include:

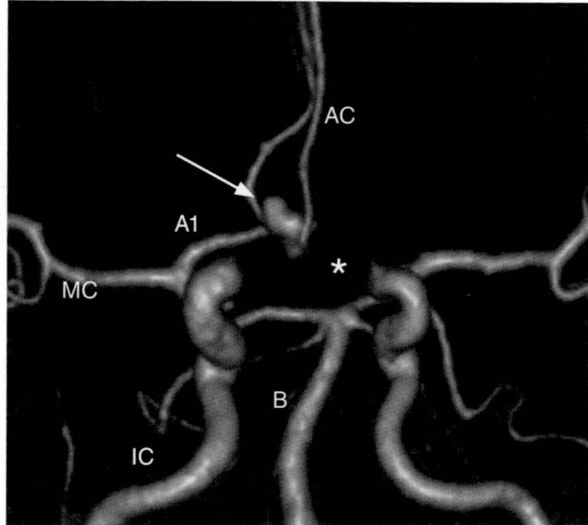

Figure 9.2 Cerebral aneurysm: CT angiogram. Three-dimensional reconstructed image shows an anterior communicating artery aneurysm (arrow). Also note anterior cerebral arteries (AC), right anterior cerebral artery pre-communicating segment (A1), right middle cerebral artery (MC), right internal carotid artery (IC), basilar artery (B). Absence of the left A1 segment (*) is an anatomical variant.

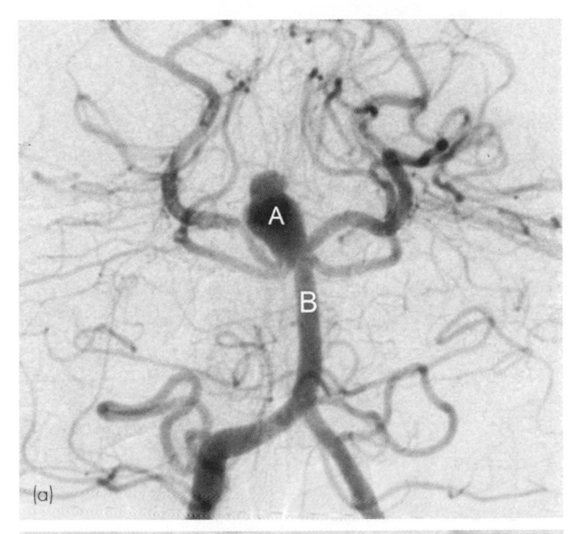

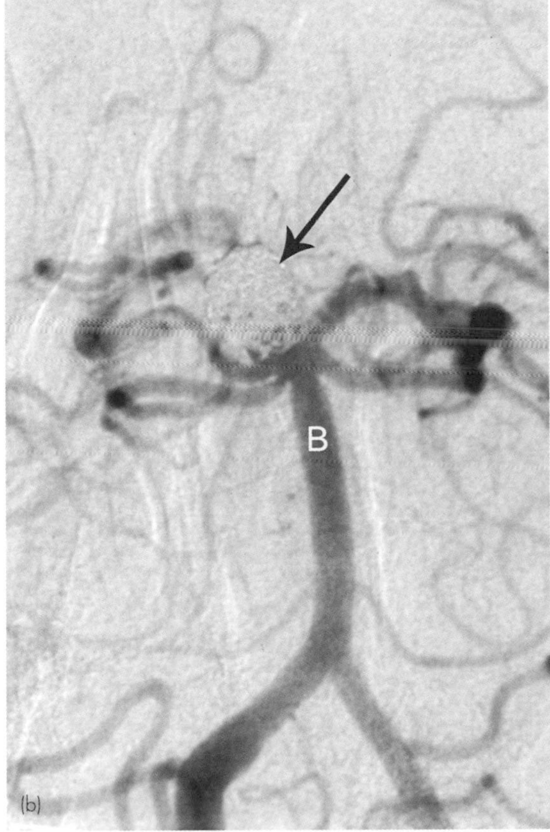

Figure 9.3 Treatment of a cerebral aneurysm: interventional neuroradiology. The aneurysm is embolized with coils via a superselective catheter. (a) A diagnostic angiogram showing an aneurysm (A) arising from the distal tip of the basilar artery (B). (b) The postprocedure subtracted angiogram image shows no blood flow into the aneurysm (arrow), indicating successful treatment.

- False positive due to a blood-stained ('traumatic') tap
- Problems with interpretation of xanthochromia
- Post-lumbar puncture headache (up to 20%).

Alternatively, in cases where there is strong clinical suspicion for SAH and CT is negative, CTA may be performed to identify a berry aneurysm.

9.1.1 SCREENING FOR CEREBRAL ARTERY ANEURYSMS

Indications for screening for intracranial artery aneurysms include:

- History of SAH or intracranial aneurysm in a first-degree relative
- Condition known to be associated with berry aneurysm, such as:
    - Coarctation of the aorta
    - Autosomal dominant polycystic kidney disease
    - Neurofibromatosis type 1
- Certain clinical presentations with a high probability of cerebral aneurysm, e.g. isolated third cranial nerve palsy, which may be caused by an aneurysm of the PComA.

CTA and magnetic resonance angiography (MRA) may be used to image the cerebral vessels. Both techniques are of comparable sensitivity to catheter angiography for displaying aneurysms of 3 mm or greater. CTA and MRA each have relative advantages and disadvantages; the choice of technique often depends on local expertise and availability.

9.2 STROKE

The generic term 'stroke' or cerebrovascular accident (CVA) refers to an acute event that causes a sudden focal neurological deficit that lasts for more than 24 hours. Stroke may be caused either by decreased blood flow to the brain (ischaemia and infarction) or by intracranial haemorrhage.

Common causes of stroke:

- Cerebral ischaemia and infarction (acute ischaemic stroke) (80%)

- Parenchymal (primary intracerebral) haemorrhage (15%)
  - Usually secondary to hypertension
  - Common sites: basal ganglia, thalamus, brainstem and cerebellum (Fig. 9.4)
- Spontaneous SAH (5%) (see section 9.1)
- Cerebral venous occlusion (<1%).

Most acute ischaemic strokes are due to acute thromboembolic occlusion of the intracranial arteries. Haemorrhagic infarction, also known as haemorrhagic transformation, refers to haemorrhage into a region of infarcted brain. Haemorrhagic transformation may occur following clearing of an arterial occlusion with restoration of blood flow to damaged brain. Acute arterial occlusion produces a central region of irreversibly infarcted brain tissue (infarct core) with a surrounding zone of hypoxic tissue.

Without restoration of blood flow, this hypoxic tissue (ischaemic penumbra) will progress to infarction.

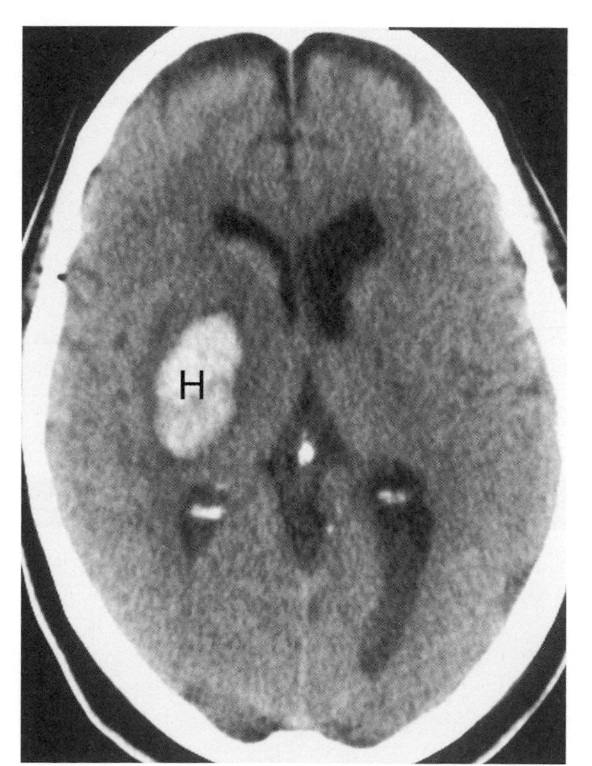

Figure 9.4 Primary hypertensive haemorrhage seen as an oval-shaped high-attenuation haematoma in the right basal ganglia (H).

However, the ischaemic penumbra is potentially salvageable with immediate management to restore flow. This can be achieved with intravenous infusion of a thrombolytic agent such as tissue plasminogen activator (tPA) within the first 4.5 hours following symptom onset. Thrombolysis with intravenous tPA is associated with improved neurological function in up to one in three patients. The risk of intracerebral haemorrhage producing an adverse outcome is about one in 30. tPA is contraindicated in the presence of haemorrhage. In the last two decades, angiographically guided mechanical thrombectomy (endovascular clot retrieval [ECR]) has become the mainstay of treatment of ischaemic stroke in patients with large-vessel occlusion.

Transient ischaemic attack (TIA) is an acute neurological deficit that resolves completely within 24 hours. TIAs are thought to be caused by a transient reduction of blood flow to the brain or eye as a result of emboli and are associated with underlying stenosis of the ICA or cerebral arteries. Patients with TIA are usually investigated with CT of the brain and carotid Doppler US (see Imaging of the carotid arteries in section 9.2.2).

9.2.1 IMAGING OF STROKE

Based on the above principles, the primary goals of acute imaging in the investigation and management of stroke/TIA are:

- Exclude haemorrhage in the acute setting (Fig. 9.5)
- Early identification of patients suitable for ECR:
  - Assessment of arterial stenosis or occlusion and cerebral collateral supply
  - Differentiate a core infarct from ischaemic penumbra
  - Confirm favourable aortic arch and neck arterial anatomy to allow endovascular access
- Selection of patients suitable for treatment with tPA.

Secondary goals of stroke imaging include:

- Identification of the source of emboli
- Identification of asymptomatic patients who may be at risk of stroke.

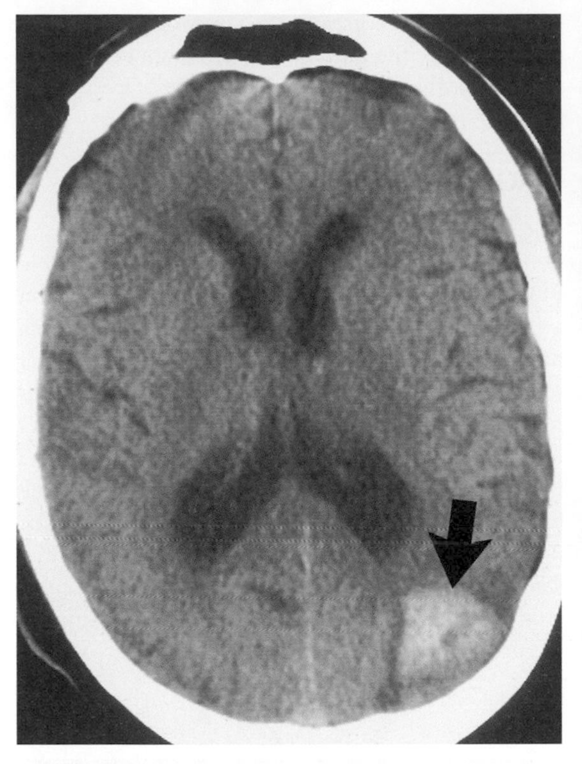

Figure 9.5 Haemorrhagic infarct seen as a peripheral wedge-shaped lesion in the left parieto-occipital region (arrow).

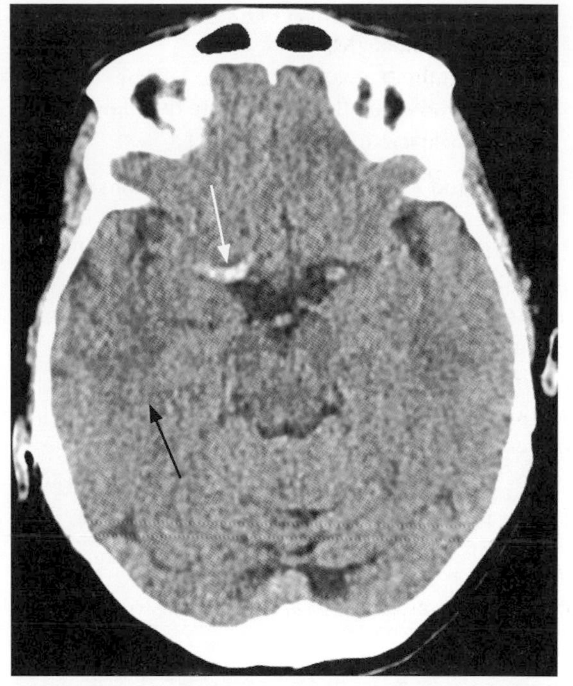

Figure 9.6 Acute stroke: CT. Hyperdense right middle cerebral artery (white arrow) due to acute thromboembolism. Note the subtle reduction in density in the right temporal lobe, indicating ischaemia (black arrow).

COMPUTED TOMOGRAPHY

CT is the investigation of choice for the initial assessment of patients with symptoms of stroke or TIA. It is widely available, highly sensitive to acute haemorrhage and studies are rapid, taking no more than a few seconds. Early subtle CT changes of acute ischaemic stroke may be recognized within 2–6 hours of the onset of symptoms (Fig. 9.6):

- Increased density of intracranial arteries as a result of thrombosis (hyperdense vessel sign):
  - May be the only CT sign in hyperacute stroke
  - Usually proximal MCA, terminal ICA and/or proximal anterior cerebral artery (ACA)
  - Basilar and vertebral arteries in posterior fossa stroke
- Decreased attenuation and loss of grey–white matter differentiation owing to cytotoxic oedema affecting an arterial territory of the brain.

From 12 to 24 hours and over the next 3 days, oedema increases with more obvious gyral swelling and mass effect. The main limitation of CT is in the delineation of very subtle changes of early ischaemia.

COMPUTED TOMOGRAPHY ANGIOGRAPHY AND PERFUSION COMPUTED TOMOGRAPHY

CTA can provide rapid assessment of the carotid arteries in the neck as well as the cerebral vessels; sites of arterial thrombosis and occlusion are clearly shown. As discussed above, CTA of the aortic arch and neck vessels is also required to 'road map' the anatomy prior to potential ECR.

Perfusion CT is achieved with sequential low-dose CT scans of the brain during intravenous contrast infusion. Computer analysis produces various colour maps based on attenuation changes in the brain, which reflect real-time perfusion. The more common parameters calculated are:

- Mean transit time (MTT)
- Time to peak (TTP)
- Cerebral blood volume (CBV)
- Cerebral blood flow (CBF; note that flow = volume per unit time).

MTT and TTP are sensitive for alterations in brain perfusion, with both parameters prolonged in ischaemic penumbra and core infarct (Fig. 9.7). CBF and CBV are used to differentiate penumbra from core infarct in the vascular territory indicated by the prolonged time parameters:

- Core infarct: markedly reduced CBF and a matched reduction in CBV
- Ischaemic penumbra: reduced CBF (but not as much as in core infarct) and normal CBV. CBV may occasionally be increased as a result of vasodilation secondary to autoregulatory mechanisms.

In general, the greater the size of the penumbra and the larger the ratio of the penumbra to the core, the greater the possible clinical benefit of ECR.

MAGNETIC RESONANCE IMAGING

MRI with diffusion-weighted imaging (DWI) and perfusion-weighted imaging (PWI) is an alternative to CT in the identification of hyperacute infarction and ischaemia. With the onset of acute ischaemia and cell death, there is increased intracellular water (cytotoxic oedema) with restricted diffusion of water molecules. An acute infarct therefore shows on DWI as an area of relatively high signal (Fig. 9.8). DWI is the most sensitive imaging test available for the diagnosis of hyperacute infarction. However, logistic difficulties with MRI, including availability, potential safety issues and time required to complete a suitable study (approximately 15 minutes), preclude its use as the primary modality in acute stroke.

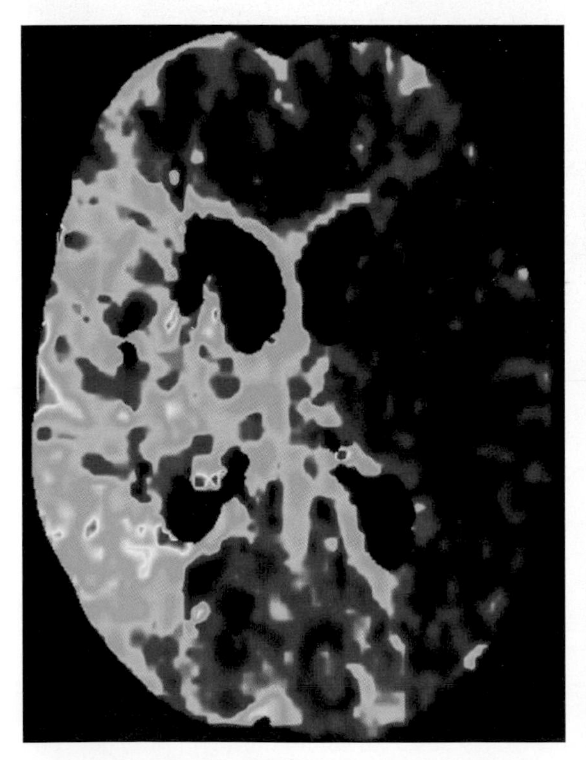

Figure 9.7 Ischaemic stroke: CT perfusion. Large wedge-shaped region of increased time to peak (TTP) in the right middle cerebral artery territory, indicating ischaemia; seen on a colour map as a region of green coloration.

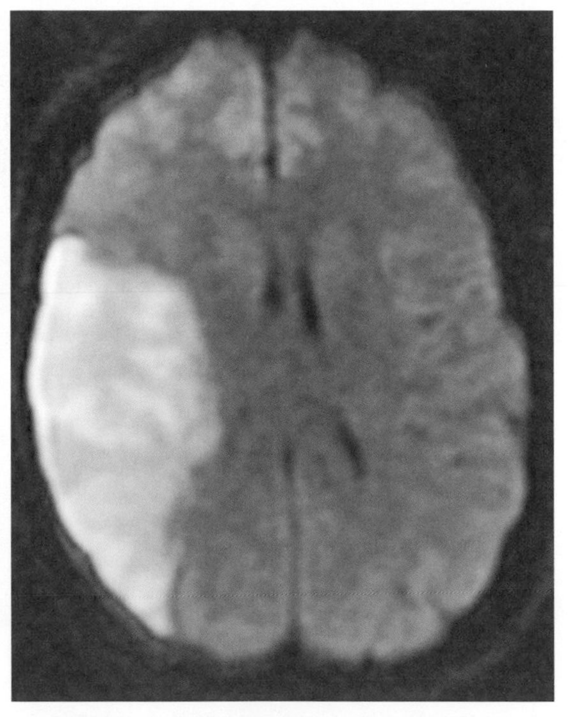

Figure 9.8 Acute cerebral infarct: MRI. Diffusion-weighted MRI shows a large area of restricted diffusion in the right middle cerebral artery territory.

INTERVENTIONAL NEURORADIOLOGY AND ENDOVASCULAR CLOT RETRIEVAL

Interventional neuroradiologists performing ECR in advanced stroke centres have revolutionized the treatment of acute ischaemic stroke in the last decade. Patient selection is critical to optimize clinical outcomes. Initially, ECR was only offered to patients within 6 hours of symptom onset for anterior circulation CVA, but this time window has extended (currently up to 24 hours). Selection criteria for ECR include:

- Large-vessel occlusion
- Adequate penumbra
- Favourable arterial anatomy
- Good premorbid function.

The procedure involves arterial access via either the femoral or radial artery. A catheter is advanced to just proximal to the occlusion and an angiogram is performed. The thrombus is removed by catheter aspiration or stent retriever (Fig. 9.9). Post-ECR angiograms demonstrate recanalization of the affected artery. Recanalization rates are over 90% in high-volume centres. Complications occur in up to 10% of cases and include reperfusion haemorrhage, dissection and distal embolization.

9.2.2 IDENTIFICATION OF ASYMPTOMATIC 'AT-RISK' PATIENTS

Identification of patients at risk for developing stroke involves identification of risk factors plus the diagnosis of structural abnormalities.

Risk factors for stroke include:

- Hypertension
- Diabetes mellitus
- Hypercholesterolaemia
- TIA: approximately 30% of patients with TIA will develop a subsequent infarct
- Coronary artery disease
- Severe peripheral artery disease.

Structural abnormalities include ischaemic changes in the brain and atheromatous disease of the carotid, vertebral and basilar arteries.

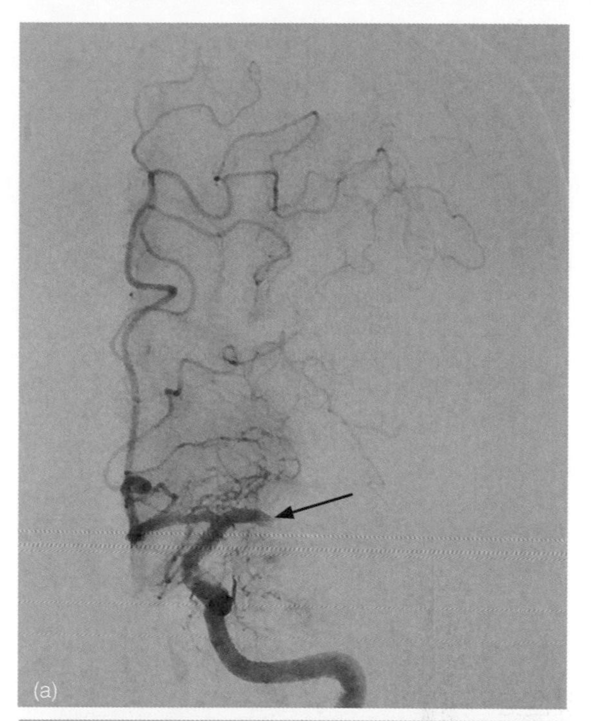

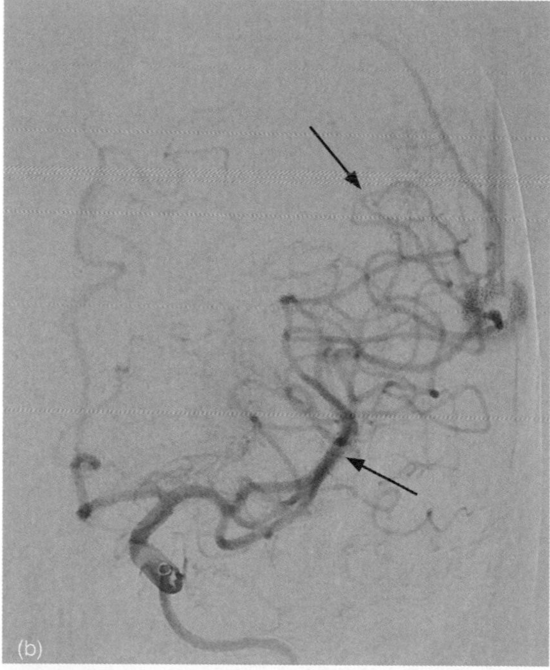

Figure 9.9 Endovascular clot retrieval (ECR): coronal digital subtraction angiography (DSA). (a) Left proximal middle cerebral artery (MCA) occlusion due to acute thromboembolism (arrow). (b) Post-ECR angiogram showing restoration of normal flow in the left MCA (arrows).

IMAGING OF THE BRAIN

CT or MRI may be used to diagnose ischaemic changes in the brain, including:

- Chronic deep white matter ischaemia
  - CT: low attenuation in the deep (periventricular and subcortical) white matter (Fig. 9.10)
  - MRI: high signal in the deep white matter on T2-weighted and fluid-attenuated inversion recovery (FLAIR) images
- Old infarcts
- Lacunar infarcts: small round infarcts in the basal ganglia and deep white matter.

IMAGING OF THE CAROTID ARTERIES

US examination of the carotid arteries is a useful screening test able to diagnose stenosis and occlusion caused by atheromatous disease. Carotid US combines direct visualization of the arterial wall, colour Doppler examination of the arterial lumen and measurement of blood flow velocity in the common carotid artery (CCA) and ICA. Blood flow velocity measurements include measurements of peak systolic velocity (PSV) and end-diastolic velocity (EDV) given in centimetres per second (cm/s). Comparison of PSV for the CCA and ICA gives the ICA/CCA ratio. Stenosis is indicated by direct visualization of arterial narrowing plus increased measured flow velocity in the ICA (Fig. 9.11).

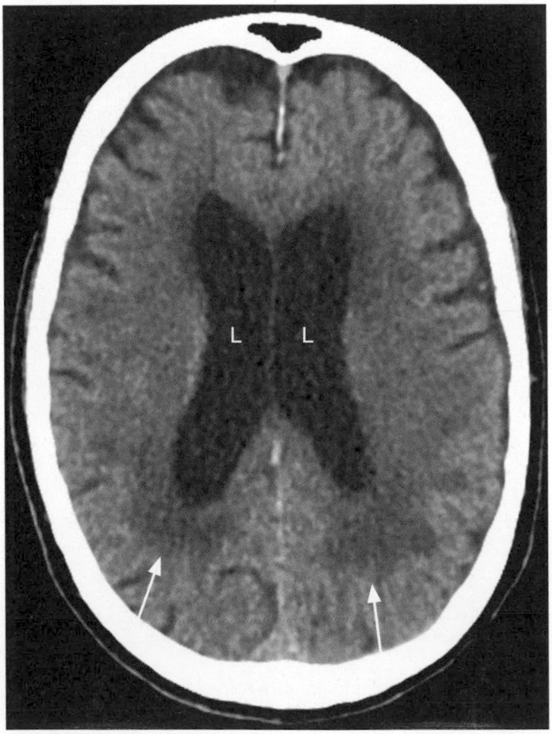

Figure 9.10 Chronic brain ischaemia: CT. CT image at the level of the lateral ventricles (L) shows multiple bilateral areas of low attenuation in the white matter (arrows).

Based on the US appearance of the carotid arteries plus the measured blood flow velocities, the degree of ICA disease may be classified as follows:

- Normal: no plaque visualized; ICA PSV less than 125 cm/s
- Less than 50% stenosis: plaque visualized; ICA PSV less than 125 cm/s
- 50–69% stenosis: plaque visualized; ICA PSV 125–230 cm/s
- 70% to near occlusion: plaque visualized; ICA PSV greater than 230 cm/s
- Near occlusion: markedly narrowed lumen visualized by colour Doppler
- Complete occlusion: no blood flow visualized by colour Doppler.

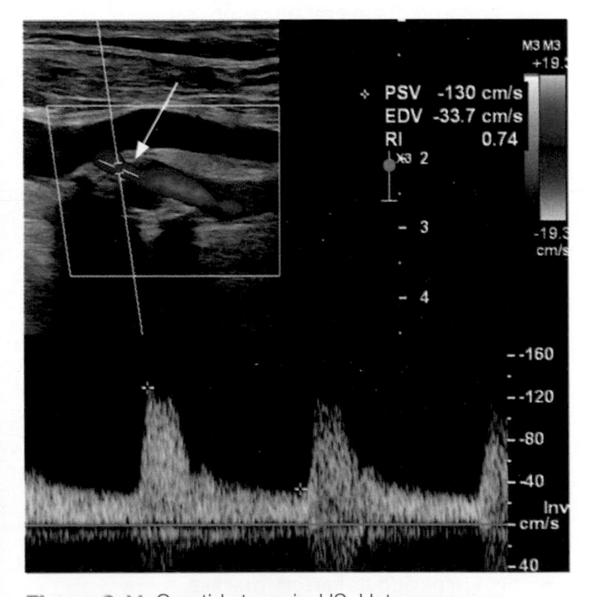

Figure 9.11 Carotid stenosis: US. Heterogeneous calcified plaque involving the proximal internal carotid artery with greater than 50% narrowing on B-mode (arrow). Corresponding mildly increased peak systolic velocity (130 cm/s) consistent with 50–69% stenosis.

This classification is clinically relevant as carotid endarterectomy is beneficial in stenosis of 70% to near occlusion, with no definite benefit shown for stenosis of less than 70%. Complete ICA occlusion is inoperable. MRA or CTA may be performed when more definitive imaging of the carotid arteries is required.

9.3 BRAIN TUMOURS

Symptoms caused by brain tumours are quite variable, as follows:

- Increased intracranial pressure caused by the tumour itself or hydrocephalus:
  - Headache
  - Nausea and vomiting
  - Irritability
- Acute presentation (may be due to haemorrhage into the tumour):
  - Sudden severe headache
  - Stroke
  - Seizure
- Focal neurological disturbance
- Cranial nerve palsy
- Hormonal effects.

9.3.1 CLASSIFICATION AND GRADING OF BRAIN TUMOURS

Primary tumours of the central nervous system (CNS) are classified and graded by the World Health Organization (WHO). Published in 2021, the fifth edition of the WHO Classification of Tumours of the CNS (WHO CNS5) introduces major changes in tumour nomenclature and classification. Newly recognized tumour types are included, and the names of some well-known tumours have been changed or modified (e.g. glioblastoma multiforme is now known as glioblastoma, IDH-wildtype), while others have stayed the same (e.g. meningioma). Details of this highly complex classification system are beyond the scope of this book; however, a few key points can be stated.

In earlier publications, the WHO classified primary tumours of the CNS into categories based on the cell or tissue of origin. WHO CNS5 emphasizes the increased importance of various molecular biomarkers in tumour classification. This may include the status of specific genes, such as isocitrate dehydrogenase (IDH). Medulloblastoma may be subclassified based on the status of the signalling pathways SHH and WNT and of the *TP53* gene into four subgroups. An increasingly relevant molecular diagnostic method is the determination of DNA methylation patterns. Known as methylome profiling, this method allows precise identification of tumour subtypes within broader groupings. In the above example, methylation profiling is leading to the description of further subgroupings within the four major types of medulloblastoma.

Previous versions of the WHO classification graded primary brain tumours into four categories of increasing malignancy and aggressiveness: WHO grades I–IV. WHO CNS5 also uses four gradings, with Arabic replacing Roman numerals. Whereas the earlier grading systems were used across all tumour types, WHO CNS5 assigns grades within individual tumour types. This reflects the fact that biologically different tumours of the same grade, e.g. grade 1 diffuse astrocytoma and grade 1 meningioma, may display different pathological behaviours with different clinical outcomes. Furthermore, specific tumours may be classified as being of different grades depending on histological and molecular factors; for example, astrocytoma, IDH mutant may be classified as CNS WHO grade 2, 3 or 4.

Relative incidences of the various types of brain tumour vary between children and adults. In adults, metastases from non-CNS primary tumours account for 50% of brain tumours. Of the primary brain tumours in adults, gliomas are the most common, followed by meningioma, pituitary adenoma and vestibular schwannoma. CNS metastases are uncommon in children. Most brain tumours in children are primary CNS lesions and are more commonly located in the posterior fossa, including astrocytomas of varying grade, medulloblastoma, ependymoma, germ cell tumour and craniopharyngioma.

9.3.2 IMAGING OF BRAIN TUMOURS

The two imaging modalities used most for the assessment of brain tumours are MRI and CT.

MRI with gadolinium is the investigation of choice in most instances as it provides more detailed anatomical information and soft-tissue characterization (Fig. 9.12). MRI of the entire neuroaxis (brain and spine) is often performed, particularly in the presence of tumours known to metastasize via CSF, e.g. medulloblastoma and germinoma. CT may be used when MRI is unavailable or for urgent clinical presentations such as sudden onset of severe headache or seizures. CT is more sensitive than MRI for the detection of calcification.

Multiparametric MRI is increasingly used in the assessment of brain tumours, combining conventional 'anatomical' sequences with more specialized sequences, including DWI and accompanying maps of apparent diffusion coefficient (ADC), PWI and MR spectroscopy (MRS) (see Fig. 3.1). These measure various parameters, including the ADC values and relative cerebral blood volume (rCBV), and levels of various metabolites, such as creatinine, choline, lactate and *N*-acetylaspartate (NAA). These parameters reflect biological features such as cellularity, angiogenesis, vascular permeability and cell membrane turnover. Multiparametric MRI is most useful in specific indications, such as the detection of malignant transformation of low-grade tumours, the selection of suitable biopsy sites in heterogeneous lesions and differentiation of tumour progression from increased size or enhancement caused by therapy (pseudoprogression of glioblastoma treated with chemoradiotherapy).

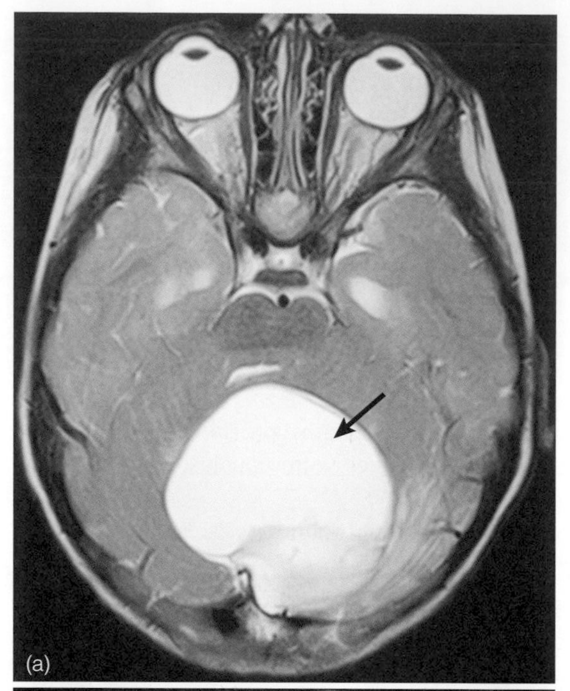

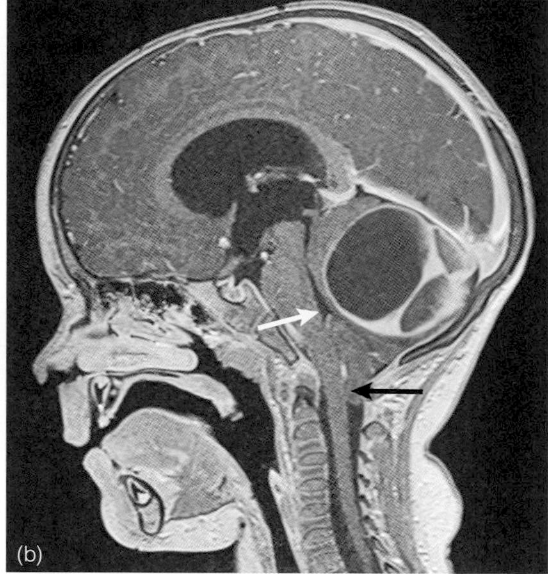

Figure 9.12 Pilocytic astrocytoma (WHO grade 1): MRI. A 4-year-old boy with headaches and ataxia. (a) Transverse T2-weighted MRI shows a large space-occupying lesion in the cerebellum. The lesion has a large cystic component (arrow). (b) Sagittal T1-weighted contrast-enhanced MRI shows enhancement of multiple septations plus the wall of the cystic component. Note that the mass effect from the tumour is causing compression and distortion of the fourth ventricle (white arrow) and downward herniation of the cerebellar tonsils (black arrow).

9.4 HEADACHE

Headache is a very common symptom. Common causes include stress or tension headache and migraine. Headache may also be a non-specific symptom of generalized malaise, such as may occur in common viral or bacterial infections. Most patients with headache can be diagnosed and treated on clinical grounds, without any need for neuroimaging. There are, however, certain specific types of headaches and associated clinical scenarios that do warrant imaging assessment, such as:

- Suspected SAH (see section 9.1):
  - Sudden onset of severe headache

  - 'Worst headache of my life'
  - Associated neck pain and stiffness
  - Investigation of choice: CT
- Suspected space-occupying lesion in a child:
  - New-onset headache, sleep related
  - No family history of migraine
  - Papilloedema
  - Investigation of choice: MRI (Fig. 9.12)
- Suspected space-occupying lesion in an adult:
  - Signs of raised intracranial pressure
  - Headache, worse in the morning
  - Confusion; focal neurology: hemiparesis, focal seizures
  - Investigation of choice: MRI
  - CT if MRI contraindicated or difficult to obtain
- Suspected dissection of carotid or vertebral artery:
  - Sudden-onset unilateral headache
  - Neck pain; ipsilateral Horner syndrome
  - History of trauma or neck manipulation
  - Investigation of choice: MRI brain and neck, CT angiogram
- Suspected temporal arteritis:
  - New headache in an elderly patient (>60 years)
  - Temporal tenderness
  - Increased erythrocyte sedimentation rate (ESR)
  - Investigation of choice: MRI
- Suspected intracranial infection:
  - New headache with fever
  - Neck stiffness with meningitis
  - Reduced consciousness with encephalitis
  - History of sinusitis or middle ear infection
  - History of immune compromise, including stem cell transplant for haematological malignancy, human immunodeficiency virus (HIV)
  - Investigation of choice: MRI with gadolinium
  - CT if MRI not available, though less sensitive than MRI for meningitis and encephalitis.

9.5 SEIZURE

Epilepsy is a common chronic condition that may be genetic or acquired and is characterized by a predisposition to recurrent seizures. Seizures are defined as abnormal electrical discharges in brain cells, producing finite events of cerebral function. The classification of seizure type is important as this will help to guide the need for further investigation and subsequent management and counselling. The two broad categories of seizure type are primary generalized and partial:

- Primary generalized seizures originate simultaneously from both cerebral hemispheres and produce bilateral clinical symptoms
- Partial seizures originate from a localized area of the brain, based on clinical manifestations and electroencephalogram (EEG) findings:
  - Clinical manifestations of partial seizures may include focal motor or sensory disturbance, psychiatric symptoms or autonomic signs or symptoms
  - Classified as simple or complex: complex partial seizures are associated with loss of consciousness; simple partial seizures are not.

Most generalized seizure disorders are idiopathic. Most patients are referred for imaging for a first generalized seizure and, in most cases, this will not show an underlying abnormality. Partial seizures are more commonly associated with an underlying structural lesion:

- Vascular malformations
- Tumours
- Brain injury
- Developmental abnormalities.

Developmental abnormalities of the temporal lobe and hippocampal formation are a common cause of partial complex seizures:

- Mesial temporal sclerosis: sclerosis and atrophy of the hippocampal formation (Fig. 9.13)
- Cortical dysplasia characterized by abnormal areas of grey matter
- Grey matter heterotopia.

MRI is the imaging investigation of choice for the assessment of seizure disorders. MRI of the brain is usually recommended in all patients presenting with a first seizure. MRI assessment should include high-resolution images of the temporal lobes in the

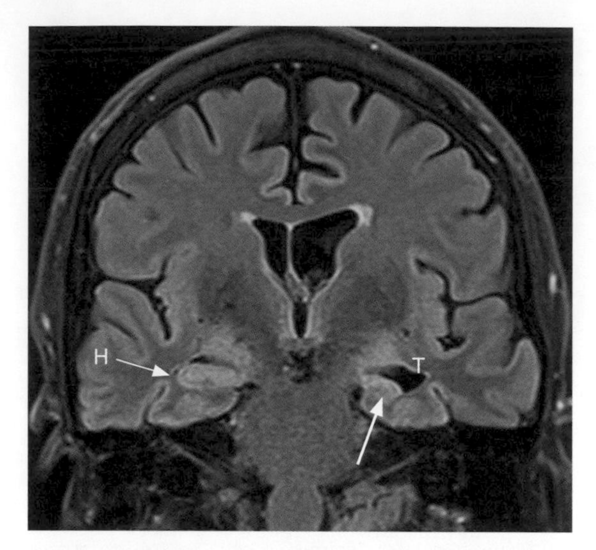

Figure 9.13 Mesial temporal sclerosis: coronal fluid-attenuated inversion recovery (FLAIR) MRI. Left hippocampal atrophy and mild T2 hyperintensity (arrow). Note the dilated temporal horn (T) of the left lateral ventricle due to hippocampal volume loss. Compare this appearance with the normal right hippocampus (H).

coronal plane to search for developmental abnormalities, some of which may be extremely subtle. Where MRI is unavailable, or in emergency situations, CT can detect surgical lesions such as haemorrhage or tumour.

9.6 DEMENTIA

The term dementia refers to deterioration of cognitive and intellectual functions not due to impaired consciousness or perception. Dementia should be differentiated clinically from delirium (acute transient confusion); psychiatric illness, such as depression; and specific brain lesions leading to restricted function, such as aphasia. Much research is currently directed at potential therapies for various types of dementia, making classification and accurate diagnosis increasingly important. Accurate diagnosis is also important for counselling of the patient and their family. The commonest causes of dementia are Alzheimer disease (up to 80% of cases) and multi-infarct dementia (10%). Alzheimer disease is suggested clinically by:

- Insidious onset of dementia after the age of 60 with progressive worsening
- Prominent loss of memory, especially of new material
- No focal neurological signs on examination.

Multi-infarct dementia occurs in patients with risk factors for atheromatous disease and stroke, such as tobacco smoking, hypertension and diabetes. Multi-infarct dementia is characterized clinically by:

- Sudden onset of cognitive decline with a stepwise deterioration in function
- Accompanying focal signs on neurological examination such as weakness of an extremity or gait disturbance.

Less commonly, dementia may be due to communicating hydrocephalus or chronic subdural haematoma, with rare causes such as frontotemporal dementia and Creutzfeldt–Jakob disease also described.

CT and MRI are the primary imaging investigations of patients with dementia. CT excludes a surgical cause of cognitive decline, such as a subdural haematoma or tumour. Following this, MRI is more accurate than CT and is the investigation of choice for underlying conditions, such as cerebral amyloid angiopathy and hippocampal abnormality. Signs of Alzheimer disease on MRI include cortical atrophy in the parietal and temporal lobes with marked volume loss of the hippocampal formation (Fig. 9.14). MRI signs of multi-infarct dementia include T2 hyperintensity in the periventricular and deep cortical white matter and lacunar or larger established infarcts in the basal ganglia, white matter and cortical grey matter. The MRI report in the context of cognitive decline may include various scores that grade the degree of cerebral atrophy (global cortical atrophy (GCA) 0–3), the extent of ischaemic changes (Fazekas score 0–3) and the severity of medial temporal lobe atrophy (MTA 0–4). The use of these scores on MRI may help in differentiating major causes of dementia, with implications for prognostication, risk factor management and possible specific therapies currently under development and investigation.

Scintigraphy may also be performed to assess focal glucose metabolism with fluorodeoxyglucose (FDG)–positron emission tomography (PET)

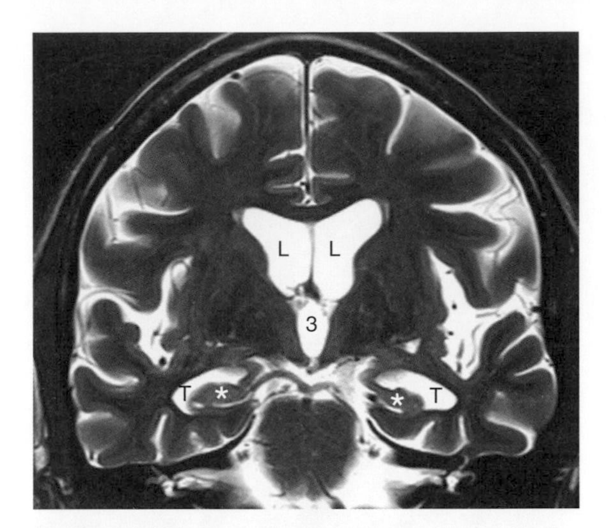

Figure 9.14 Alzheimer dementia: coronal T2-weighted MRI. Signs of diffuse cerebral atrophy include enlargement of the lateral (L) and third (3) ventricles, plus prominent cerebral sulci secondary to volume loss. In keeping with Alzheimer dementia there is bilateral hippocampal atrophy (*) and dilatation of the temporal horns (T).

or regional CBF with ^{99m}Tc-HMPAO (see Table 1.1). FDG-PET shows reduced glucose metabolism in the temporal and parietal lobes in Alzheimer disease; ^{99m}Tc-HMPAO shows reduced blood flow in these regions. In multi-infarct dementia, FDG-PET shows more widespread areas of reduced cortical and white matter metabolism. Other PET radiopharmaceuticals are undergoing development and clinical trials in the assessment of Alzheimer disease. These include agents that bind to β-amyloid fibrils and tau protein.

9.7 MULTIPLE SCLEROSIS

Multiple sclerosis (MS) is a chronic CNS disease of young adults characterized by the presence in the brain and spinal cord of focal lesions of demyelination, known as plaques. In the brain, MS has a characteristic distribution, with plaques tending to occur along the walls of the lateral ventricles, corpus callosum, subcortical white matter and posterior fossa. Plaques may also be seen in the spinal cord. The clinical presentation is extremely variable and may include diplopia or impaired vision as a result of optic neuritis, weakness, numbness and tingling in the limbs, and gait disturbance. Clinical findings on neurological examination often reflect the multifocal nature of the disease. In addition, the time course and nature of disease progression are quite variable. The most common presentation is an initial relapsing–remitting pattern characterized by episodic symptoms interspersed with periods of recovery. In most cases this develops into a secondary progressive phase. Less common presentations are a primary progressive form without relapses and a benign form in which patients may remain functionally active for many years.

MRI is the imaging investigation of choice for the diagnosis of MS. CT is not sensitive for the demonstration of MS plaques. Plaques appear on MRI as T2 hyperintense lesions, measuring more than 3 mm. Because CSF is also T2 hyperintense, small periventricular plaques may be difficult to see on T2-weighted images. FLAIR sequences show CSF as black and MS plaques as focal white lesions, and therefore provide more accurate demonstration of subtle plaques (Fig. 9.15). Chronic plaques may show on T1-weighted images as discrete low-signal lesions (black holes). DWI and gadolinium-enhanced T1-weighted images are also performed as so-called 'active' plaques may show restricted diffusion and

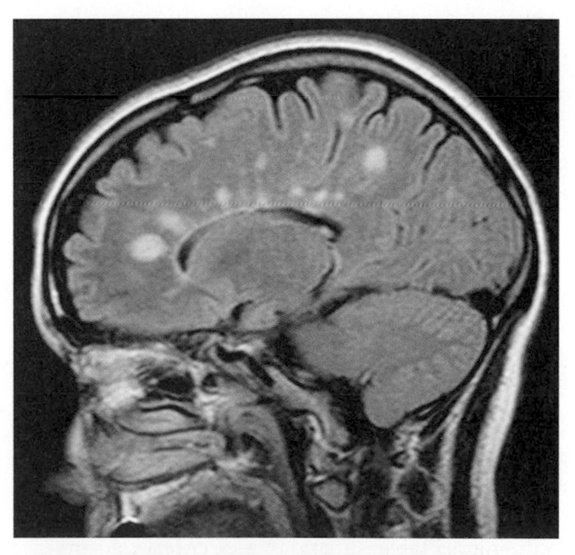

Figure 9.15 Multiple sclerosis: MRI. Sagittal fluid-attenuated inversion recovery (FLAIR) MRI shows multiple high-signal white matter lesions.

enhancement. On follow-up MRI studies the plaques may vary in appearance, with, for example, 'active' plaques becoming non-enhancing.

Because of the importance of achieving a correct diagnosis in young adults, diagnostic criteria have been developed. Known as the McDonald criteria, these were released in 2001 and revised multiple times, most recently in 2017. The McDonald criteria incorporate a combination of clinical factors, CSF findings (oligoclonal immunoglobulin G (IgG) bands) and MRI appearances to diagnose MS. The MRI components of the McDonald criteria include dissemination in space and dissemination in time. Dissemination in space refers to the lesion location and requires the presence of one or more typical lesions in two out of four typical locations: periventricular, cortical or subcortical, posterior fossa (infratentorial) and spinal cord. Dissemination in time reflects the dynamic nature of the disease and refers to the appearance of new lesions on serial imaging or the simultaneous presence of a gadolinium-enhancing lesion with a non-enhancing lesion on any single MRI study.

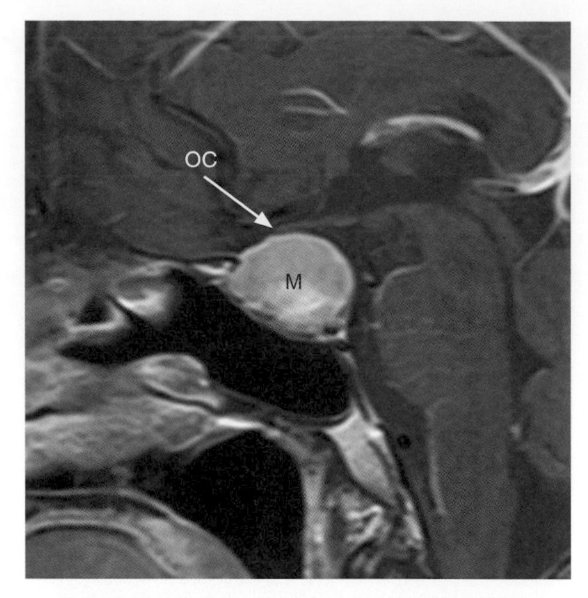

Figure 9.16 Pituitary macroadenoma: MRI. Sagittal T1-weighted contrast-enhanced MRI shows a large pituitary mass (M) expanding the pituitary fossa, with suprasellar extension contacting the optic chiasm (OC).

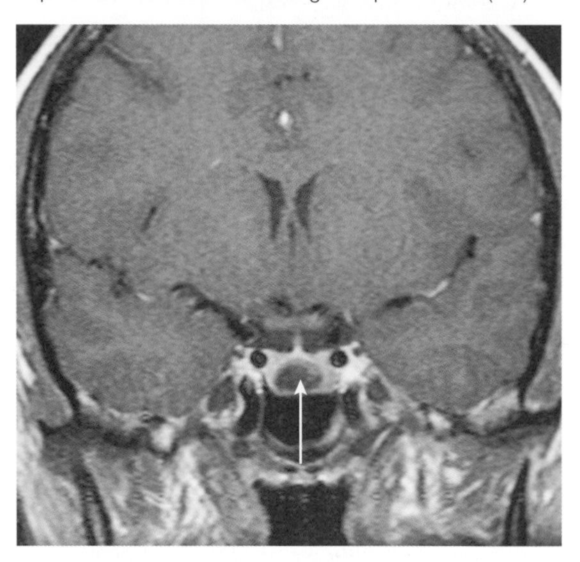

Figure 9.17 Pituitary microadenoma: MRI. Coronal T1-weighted contrast-enhanced MRI of the pituitary gland shows a small non-enhancing mass (arrow) surrounded by normally enhancing pituitary tissue.

9.8 IMAGING OF THE PITUITARY GLAND

The pituitary gland consists of two functionally separate components:

- Adenohypophysis (anterior pituitary): secretes the hormones adrenocorticotropic hormone (ACTH), thyroid-stimulating hormone (TSH), luteinizing hormone (LH), follicle-stimulating hormone (FSH), growth hormone and prolactin
- Neurohypophysis (posterior pituitary): stores hormones secreted by the hypothalamus (vasopressin and oxytocin).

The pituitary stalk connects the pituitary gland to the hypothalamus and contains axons that transport releasing hormones. Tumours of the pituitary region include:

- Pituitary adenomas, classified by hormonal status (Table 9.1) and by size criteria:
    - Macroadenoma: greater than 10 mm (Fig. 9.16)
    - Microadenoma: less than 10 mm (Fig. 9.17)
- Pituitary carcinoma (rare)
- Meningioma
- Craniopharyngioma
- Metastasis

Table 9.1 Clinical syndromes associated with pituitary adenomas.

Adenoma type	Relative incidence (%)	Hormone produced	Clinical presentation
Prolactinoma	30	Prolactin	Amenorrhoea, galactorrhoea, infertility
Corticotropic adenoma	14	ACTH	Cushing syndrome
Somatotropic adenoma	14	Growth hormone	Gigantism; acromegaly
Gonadotroph cell adenoma	7	FSH, LH	Menstrual irregularity; headache
Thyrotroph cell adenoma	1	TSH	Thyrotoxicosis
Plurihormonal adenoma	5	Multiple	Variable
Non-functioning adenoma	27	None	Pressure effects

Abbreviations: ACTH, adrenocorticotropic hormone; FSH, follicle-stimulating hormone; LH, luteinizing hormone; TSH, thyroid-stimulating hormone.

- Optic chiasm glioma
  - Commonly associated with neurofibromatosis type 1.

Pituitary region tumours may present clinically in multiple ways, depending on the size, location and hormonal status of the tumour:

- Compression of structures:
  - Pituitary: hypopituitarism
  - Optic chiasm: bitemporal hemianopia
- Raised intracranial pressure due to a large tumour or obstructive hydrocephalus:
  - Headache, nausea, vomiting
- Endocrine syndromes.

Endocrine syndromes associated with pathology of the pituitary gland and hypothalamus include:

- Pituitary dwarfism:
  - Hypoplasia of adenohypophysis
  - Ectopic neurohypophysis
  - Absent pituitary stalk
- Central diabetes insipidus:
  - Dysfunction of neurohypophysis or hypothalamus due to tumour, Langerhans cell histiocytosis, infection or trauma
- Precocious puberty:
  - Hamartoma or other neoplasm of hypothalamus
- Hypersecretion syndromes:
  - Pituitary adenomas (Table 9.1).

MRI is the investigation of choice for imaging of the pituitary gland and adjacent structures. Sagittal T1-weighted images demonstrate the lobar anatomy of the pituitary:

- Adenohypophysis of similar signal intensity to brain tissue
- Neurohypophysis seen as a posterior 'bright spot'.

Coronal T1-weighted scans with contrast enhancement are particularly useful for the diagnosis of microadenomas. Macroadenomas may involve adjacent structures, including the cavernous sinuses, cavernous segment of the ICA, sphenoid sinus and suprasellar cistern. When MRI is unavailable or contraindicated, CT may be used, though it is much less sensitive.

SUMMARY

Clinical presentation	Investigation of choice	Comment
Subarachnoid haemorrhage	CT	
Screening for cerebral artery aneurysm	CTA/MRA	
Stroke	• CT head • CT angiogram	Increasing role in stroke centres for MRI and functional studies including DWI, PWI and perfusion CT
Brain tumour (suspected space-occupying lesion)	MRI	
Carotid or vertebral artery dissection	MRI/MRA	
Intracranial infection	MRI	
Seizure	MRI	
Dementia	MRI	Scintigraphy in selected cases: FDG-PET, ^{99m}Tc-HMPAO
Multiple sclerosis	MRI	

Abbreviations: DWI, diffusion-weighted imaging; FDG, fluorodeoxyglucose; HMPAO, hexamethylpropyleneamine oxime; MRA, magnetic resonance angiography; PWI, perfusion-weighted imaging.

10 Central nervous system: spine

10.1 RADIOGRAPHIC ANATOMY OF THE SPINE

The anatomical features of each vertebral body that can be identified radiographically include (Fig. 10.1):

- Anterior vertebral body
- Posterior arch formed by the pedicles and lamina, enclosing the spinal canal
- Pedicles: posterior bony projections from the posterolateral corners of the vertebral body
- Laminae curve posteromedially from the pedicles and join in the midline at the base of the spinous process to complete the bony arch of the spinal canal

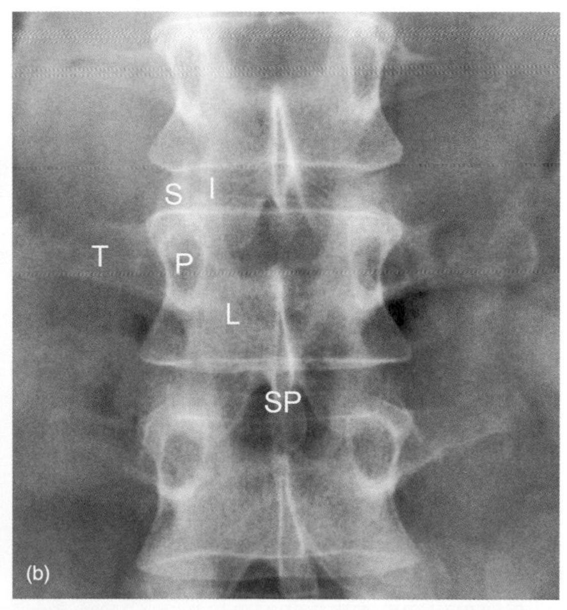

Figure 10.1 Normal lumbar spine anatomy. (a) Lateral view. (b) Frontal view. Note the following features: vertebral body (B), intervertebral disc (D), facet joint (F), intervertebral foramen (Fo), inferior articular process (I), lamina (L), pedicle (P), superior articular process (S), spinous process (SP), transverse process (T).

- Spinous process projects posteriorly
- Transverse processes project laterally from the junction of pedicle and lamina.

Articulations between adjoining vertebrae include the intervertebral disc, zygapophyseal joints and uncovertebral joints:

- Intervertebral disc:
  - Occupies the space between each vertebral body
  - Composed of a central nucleus pulposus enclosed by annulus fibrosis
- Zygapophyseal joints:
  - Commonly known as facet joints
  - Formed by articular processes that project superiorly and inferiorly from the junction of the pedicle and lamina
- Uncovertebral joints:
  - Found in the cervical spine
  - Formed by a ridge or lip of bone that projects superiorly from the lateral edge of the vertebral body and articulates with the lateral edge of the vertebral body above.

The exception to the above pattern occurs at the first and second cervical vertebrae (C1 and C2). C1, also known as the 'atlas', consists of an anterior arch, two lateral masses and a posterior arch. Lateral masses of C1 articulate superiorly with the occiput (atlanto-occipital joints) and inferiorly with the superior articular processes of C2 (atlanto-axial joints). The odontoid peg or dens is a vertical projection of bone that extends superiorly from the body of C2 and articulates with the anterior arch of C1.

See Chapter 12 for further notes on assessment of spine radiographs in a setting of trauma.

10.2 NECK PAIN

Non-traumatic neck pain is an extremely common complaint. Most cases of neck pain are due to musculoligamentous strain or injury. Seventy per cent of episodes of neck pain resolve within 1 month. Most of the remaining 30% resolve over the longer term with a small minority going on to have chronic neck problems. In the clinical assessment of neck pain there are three major sources of diagnostic difficulty:

- Multiple structures, including vertebral bodies, ligaments, muscles, intervertebral discs, vascular and neural structures, can produce pain
- Pain may be referred to the neck from other areas, such as shoulder, heart, diaphragm, mandible and temporomandibular joints
- Pain from the neck may be referred to the shoulders and arms.

10.2.1 OSTEOARTHRITIS OF THE CERVICAL SPINE

Osteoarthritis (degenerative arthropathy) is a major cause of neck pain, with increasing incidence in old age. The primary phenomenon in osteoarthritis of the spine is degeneration of the intervertebral disc, which is most common at C5/6 and C6/7. Degenerate discs may herniate into the spinal canal or intervertebral foramina, with direct compression of the spinal cord or nerve roots. More commonly, disc degeneration leads to abnormal stresses on the vertebral bodies and on the facet and uncovertebral joints. These abnormal stresses promote osteophyte growth, which may project into the spinal canal, causing compression of the cervical cord, or into the intervertebral foramina, causing nerve root compression.

Cervical cord compression presents clinically with neck pain associated with a stiff gait and brisk lower limb reflexes (myelopathy). Other causes of cervical myelopathy include:

- Syrinx
- Spinal cord tumours: ependymoma, glioma, neurofibroma, meningioma
- Vertebral body tumours: metastases, giant cell tumour, chordoma.

Nerve root compression produces local neck pain plus pain in the distribution of the compressed nerve (radiculopathy). Osteoarthritis uncomplicated by compression of neural structures may cause episodic neck pain with the following features:

- Tends to be increased by activity (mechanical)
- May be associated with shoulder pain or headache
- Usually resolves within 7–10 days.

10.2.2 IMAGING OF THE PATIENT WITH NECK PAIN

The goals of imaging of the patient with neck pain should be to exclude conditions requiring urgent attention, to diagnose a treatable condition and to direct management. With these goals in mind, and given the fact that most neck pain resolves spontaneously, it follows that most patients do not require imaging. Imaging should be reserved for those patients whose symptoms are severe and persistent, or for those who have other relevant factors on history or examination, such as trauma or a known primary tumour.

Initial imaging in most cases consists of a radiograph of the cervical spine. Radiographic signs of osteoarthritis of the cervical spine (Fig. 10.2):

- Disc space narrowing, most commonly at C5/6 and C6/7
- Osteophyte formation on the vertebral bodies and facet joints

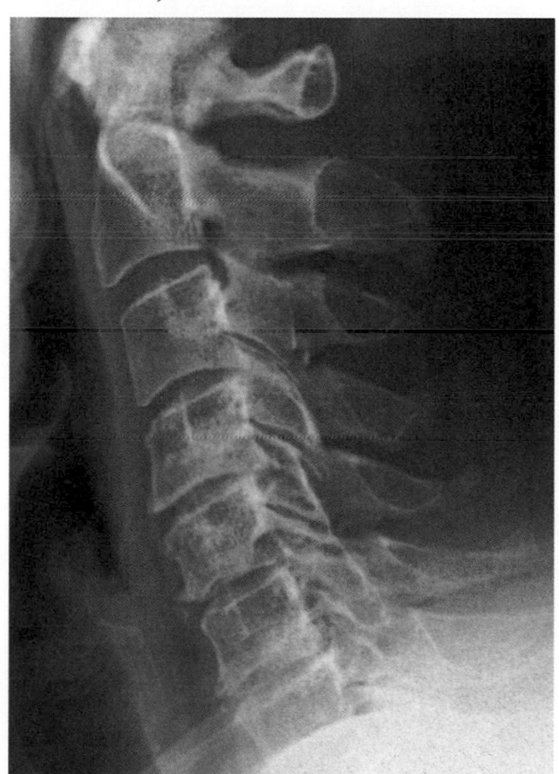

Figure 10.2 Osteoarthritis of the cervical spine. Note disc space narrowing at multiple levels.

- Osteophytes projecting into the intervertebral foramina.

Magnetic resonance imaging (MRI) is the investigation of choice when further imaging is required for persistent nerve root pain or for assessment of a possible spinal cord abnormality. Computed tomography (CT) is used in the investigation of neck pain when fine bone detail is required, such as in the assessment of a vertebral body tumour.

10.3 LOW BACK PAIN

Low back pain refers to back pain that does not extend below the iliac crests. Pain extending to the buttocks or legs is referred to as sciatica; this is a separate clinical problem from back pain and is considered in section 10.5. Low back pain may be classified into acute or chronic, with the term 'acute back pain' usually referring to pain of less than 12 weeks' duration. There are now well-developed evidence-based guidelines for the management and investigation of acute back pain from which several consistent recommendations can be identified. Primary among these is the need for diagnostic triage of patients into three major groups:

- Non-specific low back pain, acute or chronic
- Specific low back pain
- Sciatica or radiculopathy, with neurological findings such as a positive straight leg raise test.

As will be discussed in section 10.5, sciatica is best investigated with MRI or CT. Specific low back pain refers to back pain with associated clinical symptoms or signs, known as 'red flags', that may indicate an underlying problem. Examples of these 'red flags', some of which will be discussed below, include:

- Known primary tumour such as prostate or breast
- Systemic symptoms: unexplained fever or weight loss
- Recent trauma
- Known osteoporosis or prolonged steroid use
- Age at onset of pain: younger than 20 years or older than 55 years
- Thoracic pain
- Neurological changes.

10.3.1 ACUTE NON-SPECIFIC LOW BACK PAIN

All the evidence-based guidelines on acute back pain agree that imaging assessment, including radiography of the lumbar spine, is not indicated in patients with non-specific acute back pain. This reflects the fact that most cases of non-specific low back pain are due to musculoligamentous injury or exacerbation of degenerative arthropathy and will usually resolve within a few weeks. Most guidelines emphasize the importance of reassurance, discouragement of bed rest and the recognition of psychosocial risk factors that may predispose to chronic back pain.

10.3.2 CHRONIC NON-SPECIFIC LOW BACK PAIN

Most of the evidence in the medical literature dealing with the problem of chronic low back pain points to the exclusion of 'red flags' (see above). A multidisciplinary approach to therapy is often required, including exercise, education and counselling. A specific diagnosis as to the cause of pain is often not required. In some cases, however, particularly when pain is severe and debilitating or is due to other factors such as loss of employment or depression, a specific diagnosis may be required as a guide to therapy.

Most cases of chronic back pain are due to facet joint pain, sacroiliac joint (SIJ) pain or internal disruption of intervertebral discs. Imaging techniques such as radiography, CT and MRI can show changes of degenerative arthropathy in a large percentage of patients examined (Fig. 10.3). A major problem with imaging in this context is that findings are very non-specific; imaging is often unable to pinpoint the cause of pain. For example, radiographs may show a narrowed disc space; this does not mean that this is the cause of the patient's pain.

The only way to prove that a certain structure such as a facet joint is the cause of pain is to inject local anaesthetic (LA) into that structure and assess the response. Image-guided interventions are now commonplace in the management of chronic back pain and are performed under CT or fluoroscopic guidance (see section 10.6). It should be emphasized that, in the absence of 'red flags', imaging is not indicated in most patients with chronic non-specific low back pain.

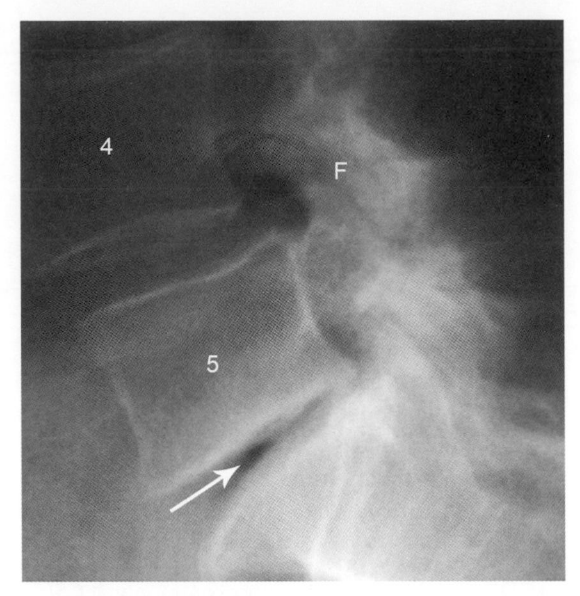

Figure 10.3 Osteoarthritis of the lumbar spine. Narrowing of the intervertebral disc space between L5 and S1 (arrow). Sclerosis of the facet joints at L4/5 (F) with degenerative spondylolisthesis at this level.

10.4 SPECIFIC BACK PAIN SYNDROMES

Imaging may be required for the assessment of back pain associated with 'red flags' as listed above. An initial radiographic examination of the lumbar spine is reasonable in these patients. This will help exclude obvious bony causes of pain, as well as delineate any other relevant factors such as scoliosis.

Limitations of radiographs of the lumbar spine:

- Soft-tissue structures such as ligaments, muscles and nerve roots are not imaged
- Relatively insensitive for many painful bone conditions such as infection
- Cross-sectional dimensions of the spinal canal are not assessed.

In many conditions such as suspected infection or suspected acute osteoporotic crush fracture, MRI is the investigation of choice. CT is highly accurate for the assessment of bony lesions such as suspected tumours or pars interarticularis defects. Scintigraphy with ^{99m}Tc-MDP (see Table 1.1) may be indicated in certain instances, such as:

- To exclude spinal metastases where there is a known primary tumour
- To pinpoint skeletal pathology as a source of severe chronic pain, e.g. selecting a specific facet joint that may be amenable to injection where there is multilevel facet osteoarthritis.

10.4.1 PARS INTERARTICULARIS DEFECTS AND SPONDYLOLISTHESIS

The pars interarticularis is the mass of bone between the superior and inferior articular processes of the vertebra. Defects of the pars interarticularis, also known as spondylolysis, may be congenital or due to trauma:

- Congenital pars interarticularis defects are often associated with other developmental anomalies of the lumbar spine, especially failure of complete bony fusion of the laminae in the midline
- Acute trauma may produce an acute fracture through the pars interarticularis, and stress fractures may occur in association with sports such as gymnastics and cricket fast bowling.

Regardless of aetiology, pars interarticularis defects may be unilateral or bilateral, and are most common at L5. Bilateral pars defects may be associated with spondylolisthesis, i.e. anterior shift of L5 on S1. Back pain in spondylolysis and spondylolisthesis may be due to several factors, including:

- The bony defects themselves
- Segmental instability
- Degenerative changes in the intervertebral disc.

Spondylolysis is suspected in otherwise healthy young adults presenting with back pain, particularly those participating in typical sporting activities. Spondylolisthesis also causes narrowing of the intervertebral foramina between L5 and S1 with compression of the exiting L5 nerve roots, producing

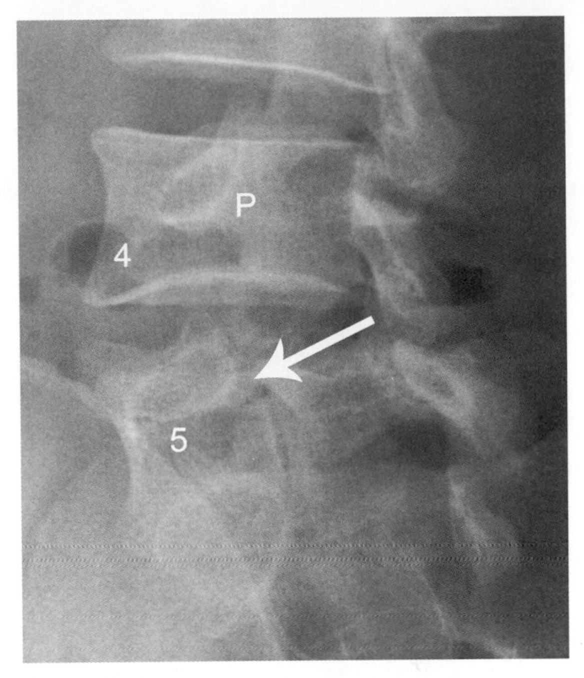

Figure 10.4 Pars interarticularis defect. Oblique view of the lower lumbar spine showing a pars interarticularis defect at L5 (arrow). Also note the intact pars interarticularis at L4 (P).

bilateral posterior leg pain and a sensation of hamstring tightness.

Radiographically, pars interarticularis defects are best seen on oblique views of the lower lumbar spine. The complex of overlapping shadows from the superior and inferior articular processes, the pars interarticularis, and the transverse process forms an outline resembling that of a Scottish terrier dog. A pars defect is seen as a line across the neck of the 'dog' (Fig. 10.4).

CT and single photon emission CT (SPECT)-CT with ^{99m}Tc-MDP may be used to diagnose spondylolysis and spondylolisthesis. These techniques are associated with exposure to ionizing radiation, a particular disadvantage in young adults. For this reason, MRI is now the investigation of choice. Dedicated MRI protocols including high-resolution short TI (inversion time) inversion recovery (STIR) and T1-weighted sequences provide detailed images of the spine. Pars defects are well demonstrated, as are foraminal stenosis and nerve root compression. A particular advantage is that STIR sequences can

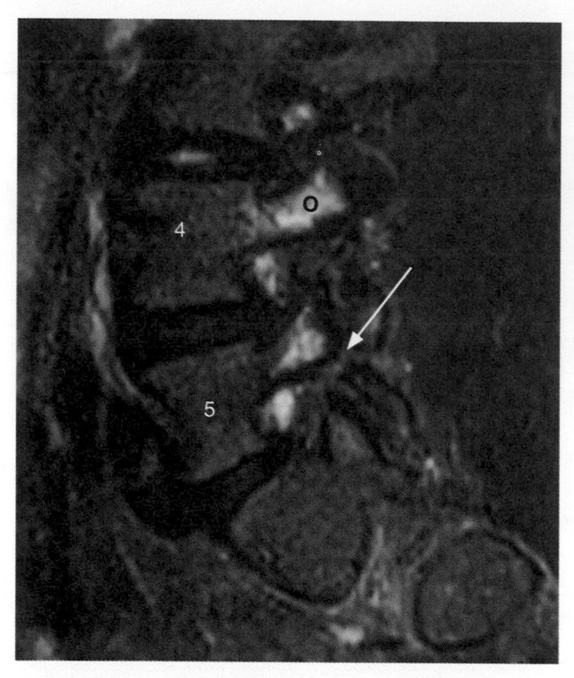

Figure 10.5 Pars defect and stress reaction: MRI sagittal short TI (inversion time) inversion recovery (STIR). A pars defect at L5 is seen as a clear break through the bone (arrow) with oedema in the pedicle indicating an acute lesion. Oedema in the L4 pedicle (O) indicates an acute stress reaction at this level.

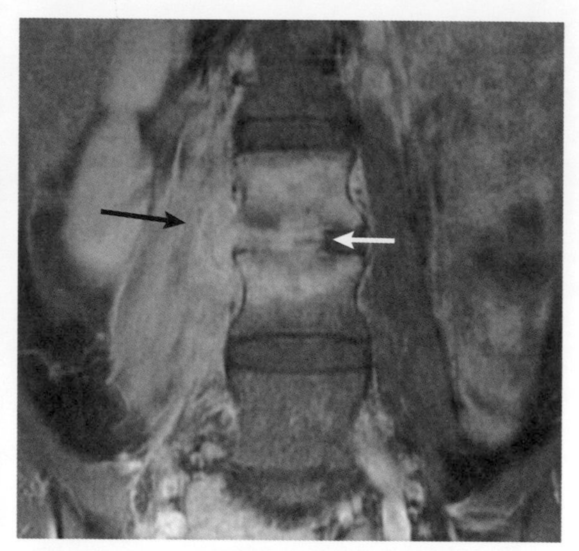

Figure 10.6 Discitis: MRI. Coronal T1-weighted, fat-saturated, contrast-enhanced MRI of the lumbar spine in a 14-year-old girl with severe back pain and fever. Enhancement of the L3/4 intervertebral disc (white arrow). Also note enhancement of the adjacent vertebral bodies and spread of infection into the right psoas muscle (black arrow).

show marrow oedema without an actual defect, indicating a stress reaction or developing stress fracture as a cause of pain (Fig. 10.5). This allows early interventions, such as bracing, that may prevent development of a defect.

10.4.2 VERTEBRAL INFECTION

Most vertebral infection commences in the intervertebral disc (discitis). Discitis may spread to involve the vertebral body, causing vertebral osteomyelitis, or may invade the spinal canal to produce an epidural abscess. Discitis is usually due to blood-borne infection, may occur in children or adults and is more common in the lower spine. Clinical features of discitis include rapid onset of back pain accompanied by fever and malaise. In young children there may be fewer specific symptoms, such as a limp or failure to weight bear.

Radiographic findings of discitis occur late in the disease process and include narrowing of the intervertebral disc with blurring of the vertebral endplates.

MRI is the investigation of choice for suspected vertebral infection. MRI is usually positive at the time of clinical presentation before radiographic signs are evident (Fig. 10.6). Infection causes oedema in the vertebral bodies and intervening disc, with extensive gadolinium enhancement. MRI is also the best imaging method for showing the full extent of infection, including epidural and psoas abscess.

10.4.3 VERTEBRAL METASTASES

Tumours with a high incidence of vertebral metastases include prostate, breast, lung, kidney and melanoma. Lymphoma and multiple myeloma may also involve the spine. Vertebral metastatic disease is suspected when back pain occurs in a patient with a known primary tumour. Other suspicious clinical factors include weight loss and raised prostate-specific antigen (PSA).

Radiographs of the spine may show focal sclerotic (dense) lesions throughout the vertebral bodies in metastases from a prostatic primary. Other primary tumours tend to produce lytic or destructive metastases that may be difficult to appreciate on radiographs (Fig. 10.7). SPECT-CT with ^{99m}Tc-MDP is generally the investigation of choice in screening for skeletal metastases, including the spine.

Occasionally, a vertebral metastasis may expand into the spinal canal and compress the spinal cord, causing an acute myelopathy. Clinical features of myelopathy include:

- Motor problems in the legs, leading to difficulty with walking
- Sensory disturbances; a band-like sensation around the abdomen
- Voiding difficulties.

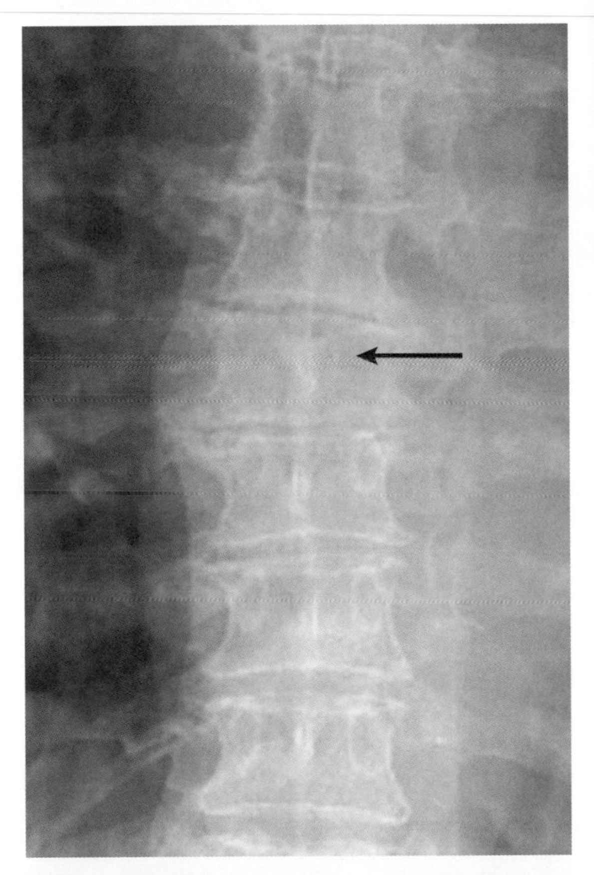

Figure 10.7 Vertebral metastasis: radiograph. Sudden-onset back pain and leg weakness in a 62-year-old woman with a history of breast cancer. Frontal radiograph shows reduced height of the T6 vertebral body. Note loss of visualization of the left pedicle due to bone destruction (arrow).

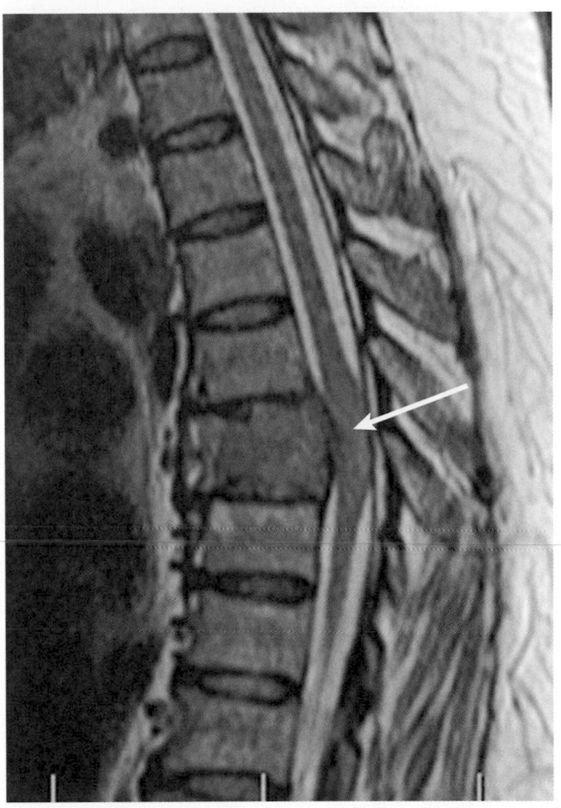

Figure 10.8 Vertebral metastasis: MRI. Same patient as in Fig. 10.7. Sagittal T2-weighted MRI shows destruction and partial collapse of T6. Neoplastic tissue is invading the spinal canal and compressing the spinal cord (arrow).

Cord compression as a result of metastatic disease is most common in the thoracic region and may require acute surgical decompression or radiotherapy. MRI is the investigation of choice for suspected spinal cord compression (Fig. 10.8).

10.4.4 ACUTE OSTEOPOROTIC CRUSH FRACTURE

Individuals with osteoporosis are at an increased risk for the development of a crush fracture of the spine. Osteoporotic crush fractures may occur at any level, though are most common in the lower thoracic and lumbar spine. The patient usually presents with acute back pain that is mechanical in type, i.e. worsened by movement or activity. There may be an associated band-like distribution of pain around the chest wall or abdomen, depending on the level involved. The pain associated with osteoporotic crush fracture usually settles in a matter of weeks. In some patients, however, the pain may persist and produce numerous complications:

- Reduced mobility
- Inhibition of respiration
- Difficulty sleeping
- Significant mortality and morbidity in elderly patients.

Radiographs of the spine will usually diagnose a crush fracture (see Fig. 12.18). Affected vertebral bodies may show a wedge shape, concavity of one or both vertebral end plates and, in more severe cases, flattening. A major limitation of radiography is that there is no reliable way to distinguish an acute crush fracture from an older healed injury. This becomes particularly relevant when percutaneous vertebroplasty is being considered and multiple crush fractures are seen radiographically. MRI can show bone marrow oedema in acutely crushed vertebral bodies (see Fig. 12.22). Older healed crush fractures show normal bone marrow signal with no evidence of oedema.

10.4.5 SCOLIOSIS

Scoliosis refers to abnormal curvature of the spine, with a lateral component of greater than 10°. Recognized causes of scoliosis include:

- Congenital as a result of abnormal vertebral segmentation (Fig. 10.9a)
- Underlying syndrome such as neurofibromatosis
- Severe degenerative disease in elderly patients

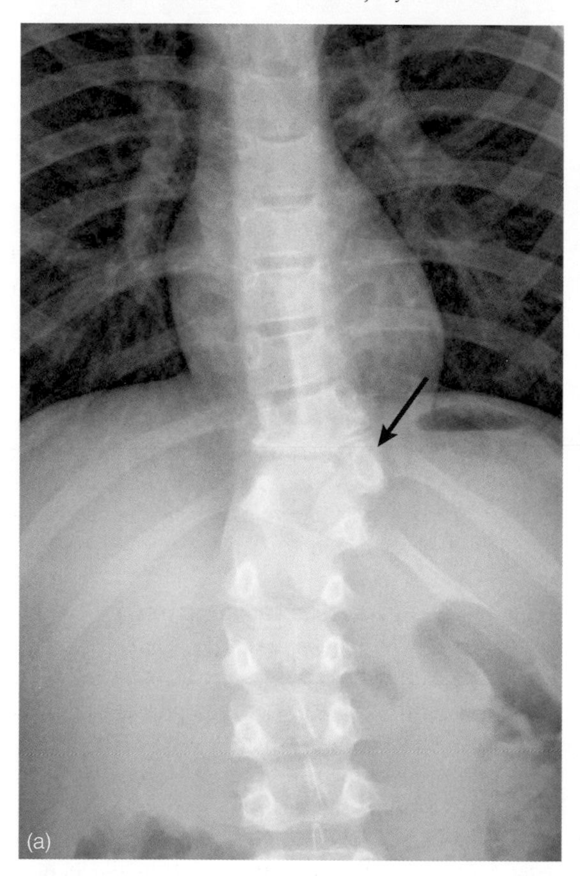

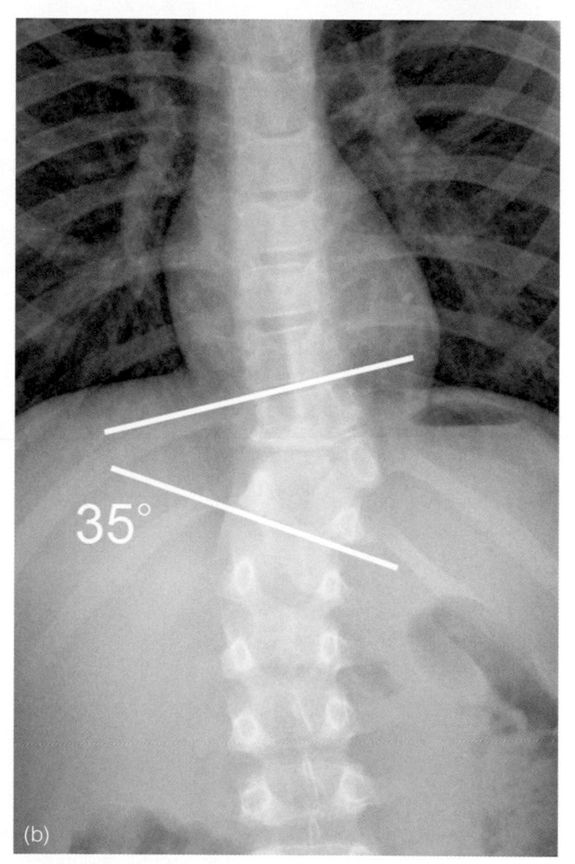

Figure 10.9 Vertebral anomaly causing scoliosis. (a) Frontal radiograph shows a left-sided hemivertebra in the lower thoracic spine (arrow). Note that the hemivertebra articulates with an unpaired left rib. (b) Cobb angle measurement: note the method of Cobb angle measurement as outlined in the text.

- Acute painful scoliosis may indicate the presence of vertebral infection or a tumour such as osteoid osteoma.

Most commonly, scoliosis is idiopathic. Idiopathic scoliosis is classified according to the age of onset with three major groups described:

- Infantile: birth to 4 years
- Juvenile: 4–10 years
- Adolescent: 10 years or older.

Adolescent idiopathic scoliosis (AIS) accounts for 90% of patients with scoliosis. The key clinical test for the diagnosis of AIS is the forward bend test. A positive forward bend test is indicated by convex bulging of the contour of the back on the side of the convexity of the spinal curve owing to rotation of the spine producing prominence of the posterior ribs on the convex side.

Patients with suspected scoliosis should be assessed radiographically with a single anteroposterior (AP) long film of the thoracic and lumbar spine taken with the patient standing erect. The key to radiographic diagnosis and follow-up is measurement of the Cobb angle, which is calculated as follows:

1. Identify the most tilted vertebral bodies above and below the apex of the curve
2. Draw a line parallel to the superior vertebral endplate of the most tilted vertebral body at the upper end of the curve
3. Draw a similar line parallel to the lower vertebral endplate of the lower most tilted vertebral body
4. The angle between these lines is the Cobb angle (Fig. 10.9b).

A Cobb angle of 10° or greater is considered abnormal. Curves are described by their region – thoracic or lumbar – and by the direction of convexity, e.g. a 'right curve' is convex to the right. The largest curve is termed the 'major' or 'primary' curve. Compensatory or secondary curves occur above and/or below the primary curve; these usually have smaller Cobb angles than the primary curve. The most common pattern in AIS is a right thoracic primary curve with a left lumbar or thoracolumbar secondary curve. A single erect radiograph is usually sufficient for the imaging assessment of AIS.

Uncommonly, further imaging with MRI may be indicated for the following:

- Neurological signs
- Certain radiographic abnormalities, e.g. bone destruction such as may indicate the presence of a vertebral tumour
- Atypical curves, such as a left thoracic primary curve may be associated with a syrinx of the cord.

10.5 SCIATICA

Radiculopathy is defined as symptoms caused by compression or inflammation of a nerve root. Nerve root distribution pain caused by cervical or thoracic spine pathology is referred to as cervical or thoracic radiculopathy. The term sciatica refers to lower limb radiculopathy, with pain affecting the lower back and buttock, hip and lower limb. Sciatica may be accompanied by other neurological symptoms, such as paraesthesia, and by signs of nerve root irritation, such as a positive straight leg raise test.

Sciatica is usually caused by herniation of an intervertebral disc or by spinal stenosis owing to degenerative disease. Each intervertebral disc is composed of a tough fibrous outer layer, the annulus fibrosis, and a softer semifluid centre, the nucleus pulposus. With degeneration of the disc, small microtears appear in the annulus fibrosis, allowing generalized bulging of the nucleus pulposus. This causes the disc to bulge beyond the margins of the vertebral bodies, causing narrowing of the spinal canal. Secondary effects of degenerative disc disease include abnormal stresses on the vertebral bodies, leading to osteophyte formation, as well as facet joint sclerosis and hypertrophy. These changes may lead to further narrowing of the spinal canal, producing spinal canal stenosis.

A common complication of disc degeneration is the occurrence of a localized tear in the annulus fibrosis through which the nucleus pulposus may herniate. Disc herniation may project into the spinal canal or posterolaterally into the intervertebral foramen, causing compression of nerve roots. 'Free fragment' or 'sequestration' are terms that refer to a fragment of disc that has broken off from the 'parent' disc; this fragment may migrate superiorly or inferiorly in the spinal canal.

10.5.1 SCIATICA SYNDROMES

Sciatica or leg pain syndromes are classified based on whether the pain is acute or chronic and whether it is unilateral or bilateral:

- Unilateral acute nerve root compression: 'classical' sciatica:
  - Usually caused by focal disc herniation
- Bilateral acute nerve root compression: cauda equina syndrome:
  - Cauda equina syndrome refers to the sudden onset of bilateral leg pain accompanied by bladder and/or bowel dysfunction
  - Usually caused by a massive disc herniation or sequestration
- Unilateral chronic nerve root compression: sciatica lasting for months:
  - Unilateral chronic sciatica may be caused by disc herniation or spinal stenosis
- Bilateral chronic nerve root compression:
  - Bilateral chronic nerve root compression refers to vague bilateral leg pain aggravated by walking and slowly relieved by rest
  - Usually caused by spinal canal stenosis
  - A common clinical difficulty is differentiating neural compression from vascular claudication:
    - Clinical pointers that indicate a vascular cause include absent peripheral pulses, pain in the exercised muscles and rapid resolution of pain with rest.

10.5.2 IMAGING OF SCIATICA

MRI is the investigation of choice for most neurological disorders of the spine, including sciatica. Advantages of MRI in this context include:

- Better soft-tissue contrast resolution than CT
- Nerve roots and the distal spinal cord and conus can be imaged without the use of contrast material
- Able to outline the anatomy of the spinal canal and the intervertebral discs
- Highly sensitive for the detection of spinal canal stenosis, disc herniation and narrowing of the intervertebral foramina (Fig. 10.10).

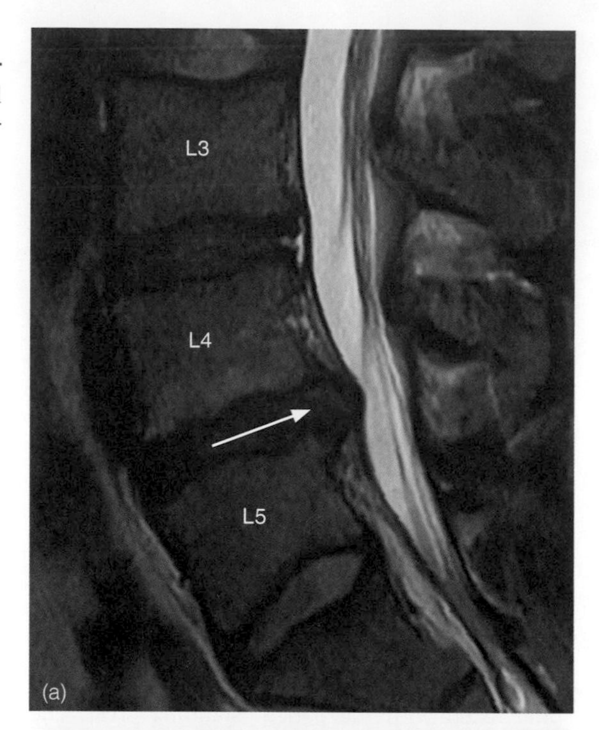

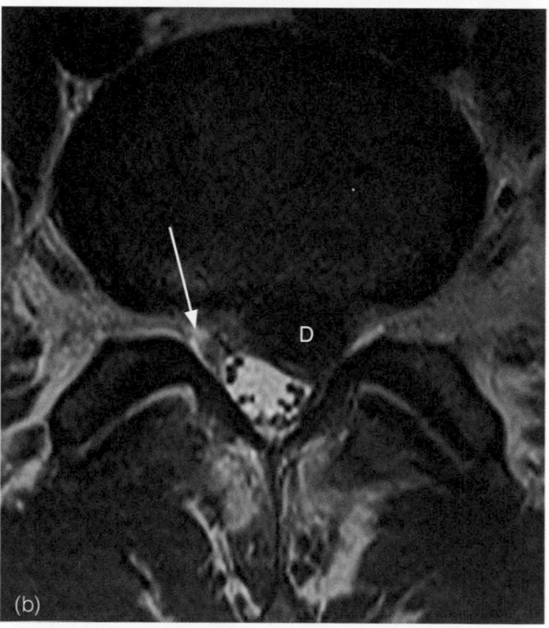

Figure 10.10 Disc herniation: MRI in a patient with left-sided sciatica. (a) Sagittal T2-weighted image shows disc herniation into the spinal canal at L4/5 (arrow). (b) Transverse T2-weighted image shows a low-signal disc protrusion (D) compressing the left side of the thecal sac and the origin of the left L5 nerve root. The right L5 nerve root is not affected (arrow).

CT is a reasonable alternative for the investigation of sciatica when MRI is not available or is contraindicated.

10.6 IMAGE-GUIDED INTERVENTIONS IN THE SPINE

Image-guided interventions are increasingly common in the management of neck and back pain, upper and lower limb radiculopathy and acute vertebral crush fracture. Most procedures outlined in this section have the following features in common:

- Performed under CT or fluoroscopic guidance
- Use of fine needles, 22–25 gauge
- Injection of local anaesthetic and corticosteroid (LACS).

Complications are very rare and may include haemorrhage or infection. A rare but devastating complication that has been encountered is embolization and occlusion of small arteries associated with particulate steroids. This has caused infarcts of the cord, brainstem and cerebellum with irreversible neurological sequalae. This complication is prevented using water-soluble steroid preparations for all procedures related to the spine. Contraindications are few and include severe coagulopathy and unsuitable anatomy.

10.6.1 FACET JOINT INJECTION

Facet joint injection (Fig. 10.11) of LACS has two roles:

- Diagnostic: confirm facet joint as pain generator
- Therapeutic.

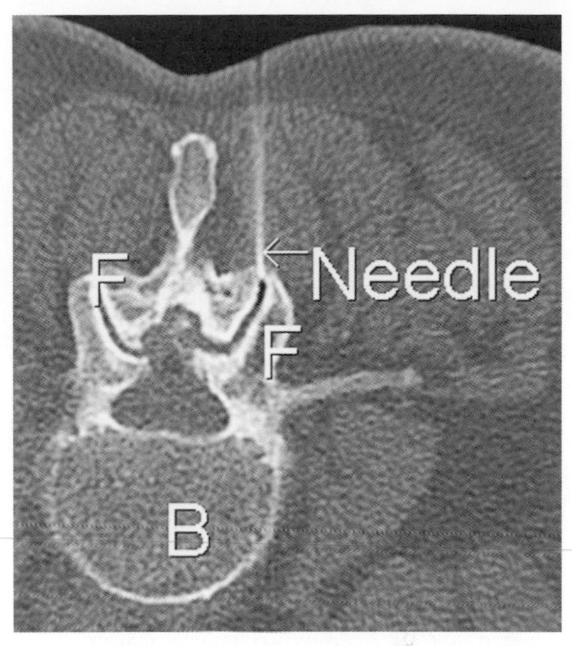

Figure 10.11 Facet joint block: CT guidance. The patient is lying prone with the vertebral body (B) towards the bottom of the image. A fine needle is inserted into the facet joint (F) for injection of local anaesthetic and steroid.

10.6.2 MEDIAL BRANCH BLOCK

Each facet joint receives dual innervation from the medial branches of two contiguous nerve roots:

- For example, each L4/5 facet joint receives innervation from medial branches of the L3 and L4 nerve roots
- These medial branches pass across the bases of the transverse processes of L4 and L5.

For medial branch block fine needles are positioned under imaging guidance at the bases of the relevant transverse processes; LACS or LA alone is injected to block the nerve supply to the facet joint. Indications for medial branch block include:

- Recurrence of symptoms following successful facet joint block
- Confirm facet joint as the pain generator
- Prior to permanent medial branch ablation.

10.6.3 MEDIAL BRANCH ABLATION

The aim of medial branch ablation is long-term pain relief from facet joint denervation.

Facet joint denervation is usually achieved by radiofrequency (RF) ablation of the medial nerve branches supplying the joint. Following injection of LA, the RF probe is placed under imaging guidance with its tip at the known position of the medial nerve branch.

Medial branch ablation is often performed with mild intravenous conscious sedation. General anaesthetic is not used as the patient must be able to respond to sensory and motor stimuli during the procedure.

10.6.4 SACROILIAC JOINT INJECTION

SIJ injection of LACS has two roles:

- Diagnostic: confirm the SIJ as the pain generator
- Therapeutic.

Each SIJ consists of two anatomically separate compartments – fibrous and synovial – and each of these compartments must be injected to maximize the procedure success.

10.6.5 SELECTIVE NERVE ROOT BLOCK

Selective nerve root block (SNRB) is used in patients with upper limb radiculopathy or sciatica as both a diagnostic tool and a means of giving temporary pain relief. SNRB is a relatively simple procedure in which a fine needle is positioned adjacent to the nerve root under CT or fluoroscopic guidance and a small volume of LACS injected. SNRB may be performed safely in the cervical, thoracic or lumbar spine. Indications for SNRB include:

- To confirm the symptomatic level when imaging findings indicate nerve root compression at multiple levels
- Lack of imaging evidence of nerve root compression despite a convincing clinical presentation
- To provide temporary pain relief from sciatica while surgery is planned
- Surgery is contraindicated because of the anaesthetic risk or other factors.

Postprocedure care:

- Some patients experience transient lower limb numbness and a subjective feeling of weakness and may need to be assisted with standing and walking following the procedure
- Patients are advised not to drive a car for a few hours following the procedure.

10.6.6 EPIDURAL INJECTION

Injection of LACS into the epidural space (Fig. 10.12) may be performed for various indications, including:

- Back pain and/or sciatica due to spinal stenosis
- 'Discogenic' back pain due to degenerative changes in the intervertebral discs.

10.6.7 DISCOGRAPHY

Discography is used to prove that pain is arising from one or more intervertebral discs. Under fluoroscopic guidance, a fine needle is positioned in the centre of the intervertebral disc. A small amount of dilute contrast material is injected to 'stress' the disc. The patient's pain response is recorded. Contrast material is used to assess the actual morphology of the disc and to diagnose annular tears.

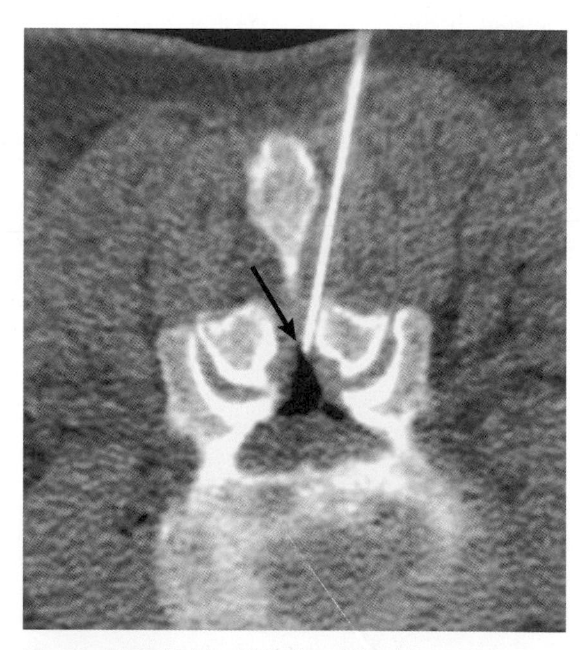

Figure 10.12 Epidural injection: CT guidance. Injection of a small amount of air confirms the needle tip position in the epidural space (arrow) prior to injection of local anaesthetic and steroid.

10.6.8 PERCUTANEOUS VERTEBROPLASTY

Percutaneous vertebroplasty (Fig. 10.13) is now a well-accepted technique for the treatment of the pain associated with acute osteoporotic crush fractures. Prior to vertebroplasty, MRI is used to define the acute level(s), and therefore assists with patient selection and procedure planning. Vertebroplasty involves insertion of a large-bore needle (11 or 13 gauge) into the vertebral body, followed by injection of bone cement. The bone cement is mixed with barium powder so that it can be visualized radiographically. Needle placement and cement injection are performed under direct fluoroscopic guidance to avoid injury to neurological structures. Vertebroplasty is a highly effective technique for reducing pain, restoring mobility and reducing dependence on analgesics. Complications of vertebroplasty are very uncommon and include:

- Haemorrhage
- Leakage of cement into the spinal canal or intervertebral foramina with impingement on the spinal cord and nerve roots
- Embolization of tiny cement fragments into the lungs: usually not clinically significant.

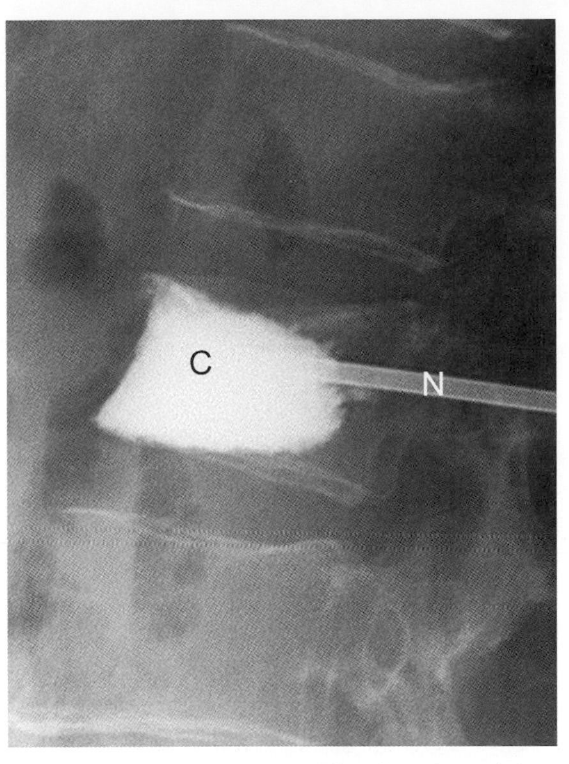

Figure 10.13 Percutaneous vertebroplasty. Lateral view showing radio-opaque bone cement (C) being injected into the vertebral body via an 11-gauge bone biopsy needle (N).

SUMMARY

Clinical presentation	Investigation of choice	Comment
Neck pain	• Imaging not indicated in most cases • Radiography • MRI/CT for radiculopathy/myelopathy	Imaging indicated in neck and back pain for chronic, relapsing or unremitting pain, or in the presence of clinical 'red flags' (see section 10.3)
Back pain	• Imaging not indicated in most cases • Radiography • MRI/CT for radiculopathy/myelopathy	
Spondylolysis and spondylolisthesis	• Radiography • MRI	MRI if sciatica is the dominant symptom
Discitis	MRI	
Vertebral metastases	Bone scintigraphy	MRI if cord compression is suspected
Acute osteoporotic crush fracture(s)	Radiography	MRI where vertebroplasty is contemplated
Scoliosis	Radiography ('long films')	MRI in selected cases
Sciatica	MRI	CT where MRI is unavailable

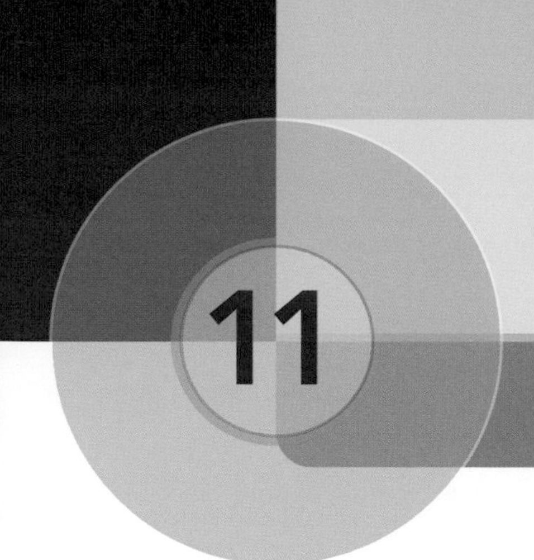

11 Head and neck

The topic of head and neck imaging covers a wide range of pathologies of the face and orbits, skull base and neck, and encompasses multiple specialties, including ophthalmology, ear–nose–throat (ENT), neurology, neurosurgery and endocrinology. The more common indications for head and neck imaging are outlined in this chapter.

11.1 IMAGING OF THE ORBIT

Imaging of orbital trauma is discussed in Chapter 12. Ophthalmologists and allied professionals diagnose most non-traumatic disorders of the eye and orbit without the need for imaging. Imaging is reserved for specific clinical indications, including:

- Sudden loss of visual acuity
- Sudden onset of diplopia
- Exophthalmos (proptosis), especially when acute and progressive, painful or pulsatile
- Diseases known to be associated with orbital pathology such as neurofibromatosis and thyroid eye disease
- To assess the extent of a known orbital tumour or vascular lesion.

Common orbital tumours include:

- Malignant tumours: retinoblastoma in children; ocular melanoma in adults; optic nerve glioma; lymphoma
- Optic nerve sheath meningioma
- Lacrimal gland tumours
- Vascular lesions: haemangioma; varix.

In many cases of suspected orbital pathology, imaging of the brain is also performed to diagnose lesions of the intracranial visual pathways or third, fourth and sixth cranial nerves. Magnetic resonance imaging (MRI) and computed tomography (CT) are the investigations of choice for orbital imaging. Both modalities have excellent natural contrast provided by the bony orbital margins and the orbital fat surrounding the optic nerve and extraocular muscles (Fig. 11.1). MRI and CT often perform complementary roles in the imaging of orbital pathology. MRI has superior soft-tissue contrast and is more accurate for delineating intracranial lesions of the visual pathways and cranial nerves. CT is more accurate for assessment of the bony margins of the orbit and for detecting calcification in vascular lesions and meningiomas.

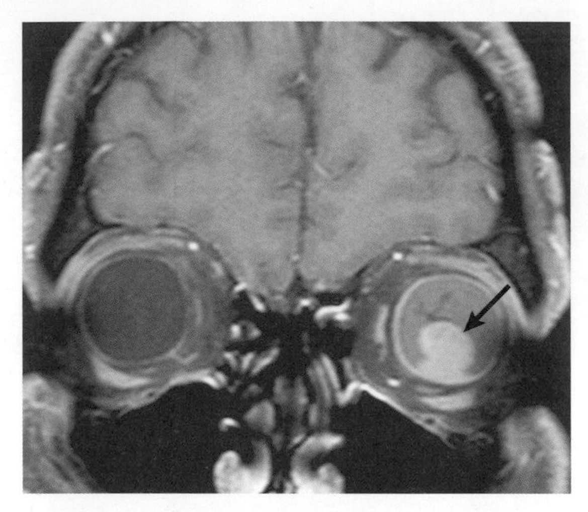

Figure 11.1 Choroidal melanoma: MRI. Coronal T1-weighted, fat-saturated, contrast-enhanced MRI shows an enhancing mass in the posterior chamber of the left eye (arrow).

11.2 IMAGING OF THE PARANASAL SINUSES

The paranasal sinuses are air-filled spaces in the medullary cavities of the skull and facial bones. Named from the bones in which they occur, the paranasal sinuses consist of the frontal, ethmoid, maxillary and sphenoid sinuses. Paranasal sinuses drain by small ostia into the nasal cavities. Mucociliary action within the sinuses pushes debris towards the draining ostia. Although a variety of congenital anomalies and tumours may affect the paranasal sinuses, the most common indication for imaging is inflammation. Paranasal sinus inflammation may be acute or chronic and is commonly associated with disease in the nasal passages, in particular nasal polyposis in association with allergic sinusitis.

11.2.1 ACUTE SINUSITIS

Acute sinusitis is usually viral or bacterial and presents clinically with facial pain and headache, nasal discharge and fever. Diagnosis is usually made on clinical grounds and may be confirmed with nasal cultures or minimally invasive procedures such as endoscopic paranasal sinus aspiration. Imaging usually is not required for acute sinusitis. Indications for imaging in suspected acute paranasal sinusitis include:

- Lack of response to antibiotic therapy
- Immunocompromised patients
- Suspected complications such as meningitis, subdural empyema or cerebral abscess.

When imaging is required in acute sinusitis, CT is the investigation of choice. Radiographs may show fluid levels in the maxillary sinuses or sinus opacification, though are much less sensitive than CT.

11.2.2 CHRONIC SINUSITIS

Chronic sinusitis is defined as sinus inflammation of over 12 weeks' duration. The clinical presentation may include facial pain, nasal obstruction and a reduced sense of smell. Chronic sinusitis may be bacterial, allergic or fungal. Functional endoscopic sinus surgery (FESS) is used to treat patients who do not respond to medical therapy. Imaging is performed to quantify disease and to define relevant underlying anatomical anomalies that may restrict sinus drainage, as well as to assist in presurgical planning and postoperative follow-up. CT is the investigation of choice. The key images in assessing chronic sinusitis and planning FESS are coronal CT scans of the ostiomeatal complex, i.e. the region of the drainage pathways of the maxillary, frontal and anterior ethmoid sinuses (Fig. 11.2).

11.3 IMAGING OF THE TEMPORAL BONE

The temporal bone is an extremely complex structure that contains the external auditory canal and the middle and inner ear structures, and transmits the seventh (facial) and eighth (vestibulocochlear) cranial nerves (CN7 and 8). Middle ear structures include the tympanic membrane, the aerated bony chambers and the three ossicles (malleus, incus, stapes) responsible for the transmission of sound vibrations to the inner ear. Inner ear structures include the cochlea (responsible for hearing), the vestibule and semicircular canals (responsible for balance), the facial nerve canal and the internal auditory canal

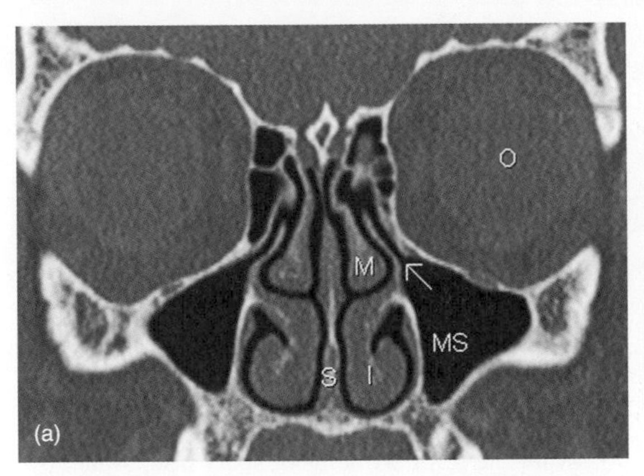

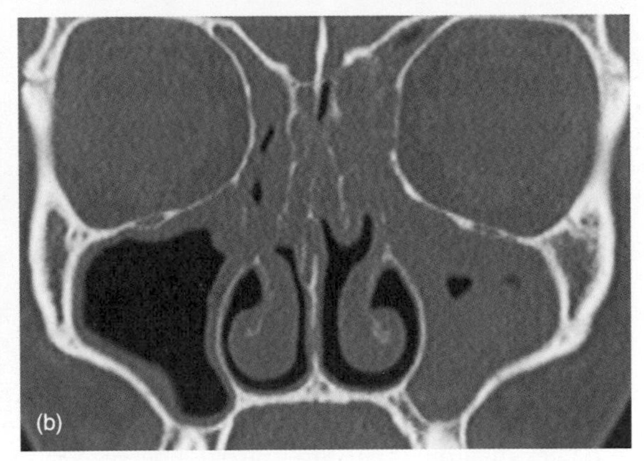

Figure 11.2 CT of the maxillary sinuses. (a) Normal sinuses: coronal CT through the ostiomeatal complex. Note: inferior turbinate (I), middle turbinate (M), maxillary sinus (MS), orbit (O), nasal septum (S), sinus drainage pathway through maxillary ostium (arrow). (b) Paranasal sinus disease: CT through the same level as in (a). Note the mucosal thickening on the right and almost complete opacification of the left maxillary sinus. Mucosal thickening is occluding both maxillary ostia.

(IAC). The IAC transmits the facial nerve and the vestibular and cochlear branches of the vestibulocochlear cranial nerve (CN8). Both these cranial nerves exit the brainstem and pass laterally across a cerebrospinal fluid (CSF)-filled space known as the cerebellopontine angle (CPA) to enter the IAC.

11.3.1 NON-TRAUMATIC TEMPORAL BONE PATHOLOGY

Temporal bone pathology includes congenital anomalies, inflammatory conditions and tumours. Symptoms referable to the temporal bone and adjacent skull base include hearing loss, vertigo and tinnitus, and may occur in isolation or in various combinations.

Hearing loss is assessed initially with audiometry. Hearing loss is classified as conductive, sensorineural or mixed and as bilateral or unilateral. Conductive hearing loss results from lesions of the external or middle ear that prevent sound waves reaching the inner ear. Sensorineural hearing loss (SNHL) is due to pathologies of the cochlea or auditory nerve that prevent the transmission of neural impulses to the auditory cortex. Unilateral SNHL may be further classified clinically with brainstem electric response audiometry (BERA) into cochlear or retrocochlear pathology. Imaging is indicated if BERA indicates a retrocochlear cause for hearing loss.

Vertigo refers to an illusion of movement such as rotation or tilt. Vertigo is classified as:

- Peripheral: due to pathology of the vestibule or semicircular canals and suggested by features such as short duration, provocation with movement and the feeling of pressure in the ear
- Central: due to pathology of the vestibular nerve or its connections in the brain, often with associated neurological symptoms, e.g. ataxia, dysarthria.

Tinnitus refers to the subjective sensation of buzzing or ringing in the ear. Tinnitus may be classified as:

- Pulsatile: repetitive sound that accompanies the patient's pulse, suggesting a vascular cause, including glomus tumour, vascular malformation or idiopathic intracranial hypertension
- Non-pulsatile: constant sound that may be due to a lesion of the CPA such as vestibular schwannoma.

Depending on clinical findings, imaging is commonly required for further assessment of hearing loss, vertigo and tinnitus. MRI with contrast is generally the imaging investigation of choice in cases of

SNHL, tinnitus and central vertigo. MRI examination includes the brain, CPAs and temporal bones. Magnetic resonance angiography (MRA) or venography may be complementary. CT may be used as the first imaging investigation for conductive hearing loss as it depicts the ossicular chain. CT assists MRI in cases where fine bone detail is required.

11.3.2 VESTIBULAR SCHWANNOMA ('ACOUSTIC NEUROMA')

One of the most common investigations in head and neck imaging is MRI to rule out a nerve sheath tumour of CN8, often referred to as 'acoustic neuroma'. These tumours are schwannomas, not neuromas, and usually involve a vestibular branch of CN8, so 'vestibular schwannoma' is a more pathologically correct term. Vestibular schwannomas usually present in adults with slowly progressive unilateral SNHL, sometimes associated with tinnitus and vertigo. Vestibular schwannomas vary in size and are often quite small. They may occur inside or outside the IAC, or both. Usually slow growing, they tend to remodel the IAC if large enough.

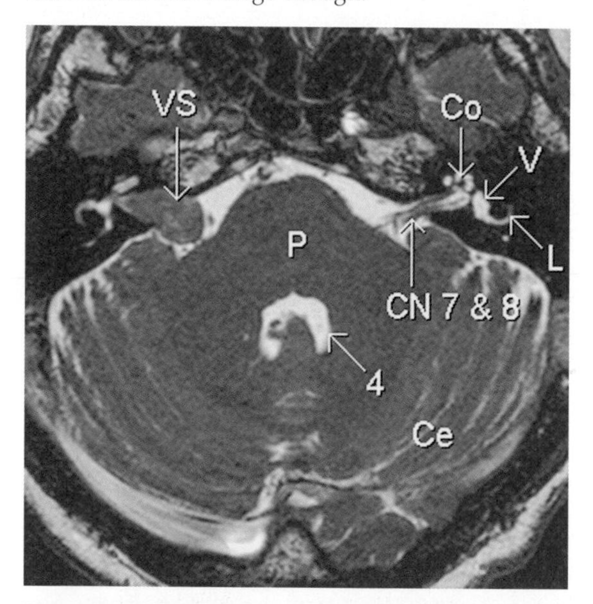

Figure 11.3 Vestibular schwannoma ('acoustic neuroma'): MRI. High-resolution T2-weighted transverse scan through the posterior fossa shows the following: fourth ventricle (4), cerebellum (Ce), normal left seventh and eighth cranial nerves (CN 7 & 8), cochlea (Co), lateral semicircular canal (L), pons (P), vestibule (V), right vestibular schwannoma (VS). (Also see Fig. 1.18.)

MRI is the imaging investigation of choice. High-definition MRI scans can display the cranial nerves and inner ear structures in exquisite detail (Fig. 11.3). When MRI is contraindicated, CT may be performed, though it is less accurate for small tumours.

11.4 NECK MASS

The anatomy of the neck is extremely complex and includes:

- Multiple compartments or spaces, separated by fat planes, some of which are bound by fascia
- Multiple muscles, blood vessels and nerves
- Airway in the midline
- Cervical spine posterior
- Salivary glands, thyroid gland and parathyroid glands
- Lymph nodes.

To make sense of this anatomy and to narrow the differential diagnosis for pathologies, the neck is divided by the hyoid bone into the suprahyoid and infrahyoid neck. The suprahyoid neck is further subdivided into various anatomical compartments, including the pharyngeal mucosal, parapharyngeal, masticator, parotid, carotid, submandibular, retropharyngeal and perivertebral spaces. Spaces of the infrahyoid neck include the visceral, anterior cervical, posterior cervical, carotid, retropharyngeal and perivertebral spaces. These anatomical spaces are all definable on CT and MRI and to a lesser extent on ultrasound (US).

The roles of imaging in the investigation of neck masses include:

- Localization
- Characterization:
  - Cystic or solid
  - Calcification or fat
  - Enhancement with intravenous contrast material
- Anatomical relations: position relative to the great vessels, thyroid gland, laryngeal cartilages
- Evidence of malignancy:
  - Invasion of surrounding structures
  - Lymphadenopathy.

US is an accurate and non-invasive screening test for the initial localization and characterization of a neck mass (Fig. 11.4). A specific diagnosis may often be made with US, particularly for cystic lesions such as a branchial cleft cyst and a thyroglossal cyst. US provides an excellent modality for the guidance of fine-needle aspiration (FNA), biopsy or cyst aspiration.

Depending on local availability and expertise, CT or MRI may be used to further delineate neck masses, particularly deep masses, or complex and multifocal pathologies, such as extensive lymphadenopathy. Both CT and MRI provide good localization of the plane of origin of a mass, plus definition of anatomical relations. Complications such as invasion of the surrounding structures and lymphadenopathy are well seen. Some of the more commonly encountered neck masses include:

- Lymph node enlargement (lymphadenopathy):
    - Infection
    - Head and neck malignancy such as squamous cell carcinoma (SCC) of the larynx, oral cavity or skin
    - Systemic malignancy, including lymphoma
- Abscess: usually occurs in close relation to the airway in the parapharyngeal or retropharyngeal spaces
- Second branchial cleft cyst: presents in young adults with a mass of the upper neck anterior to the sternocleidomastoid muscle (Fig. 11.5)
- Thyroglossal duct cyst: cyst of the remnants of the thyroglossal duct occurring anteriorly in the midline, from the foramen caecum in the posterior tongue to the hyoid bone (Fig. 11.6)
- Lymphatic malformation (previously referred to as cystic hygroma)
    - Occurs in infants and young children
    - Complex cystic mass of the lower lateral neck

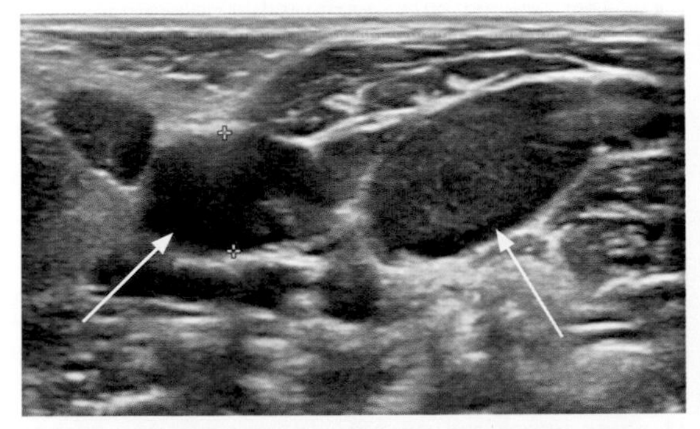

Figure 11.4 Cervical lymphadenopathy: US. Multiple enlarged cervical lymph nodes, seen on US as oval hypoechoic masses (arrows).

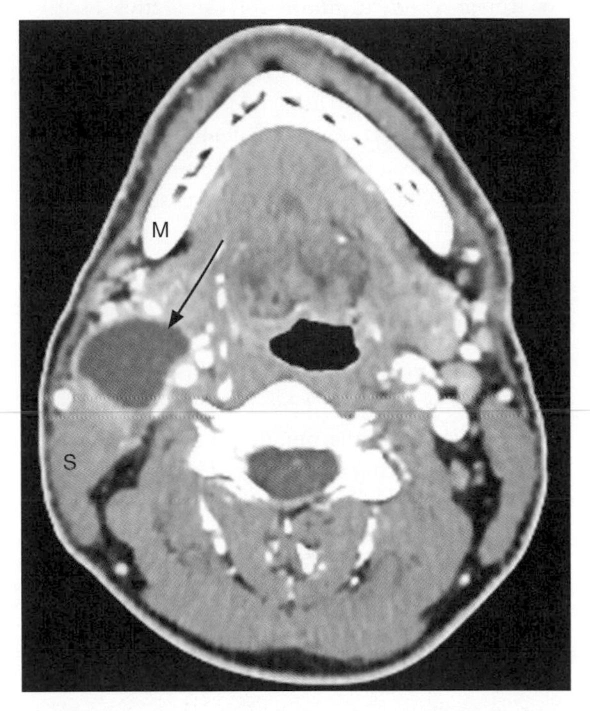

Figure 11.5 Second branchial cleft cyst: CT. Right-sided fluid density lesion (arrow) between the mandibular angle (M) and sternocleidomastoid muscle (S).

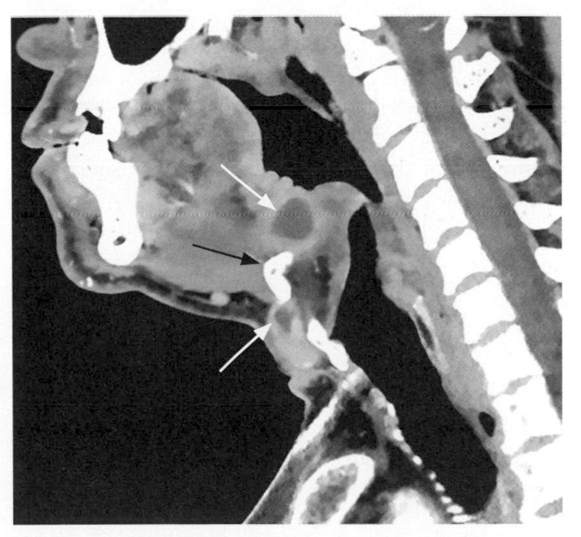

Figure 11.6 Thyroglossal duct cysts: CT. Sagittal image shows fluid density lesions (white arrows) superior and inferior to the hyoid bone (black arrow).

- Associated with various aneuploidies, most commonly Turner syndrome
- Dermoid cyst: midline cyst containing fat in the floor of the mouth
- Carotid body tumour:
  - Paraganglioma located in the bifurcation of the common carotid artery
  - Up to 10% are associated with tumour syndromes such as multiple endocrine neoplasia (MEN), neurofibromatosis type 1 and von Hippel–Lindau disease.

11.5 SALIVARY GLAND SWELLING

Focal or diffuse salivary gland swelling may be due to inflammation, systemic disease or tumour. The causes of salivary gland inflammation include bacterial or viral infection (often bilateral) and obstruction of the salivary duct by a calculus. Bilateral parotid gland swelling may be caused by various systemic diseases, including Sjögren syndrome and sarcoidosis.

Salivary gland tumours may be classified as follows:

- Benign:
  - Benign mixed tumour (pleomorphic adenoma)
  - Adenolymphoma (Warthin tumour)
- Malignant:
  - Adenoid cystic carcinoma (cylindroma)
  - Mucoepidermoid carcinoma.

Other soft-tissue tumours that may occur in the parotid gland include lipoma, neuroma and melanoma. Intraparotid lymphadenopathy also occurs. The ratio of incidences of benign and malignant tumours varies according to which salivary gland is involved:

- Parotid: 80% benign, 20% malignant
- Submandibular: 50% benign, 50% malignant
- Sublingual: 20% benign, 80% malignant.

US is the initial imaging investigation of choice for salivary gland swelling:

- Differentiates intraparotid from extraparotid masses
- Able to diagnose most parotid and submandibular calculi

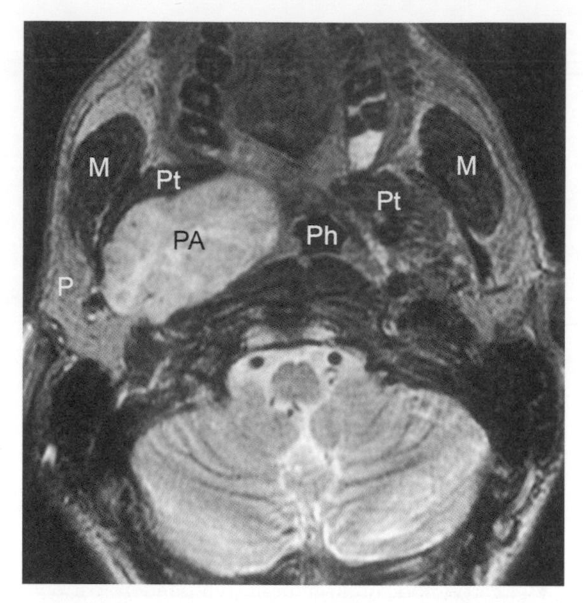

Figure 11.7 Benign mixed tumour (pleomorphic adenoma): MRI. T2-weighted transverse scan through the oropharynx shows a mass (PA) arising from the deep lobe of the right parotid gland. Also note the superficial lobe of the right parotid gland (P), masseter muscles (M), oropharynx (Ph) and pterygoid muscles (Pt), compressed on the right by the mass.

- Visualization of dilated ducts
- Guidance of FNA.

MRI may be required for the assessment of deep or large masses, particularly masses of the deep lobe of the parotid gland (Fig. 11.7).

Radiographs may be used when salivary gland calculus is suspected clinically:

- Most salivary calculi are visible on plain radiographs
- Specific views may be used for the gland of interest, such as intraoral films to show the submandibular ducts.

11.6 STAGING OF HEAD AND NECK CANCER

Head and neck cancer refers to cancers arising from the surface mucosa of four anatomical regions of the upper aerodigestive tract:

- Nasal cavity and paranasal sinuses
- Oral cavity: anterior two-thirds of the tongue, hard palate, floor of the mouth, buccal mucosa
- Pharynx:
  - Nasopharynx: posterior to the nasal cavities
  - Oropharynx: posterior one-third of the tongue, soft palate, tonsils, posterior pharyngeal wall
  - Hypopharynx: piriform sinuses, postcricoid posterior surface of the larynx
- Larynx:
  - Supraglottis: epiglottis, aryepiglottic folds, arytenoids, false vocal cords
  - Glottis: true vocal cords
  - Subglottis: from 1 cm below the true cords to the trachea.

Histologically, most head and neck cancers are SCCs. Other less commonly encountered tumour types include adenocarcinoma, sarcoma and lymphoma. The major risk factors for the development of SCC of the head and neck include tobacco use and heavy alcohol intake. Another major risk factor is infection with human papillomavirus (HPV). HPV-positive tumours have a strong association with p16 expression. p16 is a kinase inhibitor, a tumour suppression protein encoded by the *CDKN2A* gene. It is detected by immunohistochemistry and is considered a surrogate marker for HPV positivity. p16-positive tumours most commonly involve the oropharynx, including the base of the tongue. They tend to occur in younger adults and have a better prognosis than p16/HPV-negative SCC.

The clinical presentation of head and neck cancer may include a sore throat, hoarse voice or stridor. Another common presentation is with a painless neck lump due to lymph node metastasis. SCC of the head and neck spreads by local invasion through the mucosal surface to deep structures. Lymph node metastases are common. Distant metastases may also occur, most commonly in the lungs. Relevant factors for staging of head and neck cancer include the size of the primary tumour, the extent of local invasion and the presence of cervical lymphadenopathy. Further details of tumour–node–metastasis (TNM) staging of head and neck cancer may be found on the companion website.

SCC of the head and neck is assessed initially with direct clinical examination. Laryngoscopy is used for the assessment of the laryngeal mucosal surface. MRI is the investigation of choice for local staging, including assessment of local spread and cervical lymph node involvement. It is particularly useful for oral cavity and oropharyngeal assessment. It has better soft-tissue resolution than CT and is less prone to artefact from dental metalwork. CT is preferred for staging of laryngeal tumours as it is less prone to motion artefact from swallowing.

SCC of the head and neck appears on MRI as a T2 high-signal mass that enhances with gadolinium, causing asymmetry and anatomical distortion of the airway (Fig. 11.8). Invasive tumours cause obliteration of surrounding fat planes. US-guided FNA of cervical lymph nodes is useful for the assessment of nodes that are considered equivocal on CT or MRI. US-guided FNA also has an increasing role in primary diagnosis for tumours that present clinically with an enlarged lymph node and no obvious mucosal lesion.

Fluorodeoxyglucose–positron emission tomography (FDG-PET)-CT may be used to clarify local staging and to provide a baseline study for follow-up. It is most useful to assess the response to therapy, and

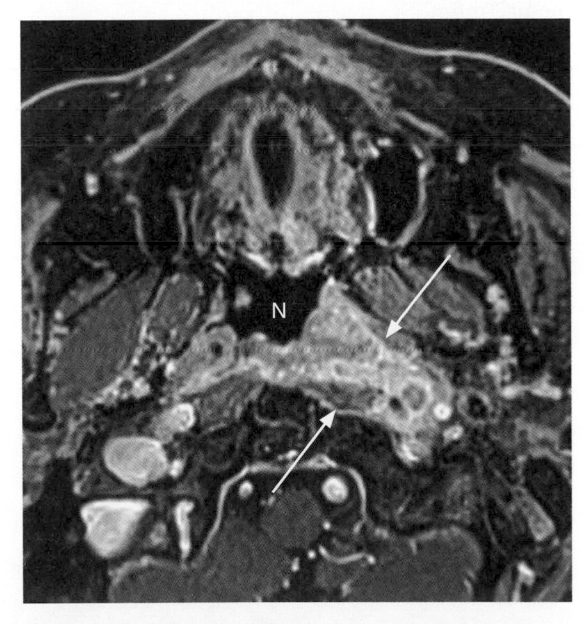

Figure 11.8 Nasopharyngeal cancer: transverse T1-weighted contrast-enhanced MRI. Note the asymmetry of the nasopharynx (N) owing to a large enhancing left nasopharyngeal mass (arrows) which extends posteriorly and laterally to the skull base.

in postoperative patients to diagnose recurrent SCC. In the context of surveillance imaging of treated head and neck cancer, the Neck Imaging Reporting and Data System (NI-RADS) is a risk classification structured reporting system proposed by the American College of Radiology (ACR). Like other RADS systems, NI-RADS uses imaging features to assess the likelihood of tumour recurrence and to make management recommendations based on the assigned category. For further details of NI-RADS, see the companion website.

11.7 THYROID IMAGING

Common clinical indications for imaging of the thyroid gland include hyperthyroidism (thyrotoxicosis), diffuse thyroid enlargement and a focal thyroid mass or nodule. The most used imaging techniques for the investigation of thyroid diseases are US, US-guided FNA and scintigraphy with ^{99m}Tc or radioiodine. CT or MRI may be used to outline the anatomy of large goitres prior to surgical removal, particularly when there is retrosternal extension into the upper mediastinum.

11.7.1 HYPERTHYROIDISM (THYROTOXICOSIS)

Thyrotoxicosis refers to a spectrum of clinical and biochemical findings that occur as a result of excess thyroid hormone:

- Heat intolerance, inability to sleep, weight loss, palpitations
- Elevated serum triiodothyronine (T_3) and/or thyroxine (T_4)
- Rarely, elevated thyroid-stimulating hormone (TSH) levels may indicate a TSH-secreting pituitary adenoma
- More commonly, TSH levels are low, indicating a thyroid problem.

In cases with a typical presentation for Graves disease, treatment may be instituted without further investigation. Where imaging is required, scintigraphy with ^{99m}Tc or radioiodine is the investigation of choice. ^{99m}Tc is more widely available than radioiodine and has a lower radiation dose. In the context of thyrotoxicosis, scintigraphy with ^{99m}Tc is useful for differentiating Graves disease from other causes of thyrotoxicosis, including subacute thyroiditis, multinodular goitre and toxic adenoma.

11.7.2 DIFFUSE THYROID ENLARGEMENT

The causes of diffuse thyroid enlargement include Graves disease, Hashimoto thyroiditis, subacute thyroiditis and multinodular goitre (Table 11.1). Diagnosis is often achieved by clinical history and examination, plus laboratory tests for thyroid function and antibodies. These may be complemented by thyroid scintigraphy with ^{99m}Tc and US with colour Doppler.

11.7.3 THYROID NODULES AND MASSES

A thyroid nodule is defined as a discrete mass lesion in the thyroid gland, distinguishable from thyroid parenchyma on US. Thyroid nodules most commonly are benign colloid nodules. Follicular adenoma is a true benign neoplasm of the thyroid gland. Thyroid

Table 11.1 Imaging appearances of common diffuse thyroid diseases.

Disease	^{99m}Tc scintigraphy	US
Graves disease	Intensely increased uptake	Enlarged, hypoechoic and hypervascular thyroid
Hashimoto thyroiditis (chronic lymphocytic thyroiditis)	Reduced uptake	Hypoechoic and hypervascular thyroid
Subacute (de Quervain) thyroiditis	Reduced uptake	Mildly enlarged and hypervascular thyroid
Multinodular goitre	Patchy uptake	Enlarged thyroid with multiple solid nodules

carcinoma is of epithelial origin and is classified into papillary, follicular, medullary and anaplastic subtypes. Papillary carcinoma is the most common type (75–80%) and has an excellent prognosis with a 30-year survival rate of 95%. Medullary carcinoma is associated with MEN and other tumour syndromes.

Thyroid nodules are extremely common: they are found in up to 40% of adults on US examination. Thyroid cancer, on the other hand, is quite uncommon. It follows that most thyroid nodules are benign. Thyroid nodules may be assessed clinically and with imaging, the aim being to identify nodules that are malignant.

Clinical factors associated with an increased likelihood of a nodule being malignant include:

- Family history of thyroid cancer
- History of irradiation to the neck
- Patient age younger than 20 years or older than 60 years
- Rapid growth of the nodule
- Fixation to adjacent structures
- Vocal cord paralysis
- Adjacent lymphadenopathy.

US is the imaging investigation of choice for the characterization of thyroid nodules. The Thyroid Imaging Reporting and Data System (TI RADS) is a reporting system for thyroid nodules that assigns points based on standardized scoring of specific US features (Fig. 11.9). The features used to grade thyroid nodules are:

- Composition: cystic, solid or mixed
- Echogenicity: hypoechoic, isoechoic or hyperechoic compared with thyroid parenchyma
- Shape: most benign lesions are oval with their long axis parallel to the skin, i.e. 'wider than tall'
- Margin: smooth, ill-defined, irregular, obvious invasion
- Echogenic foci: generally correlate with calcifications.

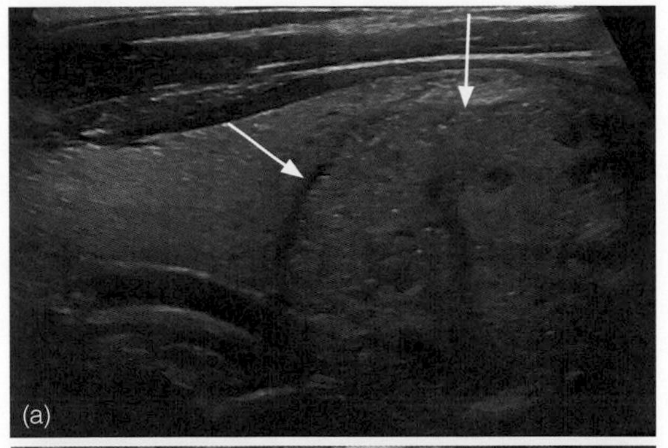

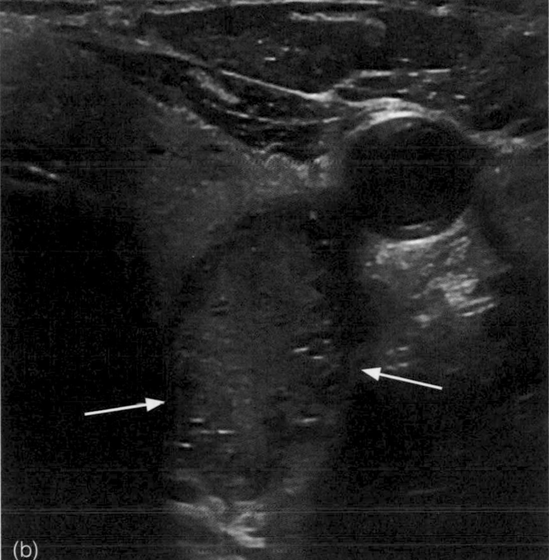

Figure 11.9 Thyroid nodules: US. (a) Longitudinal US shows a thyroid nodule (arrows) with the following features: solid, isoechoic to adjacent thyroid parenchyma, wider than tall, smooth margins and microcalcifications seen as tiny hyperechoic specks throughout the lesion. Appearance consistent with a Thyroid Imaging Reporting and Data System (TI-RADS) 4 lesion. (b) Transverse US shows a thyroid nodule (arrows) with the following features: solid, hypoechoic, taller than wide, irregular margins and microcalcifications seen as tiny hyperechoic specks throughout the lesion. Appearance consistent with a TI-RADS 5 lesion.

Depending on the total number of points based on these features, a TI-RADS score from 1 to 5 is assigned. TI-RADS 1 and 2 lesions require no further assessment. Based on size, TI-RADS 3–5 lesions are recommended for no further management, follow-up with serial US or US-guided FNA (Fig. 11.10). As with other RADS classifications, this information, including relevant clinical recommendations, is provided in a structured reporting format. Further details of TI-RADS may be found on the companion website.

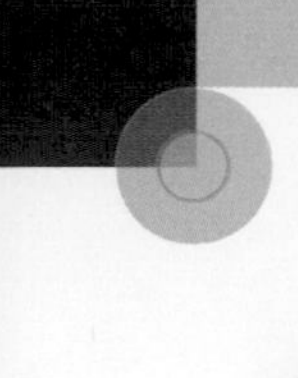

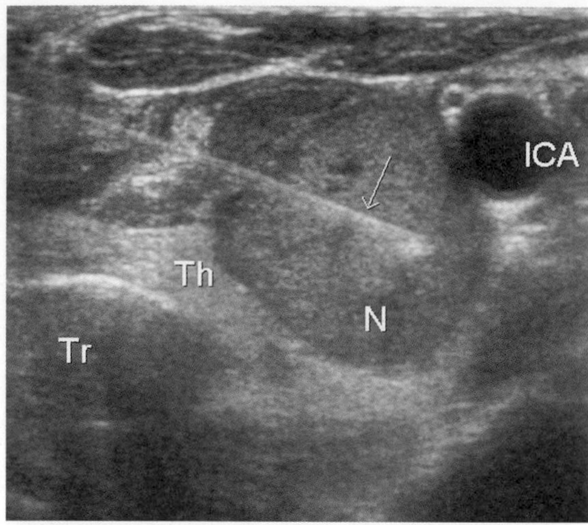

Figure 11.10 Fine-needle aspiration (FNA) of a thyroid nodule: US guidance. A transverse US image shows a fine needle (arrow) entering a nodule (N) in the left lobe of the thyroid (Th). Also note the trachea (Tr) in the midline and the internal carotid artery (ICA) lateral to the nodule.

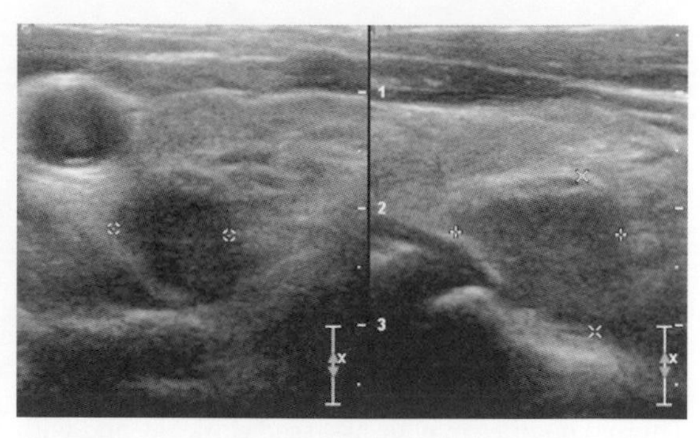

Figure 11.11 Parathyroid adenoma: US. Two US images, transverse on the left and longitudinal on the right, show a small hypoechoic nodule (+) posterior to the right lobe of the thyroid gland.

11.8 PRIMARY HYPERPARATHYROIDISM

Primary hyperparathyroidism is the most common indication for imaging of the parathyroid glands. Causes of primary hyperparathyroidism:

- Solitary parathyroid adenoma: 80%
- Multiple parathyroid adenomas: 7%
- Parathyroid hyperplasia: 10%
- Parathyroid carcinoma: 3%.

Adenomas and hyperplasia may be associated with multiple endocrine neoplasia (MEN).

Imaging is indicated in hyperparathyroidism to localize the causative lesion prior to surgery; this is relevant where minimally invasive surgery is intended. US is the investigation of first choice. US has a high sensitivity (80–90%) for the detection of parathyroid adenoma. The US appearance of parathyroid adenoma is a well-defined hypoechoic mass usually of around 1.0–1.5 cm in diameter (Fig. 11.11). Most parathyroid adenomas lie behind or immediately below the thyroid gland. The principal cause of a false-negative US is ectopic adenoma, which may be present in up to 10% of cases; ectopic sites include the mediastinum (intrathymic), the thyroid gland and the tracheal–oesophageal groove.

Where US is negative, further imaging may be performed, i.e. scintigraphy, CT or MRI. The imaging technique chosen usually reflects local expertise and availability. Scintigraphy with ^{99m}Tc-sestamibi shows a high rate of uptake in parathyroid adenoma and is especially useful for ectopic or multiple adenomas (Fig. 11.12). Postoperative imaging for recurrent or persistent hyperparathyroidism is best performed with US complemented by sestamibi scintigraphy.

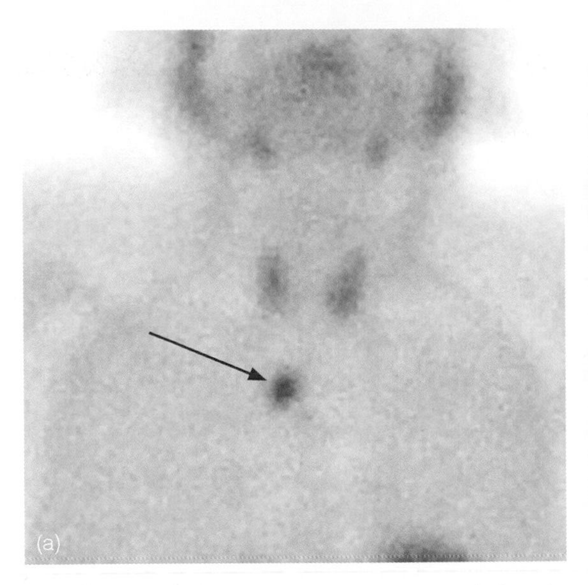

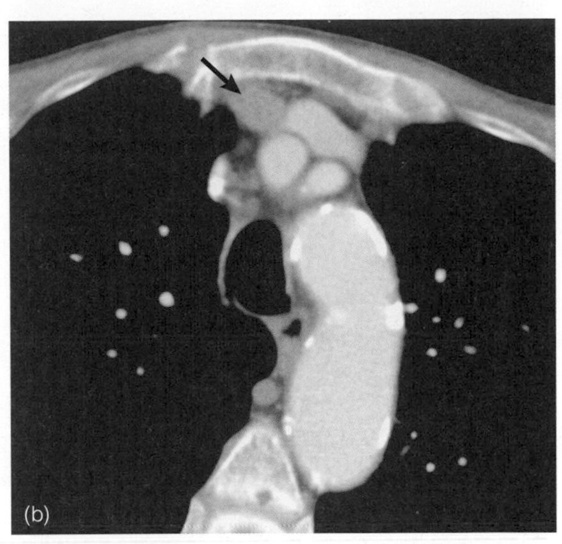

Figure 11.12 Ectopic parathyroid adenoma: scintigraphy and CT. (a) Sestamibi scan shows a small focus of increased activity in the right mediastinum (arrow) in a patient with hypercalcaemia. Note the normal physiological uptake of sestamibi by the salivary and thyroid glands. (b) Transverse contrast-enhanced CT confirms a small mass in the upper right mediastinum (arrow).

SUMMARY

Clinical presentation	Investigation of choice	Comment
Symptoms of orbital pathology, e.g. visual symptoms, proptosis	MRI/CT	MRI and CT often complementary in orbital pathology
Chronic sinusitis	CT	
Symptoms of temporal bone pathology, e.g. hearing loss, tinnitus, vertigo	MRI/CT	MRI and CT often complementary in skull base pathology
Neck mass	• US: initial assessment • MRI/CT: further definition	
Salivary gland swelling	• US: initial assessment • MRI: complex or deep lesions	
Staging of head and neck cancer	• MRI/CT • FDG-PET-CT	US-guided FNA for enlarged or equivocal lymph nodes
Surveillance head and neck cancer post therapy	• FDG-PET-CT • MRI	NI-RADS
Thyroid nodule	US	TI-RADS
Hyperparathyroidism	• US • ^{99m}Tc-sestamibi	

Abbreviations: FNA, fine-needle aspiration; NI-RADS, Neck Imaging Reporting and Data System; TI-RADS, Thyroid Imaging Reporting and Data System.

12 Non-orthopaedic trauma

Traumatic injuries are encountered daily at most medical services. Injuries can range from minor and trivial to life-threatening to fatal. Multitrauma or polytrauma are injuries of multiple body systems or regions and can be complex to manage. Blunt trauma is injury caused by a blunt force, such as a deceleration during a motor vehicle accident or a fall from a height. Penetrating trauma refers to injuries caused by objects (e.g. projectiles and knives) that enter or traverse the body; it occurs more frequently in societies where weapons are more prevalent.

Medical imaging has a fundamental and critical role in early injury diagnosis. Ultrasound (US) can be performed in the field or at the hospital bedside as a triage tool. Radiographs are performed at the bedside to provide immediate information for the trauma team. A standard trauma series includes a supine chest radiograph (chest X-ray, CXR) and a pelvic radiograph. Some centres with limited access to computed tomography (CT) may include lateral cervical spine radiographs. Following the trauma series, the investigation path of a traumatized patient depends largely on the affected body regions, clinical presentation and haemodynamic status.

Depending on the presence of other injuries and local expertise, haemodynamically unstable patients should undergo immediate surgery or may be assessed for haemoperitoneum with a specialized US technique known as a FAST scan. Focused assessment with sonography for trauma (FAST) is the rapid US assessment of the abdomen and pelvis for the presence of free fluid (Fig. 12.1). FAST has replaced peritoneal lavage in many centres and is the initial imaging investigation in patients with abdominal trauma. It may be used to help decide which patients require immediate laparotomy.

CT is the workhorse in the early accurate assessment of haemodynamically stable trauma patients.

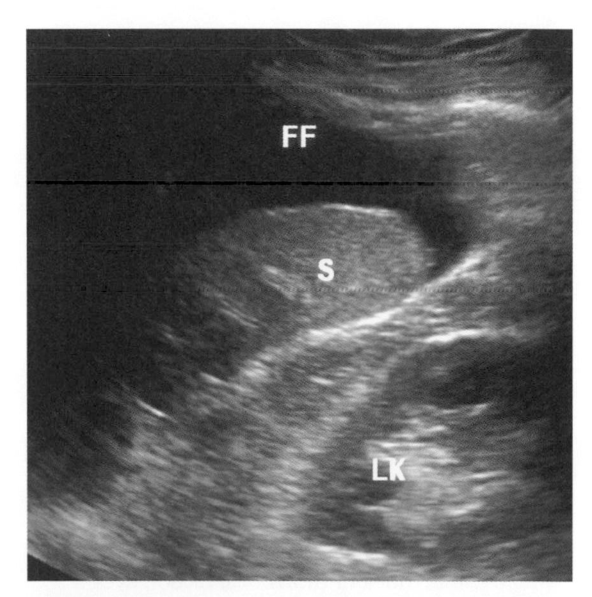

Figure 12.1 Free fluid: US (focused assessment with sonography for trauma [FAST]). Anechoic free fluid (FF) is seen in the left upper abdomen adjacent to the spleen (S) and left kidney (LK).

Most hospitals have specific trauma CT protocols tailored for assessment of life- or limb-threatening injuries. Isolated body regions can be assessed with CT or, in severely or multi-injured patients, a basic CT trauma protocol is employed. The trauma 'pan scan' assesses the head, spine and torso and typically includes non-contrast-enhanced CT of the head and cervical spine, CT angiography (CTA) of the chest and portal venous phase and contrast-enhanced CT of the abdomen and pelvis. Thoracic and lumbosacral spinal reformats are included. Rarely is oral contrast material required, but it is utilized in some trauma centres for assessment of abdominal penetrating trauma. Extra series for specific suspected injuries include CTA of the head, neck, upper or entire abdomen and pelvis, a delayed urographic phase and limb CTA.

12.1 TRAUMATIC BRAIN INJURY

Non-contrast-enhanced CT is the primary investigation for traumatic brain injury as it is rapid and accurately identifies life-threatening findings that may require immediate neurosurgical attention. Indications for brain CT following head trauma include:

- Confusion/drowsiness not improved at 4 hours
- Loss of consciousness
- Amnesia
- Glasgow Coma Scale (GCS) score of less than 15
- New focal neurological signs
- Fully conscious with:
  - Seizures
  - Nausea and vomiting
  - New and persisting headache
- Clinically obvious compound or depressed skull fracture
- Suspected skull fracture:
  - Scalp laceration to bone; boggy scalp haematoma
- Signs of skull base fracture:
  - Blood or cerebrospinal fluid (CSF) rhinorrhoea or otorrhoea; racoon eyes; Battle sign
- Penetrating head injury
- Suspected intracranial foreign body.

In all cases of major head injury, cervical spine imaging should be obtained (see section 12.3.2).

Magnetic resonance imaging (MRI) is not used in the initial assessment of traumatic brain injury; it is most useful in the assessment of an ongoing neurological or cognitive deficit. MRI is highly sensitive for diffuse axonal injury (DAI), a serious injury that is often difficult to detect on initial trauma CT.

12.1.1 COMMON COMPUTED TOMOGRAPHY FINDINGS OF TRAUMATIC BRAIN INJURY

Extradural haematoma (EDH) lies in the potential space between the dura mater and inner table of the skull. EDH is the result of tearing of the meningeal arteries and usually coexists with a skull fracture. Temporal bone fracture and middle meningeal artery injury is typical. The CT appearance of EDH includes:

- High-attenuation peripheral lesion with a convex inner margin giving a biconvex or lentiform shape (Fig. 12.2)
- Haematoma is usually limited by the cranial sutures.

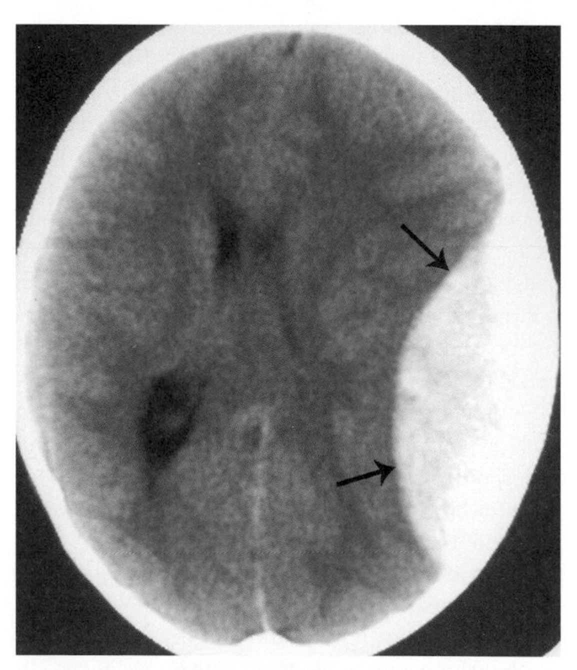

Figure 12.2 Extradural haematoma. Acute blood is of high attenuation on CT. Note the convex inner margin (arrows).

Subdural haematoma (SDH) is more common than EDH and is the result of less severe trauma. SDH occurs in the subdural space between the dura and arachnoid mater. SDH is due to bleeding from bridging veins crossing the subdural space and is usually associated with cerebral oedema. The CT appearance of SDH includes:

- High-attenuation peripheral lesion with a concave inner margin (crescent shaped), often spreading over much of the cerebral hemisphere (Fig. 12.3)
- Over 7–10 days the haematoma attenuation gradually decreases to approximate that of the adjacent brain tissue. Isodense SDH can be difficult to identify, aided by the use of blood windowing on Picture Archiving and Communication Systems (PACS)
- Over the next few weeks, attenuation decreases further to approximate that of CSF (black).

Brain parenchymal injury may take several forms, including intraparenchymal haematoma, contusion and cerebral oedema. Intracerebral haematoma is far more common than haematoma in the cerebellum and brainstem. Intraparenchymal haematomas are high-attenuation areas usually surrounded by a rim of low-attenuation oedema. Contusions are areas of mixed high and low attenuation, which may be focal or more commonly multifocal. With time, the haemorrhagic component resolves, leaving irregular areas of low attenuation. Cerebral oedema is low-attenuation parenchyma that may surround haemorrhage or be diffuse.

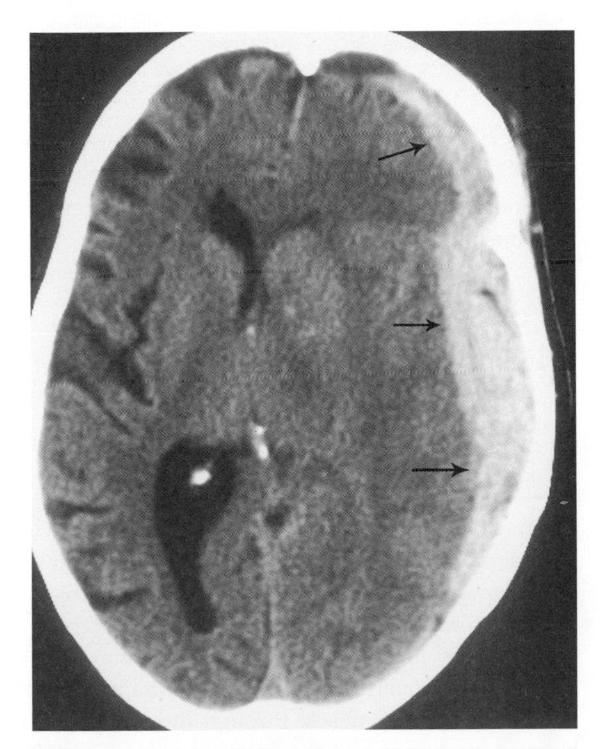

Figure 12.3 Subdural haematoma. Note the concave inner margin of the haematoma (arrows).

The above injuries often cause raised intracranial pressure, which is the secondary effect of intracranial trauma. CT signs of raised intracranial pressure:

- Midline shift: shift of the lateral/third ventricles and other midline structures away from the side of injury
- Asymmetric lateral ventricles: ipsilateral effacement and contralateral dilatation of the lateral ventricles
- Herniation:
  - Subfalcine: contralateral displacement of the cingulate gyrus under the falx
  - Uncal: inferior displacement of the hippocampus between the tentorial free edge and the brainstem
  - Tonsillar: inferior descent of the cerebellar tonsils through the foramen magnum.

Subarachnoid haemorrhage (SAH) may occur with trauma, though it is more commonly due to cerebral aneurysm rupture (see Chapter 9). SAH appears as high-attenuation material in the basal cisterns, Sylvian fissures, cerebral sulci and ventricles.

DAI is the result of rapid deceleration of the brain. Cortical grey matter slows at a different speed from underlying white matter, causing shearing of axons. DAI appears as multiple small acute haemorrhages at the grey–white matter junction, corpus callosum and brainstem. CT tends to under-represent the degree of DAI and may be normal initially. DAI is suspected when the degree of neurological compromise following injury is out of proportion to CT findings. MRI is indicated in such cases showing focal microhaemorrhages and white matter oedema (Fig. 12.4).

All the above findings can be isolated or combined. Other CT signs associated with brain trauma include:

- Fractures of skull base and calvarium

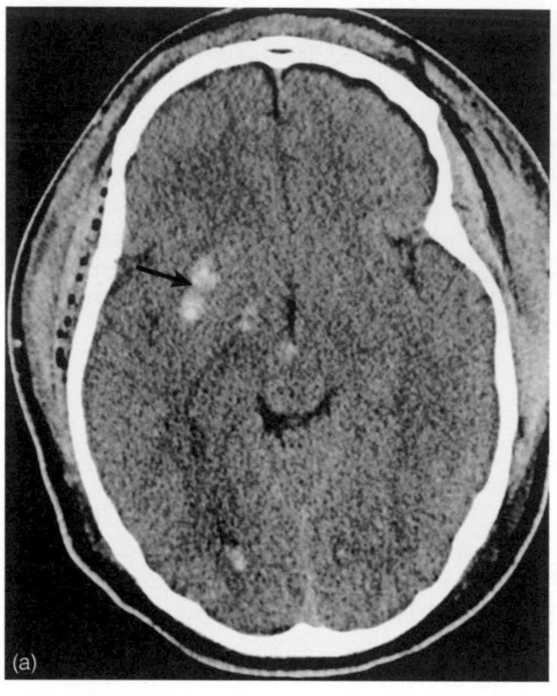

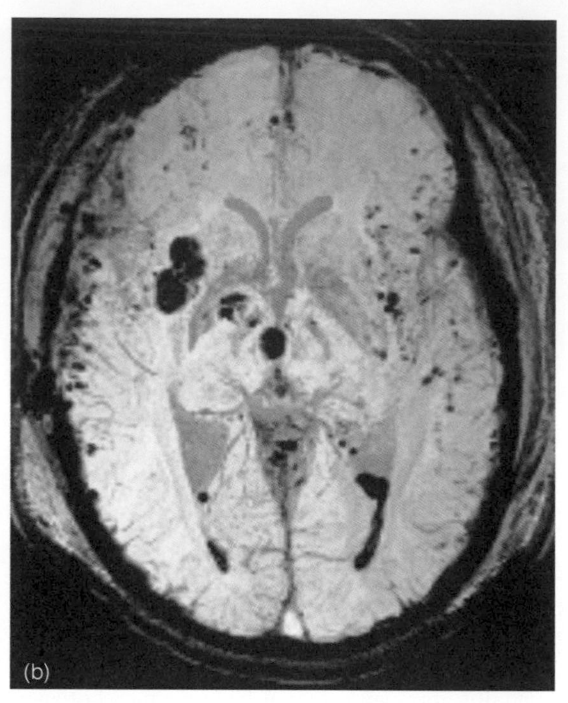

Figure 12.4 Diffuse axonal injury (DAI). Comatose 24-year-old man following head injury in a high-speed motor vehicle accident. (a) CT shows a small haemorrhage in the right basal ganglia (arrow). A couple of small haemorrhages are seen elsewhere plus a small amount of blood in the right lateral ventricle. (b) Transverse susceptibility-weighted MRI (SWI) shows the basal ganglia haemorrhage, blood in the lateral ventricles and extensive bilateral microhaemorrhages. These are seen as multiple foci of paramagnetic artefact producing small black spots. SWI is much more sensitive than CT for the detection of the microhaemorrhages associated with DAI.

- Scalp swelling, laceration and haematoma
- Intracranial air (pneumocephalus) due to penetrating injury or fractures through the paranasal sinuses and pneumatized temporal bones
- Fluid levels in the paranasal sinuses and mastoid air cells
- Foreign bodies.

12.2 FACIAL TRAUMA

Facial trauma is usually due to a direct blow to the face and has a high association with concomitant head and cervical spine injuries. Radiographic assessment has been superseded by CT, which offers greater sensitivity for injuries, improved appraisal of the involved structures and identification of possible complications. Undisplaced fractures may be subtle and indirect signs of facial fractures can aid detection, including:

- Soft-tissue swelling
- Opacification or fluid levels in the paranasal sinuses (haemosinus)
- Air within the orbit or other soft tissues.

12.2.1 ORBITAL TRAUMA

The most common type of orbital fracture is a blowout fracture of the orbital floor, which results from a direct blow causing a sudden increase of intraorbital pressure transmitted to the orbital floor. The orbital contents may herniate inferiorly into the maxillary sinus. Diplopia may occur owing to entrapment of the inferior rectus muscle through the fracture. A blowout fracture is best shown on coronal plane CT (Fig. 12.5). CT shows a soft-tissue mass in the shape

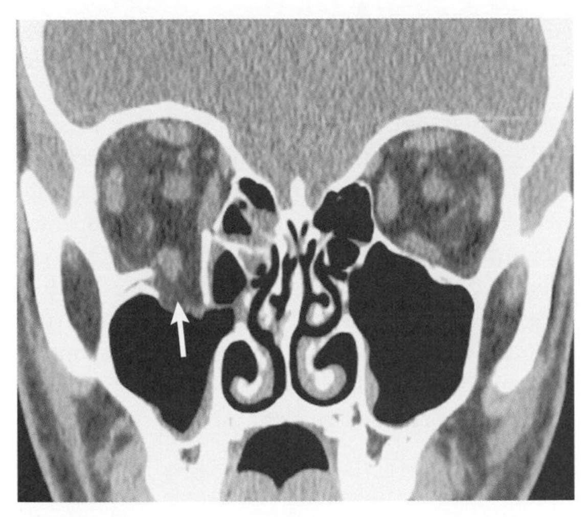

Figure 12.5 Orbital floor fracture: CT. Coronal CT images through the orbits showing a fracture of the right orbital floor with downward herniation of orbital fat and inferior rectus muscle (arrow) into the maxillary sinus.

of a 'teardrop' in the roof of the maxillary sinus, representing herniating extraconal orbital fat and possibly the inferior rectus muscle. Fracture involvement of the canal containing the infraorbital nerve may produce malar paraesthesia.

Less commonly there may be ocular injury due to blunt or penetrating trauma. CT signs of ocular injury include:

- Deformity of the eyeball
- Intraocular haemorrhage seen on CT as an irregular area of increased attenuation in the vitreous
- Dislocation of the lens
- Retinal or choroidal detachment.

12.2.2 ORBITAL FOREIGN BODIES

CT is used for the diagnosis and localization of orbital foreign bodies. Radiographs may diagnose radio-opaque foreign bodies and eye movement radiographs can determine the position of a foreign body. US can also be used in isolated cases.

12.2.3 MAXILLARY AND ZYGOMATIC FRACTURES

The zygomatic bone forms the 'cheekbone' at the inferolateral orbital margin. Zygomatic fractures typically occur from a direct blow to the malar eminence. Fractures occur in four points of relative weakness; when combined, they are termed zygomaticomaxillary complex (ZMC) fractures (Fig. 12.6):

- Inferior orbital margin
- Lateral wall of the maxillary sinus
- Zygomatic arch
- Lateral wall of the orbit (usually zygomaticofrontal suture diastasis).

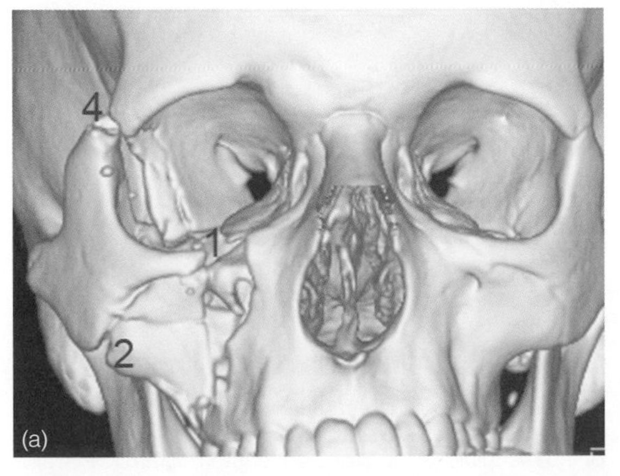

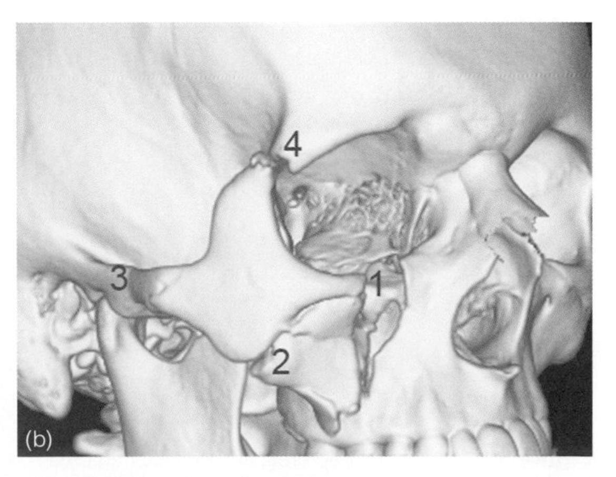

Figure 12.6 Zygomatic fracture: CT. Three-dimensional CT shows the four points of weakness at which zygomatic fractures occur: inferior orbital margin (1), lateral wall of the maxillary sinus (2), zygomatic arch (3) and zygomaticofrontal suture in the lateral wall of the orbit (4). (a) Frontal view. (b) Oblique view.

The Le Fort classification is used to describe complex midface fractures, which occur when there is partial or complete midface dissociation from the skull base. The sphenoid bone, via the pterygoid plates, joins the midface and skull base. Le Fort fractures therefore disrupt the pterygoid plates, and the three types describe the plane of injury (Fig. 12.7):

- Le Fort I: horizontal fracture lines through the lower maxillary sinuses and nasal septum with separation of the lower maxilla and teeth (floating palate)
- Le Fort II: pyramidal fracture lines extend through the lateral walls of the maxillary sinuses and the floor and medial wall of the orbits to the nasal bones and nasofrontal suture (floating maxilla)
- Le Fort III: transverse fracture lines run horizontally through the orbits and the zygomatic arches, causing complete separation of the facial bones from the cranium (floating face).

12.2.4 MANDIBULAR FRACTURES

Mandibular fractures are usually the result of direct blunt trauma. Being U-shaped, the mandible often fractures in two places and the temporomandibular joints are at risk of dislocation. Dental fractures, tooth loosening and tooth avulsion may occur in certain fractures. In isolation, mandibular injuries can be assessed with plain radiography alone. Because of the complex anatomy and overlapping structures, numerous radiographic views may be needed for full assessment of the mandible, including orthopantomogram (OPG). Used most in dentistry, the OPG is a specialized tomographic radiographic technique that gives a panoramic view of the entire mandible (Fig. 12.8). CT is used for more accurate anatomical injury assessment, especially for complex facial or major jaw trauma and preoperative planning.

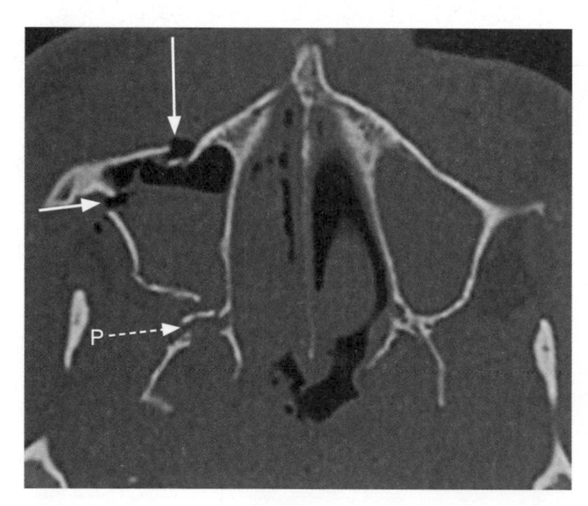

Figure 12.7 Le Fort II fractures: CT. Multiple fractures involving the right maxillary sinus (arrows) and pterygoid plates (P, dashed arrow). Also note an air–fluid level due to blood in the right maxillary sinus.

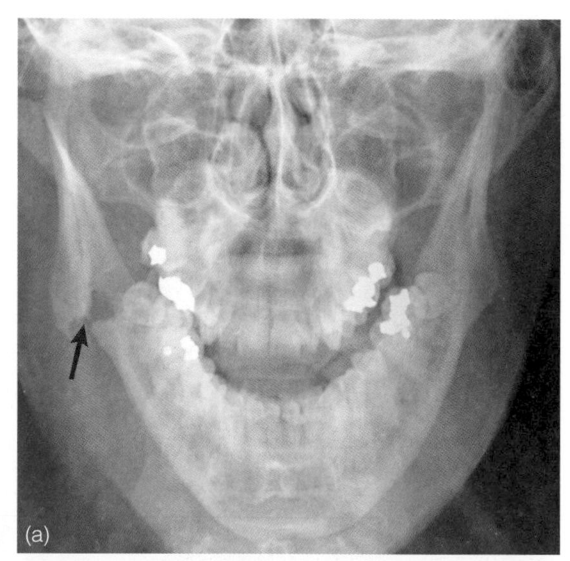

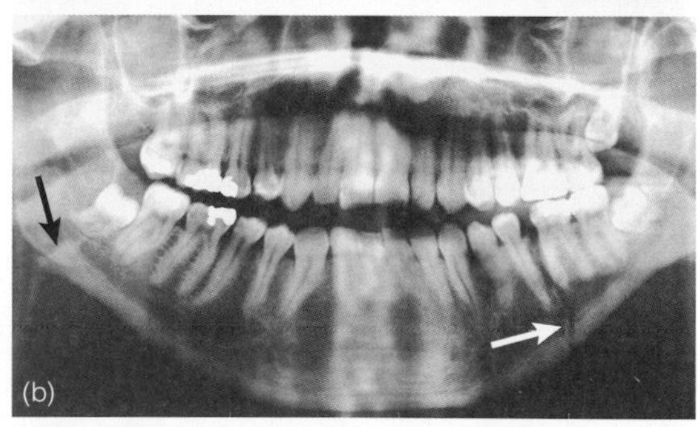

Figure 12.8 Mandible fractures: radiograph. (a) Frontal radiograph shows a displaced fracture of the right angle of the mandible (arrow). (b) Orthopantomogram (OPG) shows a fracture of the left mandibular body (white arrow) as well as a fracture of the right mandibular angle (black arrow).

12.2.5 TEMPORAL BONE FRACTURES

Fractures of the temporal bone are usually identified on CT performed for assessment of head injury. Less commonly, temporal bone fractures may present with hearing loss or CSF leak following recovery from acute head injury. Fractures have been previously classified on CT as transverse or longitudinal based on the orientation of the fracture line along the oblique temporal bone axis. Contemporary descriptions are based on the presence or absence of otic capsule involvement (Fig. 12.9). The otic capsule refers to the dense bone that surrounds the structures of the inner ear. Patients with fractures that involve the otic capsule have a higher risk of sensorineural hearing loss, facial nerve injury and CSF leak. Disruption of the middle ear ossicles in longitudinal temporal bone fractures may cause conductive hearing loss.

12.3 SPINAL TRAUMA

The roles of imaging in the assessment of spinal trauma are:

- Diagnosis of fractures/dislocation
- Assessment of stability/instability
- Diagnosis of damage to, or impingement on, neurological structures
- Follow-up:
  - Assessment of treatment
  - Diagnosis of long-term complications such as post-traumatic syrinx or cyst formation.

CT has superseded radiography as the initial investigation of spinal injury. Multiplanar and three-dimensional images greatly assist in delineation of both subtle fractures and complex injuries. CT provides accurate assessment of bony injuries, especially those of the neural arches and facet joints, and retropulsed bone fragments projecting into the spinal canal (Fig. 12.10). MRI is reserved for assessment of neural structures and ligamentous injury after CT.

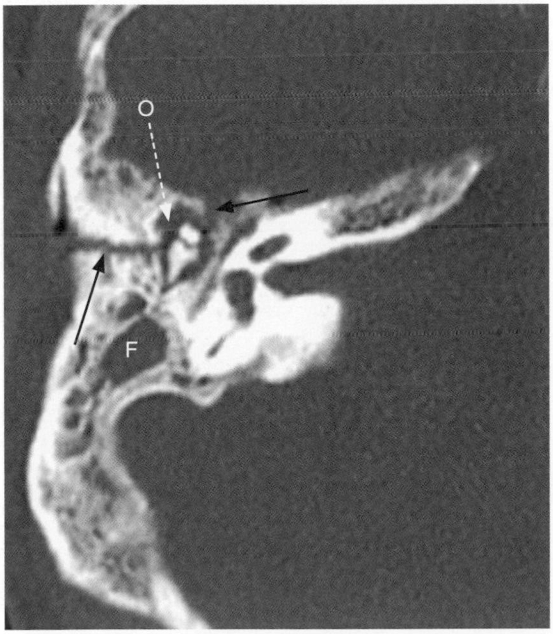

Figure 12.9 Temporal bone fracture: CT. Right temporal bone fracture extending into the middle ear (arrows). Note the fluid opacification in the mastoid air cells (F) and middle ear cavity. The ossicles are intact (O, dashed arrow).

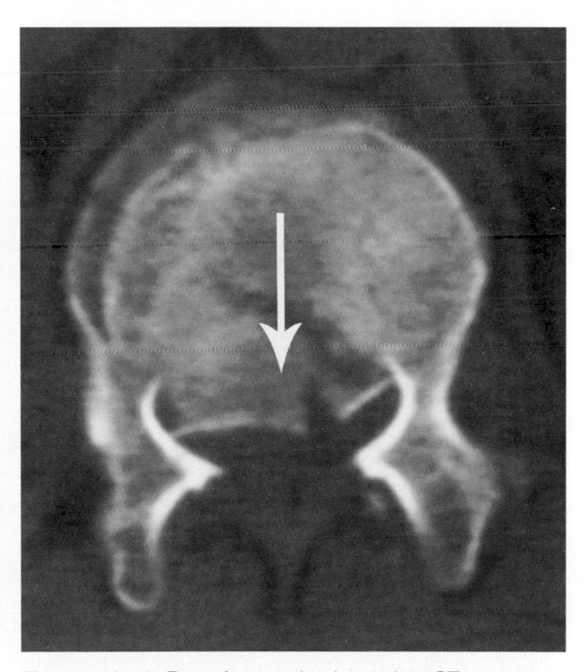

Figure 12.10 Burst fracture lumbar spine: CT. Transverse image shows a fracture of the vertebral body with a retropulsed bone fragment (arrow) extending into the spinal canal.

Cervical spine CT is often performed with head CT in the setting of head trauma or an unconscious patient. Thoracic and lumbar spine reconstructed images are obtained from CT of the torso.

12.3.1 CERVICAL SPINE TRAUMA

Indications for imaging in cervical spine trauma include:

- Neck pain or tenderness
- Other signs of direct neck injury
- Abnormal findings on neurological examination
- Severe head or facial injury
- Dangerous mechanism
- Near drowning
- Age older than 65 years
- Distracting injury or intoxication.

12.3.2 CERVICAL SPINE RADIOGRAPHY

If radiographs are performed for suspected trauma of the cervical spine, the series includes:

- Lateral view with the patient supine showing all seven cervical vertebrae:
  - o Shoulder traction may be required to assist with visualization of the lower cervical vertebrae
  - o Where the lower cervical vertebrae are obscured by the shoulders, a so-called 'swimmer's view' may be performed; this consists of a lateral view with one arm up and one down that 'uncovers' the cervicothoracic junction
  - o Traction on the head must never be used
- Anteroposterior (AP) view of the cervical spine
- AP open mouth peg view to show the C2 odontoid process and C1 lateral masses.

Cervical spine radiographs, like CT, should be assessed in a logical fashion for the following features (Figs 12.11 and 12.12):

1. Vertebral alignment:
   - o Disruption of the four curved spinal lines on lateral projection (Fig. 12.12):

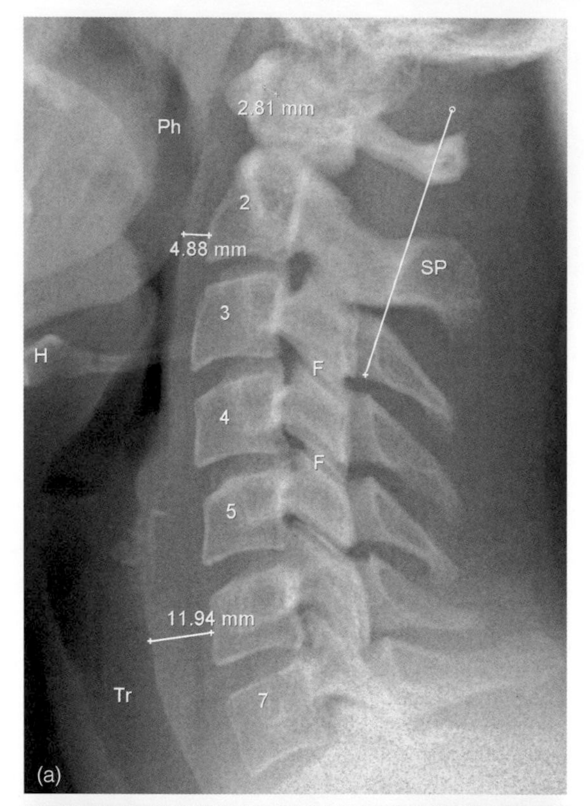

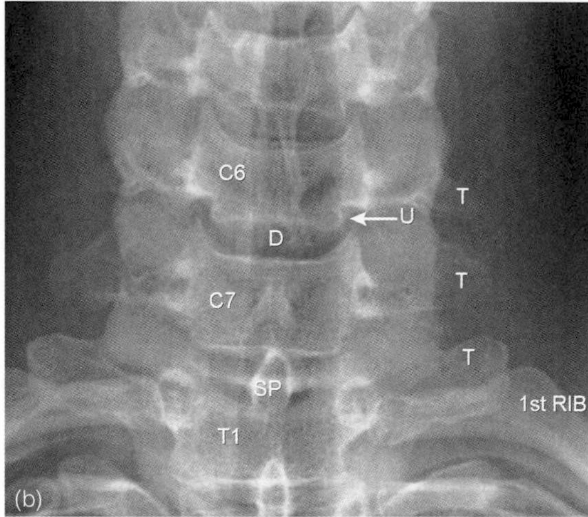

Figure 12.11 Normal cervical spine anatomy: radiograph. (a) Lateral view. Note the following: facet joint (F), hyoid bone (H), pharynx (Ph), spinous process (SP), trachea (Tr), a spinolaminar line from C1 to C3. Also note measurements of the predental space (between the anterior arch of C1 and the odontoid peg), the retropharyngeal space at C2 and the retrotracheal space at C6. (b) Frontal view of the lower cervical spine. Note the following: intervertebral disc (D), spinous process (SP), transverse process (T), uncovertebral joint (U).

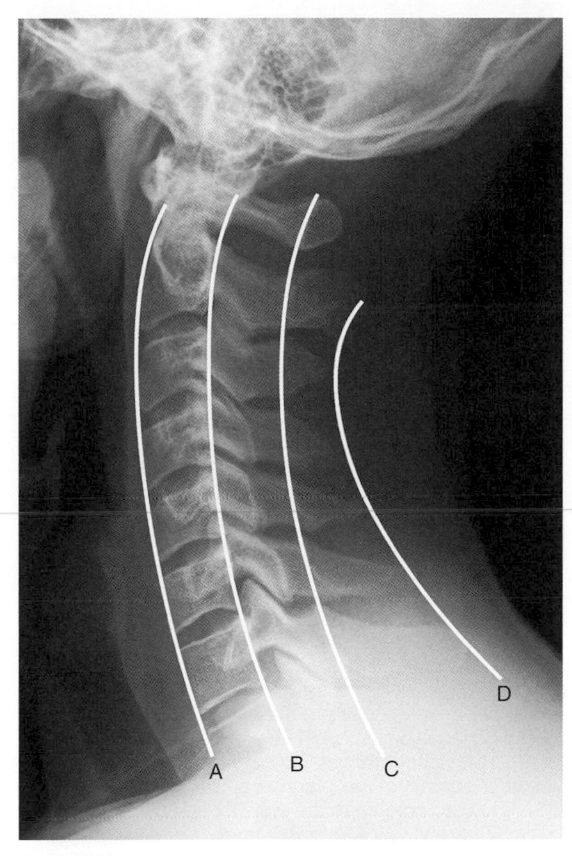

Figure 12.12 Lateral cervical spine alignment: radiograph. Anterior longitudinal line (A), posterior longitudinal line (B), spinolaminar line (C), posterior spinal line (D).

- Anterior longitudinal line joining the anterior cortical margins of the vertebral bodies
- Posterior longitudinal line joining the posterior cortical margins of the vertebral bodies
- Spinolaminar line joining the inner cortex of the laminae
- Posterior spinal line joining the posterior tips of the spinous processes

o Disruption of the coronal alignment of the vertebral bodies on the AP projection
o Facet joint alignment at all levels; abrupt disruption at one level may indicate dislocated or locked facets
o Widening of the interspinous spaces on the lateral projection
o Widening of the predental space on the lateral projection: more than 5 mm in children; more than 3 mm in adults
o Rotation of spinous processes on the AP projection

2. Bone integrity:
   o Vertebral body fractures
   o Fractures of posterior elements, i.e. pedicles, laminae, spinous processes
   o Integrity of the odontoid peg: anterior/posterior/lateral displacement
3. Disc spaces: narrowing or widening
4. Prevertebral swelling that may indicate occult fracture:
   o Widening of the retropharyngeal space: posterior aspect of pharynx to C2
     - More than 7 mm in adults and children.
   o Widening of the retrotracheal space: posterior aspect of trachea to C6
     - More than 14 mm in children
     - More than 22 mm in adults.

Erect lateral radiographs in flexion and extension (functional views) may be performed to diagnose ligamentous damage when potentially unstable fractures are found on neutral views.

12.3.3 COMMON PATTERNS OF CERVICAL SPINE TRAUMA

1. Flexion: anterior compression with posterior distraction (Fig. 12.13):
   o Vertebral body compression fracture
   o 'Teardrop' fracture, i.e. a small triangular fragment at the lower anterior margin of the vertebral body
   o Disruption of the posterior longitudinal line
   o Disc space narrowing
   o Widening of the facet joints
   o Facet joint dislocation or locking
   o Widening of the interspinous space
2. Extension: posterior compression with anterior distraction (Fig. 12.14):
   o 'Teardrop' fracture of the upper anterior margin of the vertebral body indicates severe anterior ligament damage
   o Disc space widening

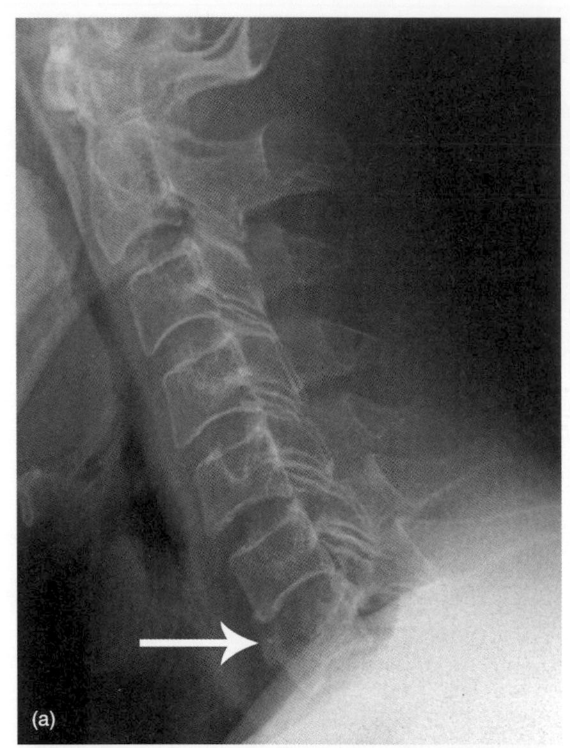

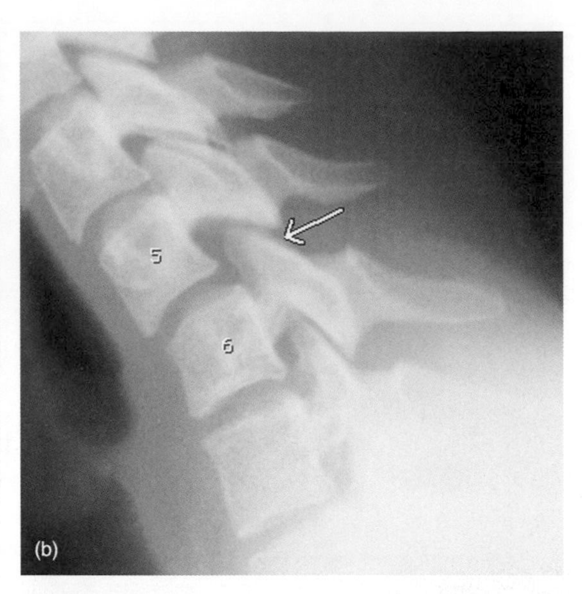

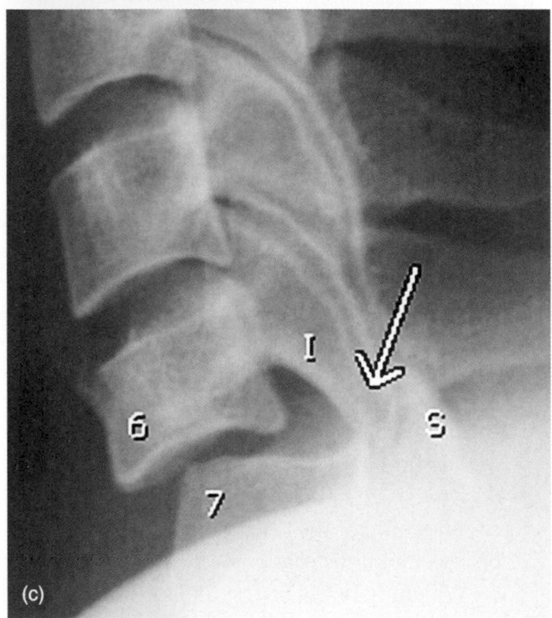

Figure 12.13 Flexion injuries of the cervical spine: radiograph of three separate examples. (a) Crush fracture of C7 (arrow). (b) Facet joint subluxation. The space between the spinous processes of C5 and C6 is widened. The inferior articular processes of C5 are shifted forwards on the superior articular processes of C6 (arrow), indicating facet joint subluxation. (c) Bilateral locked facets. Both facet joints at C6/7 are dislocated. The posterior corners of the inferior articular processes (I) of C6 are locked anterior to the superior articular processes (S) of C7 (arrow).

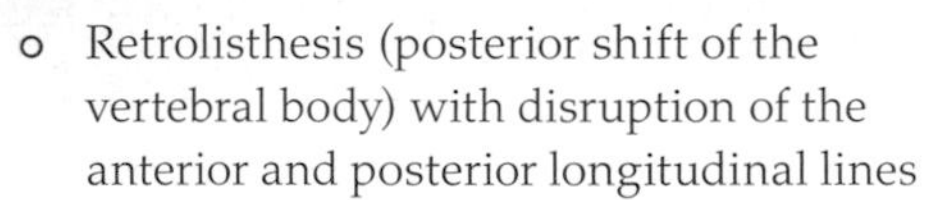

- Retrolisthesis (posterior shift of the vertebral body) with disruption of the anterior and posterior longitudinal lines
- Fractures of the posterior elements: pedicles, spinous processes, facets
- 'Hangman's' fracture: bilateral C2 pedicle fracture (Fig. 12.15)

3. Rotation (Fig. 12.16):
   - Anterolisthesis (anterior shift of the vertebral body) with disruption of the posterior vertebral line
   - Lateral displacement of the upper vertebral body on the AP view
   - Abrupt disruption of alignment of the facet joints: perched or locked facets
4. Compression:
   - Jefferson fracture: burst fracture of C1 (Fig. 12.17).

12.3.4 THORACIC AND LUMBAR SPINE RADIOGRAPHS

Assessment of radiographs of the thoracic and lumbar spine following trauma is similar to that outlined

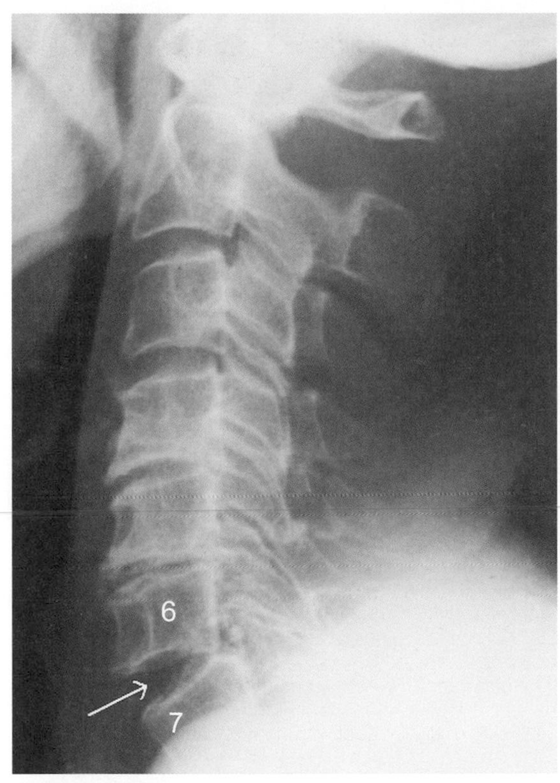

Figure 12.14 Extension injury of the cervical spine: radiograph. Note widening of the anterior disc space at C6/7 (arrow).

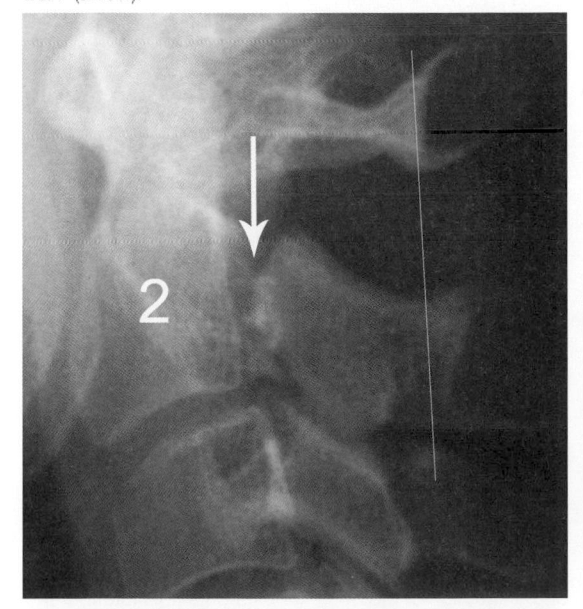

Figure 12.15 Hangman's fracture: radiograph. Fracture of the pedicles of C2 (arrow) with loss of continuity of the spinolaminar line (line).

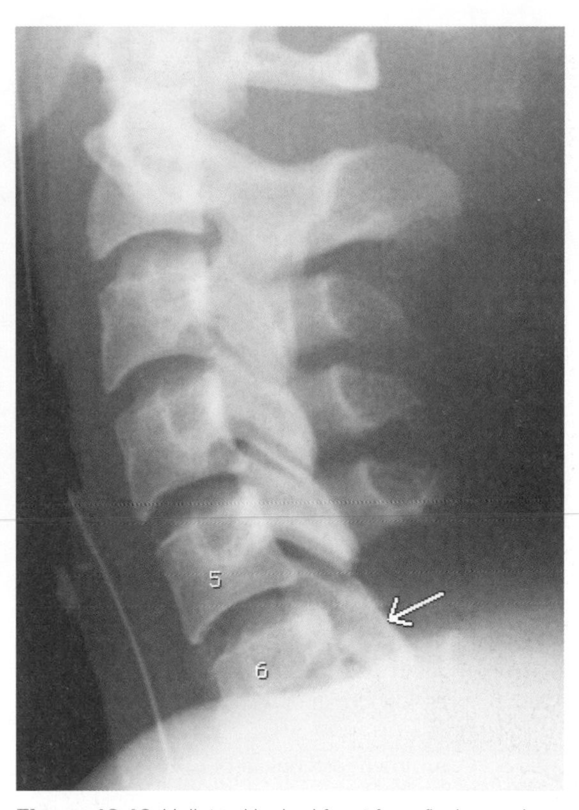

Figure 12.16 Unilateral locked facet from flexion and rotation injury of the cervical spine: radiograph. There is widening of the space between the spinous processes of C5 and C6. Only one normally aligned facet joint is seen at C5/6. Compare this with the levels above, where two normally aligned facet joints can be seen. Note the bare articular surface of one of the superior articular processes of C6 (arrow) owing to dislocation of this facet joint.

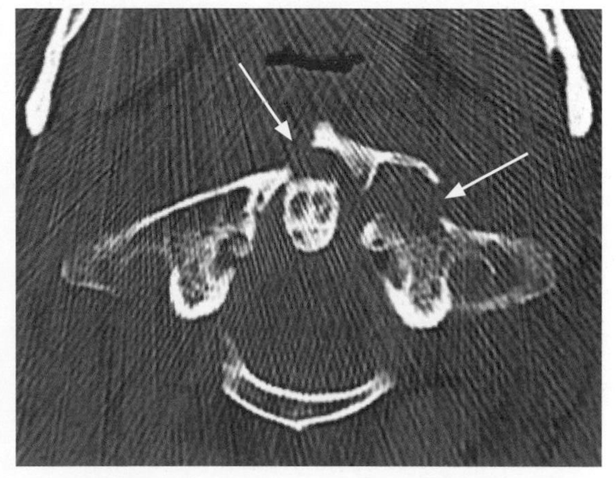

Figure 12.17 Jefferson fracture: CT. Transverse image shows fractures of C1 (arrows). The streaky appearance of the image is due to artefact from multiple metallic dental crowns.

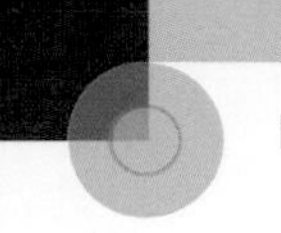

for the cervical spine, with particular attention to the following factors:

- Vertebral alignment
- Vertebral body height
- Disc space height
- Facet joint alignment
- Space between the pedicles on the AP film: widening at one level may indicate a burst fracture of the vertebral body.

12.3.5 COMMON PATTERNS OF THORACIC AND LUMBAR SPINE TRAUMA

1. Burst fracture:
    - Complex fractures of the vertebral body with a fragment pushed posteriorly (retropulsed) into the spinal canal
    - Multiple fracture lines through the vertebral endplates
2. Compression (crush or wedge) fracture (Fig. 12.18):
    - Common in osteoporosis
    - Loss of height of vertebral body most marked anteriorly, giving a wedge-like configuration
3. Fracture/dislocation:
    - Vertebral body displacement
    - Disc space narrowing or widening
    - Fractures of the neural arches, including the facet joints
    - Widening of the facet joints or interspinous spaces
4. Chance fracture, 'seatbelt fracture' (Fig. 12.19):
    - Occurs at the thoracolumbar junction from hyperflexion, usually over a lap seat belt in motor vehicle accidents
    - Horizontal fracture line through the spinous process, laminae and pedicles
    - Facet joints are often disrupted
    - Associated with abdominal injury, especially the closely located pancreas and duodenum
5. Chalkstick fracture (Fig. 12.20):
    - Fracture of a pathologically or surgically fused spine, e.g. ankylosing spondylitis, diffuse idiopathic skeletal hyperostosis (DISH)

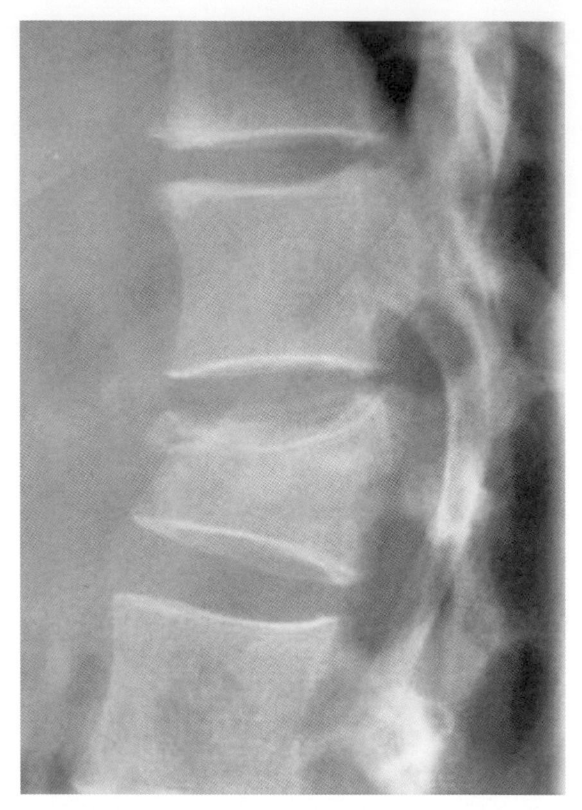

Figure 12.18 Crush fracture of the lumbar spine: radiograph. Lateral view showing a crush fracture of the upper body of L1.

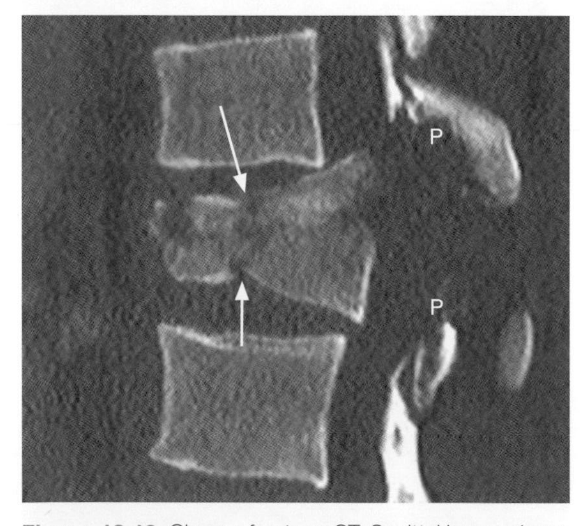

Figure 12.19 Chance fracture: CT. Sagittal image shows compression fractures of a lumbar vertebral body (arrows) and distraction of the posterior elements (P). Note that the posterior surface of the fractured vertebral body projects into the spinal canal with likely compression of neural structures.

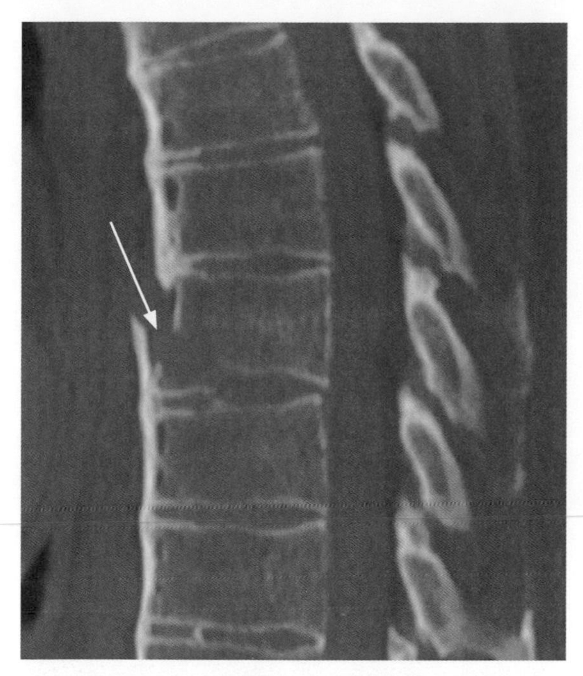

Figure 12.20 Chalkstick fracture: CT. Sagittal image shows a mid-thoracic vertebral fracture (arrow) extending into the intervertebral disc space, which is widened. The spine is fused anteriorly as a result of diffuse idiopathic skeletal hyperostosis (DISH).

- Often caused by minimal hyperextension
- Fractures typically occur in the lower cervical or upper thoracic spine and are often due to minimal hyperextension; commonly involve a disc space
- Fracture healing is often compromised in these patients
- Close surveillance for a progressive deformity is required if management is non-operative.

12.3.6 SPINAL STABILITY

As well as diagnosing and classifying spinal injuries, determining injury stability is also important. Instability implies the possibility of increased spinal deformity or neurological damage occurring with mobilization or continued stress. Viewed laterally, the spine may be divided into three columns:

- Anterior: anterior two-thirds of the vertebral body and intervertebral disc, anterior longitudinal ligament
- Middle: posterior one-third of the vertebral body and intervertebral disc and posterior longitudinal ligament
- Posterior: facet joints and bony arch of the spinal canal (pedicles, laminae and spinous process).

In general, two of these three columns must be intact for spinal stability to be maintained. Radiographic and CT signs of instability include:

- Displacement of a vertebral body
- 'Teardrop' fractures of cervical vertebral bodies
- Odontoid peg fracture
- Widening or disruption of alignment of the facet joints, including locked facets
- Widened interspinous space on the AP view
- Abnormal disc space (widened or narrowed)
- Fractures at multiple levels.

12.3.7 MAGNETIC RESONANCE IMAGING IN SPINAL TRAUMA

MRI is the primary investigation for the assessment of suspected spinal cord damage. Signs of spinal cord trauma on MRI include cord transection, cord oedema and haemorrhage (Fig. 12.21). Late sequelae of cord injury include arachnoid cyst, pseudomeningocele, myelomalacia and syrinx. Other soft-tissue changes may be seen, such as traumatic disc herniation, ligament disruption and spinal canal haematoma. Indications for MRI of the spine in the setting of trauma include:

- Known vertebral fractures: cord injury, epidural haematoma, disc integrity and ligamentous instability
- Neurological symptoms or signs (regardless of radiographic findings):
  - The phenomenon of spinal cord injury without radiographic abnormality (SCIWORA) is well described, particularly in children
  - A normal radiograph should not preclude MRI when neurological injury is clinically suspected
- Crush fractures of the thoracic and lumbar spine: differentiating acute from older healed

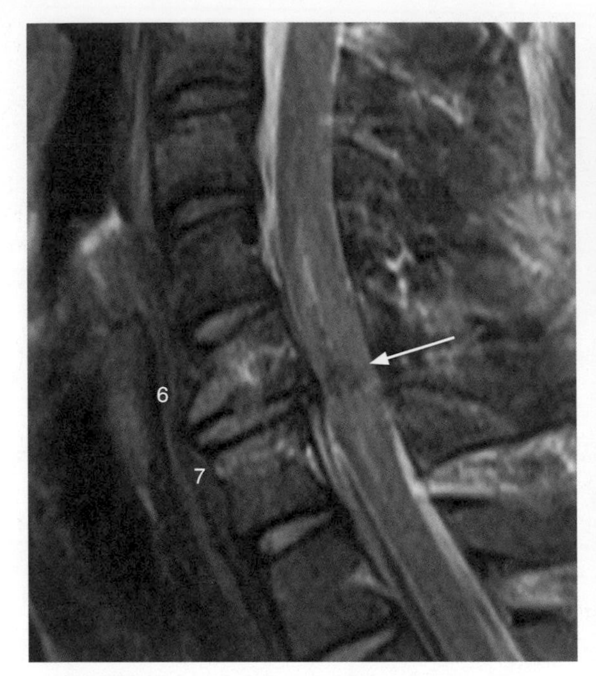

Figure 12.21 Spinal cord haematoma: sagittal T2-weighted MRI. There are fractures of the C6 and C7 vertebral bodies. A focus of low T2 signal in the central cervical cord represents haemorrhage (arrow). Thin high signal extending in the cord above and below the haematoma represents oedema.

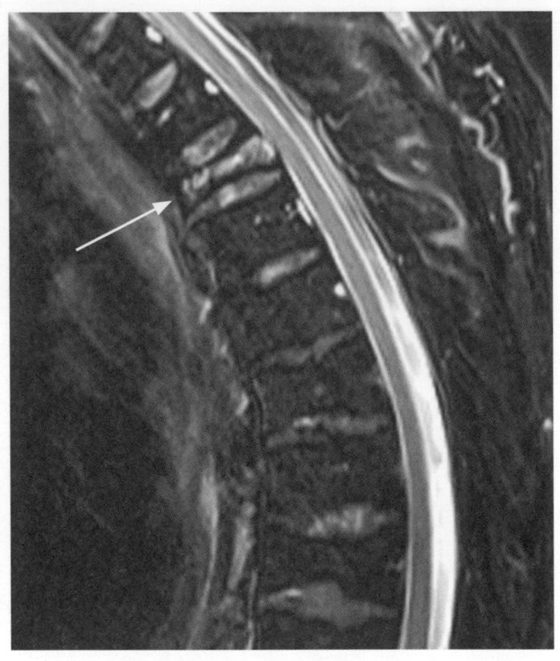

Figure 12.22 Acute vertebral crush fracture: sagittal STIR (short TI (inversion time) inversion recovery) MRI. High signal due to oedema in an upper thoracic vertebral crush fracture indicates that the fracture is acute (arrow). Note multiple other healed crush fractures that have normal low bone marrow signal.

injuries (Fig. 12.22). This has become a common indication in elderly patients with suspected osteoporotic crush fractures in whom MRI assists patient selection for percutaneous vertebroplasty (see Chapter 10).

12.4 CHEST TRAUMA

CXR is the initial imaging investigation in chest trauma. Trauma CXR is often performed with the patient supine in the trauma room, leading to several potential problems with interpretation:

- The mediastinum appears widened because of normal distension of the venous structures and magnification
- Pleural fluid may be more difficult to diagnose in the absence of a fluid level
- Pneumothorax may be more difficult to diagnose.

CXR is also used in acute settings to assess medical interventions, such as positioning of lines and tubes, and potential iatrogenic complications. CT provides more accurate assessment of thoracic injury with much greater sensitivity than CXR. CT is the investigation of choice for the assessment of chest trauma and is performed during the arterial phase of contrast enhancement. This provides a CT angiogram of the aorta as well as excellent delineation of all other chest structures. The following is a list of traumatic findings that may be seen on CXR and are better demonstrated on CT:

- Pneumothorax (see Chapter 4)
- Pneumomediastinum
- Subcutaneous emphysema (Fig. 12.23):

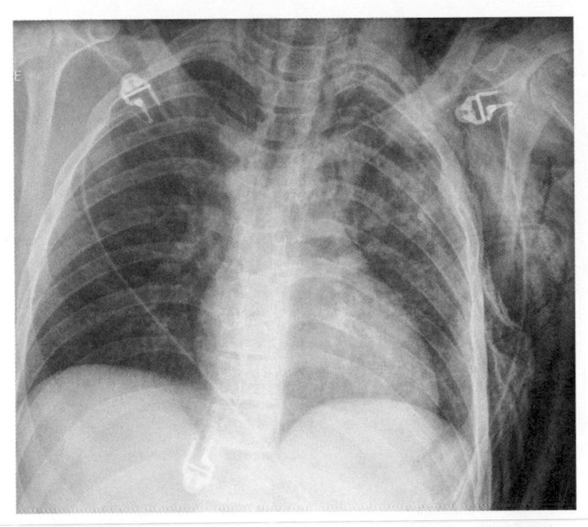

Figure 12.23 Chest trauma from a high-speed motor vehicle accident: CXR. Note multiple rib fractures, an ill-defined opacity in the left upper lobe owing to contusion, extensive subcutaneous air in the left chest wall tracking upwards into the neck.

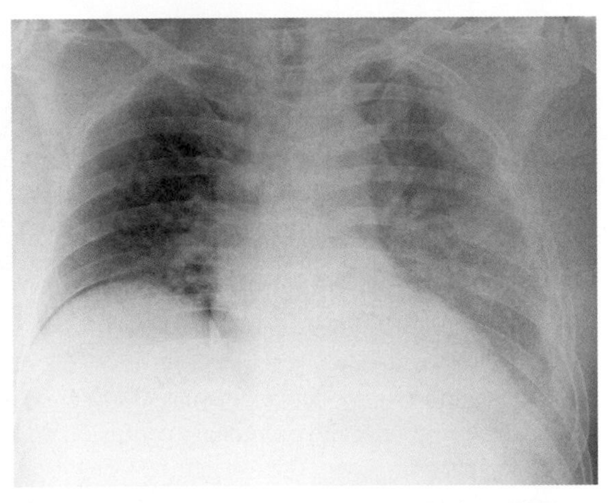

Figure 12.24 Haemothorax: supine CXR. Opacification of the left hemithorax with the ability to see the lung markings. Note multiple rib fractures.

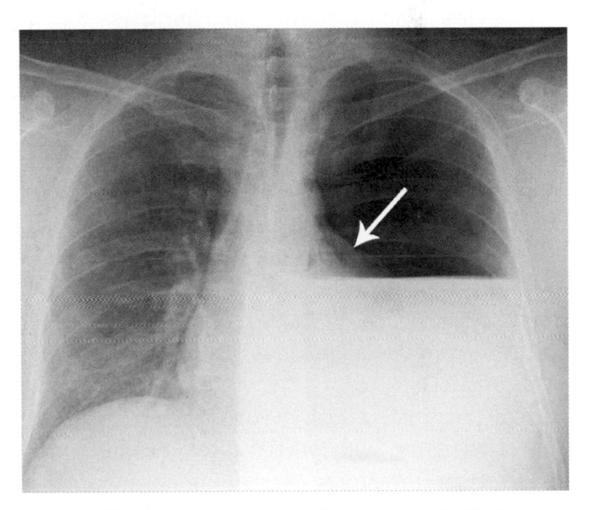

Figure 12.25 Haemopneumothorax: erect CXR. Note that a combination of air and fluid in the pleural space produces a straight line without the typical meniscus of a pleural effusion. In this case, there is also evidence of tension with increased volume on the left and marked collapse and distortion of the left lung (arrow).

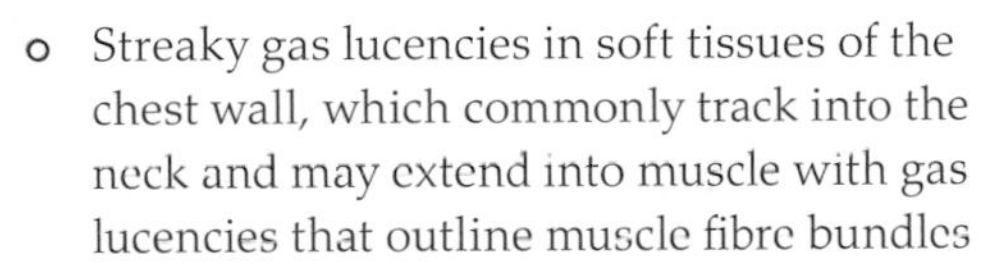

- Streaky gas lucencies in soft tissues of the chest wall, which commonly track into the neck and may extend into muscle with gas lucencies that outline muscle fibre bundles

- Haemothorax (Fig. 12.24):
  - Appearance as described for pleural effusion (see Chapter 4)
- Haemopneumothorax (Fig. 12.25):
  - Combination of fluid and air in the pleural cavity produces a sharply defined air–fluid level
  - Fluid level extends to the chest wall without forming a meniscus
- Pulmonary contusion:
  - Focal area of alveolar shadowing occurring within hours of injury that usually clears after 4 days
  - Often underlies rib fractures
- Traumatic pneumatocele:
  - Air-filled cavities formed from parenchymal laceration and tissue recoil, often surrounded by extensive contusion
  - Commonly fill with blood
- Mediastinal haematoma (see section 12.4.1)
- Ruptured diaphragm:
  - Herniation of abdominal structures into the chest
  - Contralateral mediastinal shift
- Rib fractures:
  - Fractures of the upper three ribs indicate a high level of trauma, though there is no proven increase in the incidence of great vessel damage

- Fractures of the lower three ribs are associated with upper abdominal injury (liver, spleen and kidney)
- Significant fracture displacement correlates with ventilatory difficulties
- Flail segment refers to segmental fractures of three or more adjacent ribs, which can produce segmental paradoxical movement of the chest wall with respiration
- Flail segment has a high incidence of associated injuries, including pneumothorax, subcutaneous emphysema, haemothorax and pulmonary contusion and laceration
- Adequate pain management is crucial to prevent lobar collapse and pneumonia

- Glenohumeral dislocation and fractures of the clavicle, scapula, sternum and humerus.

12.4.1 AORTIC INJURY

Rupture of the thoracic aorta is the most catastrophic injury from chest trauma. Full-thickness or complete aortic rupture (transection) is usually fatal. Up to 20% of aortic injuries are not full thickness, i.e. the adventitia is intact; if left untreated, they have a high mortality rate.

Mediastinal haematoma is the hallmark finding of traumatic aortic injury. Twenty per cent of patients with mediastinal haematoma on CXR or CT will have an aortic injury, with other causes including thoracic vertebral fractures, sternal injury and smaller vessel injury. If the aortic adventitia remains intact, mediastinal haematoma can arise from smaller vessel injury, such as the intercostal or internal thoracic vessels. CXR signs of aortic rupture result from the associated mediastinal haematoma (Fig. 12.26):

- Widened mediastinum (noting reduced sensitivity on a supine projection)
- Obscured aortic knuckle and other mediastinal structures
- Displacement of the trachea and nasogastric tube to the right
- Thickened paravertebral and paratracheal stripes
- Depression of the left main bronchus
- Loss of the aortopulmonary window
- Left haemothorax causing pleural opacification, including depression of the apex of the left lung (apical capping).

Aortic injury is confirmed by CT (Fig. 12.27). CT signs of aortic injury include:

- Periaortic haematoma

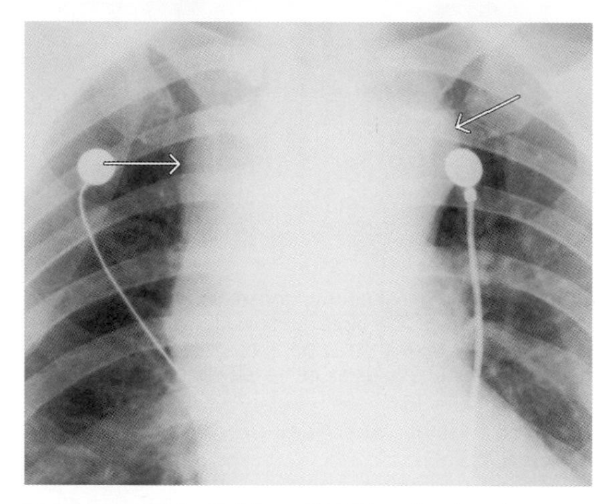

Figure 12.26 Aortic injury: CXR. Note that there is widening of the mediastinum (arrows) with loss of definition of mediastinal structures owing to mediastinal haematoma.

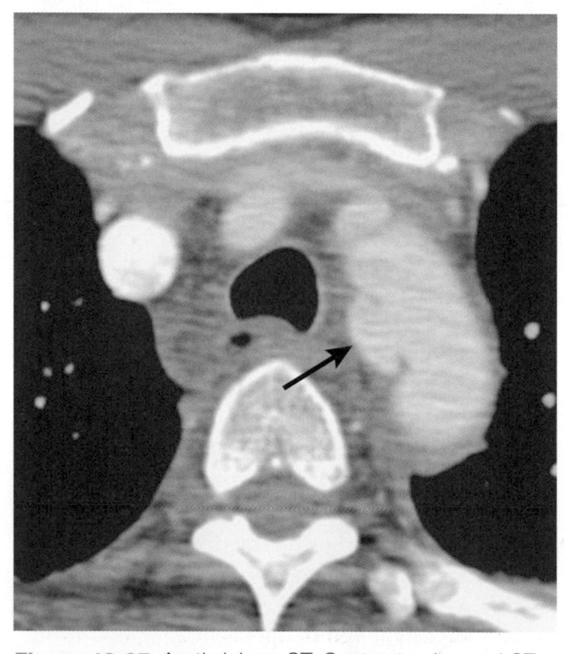

Figure 12.27 Aortic injury: CT. Contrast-enhanced CT shows a localized out-pocketing of the medial wall of the aortic arch, indicating a pseudoaneurysm (arrow). Note the periaortic haematoma.

- Abnormal aortic contour representing complete or incomplete rupture and pseudoaneurysm
- Intimal flap or intraluminal filling defect due to clot
- Contrast extravasation into the mediastinum.

Most aortic injuries occur at the aortic isthmus, just distal to the left subclavian artery origin. The attachment of the ligamentum arteriosum at this location tethers the aorta during deceleration. Minimal aortic injury (MAI) is mild vessel injury confined to the intima and/or inner media under 10 mm in size. The external aortic contour is normal and periaortic haematoma is absent. MAI can spontaneously resolve but requires close surveillance for the development of dissection or intramural haematoma. Transoesophageal echocardiography (TOE) may be used as a problem-solving tool in difficult or equivocal cases. Interventional radiology is commonly used to treat aortic rupture, with aortogram and covered stent deployment (Fig. 12.28).

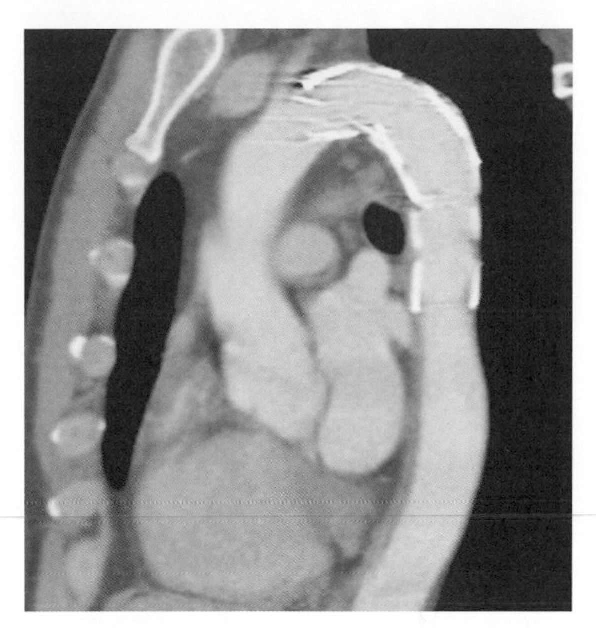

Figure 12.28 Aortic injury post repair with a covered stent: contrast-enhanced CT. The stent is seen on this sagittal image as a parallel metal density in the wall of the aorta. The aortic lumen shows normal enhancement with a smooth outline, indicating good expansion of the stent with no leakage or other complication.

12.5 ABDOMINAL AND PELVIC TRAUMA

CT provides rapid and accurate anatomical definition of abdominal and pelvic organ injury and intra-abdominal fluid. As discussed earlier, the haemodynamic status of the patient will determine the imaging path in patients with potential abdominal or pelvic trauma. Urgent life-threatening injuries of the solid organs are readily visible on CT and the presence and distribution of blood in the peritoneal cavity (haemoperitoneum) or retroperitoneum can aid in the diagnosis of more subtle visceral injuries.

12.5.1 SOLID VISCUS INJURY

The liver, spleen, kidneys, pancreas and adrenal glands may be injured by laceration, fracture, haematoma, contusion or a combination of each. The spleen is the most injured abdominal viscus and is the only organ injured in approximately two-thirds of abdominal trauma patients.

Several organ injury grading systems are employed when describing solid viscera injury; these are broadly based on injury type, size, intraparenchymal location and the presence of active parenchymal bleeding. Further details on these grading systems for specific organs may be found on the companion website. Active haemorrhage may cause a focal 'blush' of extravasated contrast material (Fig. 12.29). This sign is an indication for immediate surgery, or angiography and embolization.

Some organs have associated structures that may be injured, leading to more significant or delayed sequelae:

- Liver: inferior vena cava (IVC) producing haemorrhage, or biliary tree resulting in bile leak and biloma
- Pancreas: pancreatic duct resulting in pancreatitis and pseudocyst
- Kidneys: collecting system resulting in urine leak and urinoma.

A non-functioning kidney (non-enhancing) may be due to massive parenchymal damage (shattered kidney), vascular pedicle injury or collecting system obstruction as a result of a blood clot.

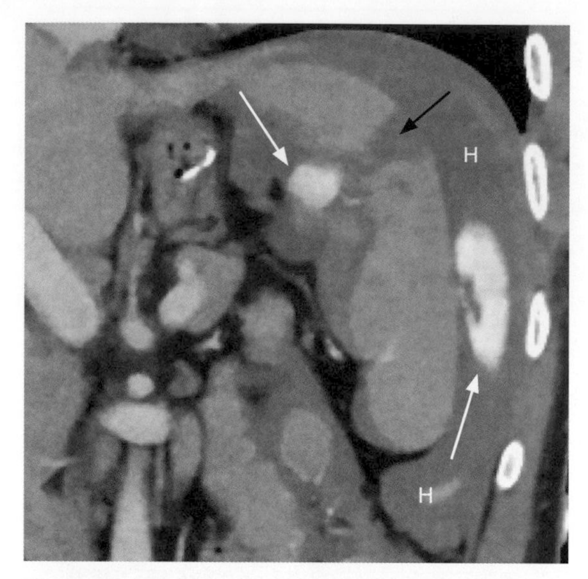

Figure 12.29 Splenic trauma: CT. Coronal image shows haematoma (H) around the spleen and a splenic upper pole laceration (black arrow). There is perisplenic contrast extravasation (white arrows) indicating active bleeding.

12.5.2 HAEMOPERITONEUM

The distribution of intraperitoneal blood can indicate the source. Blood from solid organ injury will collect in more dependent parts of the peritoneal cavity, i.e. pelvis, hepatorenal pouch and paracolic gutters. Acute clotted blood is hyperdense (30–70 HU) and a collection of higher density blood adjacent to an organ may implicate that organ as the source of bleeding (sentinel clot sign).

12.5.3 BOWEL AND MESENTERIC INJURY

Bowel and mesenteric trauma is often subtle and easily missed on CT. Free intraperitoneal and retroperitoneal gas is often absent. CT signs include blood between bowel loops or at the base of the mesentery, bowel wall haematoma and mesenteric haematoma.

12.5.4 BLADDER AND URETHRAL INJURY

Bladder injury has a high association with pelvic fractures and may be due to blunt, penetrating or iatrogenic trauma. Routine trauma CT has limited sensitivity for bladder injury. Intraperitoneal bladder rupture causes intraperitoneal leak of urine, seen as low-attenuation free fluid (approximately 10 HU). Extraperitoneal rupture is far more common and causes urine leakage into the extraperitoneal pelvic tissues. CT cystography improves sensitivity and has replaced conventional fluoroscopic cystography as it can be performed at the time of whole-body trauma CT. It is achieved with a delayed phase (10–15 minutes) after intravenous contrast administration, or by direct injection of contrast material into the bladder via a catheter. Care during catheter insertion is paramount to avoid iatrogenic urethral injury. The signs of bladder trauma on CT cystogram include bladder deformity and leakage of contrast material (Fig. 12.30).

Urethral injury complicates approximately 15% of anterior pelvic fractures or pubic symphysis diastasis in males. The most common site of injury is the proximal bulbous urethra. Signs include blood at the urethral meatus and inability to void. Retrograde urethrography is a simple procedure that can be performed quickly in the emergency department on stable patients (Fig. 12.31) and depicts contrast extravasation from the urethra.

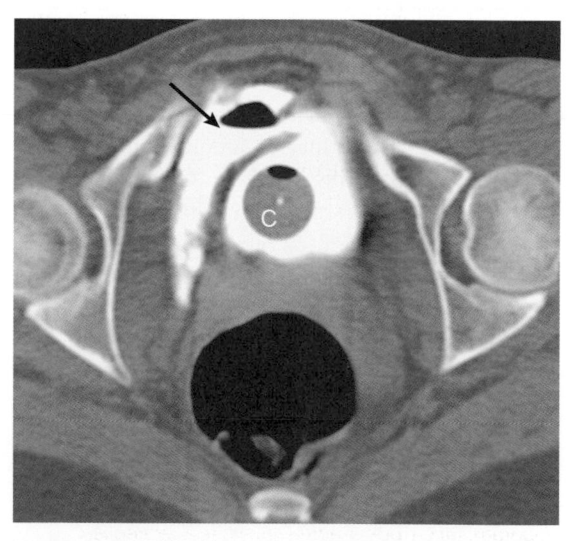

Figure 12.30 Bladder injury: CT cystogram. Transverse image following infusion of contrast material into the bladder shows extraperitoneal leakage (arrow) through a tear in the lower anterior bladder. Note the catheter balloon (C).

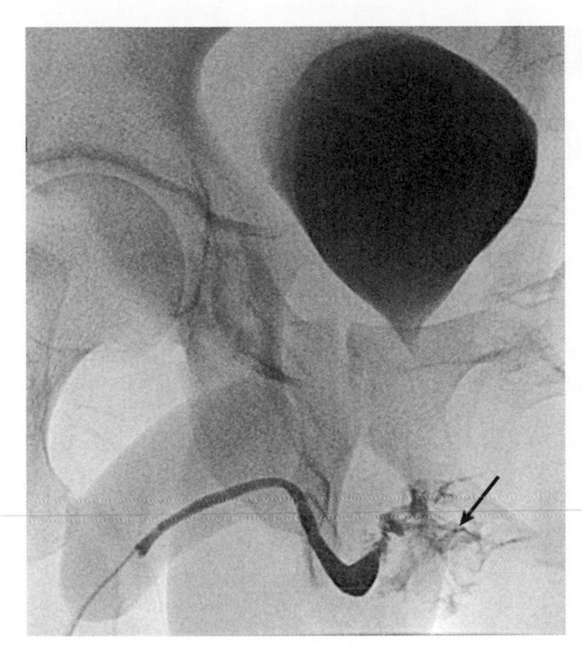

Figure 12.31 Urethral injury: urethrogram. Urethrogram outlines the bladder and urethra with leakage of contrast material (arrow), indicating a urethral tear.

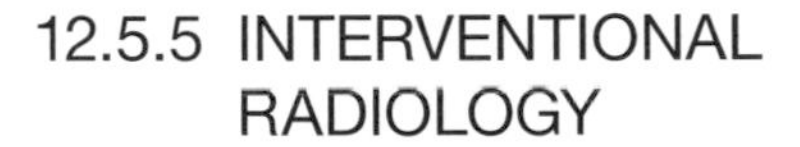

12.5.5 INTERVENTIONAL RADIOLOGY

Angiography and embolization is a successful non-operative treatment option for the management of splenic, hepatic, renal, bowel and mesenteric injuries (Fig. 12.32). It is also used as a substitute or adjunct to surgery to control active pelvic arterial bleeding associated with pelvic fractures.

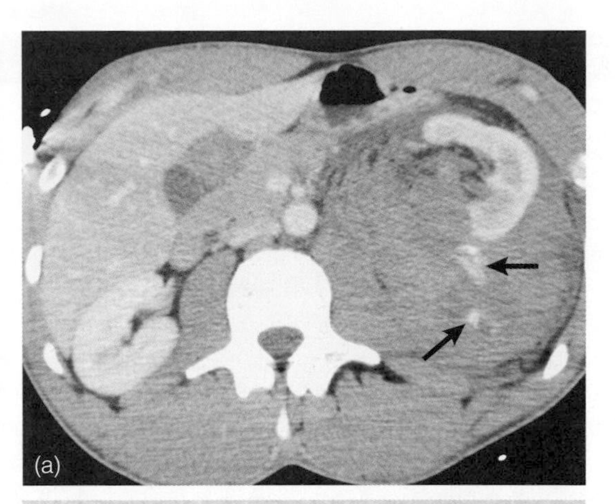

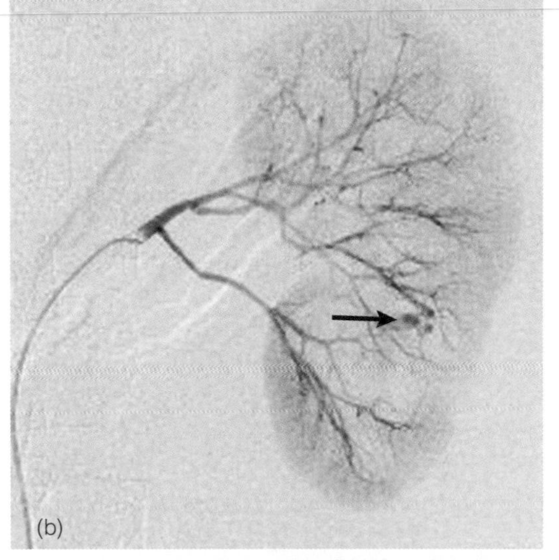

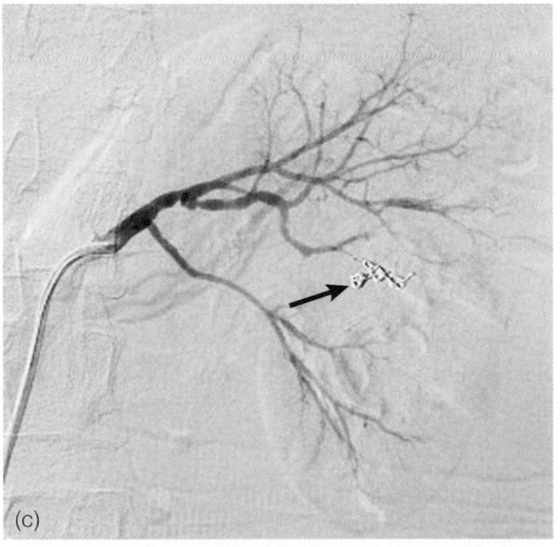

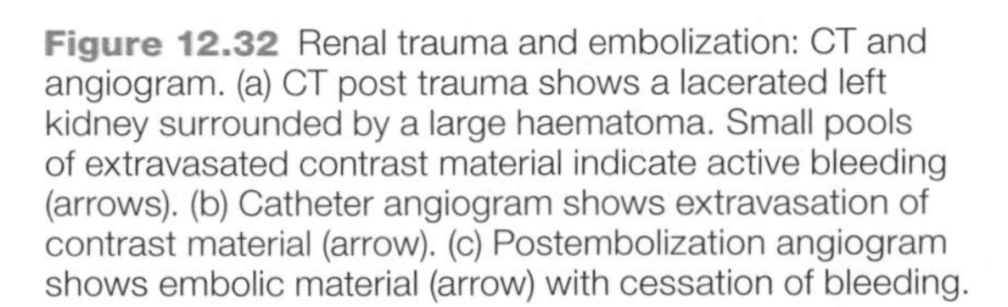

Figure 12.32 Renal trauma and embolization: CT and angiogram. (a) CT post trauma shows a lacerated left kidney surrounded by a large haematoma. Small pools of extravasated contrast material indicate active bleeding (arrows). (b) Catheter angiogram shows extravasation of contrast material (arrow). (c) Postembolization angiogram shows embolic material (arrow) with cessation of bleeding.

SUMMARY

Clinical presentation	Investigation of choice	Comment
Head trauma	• CT: initial assessment • MRI: later assessment	MRI more sensitive for DAI
Facial trauma	CT	
Spinal trauma	• CT: initial assessment • MRI: later assessment	• CTA for patients with signs or at high risk of neck vascular injury • MRI to assess cord injury and ligamentous disruption
Chest trauma	• CXR: initial bedside assessment • CT: standard assessment in arterial phase	CXR to assess for major reversible injuries and iatrogenic interventions
Abdominal trauma	• US: FAST at the bedside • CT: standard assessment in portal venous ± arterial phases	• FAST to identify those with haemoperitoneum • CT urography for upper renal tract injury
Pelvic trauma	• PXR: initial bedside assessment • CT: standard assessment • Retrograde urethrography: straddle injuries	• CT cystography for bladder injury • Retrograde urethrography for urethral injury

Abbreviations: CTA, CT angiography; DAI, diffuse axonal injury; FAST, focused assessment with sonography in trauma; PXR, pelvic radiograph.

13 Musculoskeletal system

13.1 IMAGING INVESTIGATION OF THE MUSCULOSKELETAL SYSTEM

13.1.1 RADIOGRAPHS

Radiographs are indicated in all fractures and dislocations. Radiographs are often sufficient for diagnosis in general bone conditions such as Paget disease (see section 13.8.3). Most bone tumours and other focal bone lesions are characterized by clinical history and plain radiographs. Magnetic resonance imaging (MRI), scintigraphy and computed tomography (CT) are used for staging or to assess specific complications of these lesions but usually add little to the diagnostic specificity of radiographs. A major limitation of radiography is insensitivity for early bony changes in conditions such as osteomyelitis and stress fractures.

13.1.2 MAGNETIC RESONANCE IMAGING

MRI can visualize all the different tissues of the musculoskeletal system, including cortical and medullary bone, hyaline and fibrocartilage, tendon, ligament and muscle. As such, MRI has a wide diversity of applications, including internal derangements of joints, staging of bone and soft-tissue tumours and diagnosis of early or subtle bone changes in osteomyelitis, stress fracture and trauma.

13.1.3 ULTRASOUND

Musculoskeletal ultrasound (MSUS) is used to assess the soft tissues of the musculoskeletal system, i.e. tendons, ligaments and muscles. MSUS can diagnose muscle and tendon tears. MSUS is also used to assess superficial soft-tissue masses and can provide a definitive diagnosis for common pathologies such as ganglion and superficial lipoma. MSUS is highly sensitive for the detection of soft-tissue foreign bodies, including those not visible on radiographs such as thorns, wood splinters and tiny pieces of glass. The limitations of MSUS include an inability to visualize bone pathology and most internal joint derangements.

13.1.4 COMPUTED TOMOGRAPHY

Multidetector CT is used for further delineation of complex fractures. Common indications include depressed fracture of the tibial plateau, comminuted fracture of the calcaneus and fractures involving articular surfaces. CT may also be used to diagnose complications of fractures such as non-union. CT may assist in staging bone tumours by demonstrating specific features such as soft-tissue extension and cortical destruction.

13.1.5 SCINTIGRAPHY

Bone scintigraphy, commonly known as a 'bone scan', is performed with diphosphonate-based radiopharmaceuticals such as ^{99m}Tc-MDP (see Table 1.1). MDP and similar pharmaceuticals are taken up by osteoblastic regions, where new bone is being laid down. In modern practice, bone scintigraphy is performed in combination with CT (single photon emission CT (SPECT)-CT). Bone scintigraphy is highly sensitive and therefore able to demonstrate pathologies such as subtle fractures, stress fractures and osteomyelitis prior to radiographic changes becoming apparent. Scintigraphy is also able to image the entire skeleton and is therefore the investigation of choice for screening for skeletal metastases and other multifocal tumours. The commonest exception to this is multiple myeloma, which may be difficult to appreciate on scintigraphy (see section 13.8.2).

13.2 HOW TO ASSESS A SKELETAL RADIOGRAPH

13.2.1 TECHNICAL ASSESSMENT

As is the case with a chest radiograph (chest X-ray, CXR) and an abdomen radiograph (abdomen X-ray, AXR), a skeletal radiograph should be assessed for technical adequacy. This includes appropriate centring and projections for the area to be examined, plus adequate exposure. Features of a technically adequate radiograph of a bone or joint include:

- Fine bony detail, including sharp definition of bony surfaces and visibility of bony trabeculae
- Soft-tissue detail, such as fat planes between muscles
- Where a joint is being examined, the articular surfaces should be visible with radiographs angled to show minimal overlap of adjacent bones.

Some bony overlap is unavoidable in complex areas such as the ankle and wrist, and multiple views with different angulations may be required to show the desired anatomy.

13.2.2 NORMAL RADIOGRAPHIC ANATOMY

Viewing of skeletal radiographs requires knowledge of bony anatomy. This includes an ability to name bones and joints, plus an awareness of anatomical features common to all bones. Mature bones consist of a dense cortex of compact bone and a central medulla of cancellous bone. Cortex is seen radiographically as the white periphery of a bone. The central medulla is less dense. Cancellous bone that makes up the medulla consists of a sponge-like network of thin bony plates known as trabeculae. Trabeculae support the bone marrow and are seen radiographically as a latticework of fine white lines in the medullary cavity. The cortex tends to be thicker in the shafts of long bones. Where long bones flare at their ends, the cortex is thinner and the trabeculae in the medulla are more obvious.

The anatomical features of bones that may be recognized on radiographs are listed below. These include elevations and projections that provide attachments for tendons and ligaments and various holes and depressions (Figs 13.1 and 13.2):

- Head: expanded proximal end of a long bone, e.g. humerus, radius and femur
- Articular surface: synovial articulation with other bone(s); smooth bone surface covered with hyaline cartilage
- Facet: flat articular surface, e.g. zygapophyseal joints between vertebral bodies, commonly (though strictly speaking incorrectly) referred to as 'facet joints'
- Condyle: rounded articular surface, e.g. medial and lateral femoral condyles
- Epicondyle: projection close to a condyle providing attachment sites for the collateral ligaments of the joint, e.g. humeral and femoral epicondyles

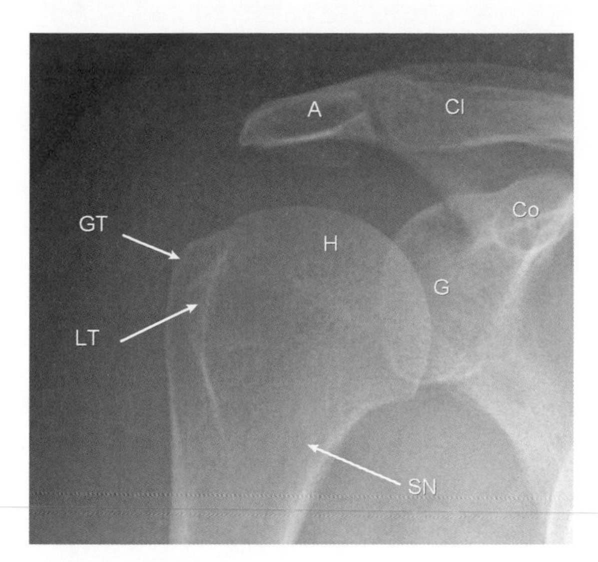

Figure 13.1 Normal shoulder. Note: acromion (A), clavicle (Cl), coracoid process (Co), glenoid (G), greater tuberosity (GT), humeral head (H), lesser tuberosity (LT), surgical neck (SN).

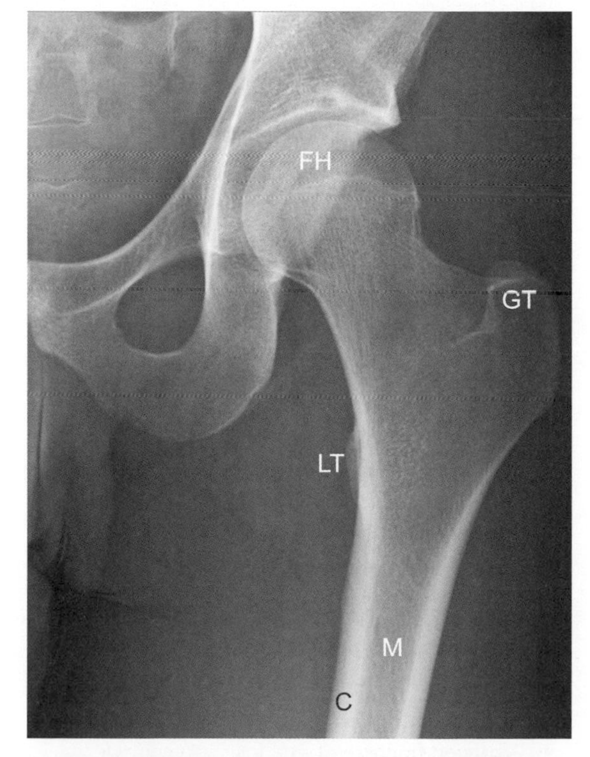

Figure 13.2 Normal upper femur. Note: cortex (C), femoral head (FH), greater trochanter (GT), lesser trochanter (LT), medulla (M).

- Process: large projection, e.g. coracoid process of the scapula
- Tuberosity: rounded projection, e.g. lesser and greater tuberosities of the humerus
- Trochanter: rounded projection, e.g. greater and lesser trochanters of the femur
- Foramen: hole in a bone that usually transmits nerve and/or blood vessels, e.g. foramen ovale in the skull base
- Canal: long foramen, e.g. infraorbital canal
- Sulcus: long depression, e.g. humeral bicipital sulcus between lesser and greater tuberosities
- Fossa: wider depression, e.g. acetabular fossa.

Cartilage is not visible on plain radiographs; cartilage disorders are best assessed with MRI. Most cartilages in the body are hyaline or fibrocartilage. Hyaline cartilage covers the articular surfaces in synovial joints. The labrum is a rim of fibrocartilage that surrounds the articular surfaces of the acetabulum and glenoid. Fibrocartilage also forms the menisci of the knee, the articular disc of the temporomandibular joint and the triangular fibrocartilage complex (TFCC) of the wrist.

13.2.3 GROWING BONES IN CHILDREN

Bones develop and grow through primary and secondary ossification centres (Fig. 13.3). Virtually all primary centres are present and ossified at birth. The part of bone ossified from the primary centre is termed the diaphysis. In long bones the diaphysis forms most of the shaft. Secondary ossification centres occur later in growing bones, most appearing after birth. The secondary centre at the end of a growing long bone is termed the epiphysis. The epiphysis is separated from the shaft of the bone by the epiphyseal growth cartilage or physis. An apophysis is another type of secondary ossification centre that forms a protrusion from the growing bone. Examples of apophyses include the greater trochanter of the femur and the tibial tuberosity. The metaphysis is that part of the bone between the diaphysis and the physis. The diaphysis and metaphysis are covered by periosteum, and the articular surface of the epiphysis is covered by articular cartilage.

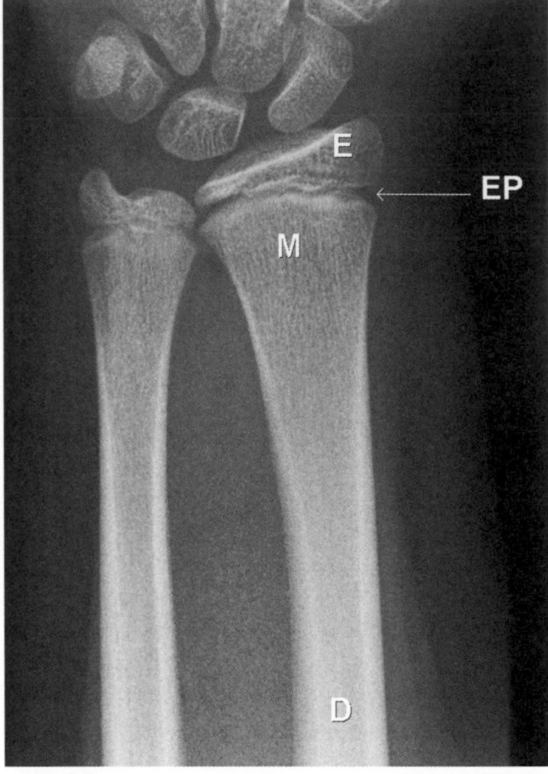

Figure 13.3 Normal wrist in a child. Note: diaphysis (D), epiphysis (E), epiphyseal plate (EP), metaphysis (M).

13.3 FRACTURES AND DISLOCATIONS: GENERAL PRINCIPLES

13.3.1 RADIOGRAPHY OF FRACTURES

- A minimum requirement for trauma radiography is that two views be taken of the area of interest
- Most trauma radiographs therefore consist of a lateral view and a front-on view, usually anteroposterior (AP)
- Where long bones of the arms or legs are being examined, the radiographs should include views of the joints at each end:
  - For example, for fractures of the midshaft radius and ulna the elbow and wrist must be included
- For suspected ankle trauma, three standard views are performed: AP, lateral and oblique
- In other areas, extra views may be requested depending on the clinical context:
  - Acromioclavicular (AC) joint: weight-bearing views
  - Elbow: oblique view for radial head
  - Wrist: angled views of the scaphoid bone
  - Hip: oblique views of the acetabulum
  - Knee: intercondylar notch view; skyline view of the patella
  - Ankle: angled views of the subtalar joint; axial view of the calcaneus
- Stress views of the ankle may rarely be performed to diagnose ligament damage, though usually not in the acute situation.

13.3.2 CLASSIFICATION OF FRACTURES

Fractures may be classified and described by using terminology that incorporates several descriptors, including fracture type, location and the degree of comminution, angulation and deformity.

FRACTURE TYPE

Complete fractures traverse the full thickness of a bone. Depending on the orientation of the fracture line, complete fractures are described as transverse, oblique or spiral. Incomplete fractures occur most commonly in children, as they have softer, more malleable bones. Incomplete fractures are classified as buckle or torus; greenstick; and plastic or bowing:

- Buckle (torus) fracture: bend in the bony cortex without an actual cortical break (Fig. 13.4)
- Greenstick fracture: only one cortex is broken with bending of the other cortex (Fig. 13.5)
- Plastic or bowing fracture: bending of a long bone without an actual fracture line (Fig. 13.6).

Other specific types of bone injury and fracture that may be seen include:

- Microfracture ('bone bruise', bone contusion)
- Avulsion fractures
- Stress fractures
- Insufficiency fractures
- Pathological fractures.

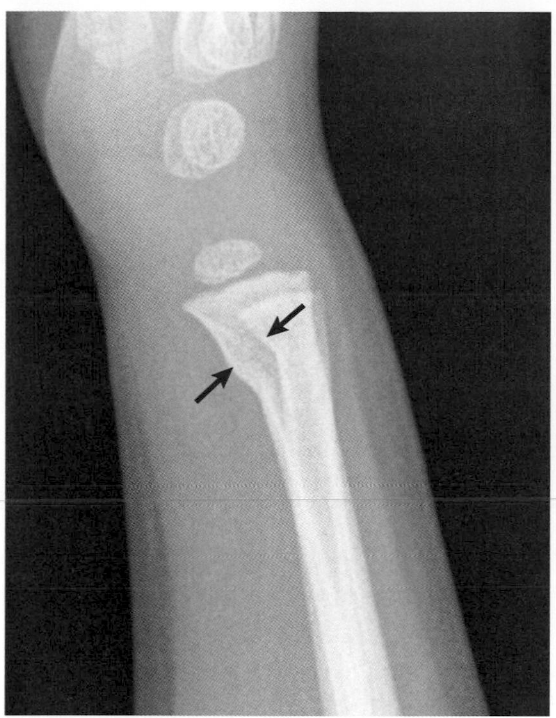

Figure 13.4 Buckle fracture of the distal radius and ulna seen as a focal bend of the volar cortex of both bones (arrows).

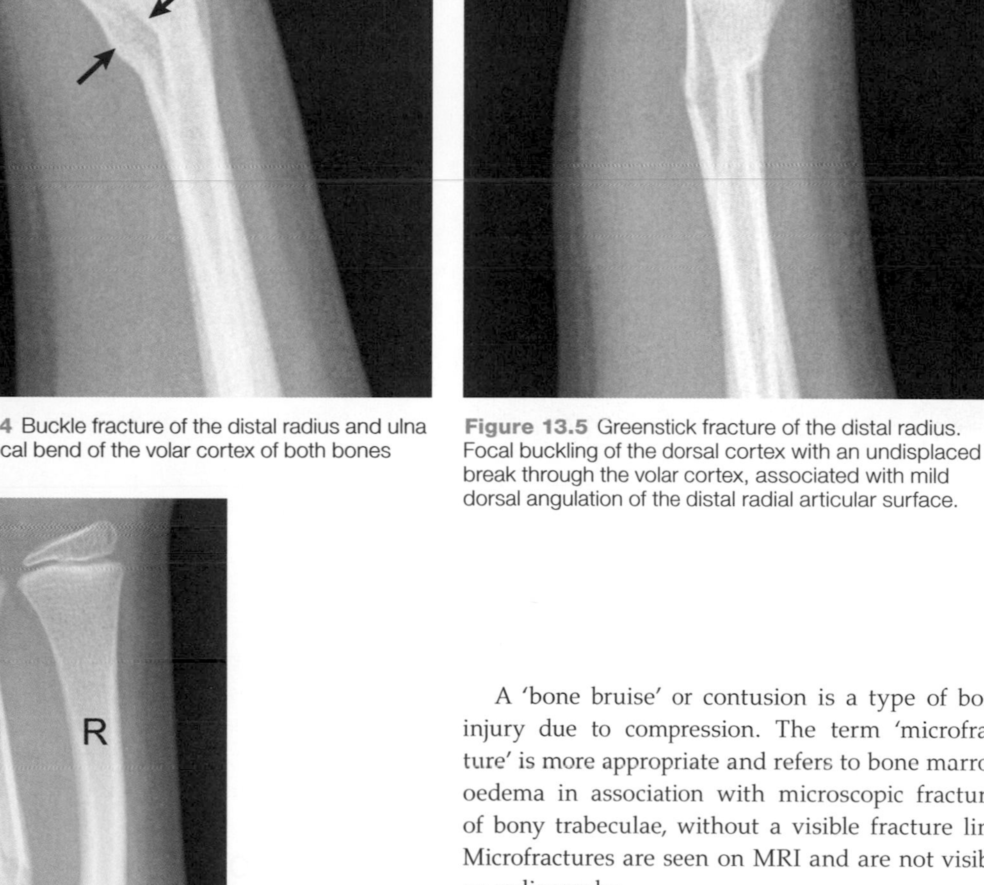

Figure 13.5 Greenstick fracture of the distal radius. Focal buckling of the dorsal cortex with an undisplaced break through the volar cortex, associated with mild dorsal angulation of the distal radial articular surface.

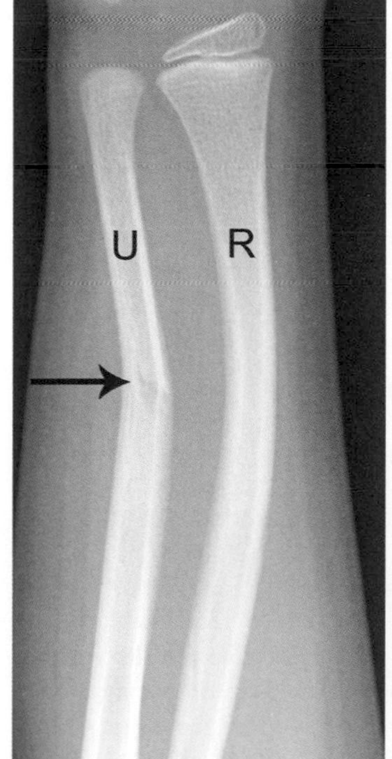

Figure 13.6 Bowing fracture. Undisplaced fracture (arrow) of the ulna (U), plus bowing of the radius (R).

A 'bone bruise' or contusion is a type of bone injury due to compression. The term 'microfracture' is more appropriate and refers to bone marrow oedema in association with microscopic fractures of bony trabeculae, without a visible fracture line. Microfractures are seen on MRI and are not visible on radiographs.

Avulsion fractures occur as a result of distraction forces at muscle, tendon and ligament insertions. Avulsion fractures are particularly common around the pelvis in athletes (Fig. 13.7). Avulsion fractures also occur in children at major ligament insertions, such as the insertion of the cruciate ligaments into the upper tibia. In children, the softer bone is more easily broken than the tougher ligament, whereas in adults the ligaments will tend to tear leaving the bony insertions intact.

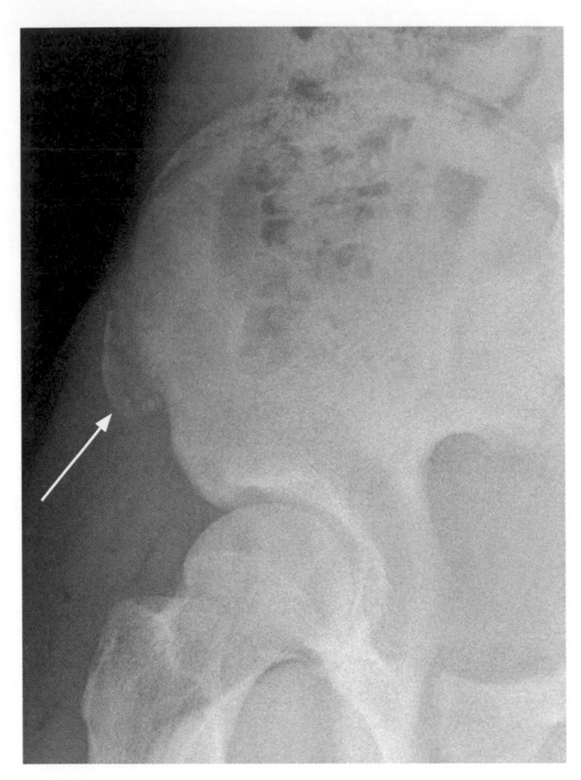

Figure 13.7 Avulsion fracture. Bone fragment adjacent to the anterior superior iliac spine indicating avulsion of the sartorius muscle origin (arrow).

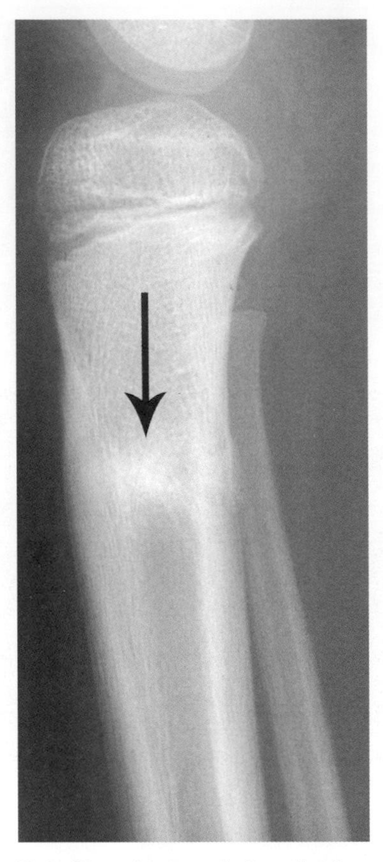

Figure 13.8 Stress fracture. A stress fracture of the upper tibia is seen as a band of sclerosis posteriorly (arrow).

Stress fractures occur as a result of repetitive trauma to otherwise normal bone and are common in athletes and other active people. Certain types of stress fracture occur in specific activities, e.g. upper tibial stress fractures in runners or metatarsal stress fractures in marchers. Radiographs are often normal at the time of initial presentation; after 7–10 days, a localized sclerotic line with periosteal thickening is usually visible (Fig. 13.8). MRI is usually positive at the time of initial presentation, as is scintigraphy with ^{99m}Tc-MDP (see Fig. 1.16).

An insufficiency fracture is a fracture of weakened bone that occurs with minor stress, e.g. insufficiency fracture of the sacrum in patients with severe systemic illnesses.

Pathological fracture is a fracture through a weak point in a bone caused by the presence of a bone abnormality. Pathological fractures may occur through benign bone lesions, such as bone cysts or Langerhans cell histiocytosis (Fig. 13.9), or with primary bone neoplasms and skeletal metastases. The clue to a pathological fracture is that the bone injury is out of proportion to the amount of trauma.

FRACTURE LOCATION

The fracture description should include the name of fractured bone(s), plus the specific part that is fractured, e.g. midshaft or distal shaft. Fracture lines involving articular surfaces are important to recognize as more precise reduction and fixation may be required.

Fractures in and around the epiphysis in children, also known as growth plate fractures, may be difficult to see and are classified by the Salter–Harris system as follows (Fig. 13.10):

- Salter–Harris 1: epiphyseal plate (cartilage) fracture
- Salter–Harris 2: fracture of metaphysis with or without displacement of the epiphysis (most common type) (Fig. 13.11)
- Salter–Harris 3: fracture of epiphysis only
- Salter–Harris 4: fracture of metaphysis and epiphysis
- Salter–Harris 5: impaction and compression of the epiphyseal plate.

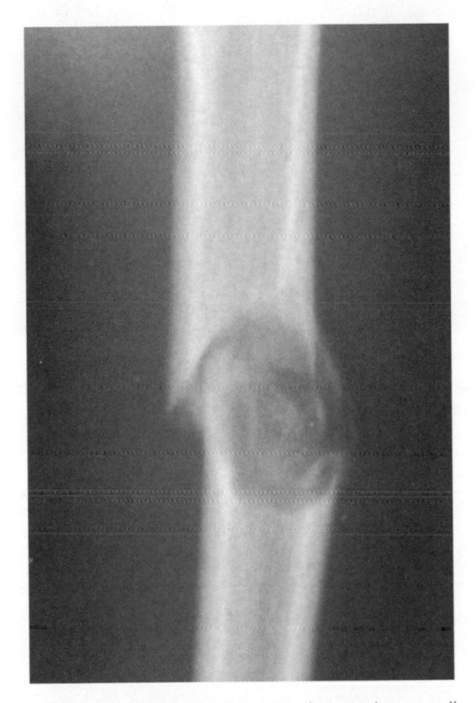

Figure 13.9 Pathological fracture: Langerhans cell histiocytosis. Acute arm pain following minimal trauma in an 8-year-old child. Radiograph shows an undisplaced fracture through a slightly expansile lytic lesion in the humeral shaft.

Salter–Harris types 1 and 5 are the most difficult to diagnose as the bones are intact and radiographic changes are often extremely subtle. Diagnosis of growth plate fractures is vital as untreated disruption of the epiphyseal plate may lead to problems with growth of the bone.

COMMINUTION

- Simple fracture: two fracture fragments only
- Comminuted fracture: fracture associated with more than two fragments.

The degree of comminution is important to assess as this partly dictates the type of treatment required. An example of this principle is fracture of the calcaneus.

Fractures with three or four major fragments are usually amenable to surgical reduction and fixation. A severely comminuted fracture of the calcaneus with multiple irregular fragments may be impossible to fix, the only option being fusion of the subtalar joint.

CLOSED OR OPEN (COMPOUND)

A compound or open fracture is usually obvious clinically. Where a bone end does not project through an open wound, air in the soft tissues around the fracture or in an adjacent joint may be a useful radiographic sign of a compound injury.

DEGREE OF DEFORMITY

The types of deformity that may occur at fractures include displacement, angulation and rotation.

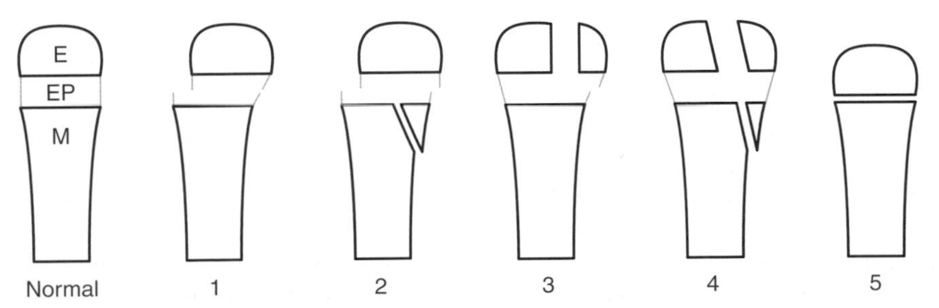

Figure 13.10 Schematic diagram illustrating the Salter–Harris classification of growth plate fractures. Note the normal anatomy: epiphysis (E), cartilage epiphyseal plate (EP), metaphysis (M).

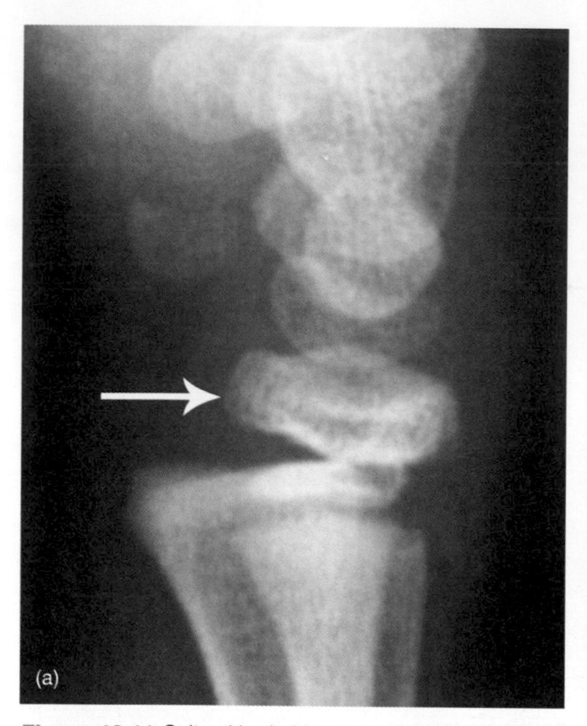

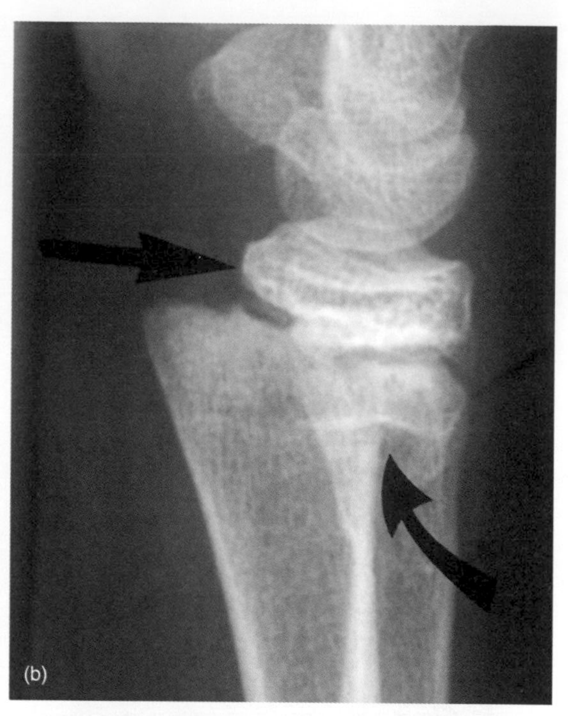

Figure 13.11 Salter–Harris fractures. (a) Salter–Harris 1 fracture of the distal radial growth plate with posterior displacement of the epiphysis but no bony fracture (arrow). (b) Salter–Harris 2 fracture of the distal radius with fracture of the metaphysis (curved arrow) and posterior displacement of the epiphysis (straight arrow).

Displacement refers to the separation of bone fragments. Undisplaced fractures are often referred to as 'hairline' fractures. Undisplaced oblique fractures of the long bones can be especially difficult to recognize, particularly in paediatric patients, e.g. undisplaced fracture of the tibia in the 1- to 3-year age group, the so-called 'toddler's fracture'. Undisplaced fractures through the waist of the scaphoid can also be difficult in the acute phase. Classification of the direction of angulation may be confusing. Angulation may be classified according to the angulation of the distal fragment *or* according to the direction of the apex of the angle formed by the bone fragments. For example, Fig. 13.12 shows a Colles fracture of the distal radius. The distal radial fragment is angled dorsally; therefore, this fracture is said to have dorsal angulation. As the apex of angulation points in a volar (anterior) direction, this may also be referred to as apex volar angulation, although this method is less commonly used in clinical practice.

13.3.3 FRACTURE HEALING

Fracture healing is also known as fracture union and occurs in three overlapping phases:

1. Inflammatory phase: haematoma and swelling at the fracture site
2. Reparative phase: proliferation of new blood vessels and increased blood flow around the fracture site. Collagen is laid down with early cartilage and new bone formation. This reparative tissue is known as callus
3. Remodelling phase: continued new bone formation bridging the fracture.

A major part of fracture management is assessing when union is sufficiently advanced to allow cessation of immobilization and resumption of unrestricted activity. The definition of 'complete union' may be quite difficult in individual cases and is usually made with a combination of clinical and

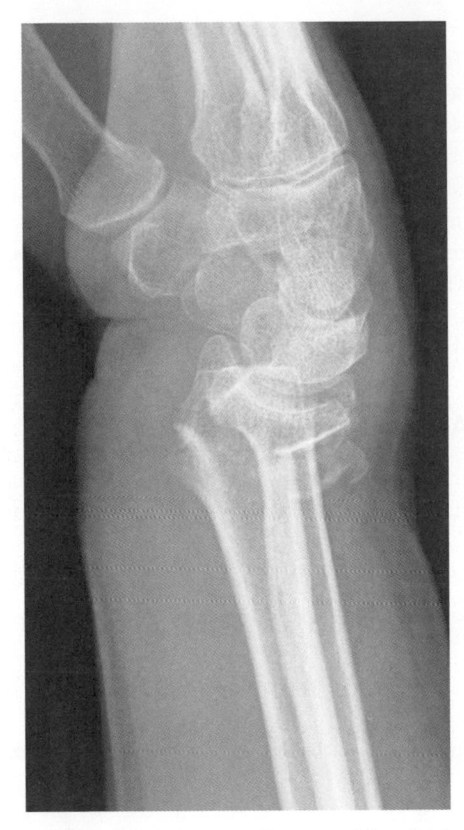

Figure 13.12 Colles fracture. Fracture of the distal radius with impaction and dorsal angulation: apex of the angle formed at the fracture site points in a volar direction.

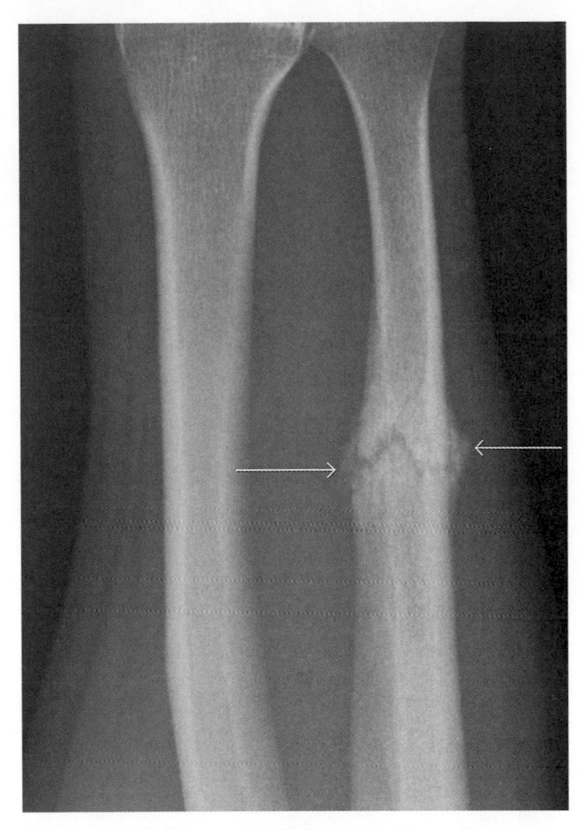

Figure 13.13 Early union. Subperiosteal new bone formation adjacent to the fracture (arrows).

radiographic assessments. Various stages of union are recognized.

Early union (incomplete repair) is indicated radiographically by densely calcified callus around the fracture with the fracture line still visible (Fig. 13.13); however, clinical assessment will usually reveal an immobile fracture site with tenderness on palpation and stress. Fracture immobilization usually can be ceased at this stage, though return to full activity is not recommended.

Late union (complete repair or consolidation) is indicated radiographically by the ossification of callus, producing mature bone across the fracture (Fig. 13.14). The fracture line may be invisible or faintly defined through the bridging bone. Clinically, the fracture is immobile with no tenderness. No further restriction of activity is necessary.

Owing to variable biological factors, it is impossible to precisely predict fracture healing times in individual cases. Some basic principles of fracture healing are as follows:

- Spiral fractures unite faster than transverse fractures
- In adults, spiral fractures of the upper limb unite in 6–8 weeks
- Spiral fractures of the tibia unite in 12–16 weeks and of the femur in 16–20 weeks
- Transverse fractures take about 25% longer to unite
- Union is much quicker in children, and slower in the elderly.

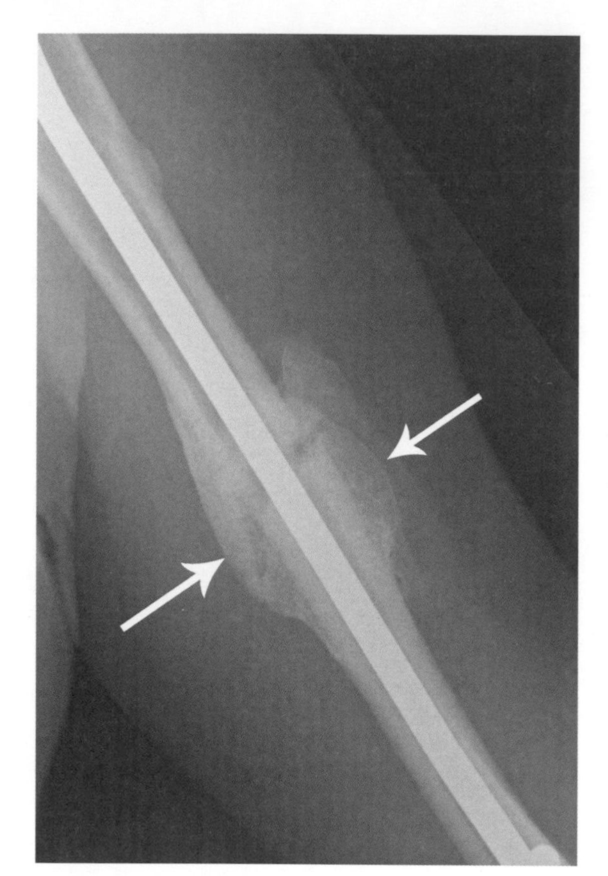

Figure 13.14 Late union. Dense new bone bridging the fracture margins (arrows). Note the intramedullary nail.

13.3.4 PROBLEMS WITH FRACTURE HEALING

DELAYED UNION

Delayed union is defined as union that fails to occur within the expected time as outlined above. Delayed union may occur in elderly patients or may be caused by incomplete immobilization, infection at the fracture site, pathological fractures or vitamin C deficiency.

NON-UNION

The term 'non-union' implies that the bone will never unite without some form of intervention. Non-union is diagnosed radiographically with visualization of sclerosis (increased density) of the bone ends at the fracture site. The fracture margins often have rounded edges and the fracture line is still clearly visible (Fig. 13.15). A variation of non-union may be encountered in which there is mature bone formation around the edge of the fracture with failure of healing centrally. This may be difficult to recognize radiographically and CT may be required for diagnosis. This form of non-union may be suspected when there is ongoing pain despite apparently solid radiographic union.

TRAUMATIC EPIPHYSEAL ARREST

Traumatic epiphyseal arrest refers to premature closure of a bony growth plate because of failure of

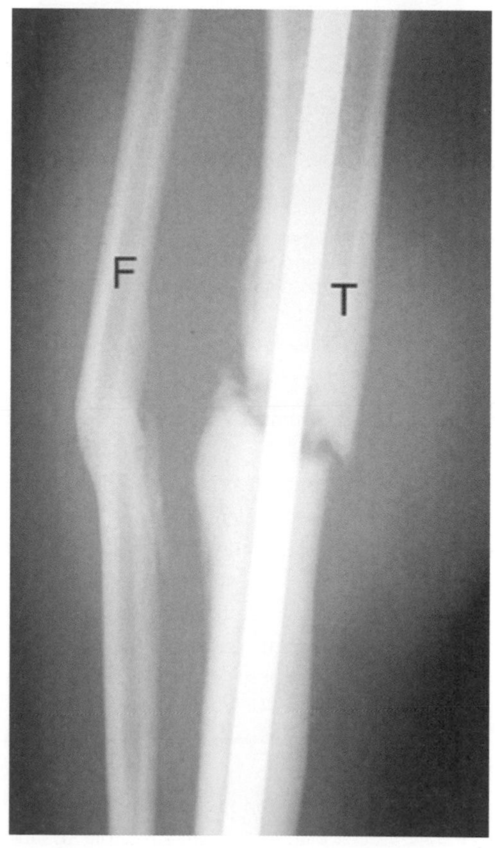

Figure 13.15 Non-union. Fracture of the tibia (T) 6 months previously. The fracture margins are rounded and sclerotic, indicating non-union. Note the intramedullary nail. The adjacent fracture of the fibula (F) has united.

recognition or inadequate management of a growth plate fracture in a child. An example of this is fracture of the lateral epicondyle of the humerus, leading to premature closure of the growth plate and alteration of the carrying angle of the elbow.

MALUNION

Malunion refers to complete bone healing in a poor position, leading to permanent bone or joint deformity and often to early osteoarthritis (OA) (Fig. 13.16).

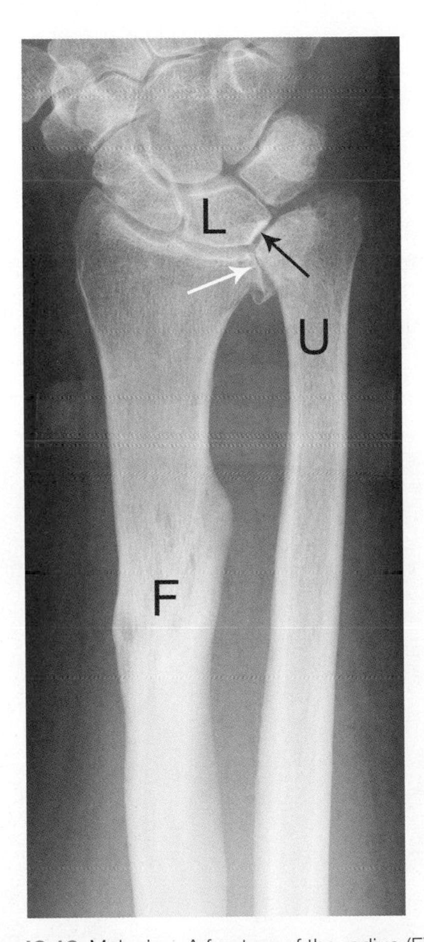

Figure 13.16 Malunion. A fracture of the radius (F) has united with shortening of the bone. As a result, the ulna (U) is relatively longer than the radius (positive ulnar variance) and is contacting the lunate (black arrow). This is known as ulnar abutment and is a cause of wrist pain. There is also secondary osteoarthritis of the distal radio-ulnar joint (white arrow).

13.3.5 OTHER COMPLICATIONS OF FRACTURES

ASSOCIATED SOFT-TISSUE INJURIES

Many examples exist of soft-tissue injuries associated with fractures:

- Pneumothorax associated with rib fractures
- Bladder injury in association with fractures of the pelvis.

These soft-tissue injuries may be of more urgent clinical significance than the bony injuries.

COMPLICATIONS OF RECUMBENCY

Complications such as pneumonia and deep vein thrombosis (DVT) are common complications of recumbency, especially in the elderly.

ARTERIAL INJURY

Arterial laceration and occlusion causing acute limb ischaemia may be seen in association with displaced fractures of the femur or tibia, and in the upper limb with displaced fractures of the distal humerus and elbow dislocation.

NERVE INJURY

Nerve injury following fracture or dislocation is a rare event; the best known examples include:

- Shoulder dislocation: axillary nerve
- Fracture of the midshaft humerus: radial nerve
- Displaced supracondylar fracture of the humerus: median nerve
- Elbow dislocation: ulnar nerve
- Hip dislocation: sciatic nerve
- Knee dislocation: tibial nerve
- Fracture of the neck of fibula: common peroneal nerve.

AVASCULAR NECROSIS

Traumatic avascular necrosis (AVN) occurs most commonly in three sites: the proximal pole of scaphoid, the femoral head and the body of talus. In these sites, AVN is due to interruption of the blood supply, as may occur in fractures of the waist of the scaphoid, the femoral neck and the neck of talus. New bone is laid down on necrosed bone trabeculae, causing the non-vascularized portion of bone to become sclerotic on radiographs over 2–3 months. Because of weight bearing, the femoral head and talus may show deformity and irregularity as well as sclerosis.

COMPLEX REGIONAL PAIN SYNDROME

Complex regional pain syndrome (also known as reflex sympathetic dystrophy or RSD) may follow trivial bone injury. It occurs in bones distal to the site of injury and is associated with severe pain and swelling. Radiographic changes include a marked decrease in bone density distal to the fracture site with thinning of the bone cortex. Scintigraphy shows increased tracer uptake in the limb distal to the trauma site.

MYOSITIS OSSIFICANS

Myositis ossificans refers to post-traumatic non-neoplastic formation of bone within skeletal muscle, usually within 5–6 weeks of trauma. Myositis ossificans may occur at any site, though the muscles of the anterior thigh are most affected. It is seen radiographically as bone formation in the soft tissues; this bone has a striated appearance conforming to the structure of the underlying muscle.

13.4 FRACTURES AND DISLOCATIONS: SPECIFIC AREAS

In the following section, radiographic signs of the more common fractures and dislocations will be discussed. Those lesions that may cause problems with diagnosis will be emphasized. Most fractures and dislocations are diagnosed with radiographs. Other imaging modalities will be described where applicable.

13.4.1 SHOULDER AND CLAVICLE

FRACTURED CLAVICLE

Fractures of the clavicle usually involve the middle third. Fractures are commonly angulated and displaced. When displaced, the outer fragment usually lies at a lower level than the inner fragment (Fig. 13.17). Less commonly, a fracture may involve the outer clavicle. In these cases, a small fragment of outer clavicle maintains normal alignment with the acromion. Because of injury of the coracoclavicular ligaments, there is variable superior displacement at the fracture site (Fig. 13.18).

STERNOCLAVICULAR JOINT DISLOCATION

Dislocation of the sternoclavicular joint is an uncommon injury usually caused by indirect trauma to the shoulder or a direct anterior blow. Anterior dislocation, in which the head of the clavicle lies anterior to the manubrium, is more common than posterior dislocation. In posterior dislocation the head of the clavicle may compress the trachea or underlying blood vessels, including the brachiocephalic veins. Because of overlapping structures, the sternoclavicular joint is difficult to see on plain radiographs. CT is the investigation of choice when sternoclavicular joint injury is suspected.

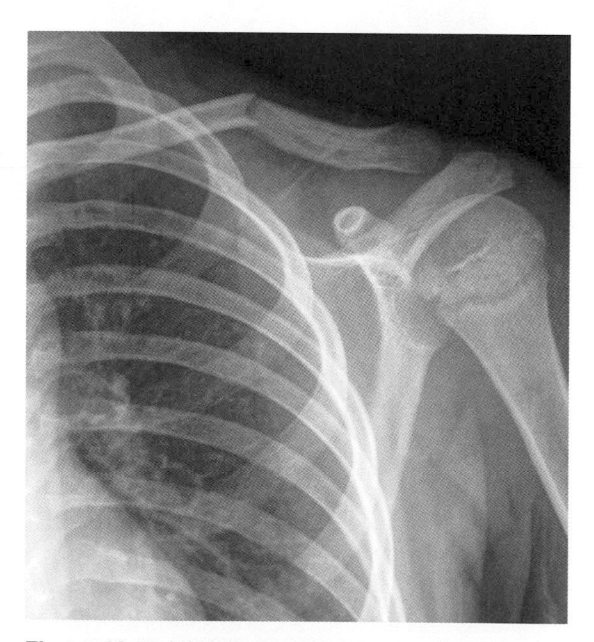

Figure 13.17 Inferiorly angulated fracture of the midshaft clavicle.

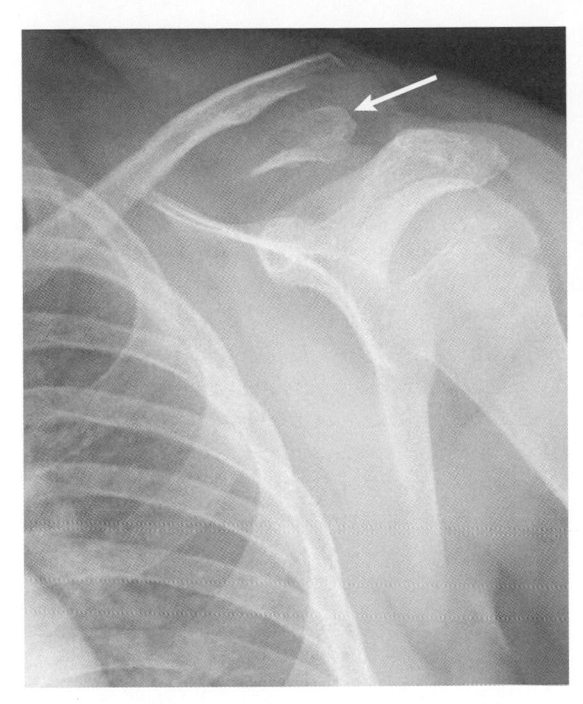

Figure 13.18 Distal clavicle fracture. Small clavicle fragment (arrow) maintains normal alignment with the acromion. The clavicular shaft is displaced superiorly owing to a tear of the coracoclavicular ligaments.

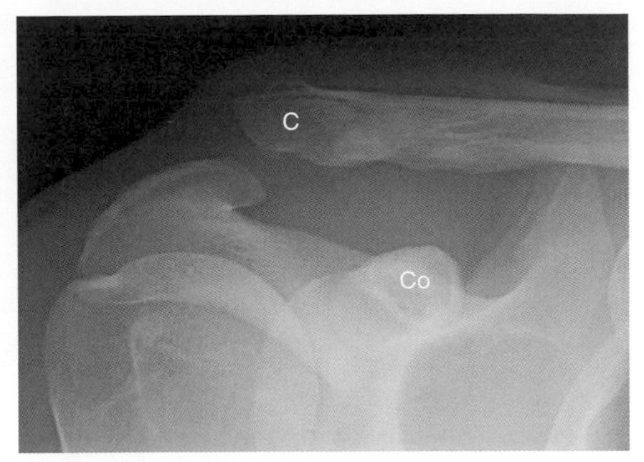

Figure 13.19 Acromioclavicular joint dislocation. Widening of the right acromioclavicular joint with superior displacement of the clavicle (C). Widening of the interval between the clavicle and coracoid process (Co) indicates rupture of the coracoclavicular ligaments.

ACROMIOCLAVICULAR JOINT DISLOCATION

AC joint dislocation produces widening of the AC joint space and elevation of the outer end of the clavicle. The underlying pathology is tearing of the coracoclavicular ligaments, seen radiographically as increased distance between the undersurface of the clavicle and the coracoid process. Radiographic signs may be subtle and a weight-bearing view may be useful in doubtful cases (Fig. 13.19).

ANTERIOR DISLOCATION OF THE SHOULDER

With anterior dislocation of the shoulder (glenohumeral joint) the humeral head is displaced anteromedially. On the lateral radiograph the humeral head lies anterior to the glenoid fossa. On the AP view the humeral head overlaps the lower glenoid and the lateral border of the scapula. Associated fractures occur commonly (Fig. 13.20):

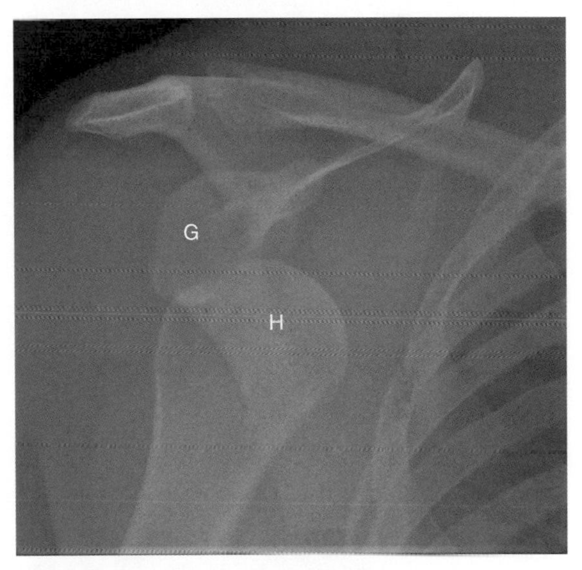

Figure 13.20 Anterior shoulder dislocation. The humeral head (H) lies anterior and medial to the glenoid articular surface (G).

- Wedge-shaped defect in the posterolateral humeral head (Hill–Sachs deformity)
- Fracture of the inferior rim of the glenoid (Bankart lesion)
- Fracture of the greater tuberosity
- Fracture of the surgical neck of the humerus.

Recurrent anterior dislocation may be seen in association with fracture of the glenoid, tear of the anterior cartilaginous labrum and laxity of the joint capsule and glenohumeral ligaments. These injuries are diagnosed with MRI (see section 13.5.2).

POSTERIOR DISLOCATION OF THE SHOULDER

Posterior dislocation is an uncommon injury, representing only 2% of shoulder dislocations. It may easily be missed on radiographic examination. Signs on the AP film are often subtle (Fig. 13.21):

- Loss of parallelism of the articular surface of the humeral head and glenoid fossa
- Medial rotation of the humerus so that the humeral head looks symmetrically rounded, like an ice cream cone or an electric light bulb.

On the lateral film, the articular surface of the humeral head is seen rotated posterior to the glenoid fossa.

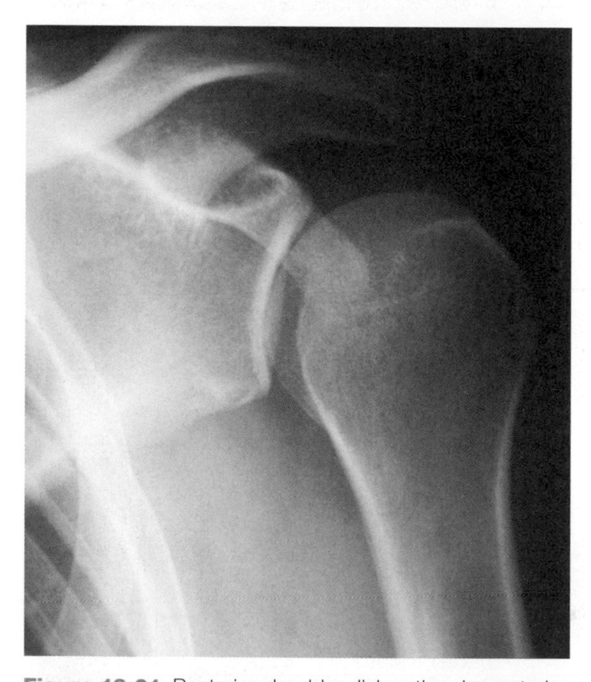

Figure 13.21 Posterior shoulder dislocation. In posterior dislocation the humeral head is internally rotated with the articular surface of the humerus facing posteriorly. As a result, the humeral head has a symmetric round configuration likened to a light bulb or ice cream cone. Compare this with the normal appearance in Fig. 13.1.

13.4.2 HUMERUS

Fractures of the proximal humerus are common in the elderly. Proximal humeral fractures commonly involve the surgical neck, greater tuberosity, lesser tuberosity and anatomical neck, causing separation of the humeral head. Surgical neck fractures are often undisplaced, although significant angulation or impaction may occur. For the purposes of classification, the proximal humerus can be thought of as four parts or segments: the humeral head including the articular surface, the greater tuberosity, the lesser tuberosity and the humeral shaft. Displacement of upper humoral fractures is defined as greater than 1 cm displacement of a segment or more than 45° angulation. Proximal humeral fractures are classified according to the number of separate bone parts and the degree of displacement:

- one-part fracture: no significant displacement or angulation of any segments
- two-part fracture: displacement of one segment
- three-part fracture: non-impacted fracture of the surgical neck and displacement of two segments
- four-part fracture: displacement of all four segments.

Humeral shaft fractures may be transverse, oblique, simple or comminuted.

13.4.3 ELBOW

ELBOW JOINT EFFUSION

Fat pads lie on the anterior and posterior surfaces of the distal humerus at the attachments of the elbow joint capsule. On a lateral radiograph of the elbow these fat pads are usually not visualized; occasionally, the anterior fat pad may be seen lying on the anterior surface of the humerus. In the presence of an elbow joint effusion the fat pads are seen on lateral radiographs as dark grey triangular structures lifted off the humeral surfaces; this is sometimes referred to as the 'fat pad' sign (Fig. 13.22). There is a high rate of association of elbow joint effusion with fracture. Where an elbow joint effusion is present in a setting of trauma and no fracture can be seen on standard elbow radiographs, consider an undisplaced fracture

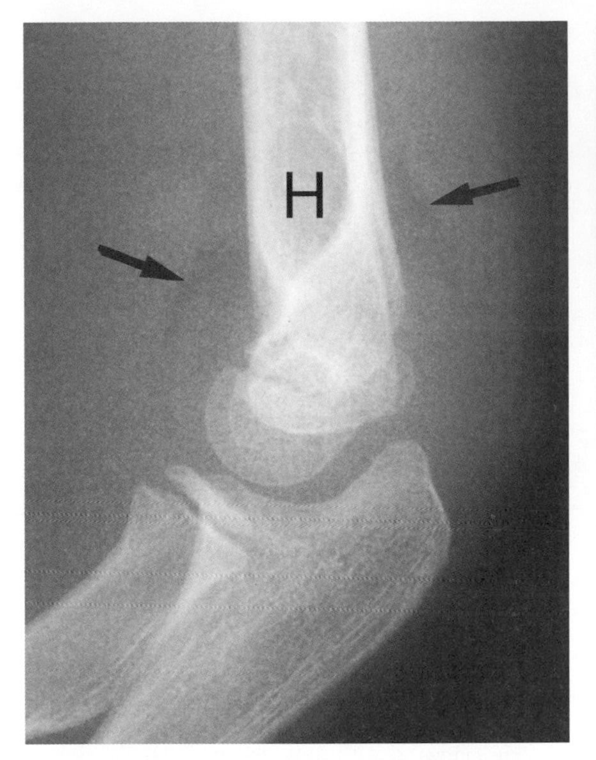

Figure 13.22 Elbow joint effusion. Elbow joint effusion causes elevation of the anterior and posterior fat pads, producing triangular lucencies (arrows) anterior and posterior to the distal humerus (H).

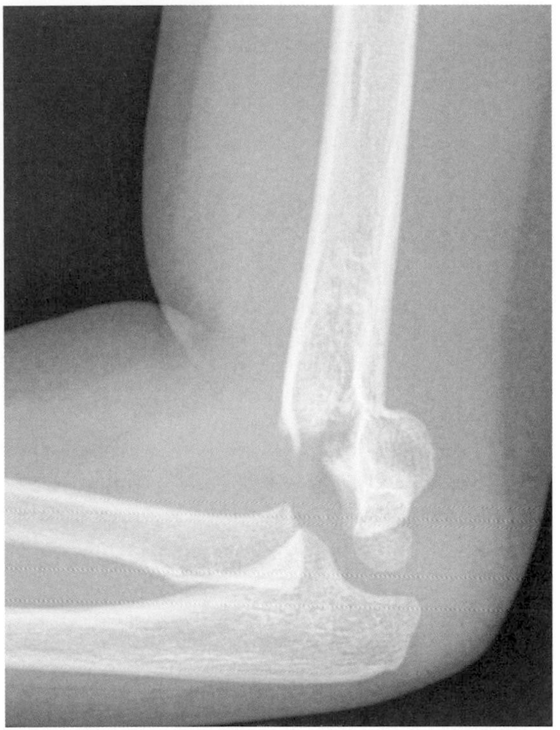

Figure 13.23 Supracondylar fracture of the distal humerus. The distal fragment is angulated though not displaced.

of the radial head or a supracondylar fracture of the distal humerus. In this situation, either perform further oblique views or treat and repeat radiographs in 7–10 days.

SUPRACONDYLAR FRACTURE

Supracondylar fracture of the distal humerus is a common injury in children (Fig. 13.23). Supracondylar fracture may be undisplaced or the distal fragment may be displaced anteriorly or posteriorly. Posterior displacement is the most common; when severe, it may be associated with injury to the brachial artery and median nerve (Fig. 13.24).

FRACTURE AND SEPARATION OF THE LATERAL CONDYLAR EPIPHYSIS

Fracture of the lateral humeral epicondyle in children may be difficult to see on radiographs. Because

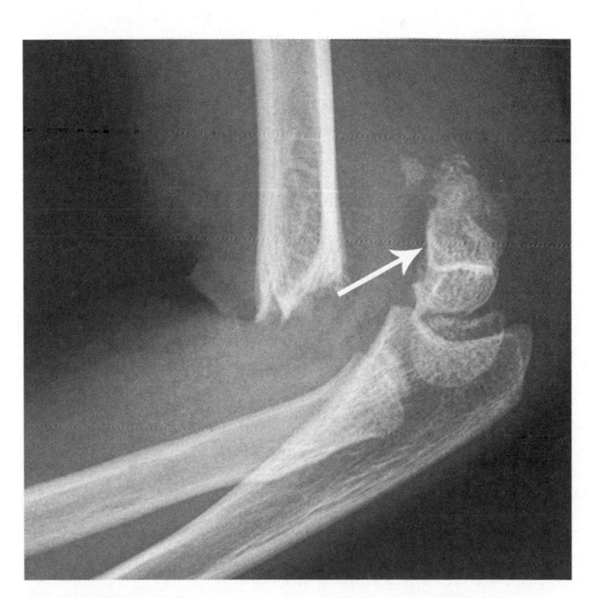

Figure 13.24 Supracondylar fracture of the distal humerus. The distal fragment is displaced posteriorly (arrow).

the growth centre is predominantly cartilage the bony injury may look deceptively small (Fig. 13.25). Adequate treatment is vital as this fracture may damage the growth plate and the articular surface, leading to deformity.

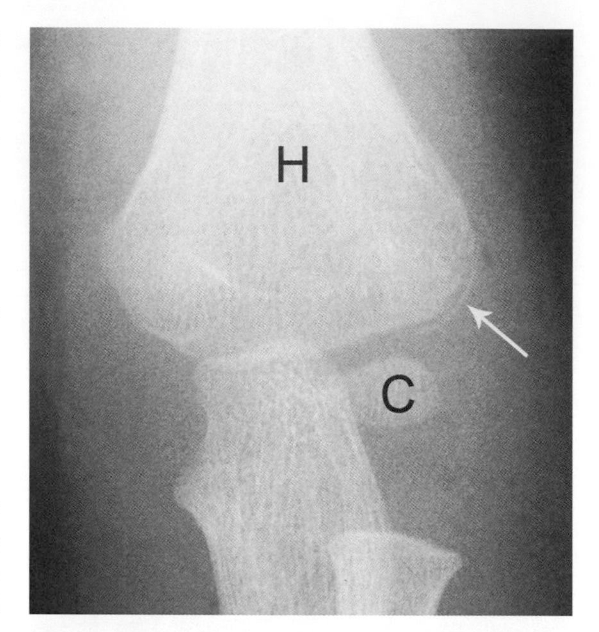

Figure 13.25 Lateral epicondyle fracture of the distal humerus. Note the normal appearance of the humerus (H) and growth centre for the capitulum (C) in an 18-month-old child. A fracture of the lateral humeral epicondyle is seen as a thin sliver of bone adjacent to the distal humerus (arrow).

FRACTURE OF THE HEAD OF THE RADIUS

Three patterns of radial head fracture are commonly seen:

1. Vertical split (Fig. 13.26)
2. Small lateral fragment
3. Multiple fragments.

Radial head fracture may be difficult to visualize radiographically, and elbow joint effusion may be the only radiographic sign on initial presentation. In such cases the arm is usually placed in a sling and radiographs repeated in a few days.

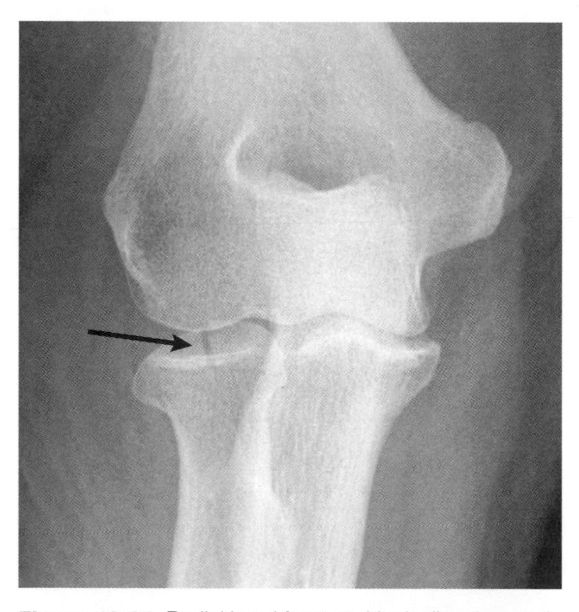

Figure 13.26 Radial head fracture. Vertically orientated split of the articular surface of the radial head (arrow).

FRACTURE OF THE OLECRANON

Two patterns of olecranon fracture are commonly seen:

1. Comminuted fracture
2. Single transverse fracture line with separation of the fragments owing to unopposed action of the triceps muscle (Fig. 13.27).

OTHER ELBOW FRACTURES

Other less commonly encountered elbow fractures include:

- 'T'- or 'Y'-shaped fracture of the distal humerus with separation of the humeral condyles
- Fracture and separation of the capitulum usually results in the capitulum being sheared off vertically
- Fracture and separation of the medial epicondylar apophysis (Fig. 13.28).

13.4.4 RADIUS AND ULNA

MIDSHAFT FRACTURES

Midshaft fractures of the radius and ulna usually involve both bones and may be transverse or oblique

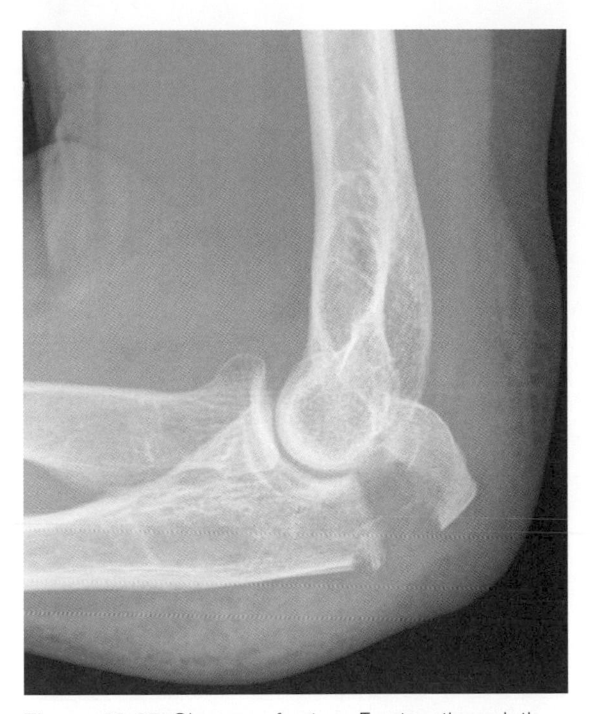

Figure 13.27 Olecranon fracture. Fracture through the articular surface of the olecranon with wide separation of bone fragments. The proximal fragment is displaced proximally because of unopposed action of the triceps muscle.

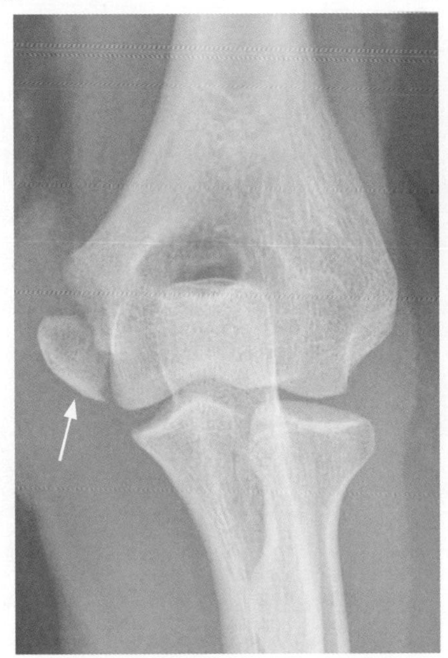

Figure 13.28 Medial epicondyle fracture. Bone fragment separated from the medial humeral epicondyle, indicating avulsion of the common flexor tendon origin (arrow).

with varying degrees of angulation and displacement. A 'nightstick' fracture of the ulnar midshaft may occur in isolation when caused by a direct blow to the forearm.

Commonly, though, isolated fracture of the midshaft of either the radius or ulna is associated with disruption of the wrist or elbow joint:

- Monteggia fracture: anteriorly angulated fracture of upper third of the shaft of the ulna associated with anterior dislocation of the radial head (Fig. 13.29)
- Galeazzi fracture: fracture of the lower third of the shaft of the radius associated with subluxation or dislocation of the distal radio-ulnar joint.

FRACTURE OF THE DISTAL RADIUS

The distal radius is the most common site of radial fracture. The distal radius is a common fracture site in children with buckle, greenstick or Salter–Harris type 2 fractures being particularly common. Distal radial fractures are also common in elderly patients, particularly those with osteoporosis. Classical Colles fracture consists of a transverse fracture of the distal radius with dorsal angulation (Fig. 13.12). The distal fragment is angulated and/or displaced posteriorly, often with a degree of impaction. Distal radial fractures are commonly associated with avulsion of the tip of the ulnar styloid process. Volar angulated fracture of the distal radius, commonly known as a Smith fracture, is less common than Colles fracture.

Comminuted fracture of the distal radius is a common injury in adults. Fracture lines may extend into the articular surfaces of the radiocarpal and

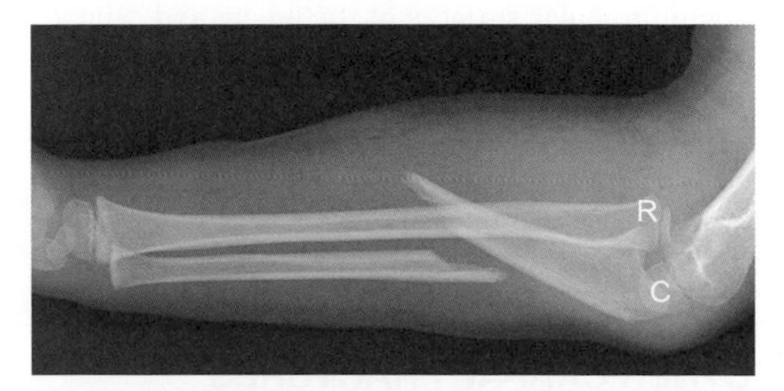

Figure 13.29 Monteggia fracture/dislocation. Fracture of the ulnar shaft. The head of the radius (R) is displaced from the capitulum (C), indicating dislocation.

distal radio-ulnar joints. CT may be used for planning of surgical fixation of these complex fractures.

13.4.5 WRIST AND HAND

SCAPHOID FRACTURE

Two types of scaphoid fracture are encountered commonly:

1. Transverse fracture of the waist of the scaphoid
2. Fracture and separation of the scaphoid tubercle.

Undisplaced fracture of the waist of the scaphoid may be difficult to see on radiographs at initial presentation, even on dedicated oblique views (Fig. 13.30). Further investigation may be required to confirm the diagnosis. This usually consists of a repeat radiograph after 7–10 days of immobilization. If immediate diagnosis is required MRI is the investigation of choice.

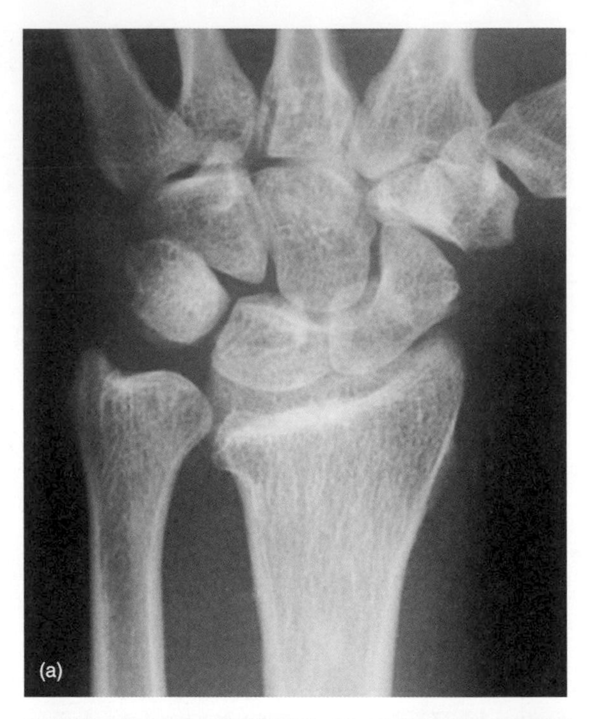

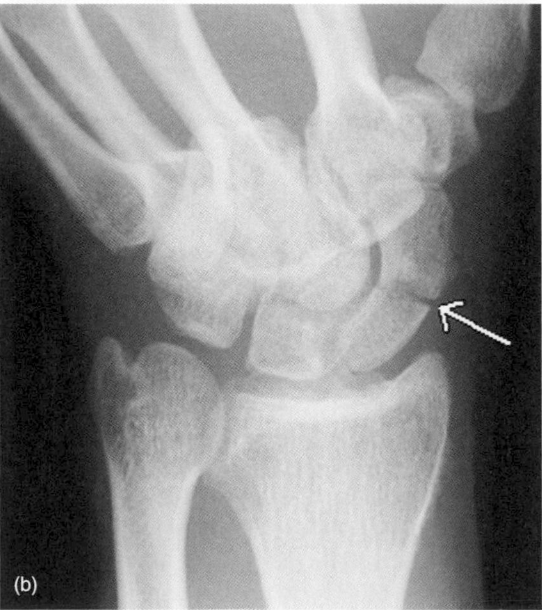

Figure 13.30 Scaphoid fracture. (a) Frontal radiograph of the wrist shows no visible fracture. (b) Oblique ulnar deviation view of the scaphoid shows an undisplaced fracture (arrow). This example demonstrates the need to obtain dedicated scaphoid views where scaphoid fracture is suspected.

LUNATE DISLOCATION

Lunate dislocation refers to anterior dislocation of the lunate. This may be difficult to appreciate on the frontal film, though it is easily seen on the lateral view with the lunate rotated and displaced anteriorly (Fig. 13.31).

PERILUNATE DISLOCATION

In perilunate dislocation, the lunate articulates normally with the radius and other carpal bones are displaced posteriorly. On the frontal radiograph there is abnormal overlap of bone shadows, with dissociation of articular surfaces of the lunate and capitate. The lateral film shows minimal, if any, rotation of the lunate and posterior displacement of the remainder of the carpal bones (Fig. 13.32). Perilunate dislocation may be associated with scaphoid fracture (trans-scaphoid perilunate dislocation) or fracture of the radial styloid.

OTHER CARPAL FRACTURES

Avulsion fracture of the triquetral is seen on the lateral view as a small fragment of bone adjacent to the

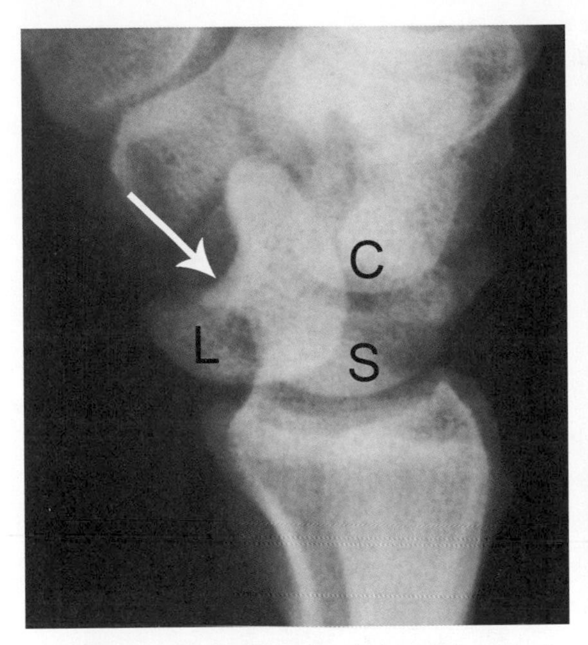

Figure 13.31 Lunate dislocation. Lateral radiograph of the wrist showing the capitate (C) and scaphoid (S) in the normal position with the lunate (L) displaced anteriorly. Note the distal articular surface of the lunate (arrow). This would normally articulate with the capitate.

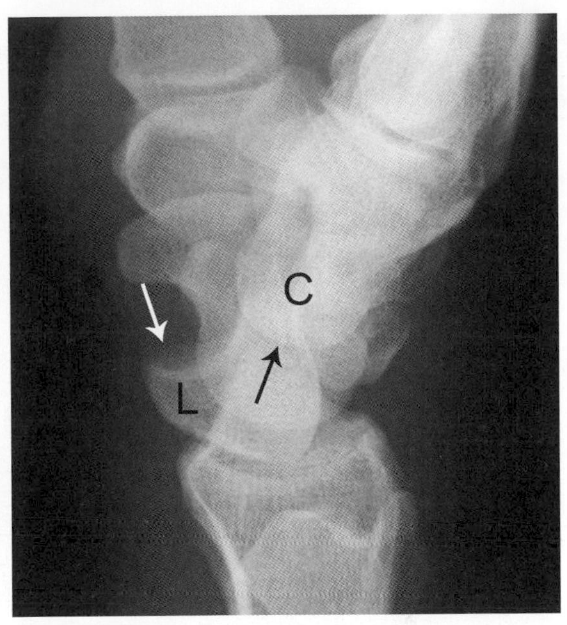

Figure 13.32 Perilunate dislocation. Lateral radiograph of the wrist showing the lunate (L) in the normal position with the capitate (C) and other carpal bone displaced posteriorly. Note the separation of the distal articular surface of the lunate (white arrow) from the proximal articular surface of the capitate (black arrow).

posterior surface. Fracture of the hook of hamate is a common injury in golfers and tennis players. Because of overlapping structures, this fracture is difficult to diagnose on radiographs unless dedicated views are performed. CT or MRI may be required to confirm the diagnosis.

HAND FRACTURES

Fractures of the metacarpals and phalanges are common. Fracture through the neck of the fifth metacarpal is the classic 'punching injury'. Fractures of the base of the first metacarpal are usually unstable.

Two types of proximal first metacarpal fracture are seen:

1. Transverse fracture of the proximal shaft with lateral bowing
2. Oblique fracture extending to the articular surface at the base of the first metacarpal (Fig. 13.33).

Avulsion fracture of the distal extensor tendon insertion at the base of the distal phalanx, known as a mallet fracture, may result in a flexion deformity of the distal interphalangeal joint (Fig. 13.34).

13.4.6 PELVIS

PELVIC RING FRACTURE

Pelvic ring fractures are most commonly the result of significant trauma, such as motor vehicle and cycling accidents. In general, fractures of the pelvic ring occur in two separate places, though there are exceptions. Isolated fractures of the ischium and pubic rami may occur as a result of a minor fall in elderly patients.

Three common patterns of anterior pelvic injury are seen:

1. Separation of the pubic symphysis
2. Bilateral fractures of the pubic rami
3. Unilateral fractures of the pubic rami.

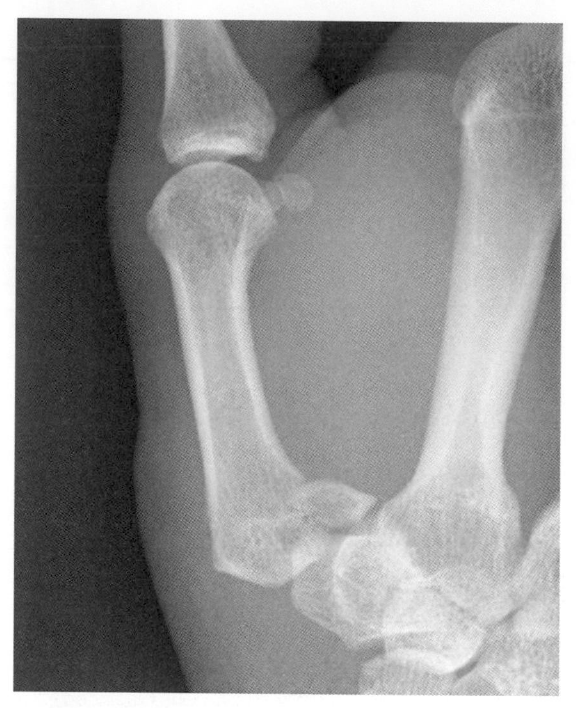

Figure 13.33 First metacarpal fracture. Fracture of the ulnar side of the base of the first metacarpal; the fracture involves the articular surface.

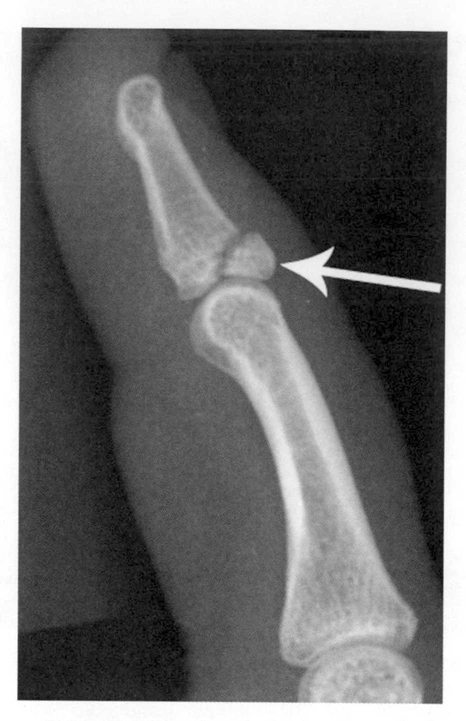

Figure 13.34 Mallet fracture. Lateral radiograph shows an avulsion fracture (arrow) at the dorsal base of the distal phalanx at the distal attachment of the extensor tendon. As a result, the distal interphalangeal joint cannot be extended.

These anterior fractures are often associated with posterior injuries:

- Widening of sacroiliac joint
- Unilateral vertical sacral fracture
- Fracture of iliac bone
- Combinations of the above.

Pelvic ring fractures have a high rate of association with urinary tract injury (see Chapter 12) and with arterial injury, causing severe blood loss. Angiography and embolization may be required in such cases. Because of overlapping structures, pelvic ring fractures may be difficult to define accurately with plain films and CT is often indicated (Fig. 13.35).

AVULSION FRACTURES

Multiple large muscles attach to the pelvic bones. Sudden applied stress to the muscle insertion may result in avulsion, i.e. separation of the bony attachment. Commonly avulsed muscle insertion sites include:

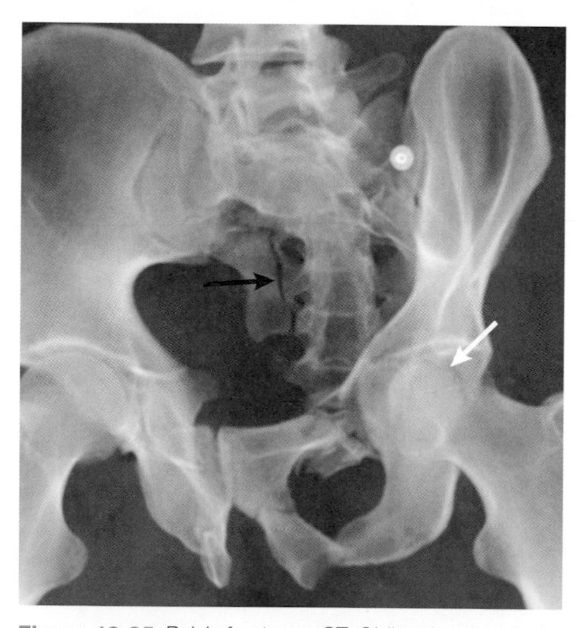

Figure 13.35 Pelvis fractures: CT. Obliquely orientated three-dimensional CT reconstruction demonstrates multiple pelvic fractures, including bilateral superior and inferior pubic rami, left acetabulum (white arrow) and right sacrum (black arrow).

- Anterior inferior iliac spine: rectus femoris
- Anterior superior iliac spine: sartorius (Fig. 13.7)
- Ischial tuberosity: hamstrings
- Lesser trochanter: iliopsoas
- Greater trochanter: gluteus medius and minimis.

HIP DISLOCATION

Anterior hip joint dislocation is a rare injury easily recognized radiographically and is usually not associated with fracture.

Posterior dislocation is the most common form of hip dislocation. The femoral head dislocates posteriorly and superiorly. Posterior dislocation is usually associated with fractures of the posterior acetabulum and occasionally with fractures of the femoral head.

FRACTURES OF THE ACETABULUM

Three common acetabular fracture patterns are seen:

1. Fracture through the anterior acetabulum, associated with fracture of the inferior pubic ramus
2. Fracture through the posterior acetabulum extending into the sciatic notch, associated with fracture of the inferior pubic ramus
3. Horizontal fracture through the acetabulum.

Combinations of the above fracture patterns may be seen, as well as extensive comminution and central dislocation of the femoral head. Acetabular fractures are difficult to define radiographically owing to the complexity of the anatomy and overlapping bony structures (Fig. 13.36). CT is useful for the definition of fractures and for planning of operative reduction (Fig. 13.37).

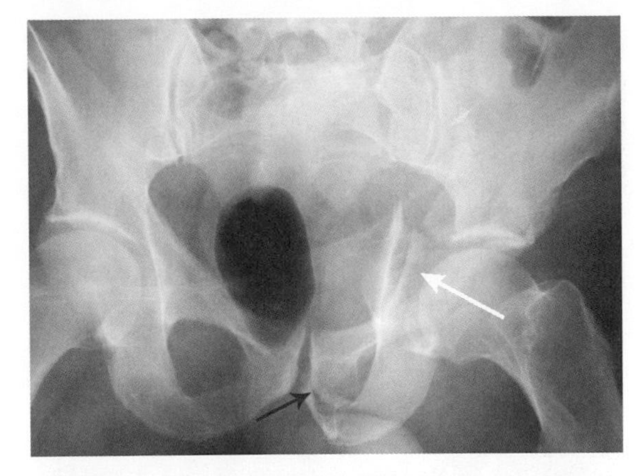

Figure 13.36 Acetabulum fracture. A comminuted fracture of the acetabulum with central impaction of the femoral head (white arrow). Also note a fracture of the pubic bone (black arrow).

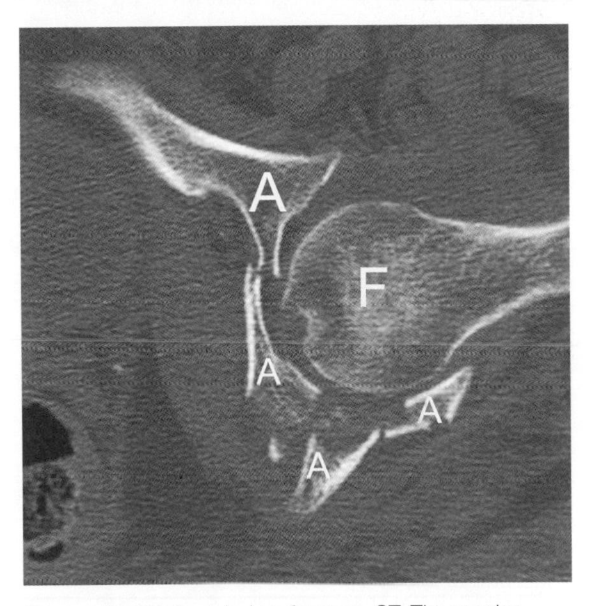

Figure 13.37 Acetabulum fracture: CT. The precise anatomy of an acetabular fracture is demonstrated with CT. Note the multiple acetabular fragments (A) and the femoral head (F).

13.4.7 FEMUR

UPPER FEMUR ('HIP FRACTURE')

Fractures of the upper femur (also known as hip fractures) are common, particularly in the elderly, and have a strong association with osteoporosis. Fractures are classified anatomically as femoral neck, intertrochanteric and subtrochanteric.

Femoral neck fractures are classified according to location:

- Subcapital: junction of the femoral neck and head
- Transcervical: middle of the femoral neck
- Basilar: junction of the femoral neck and intertrochanteric region.

Femoral neck fractures display varying degrees of angulation and displacement. These may be underestimated on a frontal view and a lateral view should be obtained when possible. The lateral view may be difficult to obtain owing to pain and difficult to interpret owing to overlapping soft-tissue density. Despite these limitations, the lateral view often provides invaluable information in the setting of femoral neck fracture (Fig. 13.38). Undisplaced or mildly impacted femoral neck fracture may be difficult to recognize radiographically. These fractures may be seen as a faint sclerotic band passing across the femoral neck (Fig. 13.39).

Fracture of the femoral neck is complicated by AVN in 10% of cases, with a higher incidence in severely displaced fractures.

Intertrochanteric fractures involve the greater and lesser trochanters and the bone in between. Intertrochanteric fractures vary in appearance from undisplaced oblique fractures to comminuted fractures with displacement of the lesser and greater trochanters (Fig. 13.40). Subtrochanteric fractures involve the upper femur below the lesser trochanter (Fig. 13.41).

SHAFT OF THE FEMUR

Fractures of the femoral shaft are easily recognized radiographically. Common patterns include transverse, oblique, spiral and comminuted fractures with varying degrees of displacement and angulation. Femoral shaft fractures are often associated with severe blood loss and occasionally with fat embolism.

13.4.8 KNEE

LOWER FEMUR

Three types of distal femoral fracture are seen:

1. Supracondylar fracture of the distal femur usually consists of an anteriorly angulated transverse fracture above the femoral condyles
2. Isolated fracture and separation of a femoral condyle
3. 'T'- or 'Y'-shaped distal femoral fracture with a vertical fracture line extending upwards from the articular surface causing separation of the femoral condyles.

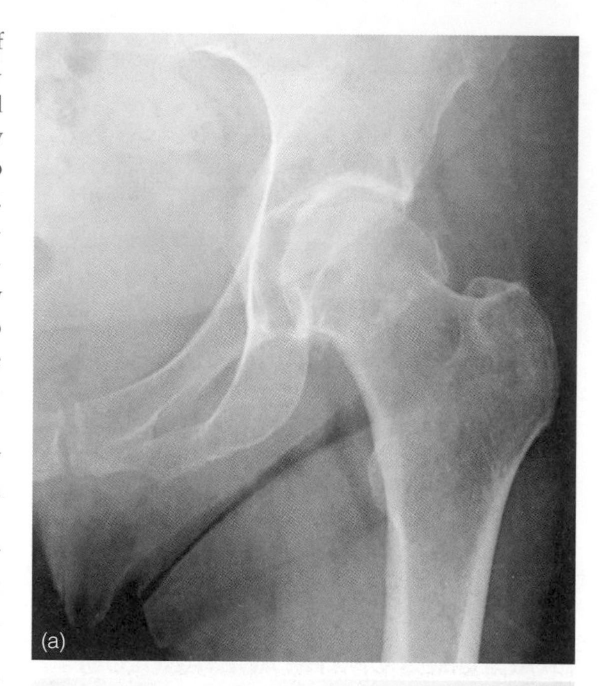

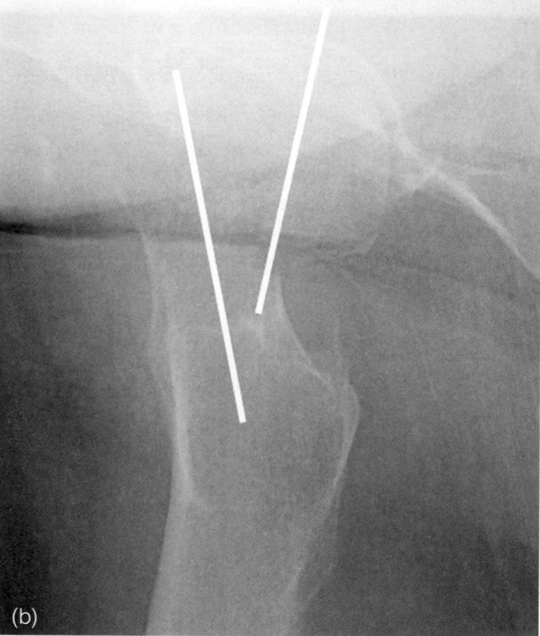

Figure 13.38 Subcapital neck of femur fracture. (a) The frontal view underestimates the degree of deformity. (b) The lateral view shows considerable angulation and displacement. The lines show the axes of the femoral neck and head.

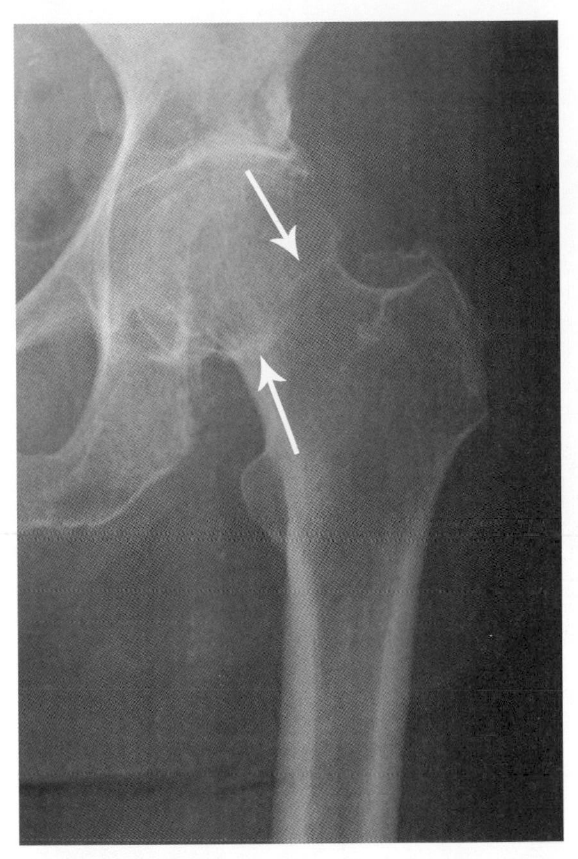

Figure 13.39 Subcapital neck of femur fracture. Undisplaced minimally impacted fracture seen as a sclerotic line (arrows).

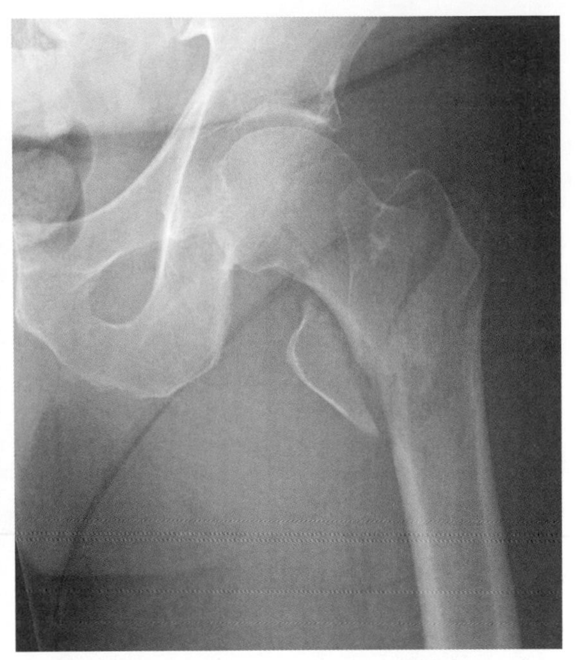

Figure 13.40 Intertrochanteric fracture. Complex intertrochanteric fracture that includes separation of the lesser trochanter.

PATELLA

Three types of patellar fracture are seen:

1. Undisplaced simple fracture
2. Displaced transverse fracture (Fig. 13.42)
3. Complex comminuted fracture.

Fracture of the patella should not be confused with bipartite patella. Bipartite patella is a common anatomical variant with a fragment of bone separated from the superolateral aspect of the patella. Unlike an acute fracture, the bone fragments in bipartite patella are corticated (well-defined margin) and rounded.

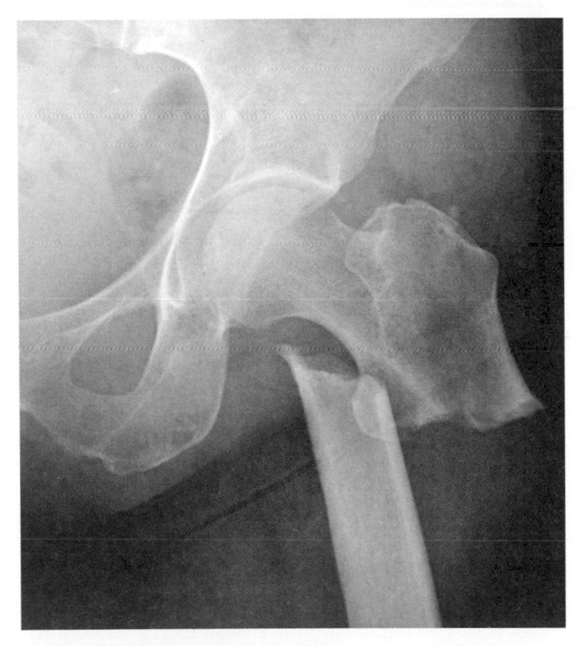

Figure 13.41 Subtrochanteric fracture. Markedly displaced fracture of the upper femur just below the level of the lesser trochanter.

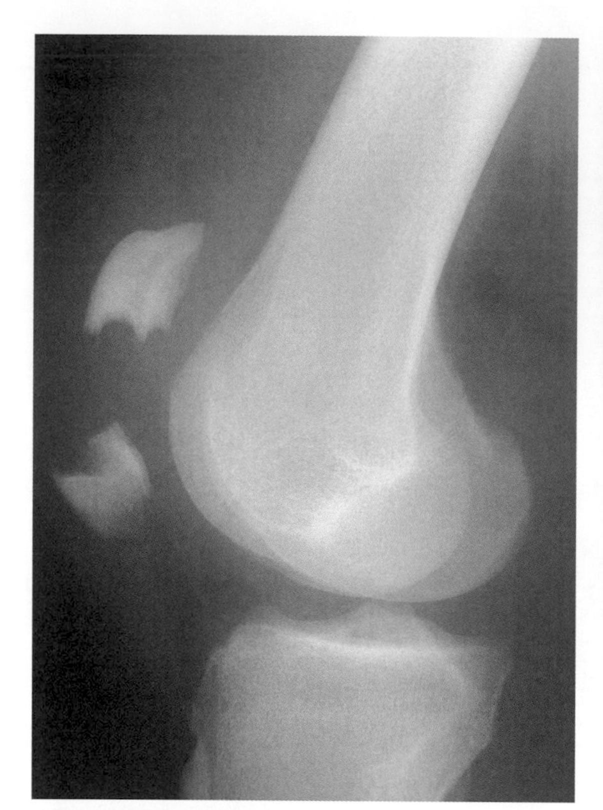

Figure 13.42 Transverse fracture of the patella. Bone fragments are markedly displaced because of unopposed action of the quadriceps muscle.

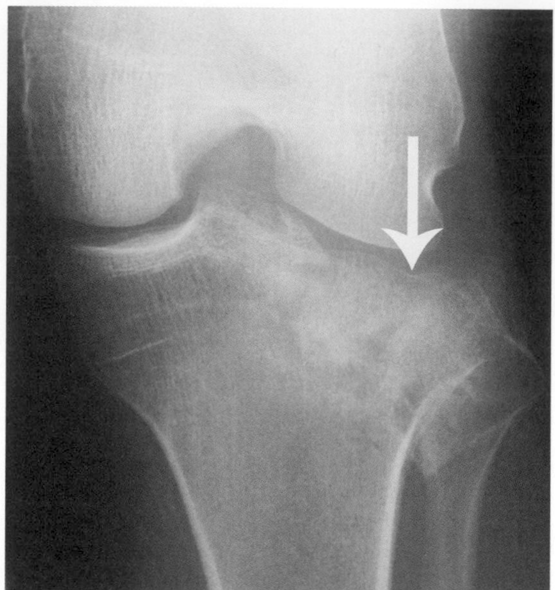

Figure 13.43 Tibial plateau fracture. Note an inferiorly impacted fracture of the lateral tibial plateau (arrow).

TIBIAL PLATEAU

Common patterns of upper tibial injury include:

- Crush fracture of the lateral tibial plateau (Fig. 13.43)
- Fracture and separation of one or both tibial condyles
- Complex comminuted fracture of the upper tibia.

Minimally crushed or displaced fractures of the upper tibia may be difficult to recognize radiographically. Often, the only clue is the presence of a knee joint effusion or lipohaemarthrosis. Knee joint effusion is best recognized on a lateral view. Fluid distension of the suprapatellar recess of the knee joint produces an oval-shaped opacity between the quadriceps tendon and the anterior surface of the distal femur (Fig. 13.44). With lipohaemarthrosis, a fluid–fluid level may be seen in the distended suprapatellar

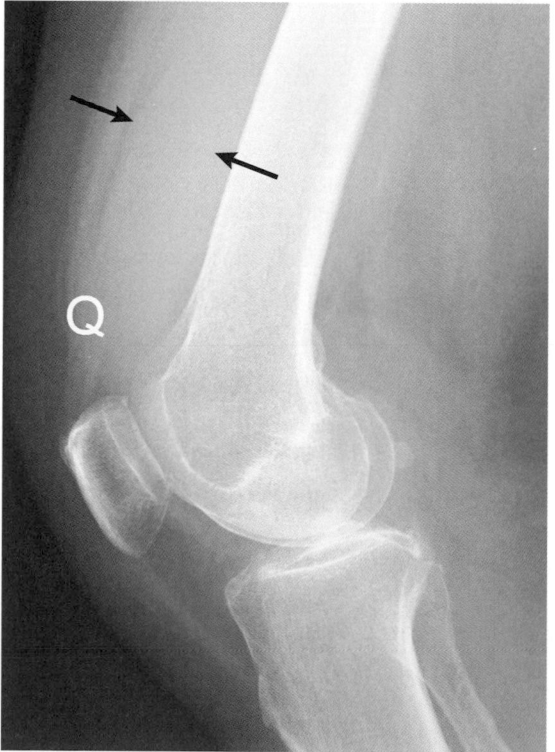

Figure 13.44 Knee joint effusion. Lateral radiograph shows fluid distending the suprapatellar recess of the knee joint (arrows) between the quadriceps tendon (Q) and the femur.

recess because of low-density fat 'floating' on blood in the knee joint (Fig. 13.45). Lipohaemarthrosis is due to release into the knee joint of fatty bone marrow and is almost always associated with an intra-articular fracture. Oblique views may be required to diagnose subtle fractures. CT is often performed to assist in the planning of surgical management (Fig. 13.46). Three-dimensional CT views are used to assess the degree of comminution and depression of the articular surface.

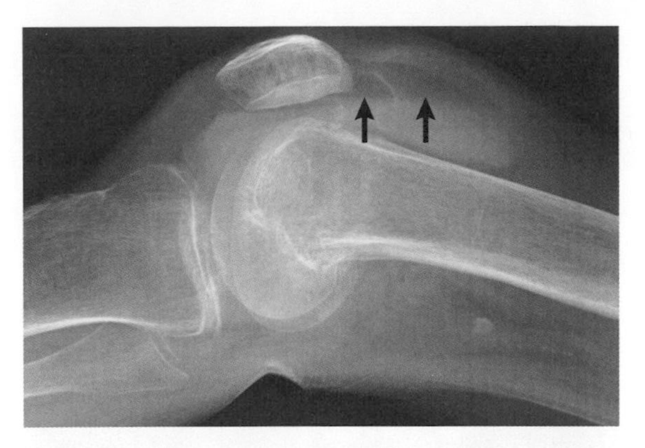

Figure 13.45 Lipohaemarthrosis. Lateral radiograph obtained with the patient supine shows a fluid–fluid level (arrows) in the distended suprapatellar recess of the knee joint. Lipohaemarthrosis is virtually always associated with an intra-articular fracture, in this case an undisplaced supracondylar fracture of the distal femur.

13.4.9 TIBIA AND FIBULA

Fracture of the tibial shaft is often associated with fracture of the fibula. Fractures may be transverse, oblique, spiral or comminuted, with varying degrees of displacement and angulation. Fractures of the tibia are often open (compound) with an increased incidence of osteomyelitis. Displaced upper tibial fractures may be associated with injury to the popliteal artery and its major branches, requiring emergency angiography and treatment.

Isolated fracture of the tibia is a relatively common injury in children aged 1–3 years (toddler's fracture). These fractures are often undisplaced and therefore very difficult to see. They are usually best seen as a thin oblique lucent line on the lateral radiograph (Fig. 13.47). Scintigraphic bone scan or MRI may be useful in difficult cases.

Isolated fracture of the shaft of the fibula may occur secondary to direct trauma. More commonly, fracture of the upper fibula is associated with disruption of the syndesmosis between the distal tibia and fibula (Maisonneuve fracture).

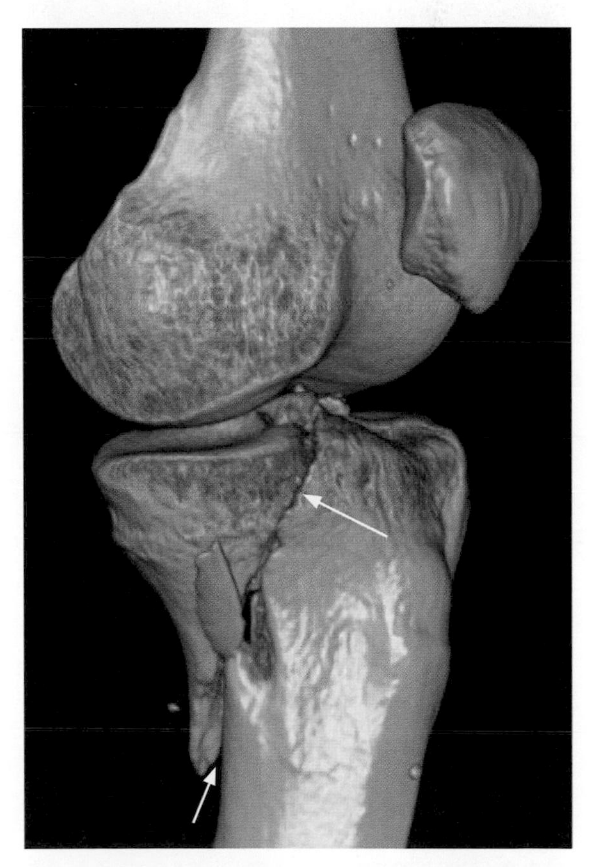

Figure 13.46 Tibial plateau fracture: CT. Three-dimensional reconstruction of an oblique impacted fracture of the medial tibial plateau (arrows) extending into the intercondylar eminence.

13.4.10 ANKLE AND FOOT

COMMON ANKLE FRACTURES

Ankle injuries may include fractures of the distal fibula (lateral malleolus), medial distal tibia (medial malleolus) and posterior distal tibia; talar shift and displacement; fracture of the talus; separation of the distal tibiofibular joint (syndesmosis injury); and ligament rupture with joint instability. Salter–Harris fractures of the distal tibia and fibula are common in children.

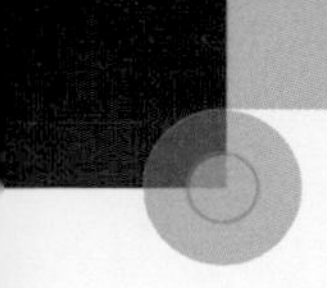

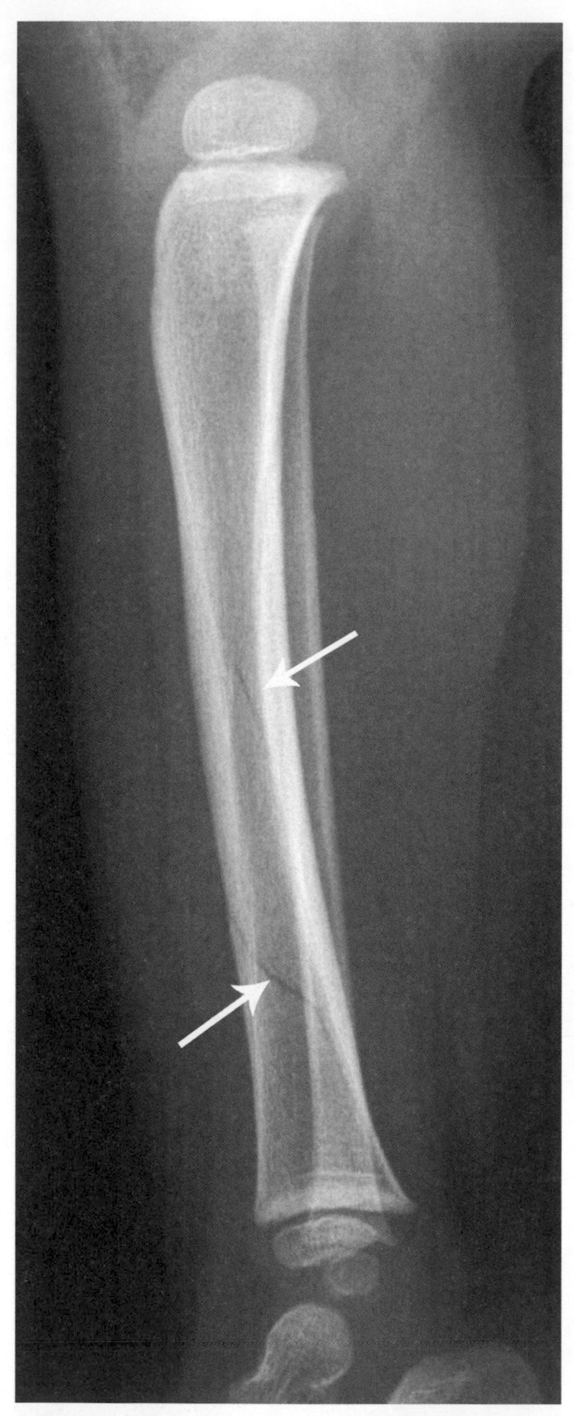

Figure 13.47 Toddler's fracture. Undisplaced spiral fracture of the tibia (arrows).

The types of fracture seen radiographically depend on the mechanism of injury:

- Adduction (inversion): vertical fracture of the medial malleolus, avulsion of the tip of the lateral malleolus, medial tilt of the talus
- Abduction (eversion): fracture of the lateral malleolus, avulsion of the tip of the medial malleolus, separation of the distal tibiofibular joint
- External rotation: spiral or oblique fracture of the lateral malleolus, lateral shift of the talus (Fig. 13.48)
- Vertical compression: fracture of the distal tibia posteriorly or anteriorly, separation of the distal tibiofibular joint.

FRACTURES OF THE TALUS

Small avulsion fractures of the talus are commonly seen in association with ankle fractures and ligament damage.

Osteochondral fracture of the upper articular surface of the talus (talar dome) is a common cause of

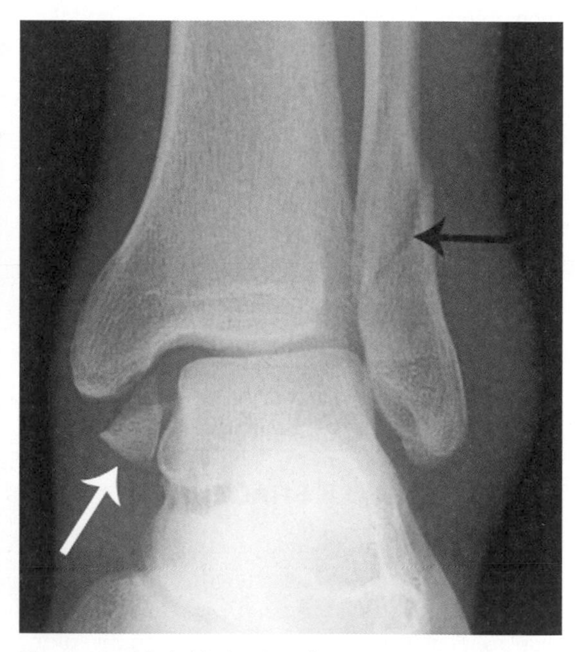

Figure 13.48 Ankle fracture due to external rotation. Note: spiral fracture of the distal fibula (black arrow), avulsion of the medial malleolus (white arrow), lateral shift of the talus, widening of the space between the distal tibia and fibula indicating syndesmosis injury.

persistent pain following an inversion ankle injury. Osteochondral fractures of the medial talar dome tend to be rounded defects in the cortical surface, often with loose bone fragments requiring surgical fixation. Osteochondral fractures of the lateral talar dome are usually small bone flakes. Osteochondral fractures may be difficult to see on radiographs and often require CT or MRI for diagnosis (Fig. 13.49).

Fracture of the neck of the talus may be widely displaced, associated with disruption of the subtalar joint and complicated by AVN.

FRACTURES OF THE CALCANEUS

Fractures of the calcaneus may show considerable displacement and comminution and may involve the subtalar joint. The Böhler angle is the angle formed by a line tangential to the superior extra-articular portion of the calcaneus and a line tangential to the superior intra-articular portion. The Böhler angle normally measures 25–40°. Reduction of the Böhler angle in a setting of trauma is a useful sign of a displaced intra-articular fracture of the calcaneus; these fractures may otherwise be difficult to see on radiographs (Fig. 13.50).

CT is useful for the assessment of calcaneal fractures and to assist in planning of surgical reduction. Calcaneal fractures, particularly when bilateral, have a high association with spine and pelvis fractures.

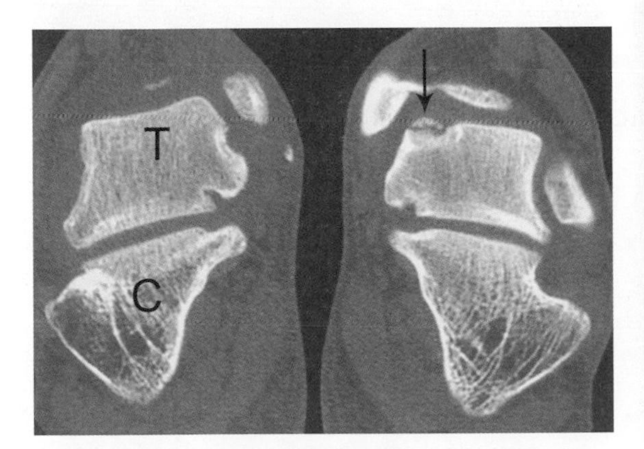

Figure 13.49 Osteochondral fracture of the talus: coronal CT of both ankles. Note the normal appearance of right talus (T) and calcaneus (C). A defect in the cortical surface of the left talar dome is associated with a loose bone fragment (arrow).

OTHER FRACTURES OF THE FOOT

Any of the tarsal bones may be fractured. With major trauma, dislocation of intertarsal or tarsometatarsal joints may occur. Lisfranc fracture/dislocation refers to disruption of the Lisfranc ligament, with midfoot instability. The Lisfranc ligament joins the distal

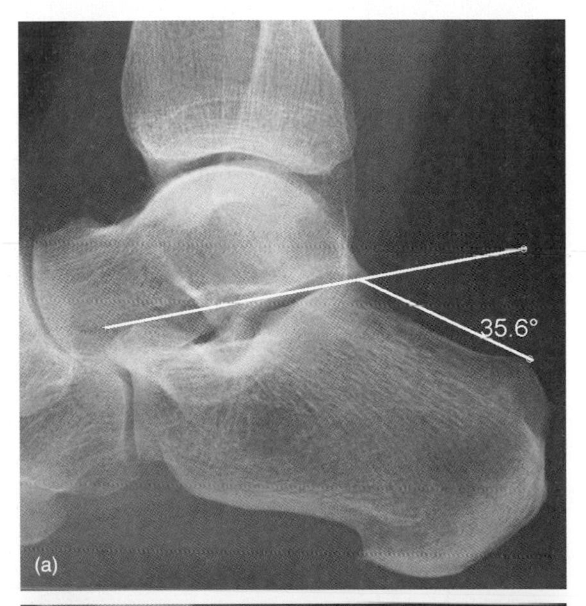

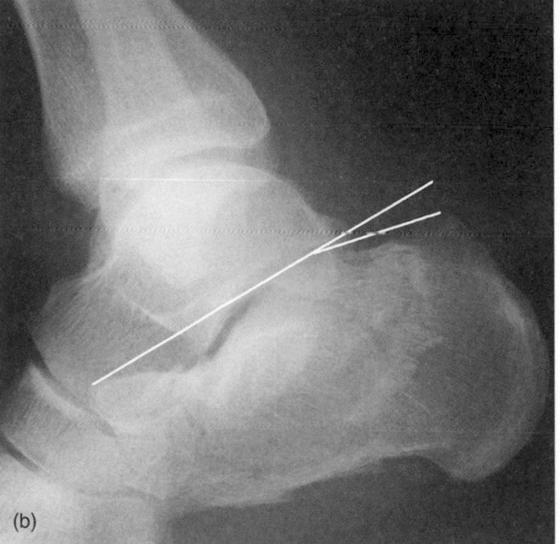

Figure 13.50 Calcaneus fracture. (a) Note the method of determining the Böhler angle. (b) In this example, there is a reduction of the Böhler angle associated with multiple displaced fractures of the calcaneus.

lateral surface of the medial cuneiform to the base of the second metatarsal and is a major stabilizer of the midfoot. Radiographic signs of Lisfranc ligament disruption may be difficult to appreciate and include widening of the space between the bases of the first and second metatarsals and associated fractures of the metatarsals, cuneiforms and other tarsal bones (Fig. 13.51). CT or MRI may be required to confirm the diagnosis.

Metatarsal fractures are usually transverse. The growth centre at the base of the fifth metatarsal lies parallel to the shaft and should not be mistaken for a fracture; fractures in this region usually lie in the transverse plane (Fig. 13.52).

Stress fractures of the foot are common, particularly those involving the metatarsal shafts and less commonly the navicular and talus bones.

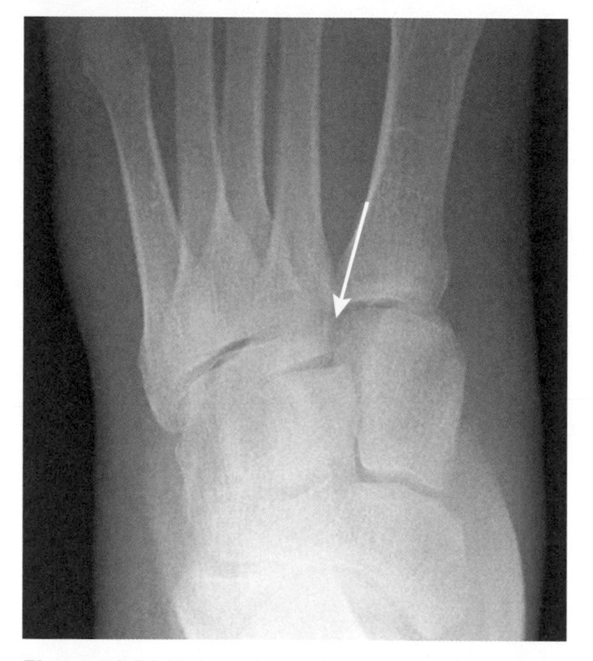

Figure 13.51 Lisfranc ligament tear. Severe foot pain following major trauma. No obvious fracture on initial inspection of the radiographs. Note: widening of the gap between the base of the second metatarsal and medial cuneiform (arrow) and malalignment of the second tarsometatarsal joint. These signs indicate a tear of the Lisfranc ligament.

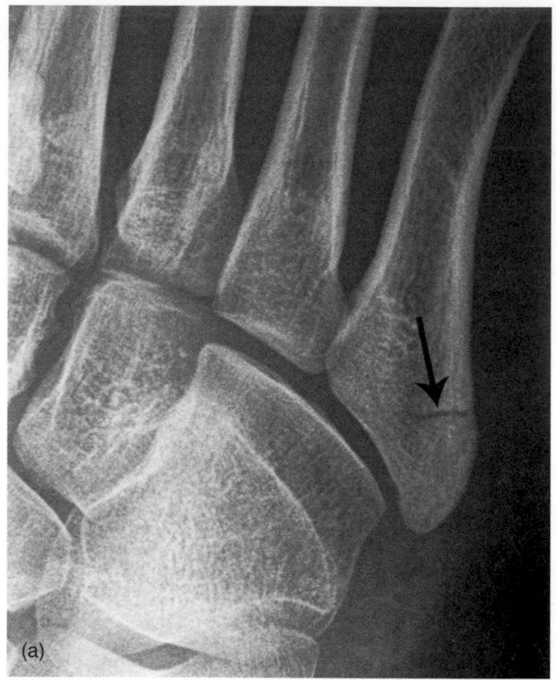

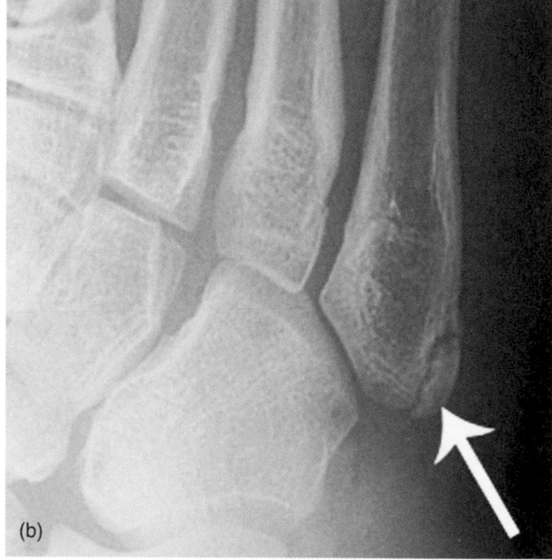

Figure 13.52 Fifth metatarsal fracture. (a) Transverse fracture of the base of the fifth metatarsal (arrow). (b) Normal growth centre at the base of the fifth metatarsal (arrow). This is aligned parallel to the long axis of the bone and should not be confused with a fracture.

13.5 INTERNAL JOINT DERANGEMENT: METHODS OF INVESTIGATION

Internal joint derangements refer to the disruption of supporting structures, such as ligaments and articular cartilages, and fibrocartilage structures, such as the menisci of the knee and the hip and shoulder labra. Causes of internal joint derangements:

- Trauma, including sporting injuries
- Overuse syndromes, as may occur in occupational or athletic settings
- Secondary to degenerative or inflammatory arthropathies.

13.5.1 WRIST

The wrist is an anatomically complex area with several important ligaments and cartilages supporting the carpal bones. Persistent wrist pain following trauma or post-traumatic carpal instability may be due to ligament or cartilage tears. The two most commonly injured internal wrist structures are the scapholunate ligament and the TFCC. The scapholunate ligament is a strong 'C'-shaped ligament that stabilizes the joint between the scaphoid and lunate. The TFCC consists of a fibrocartilage disc and adjacent ligaments joining the distal radius to the base of the ulnar styloid; it is a major stabilizer of the ulnar side of the wrist joint.

Radiographs of the wrist including stress views may be useful to confirm carpal instability, such as widening of the space between the scaphoid and lunate with disruption of the scapholunate ligament. MRI is the investigation of choice to confirm tears of the internal wrist structures (Fig. 13.53).

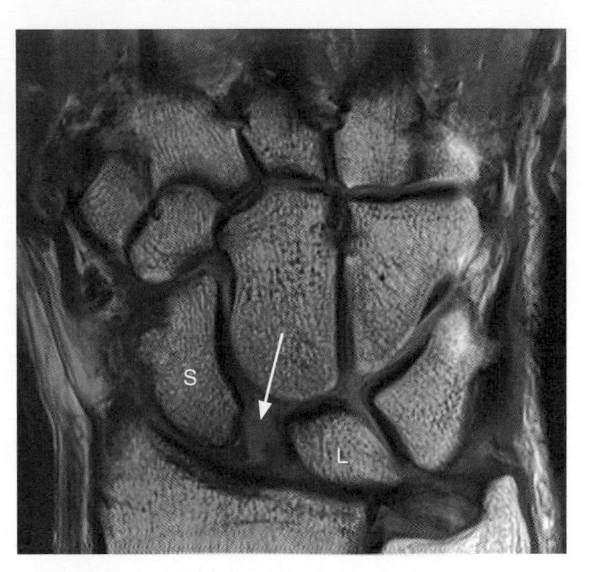

Figure 13.53 Scapholunate ligament tear: MRI. Coronal proton density image shows separation of the scaphoid (S) and lunate (L), with a fluid-filled gap in the position of the torn scapholunate ligament (arrow).

13.5.2 SHOULDER

ROTATOR CUFF DISEASE

Two types of rotator cuff disorder are common causes of shoulder pain:

1. Calcific tendinosis
2. Degenerative tendinosis and rotator cuff tear.

Calcific tendinosis due to hydroxyapatite crystal deposition is particularly common in the supraspinatus tendon and occurs in young to middle-aged adults. Calcific tendinitis (tendinosis) usually presents with acute shoulder pain accentuated by abduction. Tears of the rotator cuff most commonly involve the supraspinatus tendon and are usually caused by tendon degeneration ('wear and tear') encountered in elderly patients. Clinical presentation is with persistent shoulder pain worsened by abduction. The pain is often worse at night, with interruption of sleep a common complaint.

For suspected rotator cuff disease, radiographs of the shoulder are used to diagnose calcific tendinitis and to exclude underlying bony pathology as a cause of shoulder pain (Fig. 13.54). Ultrasound (US) is the investigation of choice for suspected rotator cuff tear (Fig. 13.55). MRI is used as a problem-solving tool for difficult or equivocal cases.

GLENOHUMERAL JOINT INSTABILITY (RECURRENT DISLOCATION)

Dislocation of the glenohumeral (shoulder) joint is a common occurrence and, in most cases, recovery

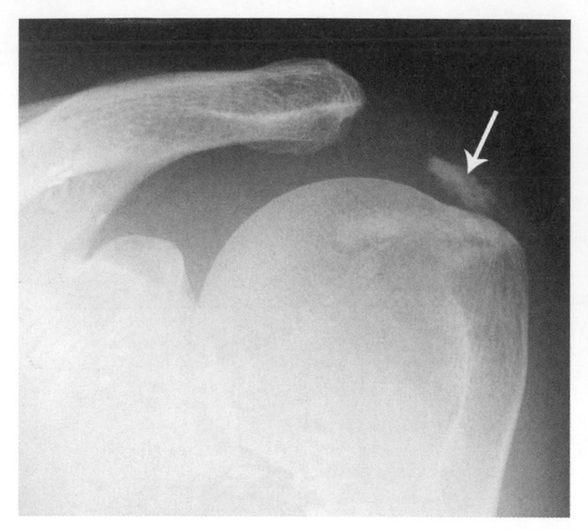

Figure 13.54 Calcific tendinitis. A focal calcification is seen as an oval-shaped opacity above the humeral head in the supraspinatus tendon (arrow).

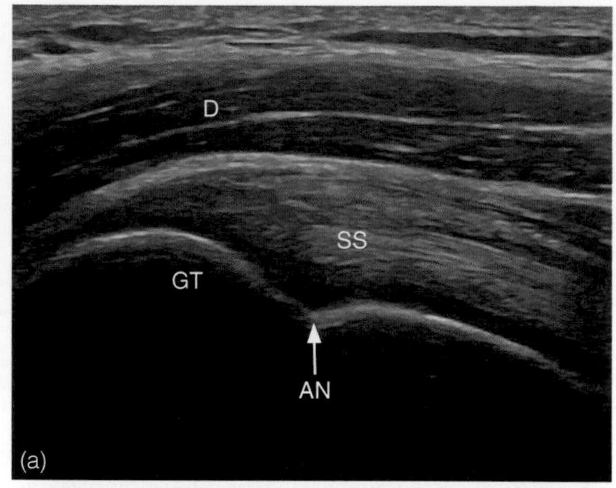

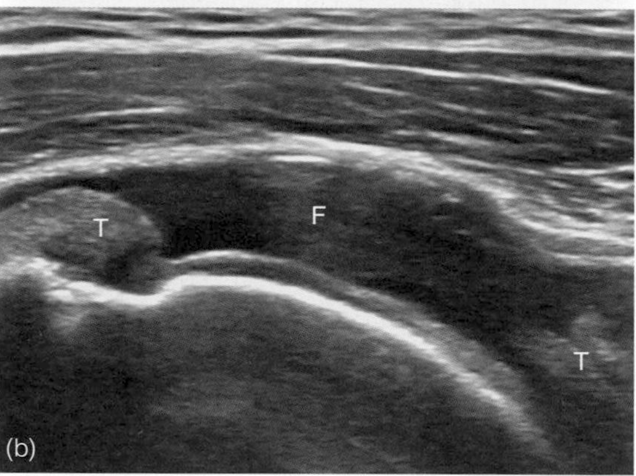

Figure 13.55 US of the rotator cuff. (a) Normal study showing the following features: anatomical neck (AN), deltoid muscle (D), greater tuberosity (GT), supraspinatus tendon (SS). (b) Supraspinatus tendon tear. Torn tendon ends (T) separated by a fluid-filled defect (F). The thin hypoechoic layer on the surface of the humeral head is articular cartilage.

is swift and uncomplicated. In a small percentage of cases, tearing of the stabilizing structures such as the labrum and glenohumeral ligaments may cause glenohumeral instability and recurrent dislocation. MRI is the investigation of choice for assessment of glenohumeral instability. The accuracy of MRI may be enhanced by the intra-articular injection of a dilute solution of gadolinium (magnetic resonance (MR) arthrogram); this is done under fluoroscopic or US guidance (Fig. 13.56).

13.5.3 HIP

Hip pain is a widespread problem and may occur at any age. Hip disorders in children are discussed in Chapter 16. In elderly patients, OA is a common cause of hip pain. Radiographs are usually sufficient for the diagnosis of OA of the hip. In young active adults a tear of the fibrocartilaginous labrum may present with hip pain plus an audible 'clicking'. Less commonly, hip pain may be due to bone disorders such as AVN, and a history of relevant risk factors such as steroid use may be relevant. MRI is the investigation of choice for suspected labral tear, AVN and other hip joint disorders.

13.5.4 KNEE

Radiographs are performed for the assessment of most causes of knee pain. MRI is the investigation of choice in the assessment of most internal knee derangements, including meniscus injury (Fig. 13.57), cruciate ligament tear, collateral ligament tear, osteochondritis dissecans, etc. MSUS is useful in the assessment of periarticular pathology such as popliteal cysts and patellar tendinopathy. MSUS cannot be used to reliably diagnose other internal derangements.

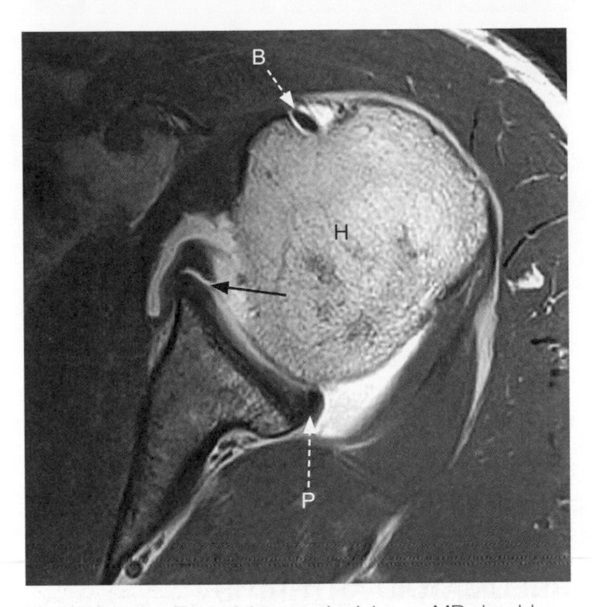

Figure 13.56 Tear of the anterior labrum: MR shoulder arthrogram. T1-weighted transverse image shows the shoulder joint filled with contrast-enhanced fluid. Note a layer of joint fluid between the torn anterior labrum and the underlying anterior glenoid (arrow). Also note: humerus (H), biceps tendon (B, dashed arrow), posterior labrum (P, dotted arrow).

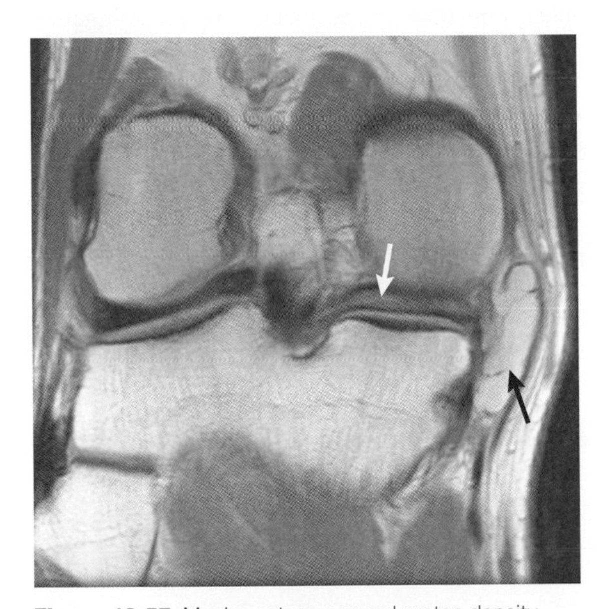

Figure 13.57 Meniscus tear: coronal proton density MRI of the knee. A horizontal tear of the medial meniscus, seen as a high-signal line (white arrow), is associated with formation of a lobulated parameniscal cyst (black arrow).

13.5.5 ANKLE

Persistent ankle pain post trauma may be due to delayed healing of ligament tears or osteochondral fracture of the articular surface of the talus. MRI is the investigation of choice in the assessment of persistent post-traumatic ankle pain. Tendinopathy and tendon tears are common around the ankle joint. The most commonly involved tendons are the Achilles tendon, tibialis posterior and peroneus longus and brevis. These tendons are well assessed with US and MRI.

13.6 APPROACH TO ARTHROPATHIES

In the diagnosis of arthropathies it is most useful to decide first whether there is involvement of a single joint (monoarthropathy) or multiple joints (polyarthropathy). One must remember though that a polyarthropathy may present early with a single painful joint.

Polyarthropathies may be divided into three large categories:

1. Inflammatory
2. Degenerative
3. Metabolic.

Various clinical features and biochemical tests may be used for further assessment of arthropathies. Biochemical tests may include:

- Erythrocyte sedimentation rate (ESR)
- C-reactive protein (CRP)
- Rheumatoid factor (RhF)
- Antinuclear antibody (ANA)
- Uric acid
- Human leukocyte antigen B27 (HLA-B27).

Radiographs are usually sufficient for the imaging assessment of suspected arthropathy. Certain radiographic features of affected joints may assist in the diagnosis:

- Distribution
  - Symmetrical or asymmetrical
  - Small joints or large, weight-bearing joints

- Erosions
- Joint space narrowing
- Osteophytes.

Occasionally, MRI may be useful to detect early signs of joint inflammation when radiographs are normal or equivocal. MRI can detect synovial inflammation as well as bone changes such as marrow oedema and small erosions (Fig. 13.58).

Below is a summary of radiographic manifestations of the more commonly encountered arthropathies.

13.6.1 MONOARTHROPATHY

A common cause for a single painful joint is trauma. In most cases, diagnosis is obvious from the clinical history and radiographs are usually sufficient for diagnosis. In cases of septic arthritis, the affected joint may be radiographically normal at the time of initial presentation. After a few days, radiographic signs such as periarticular bone erosions and destruction may occur. MRI or scintigraphy with ^{99m}Tc-MDP are usually positive at the time of presentation. The other major category of monoarthropathy is polyarthropathy presenting initially in a single joint, e.g. OA, gout and rheumatoid arthritis (RA).

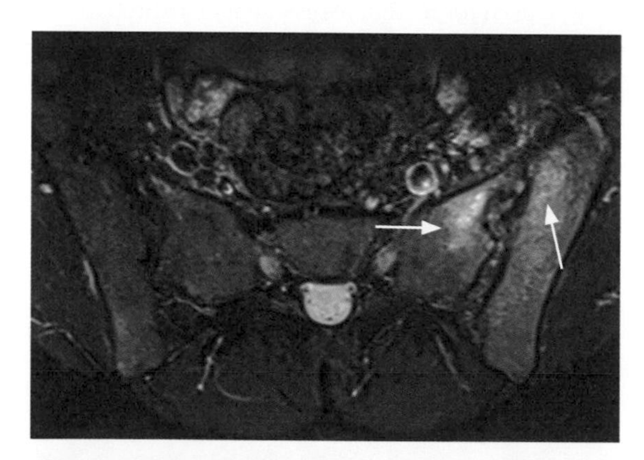

Figure 13.58 Sacroiliitis: MRI. Transverse sagittal STIR (short TI (inversion time) inversion recovery) image shows high signal, indicating oedema on both sides of the left sacroiliac joint (arrows). Note the normal appearance of the right sacroiliac joint.

13.6.2 INFLAMMATORY POLYARTHROPATHY

Inflammatory arthropathies present with painful joints and associated soft-tissue swelling. Inflammatory joint pain is usually non-mechanical in nature, i.e. not related to movement and not relieved by rest. Pain is often worse on waking, and 'morning stiffness' is a common complaint. Inflammatory polyarthropathies are classified into seropositive and seronegative arthropathies. The term 'seropositive' means that RhF is present in the blood. RhF is an autoantibody against the Fc portion of immunoglobulin G (IgG). It is present in the blood of most, though not all, patients with RA and other seropositive arthropathies associated with connective tissue disorders.

RHEUMATOID ARTHRITIS

The fundamental pathological process in RA is inflammation of the synovium. Synovial inflammation leads to joint swelling and formation of synovial inflammatory masses (pannus). Pannus may cause bone erosions and lead to joint deformity. RA is usually symmetrical in distribution and predominantly affects the small joints, especially metacarpophalangeal (MCP), metatarsophalangeal (MTP), intercarpal and proximal interphalangeal joints. Spinal involvement is rare, apart from erosion of the odontoid peg of C2.

Radiographic signs of RA (Fig. 13.59):

- Soft-tissue swelling overlying joints
- Bone erosions occur in the feet and hands, best demonstrated in the metatarsal and metacarpal heads, articular surfaces of phalanges and carpal bones
- Reduced bone density adjacent to joints (periarticular osteoporosis)
- Abnormalities of joint alignment with subluxation of MCP joints causing ulnar deviation of the fingers and subluxation of MTP joints producing lateral deviation of the toes.

OTHER CONNECTIVE TISSUE (SEROPOSITIVE) ARTHROPATHIES

Other ('non-RA') seropositive arthropathies include systemic lupus erythematosus (SLE), systemic

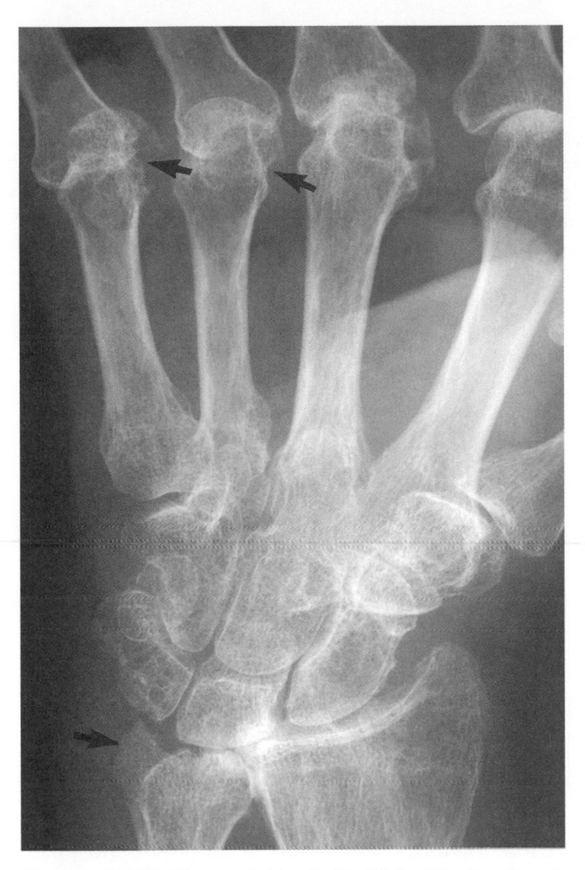

Figure 13.59 Rheumatoid arthritis (RA) of the hand and wrist. Bone erosions are seen involving the metacarpals and the ulnar styloid process (arrows).

sclerosis, CREST (calcinosis, Raynaud's phenomenon, (o)esophageal dysmotility, sclerodactyly and telangiectasia), mixed connective tissue disease, polymyositis and dermatomyositis. These arthropathies tend to present with symmetrical arthropathy involving the peripheral small joints, especially the MCP and proximal interphalangeal joints. Radiographic signs of non-RA seropositive arthropathies may be subtle and include:

- Soft-tissue swelling
- Periarticular osteoporosis
- Soft-tissue calcification is common, especially around joints
- Bone erosions are less common than with RA
- Resorption of distal phalanges and joint contractures are prominent features of systemic sclerosis.

SERONEGATIVE SPONDYLOARTHROPATHY

The spondyloarthropathies (SpAs) are asymmetrical polyarthropathies, usually involving only a few joints. SpAs have a predilection for the spine and sacroiliac joints. Five subtypes of SpA are described with shared clinical features, including association with HLA-B27:

- Ankylosing spondylitis
- Reactive arthritis
- Arthritis spondylitis with inflammatory bowel disease
- Arthritis spondylitis with psoriasis
- Undifferentiated spondyloarthropathy (uSpA).

Clinical features of SpA may include inflammatory back pain, positive family history, acute anterior uveitis and inflammation at tendon and ligament insertions (enthesitis).

Enthesitis most commonly involves the distal Achilles tendon insertion and the insertion of the plantar fascia on the undersurface of the calcaneus. Features of inflammatory back pain include insidious onset, morning stiffness and improvement with exercise. Ankylosing spondylitis is the most common SpA.

Radiographic findings of ankylosing spondylitis (Fig. 13.60) are:

- Vertically orientated bony spurs arising from vertebral bodies (syndesmophytes)

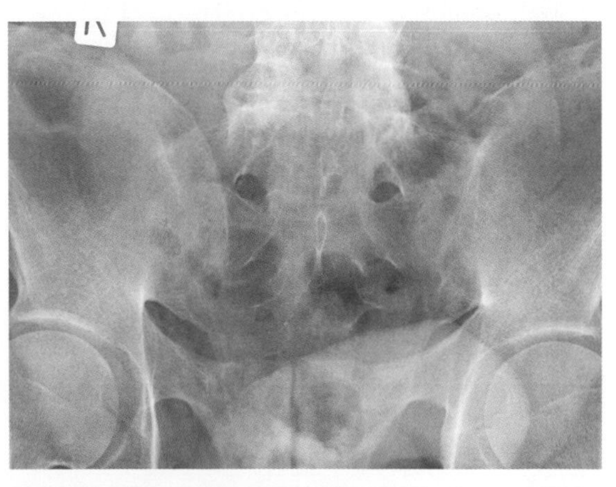

Figure 13.60 Ankylosing spondylitis. Frontal view of the pelvis showing fused sacroiliac joints.

- Fusion or ankylosis of the spine giving the 'bamboo spine' appearance
- Sacroiliac joint changes, including erosions producing an irregular joint margin
- Sclerosis and fusion of sacroiliac joints later in the disease process.

Psoriatic arthropathy is an asymmetrical arthropathy affecting the small joints of the hands and feet. Radiographic changes of psoriatic arthropathy include periarticular erosions and periosteal new bone formation in peripheral joints.

13.6.3 DEGENERATIVE ARTHROPATHY: OSTEOARTHRITIS

Primary OA refers to degenerative arthropathy with no apparent underlying or predisposing cause. Primary OA is an asymmetric process involving the large weight-bearing (mainly the hips and knees), lumbar and cervical spine (see Chapter 10), distal interphalangeal, first carpometacarpal and lateral carpal joints. Secondary OA refers to degenerative changes complicating underlying arthropathy such as RA, trauma or Paget disease (see section 13.8.3). The fundamental pathological process in OA is the loss of articular cartilage. Loss of articular cartilage results in joint space narrowing and abnormal stresses on joint margins; these abnormal stresses lead to the formation of bony spurs (osteophytes) at the joint margins.

Radiographic changes of OA (Fig. 13.61):

- Joint space narrowing
- Osteophytes
- Sclerosis of joint surfaces
- Periarticular cyst formation
- Loose bodies in joints due to detached osteophytes and ossified cartilage debris.

13.6.4 METABOLIC ARTHROPATHIES

GOUT

Gout is caused by uric acid crystal deposition in soft tissues and articular structures. Acute gout refers to soft-tissue swelling, with no visible bony changes. Chronic gouty arthropathy occurs with recurrent acute gout. Gouty arthropathy is usually asymmetric in distribution and often monoarticular. Gouty arthropathy involves the first MTP joint in 70% of cases. Other commonly affected joints include ankles, knees and intertarsal joints.

Radiographic features of gouty arthropathy (Fig. 13.62):

- Bone erosions: usually set back from the joint surface (para-articular)
- Calcification of articular cartilages, especially the menisci of the knee
- Tophus: soft-tissue mass in the synovium of joints, the subcutaneous tissues of the lower leg, Achilles tendon, olecranon bursa at the elbow, helix of the ear
- Calcification of tophi is an uncommon feature.

The diagnosis of gout may be confirmed with spectral CT, which can display deposition of sodium urate crystals in and around joints (Fig. 13.63).

CALCIUM PYROPHOSPHATE DEPOSITION DISEASE

Also known as pseudogout, calcium pyrophosphate deposition disease (CPPD) may occur in young adults as an autosomal dominant condition or sporadically in older patients. CPPD presents clinically with intermittent acute joint pain and swelling. CPPD may affect any joint, most commonly the knee, hip, shoulder, elbow, wrist and ankle. Radiographic signs of CPPD include calcification of intra-articular cartilages, especially the menisci of the knee and the TFCC of the wrist. Secondary OA may occur with subchondral cysts and joint space narrowing.

CALCIUM HYDROXYAPATITE CRYSTAL DEPOSITION DISEASE

Calcium hydroxyapatite crystal deposition usually manifests as with calcific tendinosis of the supraspinatus tendon (Fig. 13.54). Clinical presentation consists of severe shoulder pain and limitation of movement in patients aged 40–70 years. Virtually any other tendon in the body may be affected, though much less commonly than supraspinatus.

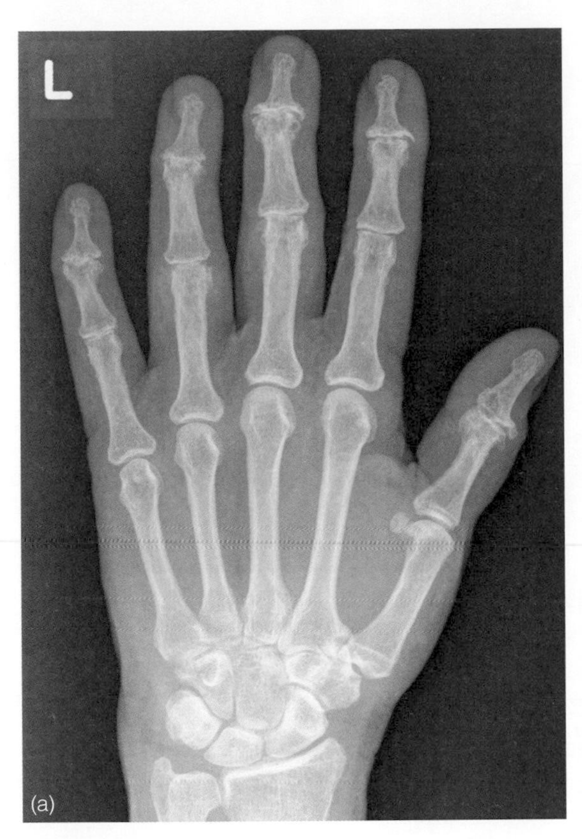

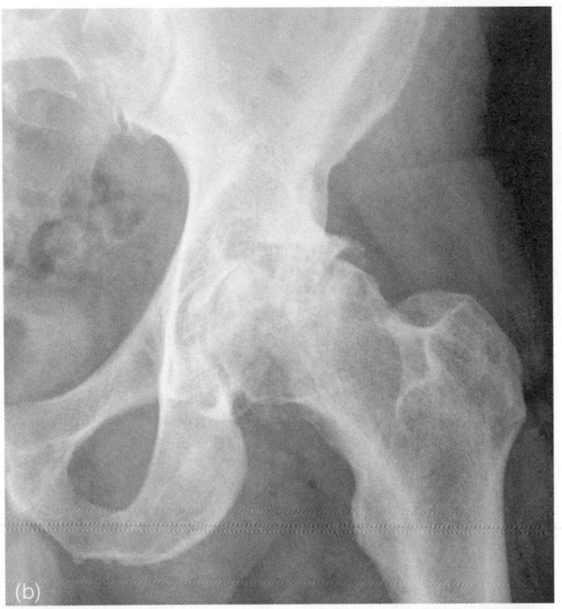

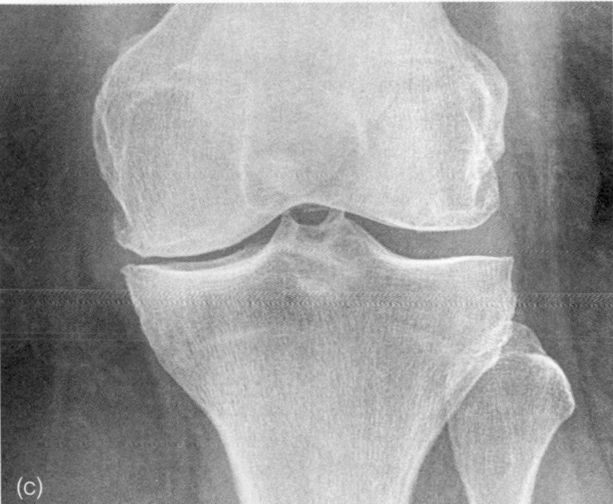

Figure 13.61 Osteoarthritis (OA). (a) Hands: joint space narrowing, articular surface irregularity and osteophyte formation involving interphalangeal joints. (b) Hip: joint narrowing, most marked superiorly; articular surface sclerosis and irregularity; lucencies in the acetabulum and femoral head due to subcortical cyst formation. (c) Knee: narrowing of the medial joint compartment due to thinning of the articular cartilage.

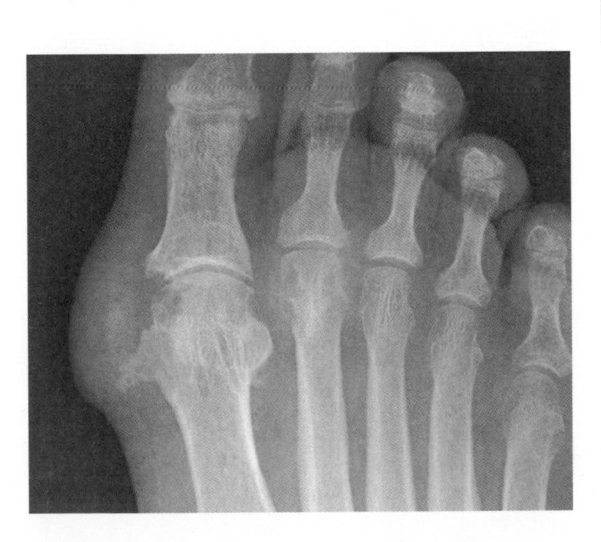

Figure 13.62 Chronic gouty arthropathy of the first metatarsophalangeal (MTP) joint. Bone erosions adjacent to, but not directly involving, articular surfaces (juxta-articular). Soft-tissue swelling and calcification is seen medial to the joint.

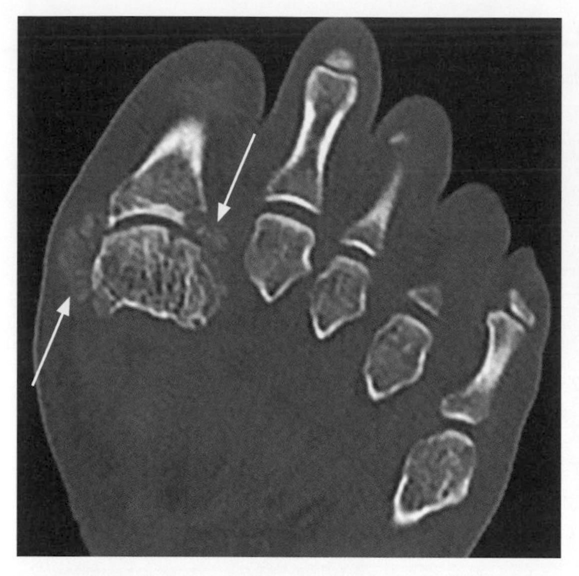

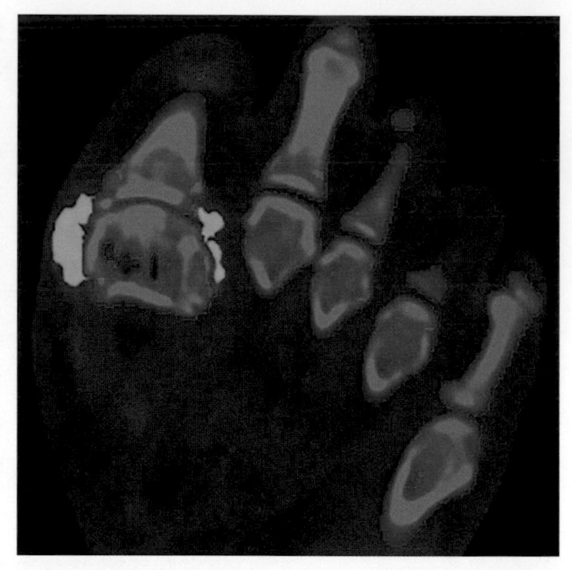

Figure 13.63 Gouty arthropathy and monosodium urate crystal deposition: spectral CT. (a) CT shows faint calcification around the first metatarsophalangeal (MTP) joint (arrows). (b) Uric acid colour map displays monosodium urate crystals as green deposits around the joint.

The classical radiographic sign of calcium hydroxyapatite deposition is calcification in the supraspinatus tendon. In acute cases, the calcification may be semiliquid and difficult to see radiographically. Calcific tendinosis may also be diagnosed with US. US-guided aspiration of calcification and steroid injection may be curative.

13.7 APPROACH TO PRIMARY BONE TUMOURS

Primary bone tumours (Table 13.1) are relatively rare, representing less than 1% of all malignancies. Imaging, particularly radiographic assessment, is vital to the diagnosis and delineation of bone tumours and a basic approach is outlined here, along with a summary of the roles of the various modalities. Remember that in adult patients a solitary bone lesion is more likely to be a metastasis than a primary bone tumour.

Remember also that in children and adults several conditions may mimic bone tumour, including:

- Benign fibroma (fibrous cortical defect)
- Simple (unicameral) bone cyst
- Osteomyelitis
- Fibrous dysplasia
- Langerhans cell histiocytosis.

The clinical history is often extremely helpful, especially the age of the patient and the location of the lesion.

Multiple parameters are assessed on examination of the radiograph:

- Location of the tumour within the bone, for example:
  - Diaphysis: Ewing sarcoma
  - Metaphysis: osteogenic sarcoma
  - Epiphysis: chondroblastoma and giant cell tumour
- Matrix of the lesion, i.e. the appearance of material within the tumour:
  - Lytic, i.e. lucent or dark
  - Sclerotic, i.e. dense or white
- Zone of transition, i.e. the margin between the lesion and normal bone
  - Thin, sclerotic rim: more likely benign
  - Wide and irregular: more likely malignant

Table 13.1 Features of common bone tumours and 'mimics'.

Diagnosis	Age (years)	Site	Matrix	Margin	Effect on bone
Simple bone cyst	5–15	Proximal metaphysis femur and humerus	Lucent	Thin, sclerotic	Mild expansion, thin cortex
Fibroma	10–20	Femur and tibia	Lucent	Thin, sclerotic	Mild expansion of cortex
Osteoid osteoma	10–30	Femur, tibia	Lucent nidus	Thick, sclerotic	Mild eccentric expansion
Osteosarcoma	10–25	Metaphysis femur, tibia, humerus	Lytic or mixed lytic and sclerotic	Wide	Eccentric expansion, cortical destruction, spiculated periosteal new bone
Enchondroma	10–50	Hands; metaphysis humerus and femur	Lytic with focal calcifications	Thin, sclerotic	Mild expansion, thin cortex
Chondrosarcoma	30–60	Pelvis and shoulder; metaphysis humerus and femur	Lytic with focal calcifications	Irregular, sclerotic	Expansion and cortical destruction
Giant cell tumour	20–40	Subarticular ends of long bones	Lucent	Thin, ill-defined	Eccentric expansion, thin or destroyed cortex
Ewing sarcoma	5–15	Diaphysis of femur; pelvis	Lytic	Wide	Layered or spiculated periosteal new bone

- Effect on surrounding bone:
  - Expansion and thinning of cortex: more likely benign
  - Penetration of cortex: more likely malignant
  - Periosteal reaction and new bone formation: osteogenic sarcoma, Ewing sarcoma
- Associated features:
  - Soft-tissue mass
  - Pathological fracture.

Most diagnostic information as to tumour type comes from clinical assessment and radiographic appearances (Fig. 13.64). Other imaging modalities add further, often complementary, information on staging and complications. MRI is used to assess tumour extent within the marrow cavity of the bone and associated soft-tissue mass (Fig. 13.65). CT is more sensitive than MRI in the detection of calcification; it may be used in specific instances where accurate characterization of the tumour matrix may be diagnostic, such as suspected cartilage tumour. Scintigraphy with ^{99m}Tc-MDP (bone scan) may be used to assess the activity of the primary bone lesion and to detect multiple lesions. In modern practice, bone tumours are commonly treated with chemotherapy or radiotherapy prior to surgery. MRI and/or positron emission tomography (PET)-CT may be used to assess the response to therapy.

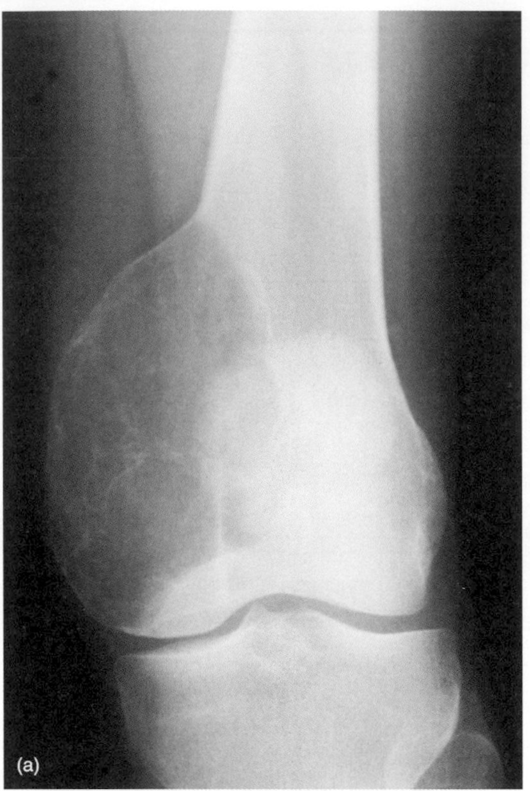

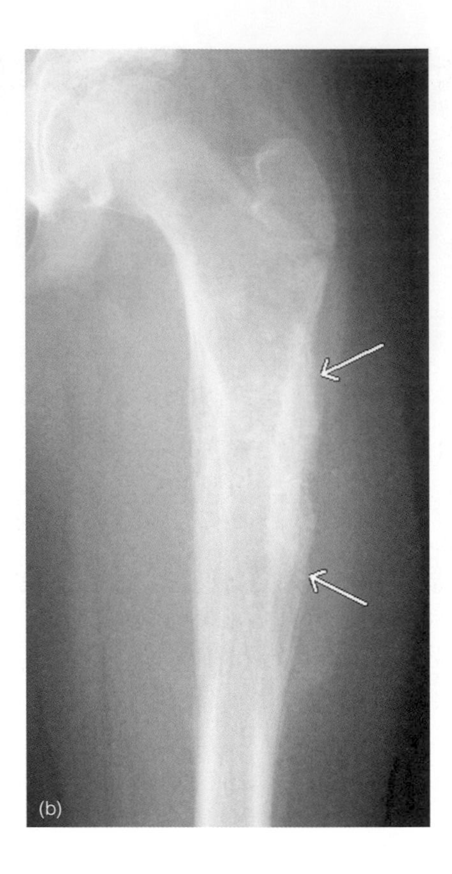

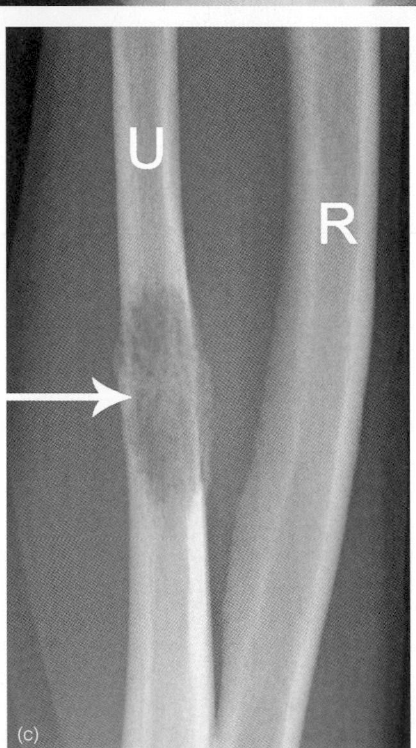

Figure 13.64 Bone tumours; three examples. (a) Giant cell tumour of the distal femur seen as an eccentric lytic expanded lesion with a well-defined margin. (b) Osteosarcoma of the upper femur. Note the irregular cortical thickening with new bone formation beneath the elevated periosteum (arrows). (c) Metastasis (arrow) from non-small cell carcinoma of the lung in the ulna (U) seen as a lytic lesion with irregular margins. Note the normal radius (R).

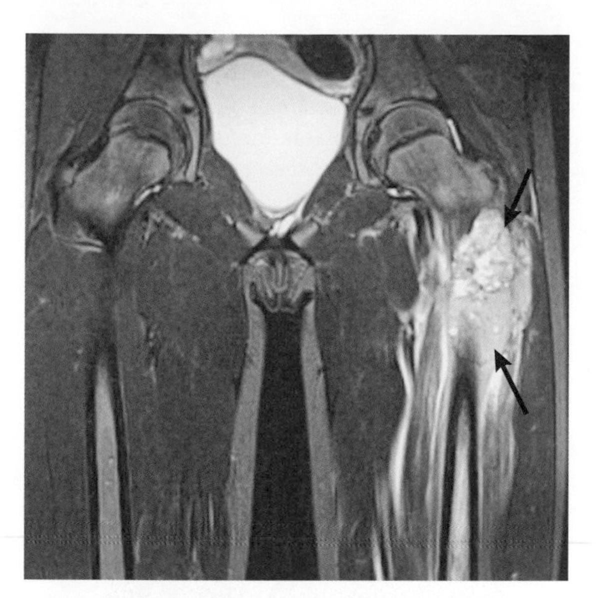

Figure 13.65 Ewing sarcoma: MRI. Thigh pain and swelling in a 13-year-old girl. Coronal STIR (short TI (inversion time) inversion recovery) image of the thighs and pelvis show a lesion with a large soft-tissue component (arrows) arising from the left upper femur.

13.8 MISCELLANEOUS COMMON BONE CONDITIONS

13.8.1 SKELETAL METASTASES

Almost any primary tumour may metastasize to bone, including breast, prostate, kidney, lung, gastrointestinal tract, thyroid and melanoma. Skeletal metastases are often clinically occult or they may present with bone pain, pathological fracture or hypercalcaemia. Radiographically, skeletal metastases are most commonly lytic, producing focal lesions of bone destruction (Fig. 13.64c). Sclerotic metastases occur with prostate, stomach and carcinoid tumour. Skeletal metastases most commonly involve spine, pelvis, ribs, proximal femur and proximal humerus, and are uncommon distal to the knee and elbow. Skeletal metastases are usually detected on PET-CT tumour staging studies, including scans with fluorodeoxyglucose (FDG) for various primaries and prostate-specific membrane antigen (PSMA) for prostate. These studies may be complemented by scintigraphy with ^{99m}Tc-MDP (bone scan) on which skeletal metastases usually show as multiple areas of increased tracer uptake (Fig. 13.66).

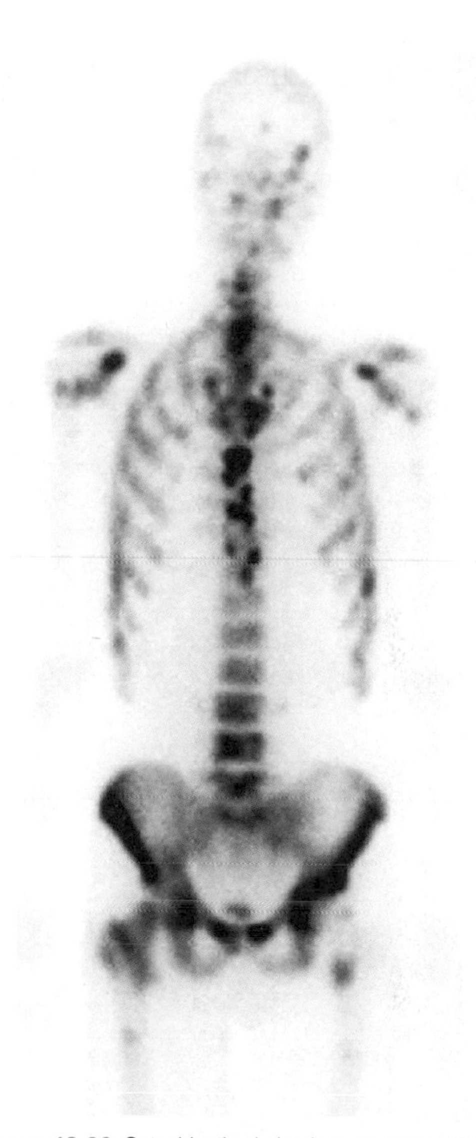

Figure 13.66 Osteoblastic skeletal metastases: HDP single photon emission CT (SPECT) (see Table 1.1). Diffuse increase in radiotracer uptake throughout the axial and proximal appendicular skeleton, with several superimposed regions of more intense uptake, particularly within the skull, sternum, ribs, spine, bony pelvis and bilateral proximal femora.

13.8.2 MULTIPLE MYELOMA

Multiple myeloma is a common malignancy of plasma cells characterized by diffuse bone marrow infiltration or multiple nodules in bone. It occurs in elderly patients and is rare below the age of 40 years. Multiple myeloma may present clinically in several non-specific ways, including bone pain, anaemia, hypercalcaemia or renal failure. Unlike most other bone malignancies, bone scintigraphy is insensitive in the detection of multiple myeloma. Therefore, radiography, whole-body MRI or low-dose CT may be used for the detection and staging of multiple myeloma. Common sites of involvement include spine, ribs, skull (Fig. 13.67), pelvis and long bones.

Radiographic appearances of multiple myeloma include:

- Generalized severe osteoporosis
- Multiple lytic, punched-out defects
- Multiple destructive and expansile lesions.

13.8.3 PAGET DISEASE

For reasons that are unclear, Paget disease of bone has become much less common. It occurs in elderly patients and is characterized by increased bone resorption followed by new bone formation. The new bone thus formed has thick trabeculae and is softer and more vascular than normal bone. Common sites include the pelvis and upper femur, spine, skull, upper tibia and proximal humerus. Paget disease is often asymptomatic and seen as an incidental finding on radiographs performed for other reasons.

Radiographic changes of Paget disease are variable depending on the phase of the disease process:

- Early active phase of bone resorption:
  - Well-defined reduction in density of the anterior skull: osteoporosis circumscripta
  - V-shaped lytic defect in the long bones extending into the shaft of the bone from the subarticular region
- Later phase of sclerosis and cortical thickening, or mixed lytic and sclerotic change:
  - Thick cortex and coarse trabeculae with enlarged bone (Fig. 13.68)
  - Bowing of long bones.

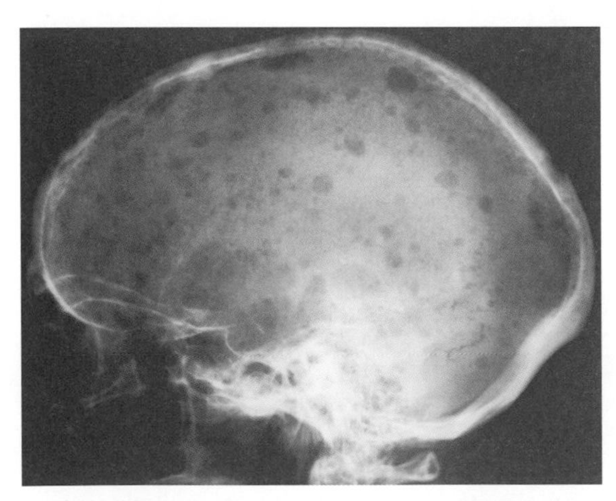

Figure 13.67 Multiple myeloma. Note the presence of multiple lucent 'punched-out' defects throughout the skull.

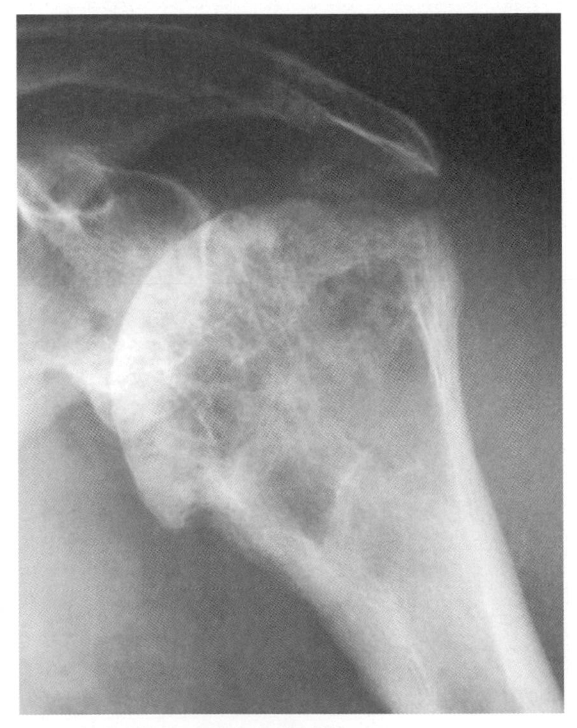

Figure 13.68 Paget disease of the humerus. Note the coarse trabecular pattern in the humeral head and thickening of the bony cortex.

13.8.4 FIBROUS DYSPLASIA

Fibrous dysplasia is a common condition characterized by single or multiple benign bone lesions composed of islands of osteoid and woven bone in a fibrous stroma. Fibrous dysplasia may occur up to the age of 70 years, although the peak age of incidence is from 10 to 30 years. It most commonly involves the lower extremity or skull and presents with local swelling, pain or pathological fracture. Bone lesions are solitary in 75% of cases.

Radiographic features of fibrous dysplasia (Fig. 13.69):

- Expansile lytic lesion
- Cortical thinning
- Areas of homogeneous grey hazy density usually described as 'ground glass': characteristic radiographic feature that differentiates fibrous dysplasia from other pathologies.

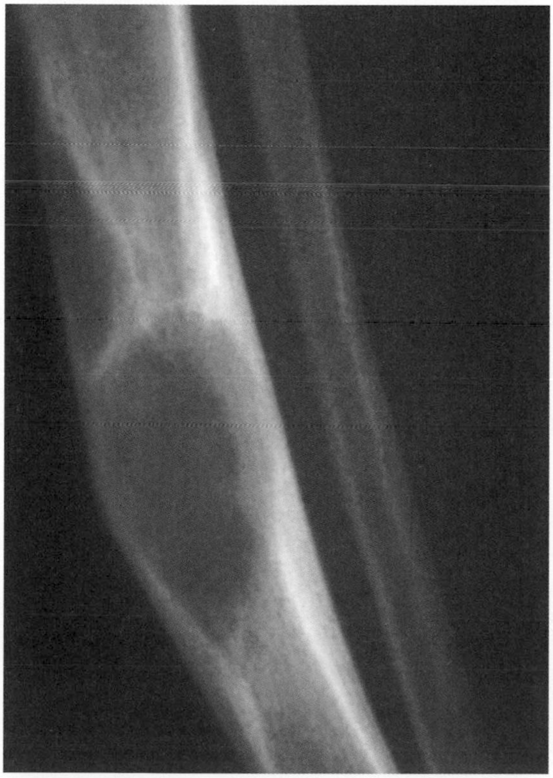

Figure 13.69 Fibrous dysplasia of the tibia. Well-defined lucent lesion with 'ground glass' density expanding the midshaft of the tibia.

CT in fibrous dysplasia shows an expansile lesion with ground glass density, based in the medullary cavity of the affected bone.

Associated syndromes:

- McCune–Albright syndrome: polyostotic fibrous dysplasia, patchy cutaneous pigmentation and sexual precocity
- Leontiasis ossea ('lion's face'): asymmetric sclerosis and thickening of the skull and facial bones.

Cherubism, a rare condition characterized clinically by symmetrical swelling of the face, is often described incorrectly as a form of fibrous dysplasia. Cherubism is an autosomal dominant disorder presenting in early childhood. Facial swelling increases to puberty, followed by spontaneous regression. Imaging with radiography and CT shows symmetrical expansion of the mandible and maxilla with multiloculated osteolytic lesions.

13.8.5 OSTEOCHONDRITIS DISSECANS

Osteochondritis dissecans is a traumatic bone lesion that affects males more than females, most commonly in the 10- to 20-year age group. The knee is most affected; other less common sites include the dome of the talus and the capitulum. In the knee the lateral aspect of the medial femoral condyle is involved in 75–80% of cases, with the lateral femoral condyle in 15–20% and the patella in 5%. Trauma is thought to be the underlying cause in most cases. Subchondral bone is first affected, then overlying articular cartilage. Subsequent revascularization and healing occur, though a necrotic bone fragment may persist. This bone fragment may become separated and displaced as a loose body in the joint.

Radiographs show a lucent defect on the cortical surface of the femoral condyle, often with a separate bone fragment (Fig. 13.70). MRI is the investigation of choice to further define the bone and cartilage abnormality. MRI helps to establish the prognosis, guide management and confirm healing.

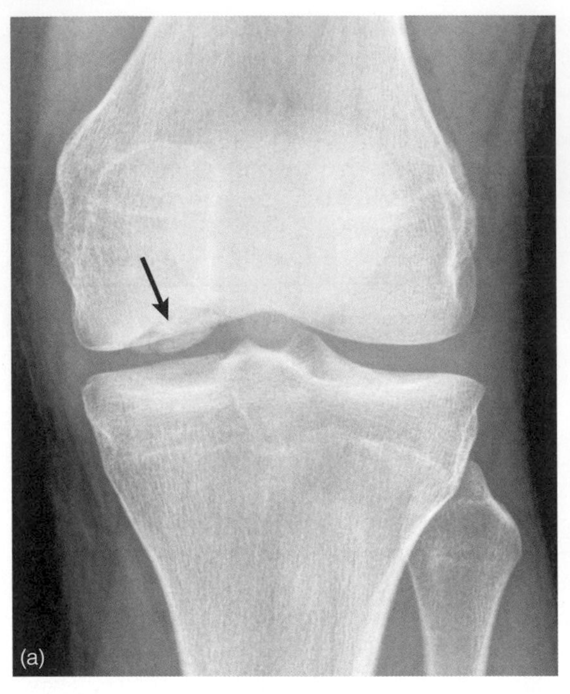

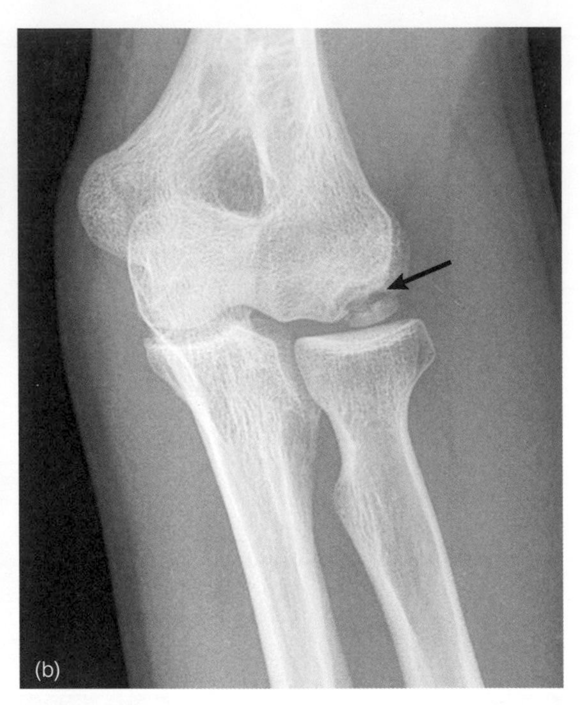

Figure 13.70 Osteochondritis dissecans: concave defect in the articular surface with a loose bone fragment. (a) Knee: medial femoral condyle (arrow). (b) Elbow: capitulum (arrow).

13.8.6 OSTEOPOROSIS

Osteoporosis may be defined as a condition in which the quantity of bone per unit volume or bone mineral density (BMD) is decreased. Osteoporosis is an enormous public health issue, increasing in incidence with the gradual ageing of the population. It leads to fragility of bone with an increased incidence of fracture, particularly crush fractures of the vertebral bodies and hip and wrist fractures. Treatment of osteoporosis can help to prevent further bone loss and reduce the incidence of fragility fractures. The three key factors in the decision to treat osteoporosis are:

1. the age of the patient
2. the presence of a previous fragility fracture
3. the BMD.

Accurate measurement of the BMD is the key to the diagnosis of osteoporosis and the decision to institute treatment. Dual X-ray absorptiometry (DEXA) is widely accepted as a highly accurate, low radiation dose technique for measuring BMD. DEXA uses an X-ray source, which produces X-rays of two different energies. The lower of these energies is absorbed almost exclusively by soft tissue. The higher energy is absorbed by bone and soft tissue. Calculation of the two absorption patterns gives an attenuation profile of the bone component from which the BMD may be estimated. Measurements are usually taken from the lumbar spine (L2–L4) and the femoral neck. The DEXA report gives an absolute measurement of BMD expressed as grams per centimetre squared (g/cm^2). This value is compared with a normal young adult population to give a 'T score', which is expressed as the number of standard deviations from the mean (Fig. 13.71).

Osteoporosis is defined as a BMD of 2.5 standard deviations below the young normal adult mean, i.e. a T score of equal to or less than –2.5. A T score of –1 to –2.5 is defined as osteopenia, with normal being a T score of more than –1.

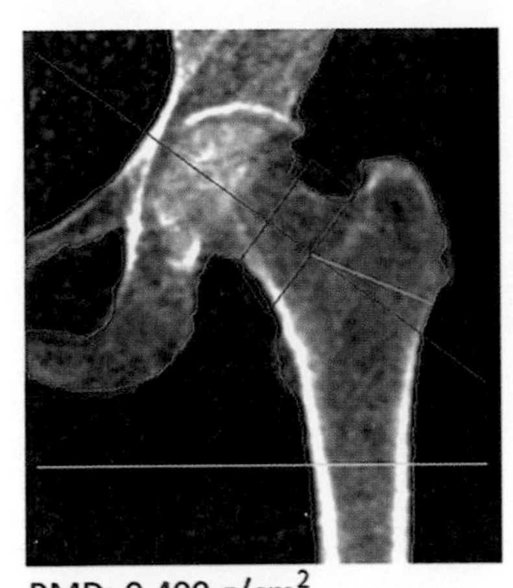

Figure 13.71 Osteoporosis. Bone mineral density (BMD) of the left femoral neck in an 82-year-old woman shows a bone density of 0.499 g/cm^2, with a T score of –3.6.

Treatment of osteoporosis includes bisphosphonates, hormone replacement therapy and weight-bearing exercise. There is good evidence for the following treatment guidelines based on the BMD as calculated with DEXA:

- T score greater than –1: no treatment
- T score –1 to –2.5: treatment if there is a previous fragility fracture
- T score less than –2.5: treatment recommended whether there is a previous fracture or not.

SUMMARY

Clinical presentation	Investigation of choice	Comment
Trauma: suspected fracture or dislocation	Radiography	• CT in selected cases for further definition of anatomy • MRI in selected cases for detection of subtle fractures not shown on radiographs, e.g. scaphoid
Arthropathy/painful joint(s)	Radiography	MRI in selected cases to detect synovial or bony inflammation
Primary bone tumour	Radiography	Bone scintigraphy, CT and MRI for further characterization and staging
Skeletal metastases	Bone scintigraphy	
Multiple myeloma	Radiography (skeletal survey)	Increasing role for whole-body MRI
Paget disease	Radiography	
Fibrous dysplasia	Radiography	CT for complex areas, e.g. craniofacial
Osteochondritis dissecans	• Radiography • MRI	
Osteoporosis	DEXA	

Abbreviation: DEXA, dual X-ray absorptiometry.

Breast imaging

14.1 BREAST CANCER

Breast cancer is the commonest malignancy in women. The overall lifetime risk of development of breast cancer in women is one in eight by age 85 years. The factors associated with a higher risk of breast cancer include:

- First-degree relatives diagnosed with breast or ovarian cancer
- Genetic predisposition in 5–10% of cases, most commonly mutation of *BRCA1*/*BRCA2*
- Cancer predisposition syndromes, e.g. Cowden syndrome, Li–Fraumeni syndrome
- Large-dose radiation exposure under the age of 30, most commonly radiotherapy of the chest for Hodgkin lymphoma
- Hormonal: early menarche, nulliparity, late menopause.

Most breast cancers arise from tissues in the terminal ductal/lobular units of the breast. The term *'in situ'* refers to tumours confined within the lumen of lobules or ducts. 'Invasive' or 'infiltrating' refers to tumours that have breached the basement membrane. Multiple factors are relevant in the classification, prognosis and treatment of breast cancer:

- Histological type
- Histological grades 1–3: low, intermediate and high
- Tumour–node–metastasis (TNM) stage
- Biomarkers:
  - Receptor status
    - Oestrogen receptor
    - Progesterone receptor
    - Human epidermal growth factor receptor 2 (HER2) status
  - E-cadherin expression.

Almost all breast cancers are adenocarcinomas, most commonly:

- Ductal:
  - Ductal carcinoma *in situ* (DCIS): 20–25% of breast cancers
  - Invasive ductal carcinoma of no specific type: 40–75% of breast cancers
- Lobular: invasive lobular carcinoma: 5–15% of breast cancers.

Less common types of breast cancer may be encountered, such as adenoid cystic and apocrine carcinoma, lymphoma and sarcoma, as well as rare subtypes of invasive ductal carcinoma.

Breast cancer may present clinically as a palpable breast mass or less commonly with nipple discharge, change in breast shape, palpable axillary lymph nodes or symptoms related to metastatic disease such as bone pain. Increasingly, breast cancer is detected in asymptomatic women through breast screening programmes. The main goal of breast imaging, whether it is in women with specific symptoms or in screening of asymptomatic women, is early diagnosis of breast cancer. Diagnosis at an earlier stage may result in less radical therapy with a reduced risk of metastatic disease and local recurrence.

Treatment of breast cancer consists of one, or a combination, of the following:

- Surgery for optimal tumour control in the breast and axillary lymph nodes
- Postoperative radiotherapy to reduce the risk of local recurrence
- Systemic chemotherapy and hormonal therapy to treat undetectable micrometastases.

The current trend towards less radical surgery requires accurate preoperative imaging to provide the following information:

- Precise site of the tumour in the breast, including the relationship to the nipple and chest wall
- Presence of adjacent DCIS
- Presence of multifocal or bilateral disease.

14.2 BREAST IMAGING TECHNIQUES

14.2.1 MAMMOGRAPHY AND DIGITAL BREAST TOMOSYNTHESIS

Mammography is a radiographic examination of the breast. Digital mammography (DM) uses digital radiographic systems, as described in Chapter 1. Digital breast tomosynthesis (DBT) is an extension of DM, in which multiple projection exposures are obtained from a mammographic X-ray source that moves over a limited arc. By obtaining a series of tomographic images of the breast, DBT increases the sensitivity for detection of masses and microcalcifications by removing the overlying parenchymal density. As it is now in widespread use, for the remainder of this chapter the term 'mammography' is used to mean DM and DBT. Sensitivity for the presence of an abnormality may be further enhanced with the use of computer-aided detection (CAD), in which a computer 'flags' potential abnormalities, which are then assessed by a radiologist.

Mammography is performed in two circumstances: diagnostic and screening. Diagnostic mammography is the first investigation of choice for a breast lump in women over 35 years of age. Diagnostic mammography may also be performed for other reasons, such as nipple discharge or to search for a primary breast tumour when metastases are found elsewhere. Screening mammography is performed to identify early cancers in asymptomatic women (see section 14.6).

The standard mammography examination consists of images obtained with two projections: craniocaudal (CC) and mediolateral oblique (MLO) (Fig. 14.1). A range of further views, including spot

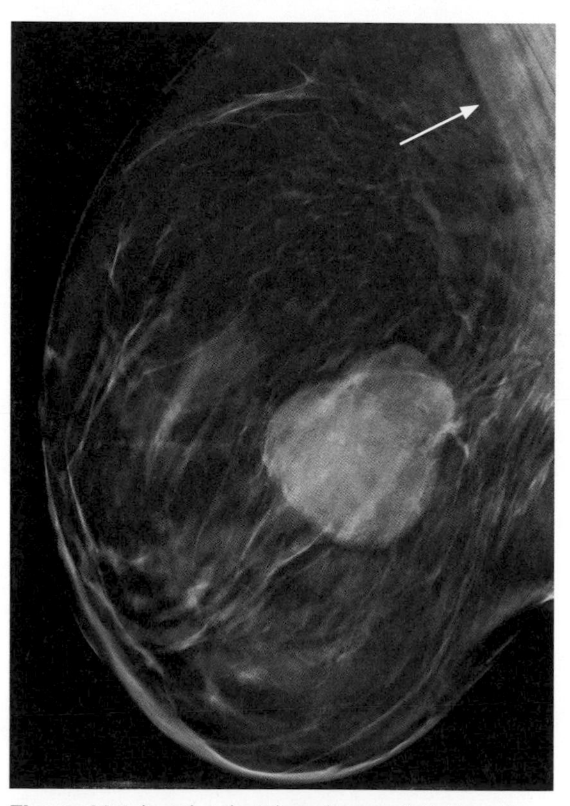

Figure 14.1 Invasive ductal carcinoma: digital breast tomosynthesis (DBT). Mediolateral oblique (MLO) projection shows a large well-circumscribed mass. The breast in this case is almost entirely fatty, which makes the mass easy to see. The oblique opacity at the upper right corner of the image is the pectoralis muscle (arrow).

compression, magnification and angulated views, may be used to delineate an abnormality seen on the two standard views. Abnormalities seen on mammography include soft-tissue masses, asymmetric densities, calcifications and secondary signs such as distortion of breast architecture and skin thickening.

A key mammographic finding in breast cancer is a stellate mass, i.e. a soft-tissue density with irregular margins visible on both mammographic projections. Benign breast lesions, including cyst, fibroadenoma, lipid cyst and galactocele, tend to produce well-defined masses on mammography. Certain types of breast cancer, such as colloid and medullary cancers, may produce well-defined masses and therefore mimic benign pathology.

Calcification is a primary mammographic sign of early cancer, particularly DCIS. Most calcifications are small and therefore the term microcalcification is used. Malignant calcifications tend to occur in clusters, and are usually of variable size and density, often with a branching configuration. Causes of benign microcalcification include arterial calcification, calcification in cysts and calcification of benign masses such as fibroadenoma (Fig. 14.2).

Mammography may be used to guide various procedures, including:

- Biopsy of a mammographically visible mass
- Biopsy of microcalcification
- Hookwire localization of a non-palpable abnormality prior to surgical biopsy and removal (Fig. 14.3).

The principal disadvantage of mammography is its inherent false-negative rate. The overall sensitivity of mammography for detection of breast cancer is 85%; however, this varies with background breast stromal density. In breasts that are composed primarily of fatty tissue, the sensitivity of mammography may approach 95%. In younger patients in whom dense breast tissue may obscure a focal abnormality, the sensitivity of mammography is much lower. For this reason, ultrasound (US) is generally preferred in women younger than 35 years. Another disadvantage is relatively poor specificity due to the considerable overlap in appearances between malignant and benign pathologies. Fine-needle aspiration (FNA), core biopsy or surgical removal are commonly required for assessment of mammographic abnormalities. Breast magnetic resonance imaging

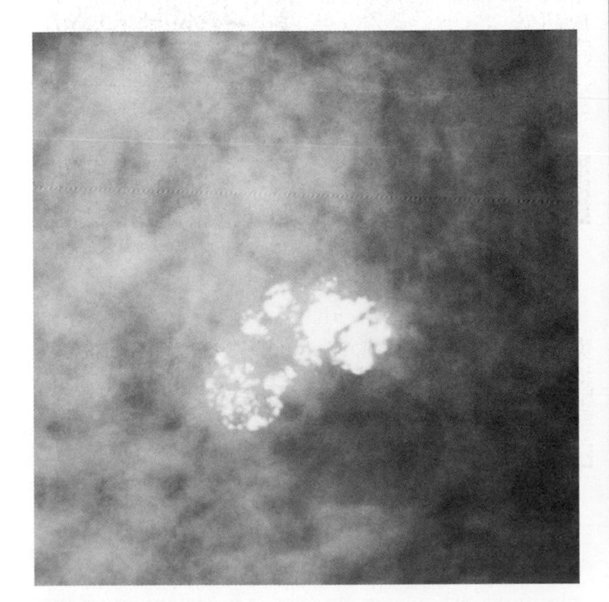

Figure 14.2 Fibroadenoma: mammogram. Small mass containing popcorn-like calcifications.

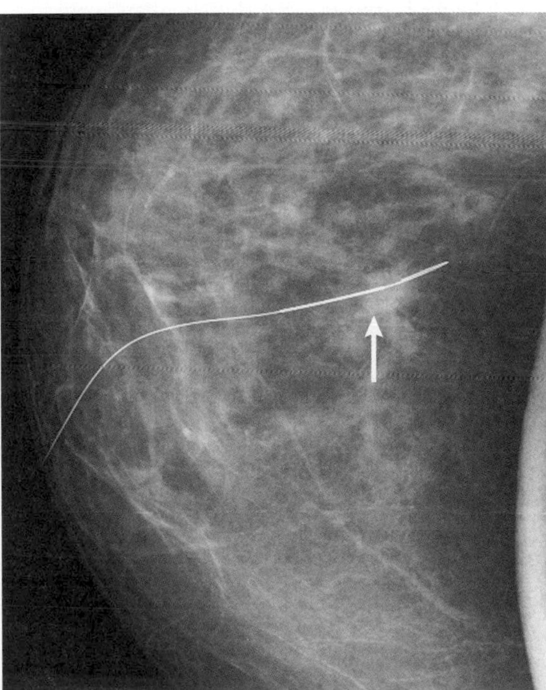

Figure 14.3 Hookwire localization: mammogram. Craniocaudal (CC) view showing a fine hookwire passing through a small mass (arrow). Histology confirmed invasive ductal carcinoma.

(MRI) may be helpful in some instances and is in widespread use for certain indications.

14.2.2 ULTRASOUND

US is the first investigation of choice for a palpable breast lump in a woman under 35 years of age and in women who are pregnant or lactating. US also complements mammography, particularly for differentiating cysts from solid masses and for the assessment of mammographically dense breasts in which small masses or cysts may be obscured by overlying breast tissue (Fig. 14.4). As well as being used to diagnose cysts, breast US is useful for providing further definition of solid masses, specifically for differentiating benign and malignant lesions. Depending on the experience and expertise of the operator, a limitation of US is the lack of sensitivity and specificity for the detection and characterization of microcalcifications.

US may be used to guide various procedures, including:

- Cyst aspiration
- Lesion diagnosis: FNA (Fig. 14.5) and core biopsy
- Preoperative localization: hookwire and radioactive seed (radio-guided occult lesion localization using iodine-125 seeds [ROLLIS])

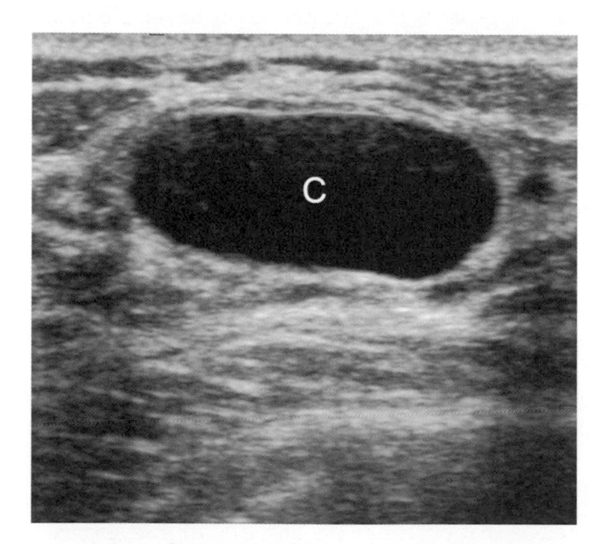

Figure 14.4 Simple cyst of the breast: US. Note the US features of a simple cyst (C): anechoic contents, smooth wall, no soft-tissue components and posterior acoustic enhancement.

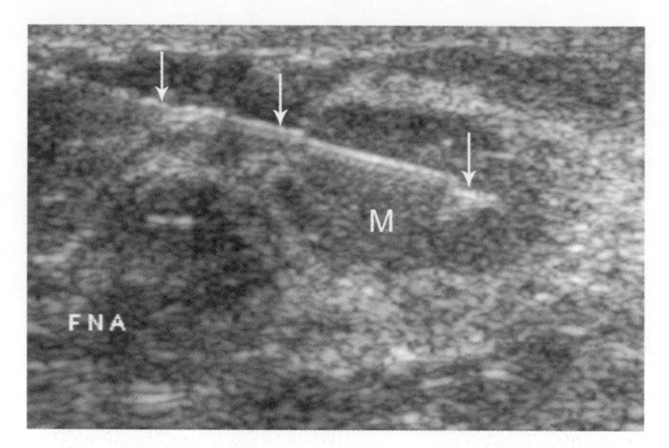

Figure 14.5 Fine-needle aspiration (FNA) of a breast mass under US guidance. The needle is seen as a hyperechoic line (arrows) passing into a hypoechoic mass (M). Cytology confirmed a fibroadenoma.

- Drainage of fluid collections, such as postoperative seroma or abscess complicating mastitis.

14.2.3 MAGNETIC RESONANCE IMAGING

MRI using specifically designed breast coils and intravenous gadolinium is used for the detection and staging of breast cancer. Sequences performed include:

- Fat-saturated T2-weighted or short TI (inversion time) inversion recovery (STIR)
- Diffusion-weighted imaging (DWI)
- T1-weighted
- T1-weighted dynamic contrast enhanced (DCE) imaging.

MRI detection of breast cancer relies on malignant neovascularity, with 'leaky' capillaries allowing intense rapid enhancement with gadolinium, followed by rapid reduced enhancement ('washout') or, less commonly, prolonged enhancement. Contrast enhancement kinetics may be represented by time of enhancement curves. MRI has high sensitivity for all forms of breast cancer, including invasive cancer and DCIS (Fig. 14.6).

MRI is usually used as an adjunct to mammography and US; however, its roles in breast imaging continue to evolve. Current roles for breast MRI include:

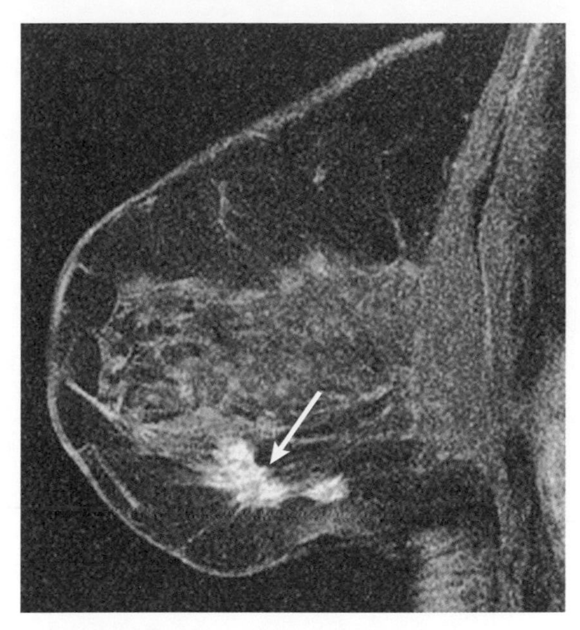

Figure 14.6 Invasive ductal carcinoma: breast MRI. Sagittal T1-weighted, fat-saturated, contrast-enhanced MRI. Note in the inferior breast an intensely enhancing complex mass with a spiculated margin (arrow).

- Problem solving for indeterminate findings on mammography or US
- Assessment of lobular carcinoma *in situ* due to a high incidence of multicentric and bilateral disease
- Assessment for tumour recurrence following lumpectomy
- Screening in young high-risk women (e.g. *BRAC1*/*BRAC2* mutations)
- Evaluation of nipple discharge
- Assessment of complications related to breast implants, e.g. breast implant-associated anaplastic large cell lymphoma (BIA-ALCL).

14.2.4 LYMPHOSCINTIGRAPHY (SENTINEL NODE DETECTION)

The prognosis of breast cancer is greatly affected by the axillary lymph node status at the time of diagnosis. Axillary lymph node dissection (ALND) is definitive in classifying axillary node status; however, it is associated with complications, including lymphoedema, pain and reduced shoulder movement. Sentinel lymph node biopsy (SLNB) is much less traumatic than ALND. The sentinel lymph node is the first axillary lymph node on the lymphatic drainage pathway from the tumour; therefore, it is the first node to receive tumour cells if lymphatic metastatic spread has occurred. If the sentinel axillary lymph node can be identified and shown to be tumour free, then spread to any other axillary nodes is excluded with a high degree of accuracy.

For lymphoscintigraphy, ^{99m}Tc-labelled colloid particles are injected prior to surgery. Injection may be perilesional, in the skin over the lesion, at the areola or directly into the lesion. The surgeon localizes the sentinel node in theatre with a hand-held gamma-detecting probe. The node is removed and examined by a pathologist:

- Sentinel node positive = 40% chance of spread to other axillary nodes and ALND is usually performed
- Sentinel node negative = 98% chance of no further lymph node spread and ALND is not required.

14.2.5 BREAST BIOPSY

Cyst aspiration under US control may be done to drain large cysts that are painful or to sample fluid from atypical cystic lesions. Breast biopsy is usually performed under imaging guidance, either mammography or US. For most masses, US is the quickest and most accurate method. US cannot be used to accurately visualize microcalcification; therefore, for biopsy of microcalcification mammographic guidance is required. Several biopsy methods are used, including FNA, core biopsy, vacuum-assisted core biopsy and open surgical biopsy requiring preoperative localization. FNA is usually performed with US guidance (Fig. 14.5), is minimally invasive using 21- to 25-gauge needles and requires an experienced cytopathologist for interpretation.

Core biopsy may be performed under US or mammographic guidance with 14- to 18-gauge cutting needles that obtain a core of tissue for histological diagnosis. A variation of core biopsy is vacuum-assisted core biopsy (Mammotome®), which consists of an 11-gauge probe that is positioned under mammographic control. A vacuum pulls a small sample of breast tissue into the probe; this is then cut off and transported back through the probe into a specimen chamber. This technique is particularly useful for microcalcifications.

For open surgical biopsy non-palpable masses may be localized under US or mammographic control prior to surgery. Suspicious microcalcifications may be localized under mammographic control. A needle containing a hook-shaped wire is positioned in or near the breast lesion. Once correct positioning is attained, the needle is withdrawn, leaving the wire in place. US or mammography of the excised specimen is performed to ensure that the mass or calcification has been removed.

14.3 INVESTIGATION OF A BREAST LUMP

Palpable breast masses may be discovered by self-examination or clinical examination. Prominent glandular tissue may commonly mimic a breast mass in younger women. Benign lesions tend to be mobile with well-defined smooth margins. Malignant masses tend to be firm to palpation with irregular margins and possible tethering to skin or deep structures.

14.3.1 MAMMOGRAPHY

Mammography is the first investigation of choice for a breast lump in women over 35 years of age.

Mammographic features of a benign mass, e.g. cyst or fibroadenoma:

- Tend to compress but not invade adjacent tissue
- Round or oval
- Well circumscribed, often with a surrounding dark halo due to compressed fat
- Various patterns of calcification may occur in benign masses:
    - Large cyst: thin peripheral rim of wall calcification
    - Fibroadenoma: dense, coarse, 'popcorn' calcification (Fig. 14.2)
    - Small cysts, adenosis and hyperplasia: multiple, tiny, pinpoint calcifications; milk of calcium in tiny cysts with layering ('fluid levels') on the MLO images ('tea cupping').

Mammographic features of a malignant mass:

- Tend to invade adjacent tissue and often cause an irregular desmoplastic or fibrotic reaction
- Carcinomas therefore tend to have irregular or indistinct margins, often described as spiculated or stellate (Fig. 14.7)
- Distortion of surrounding breast tissue (architectural distortion)
- Secondary signs such as skin thickening and nipple retraction.

Malignant microcalcification is commonly seen in association with a mass, or without a mass in the case of DCIS (Fig. 14.8). Malignant microcalcification has the following features:

- Irregular
- Variable shape and size (pleomorphism)

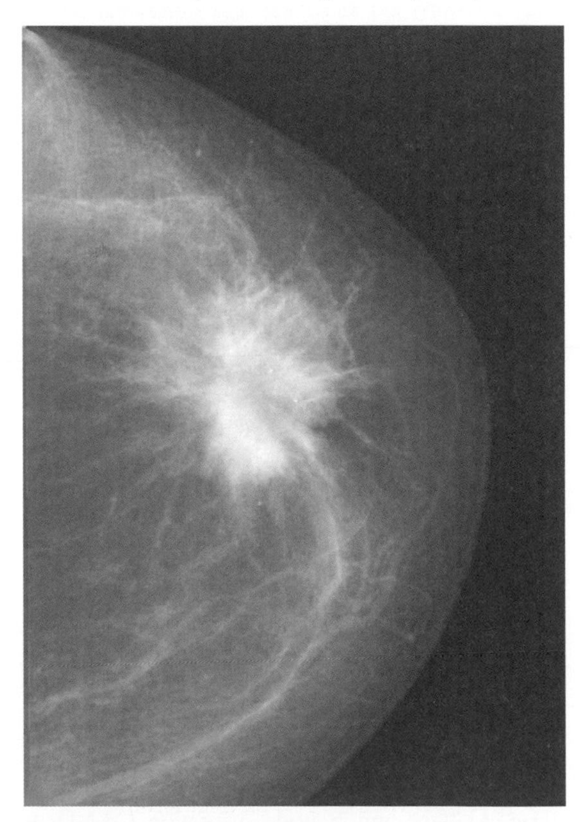

Figure 14.7 Invasive ductal carcinoma: mammogram. Craniocaudal (CC) view shows a large spiculated breast mass.

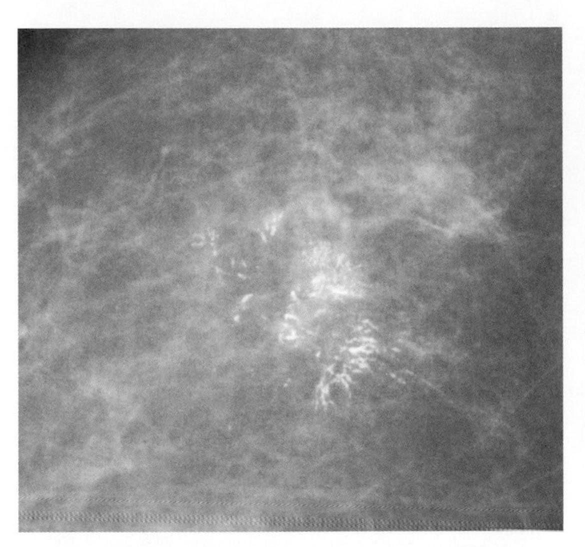

Figure 14.8 Ductal carcinoma *in situ*: mammogram. Note the typical features of malignant microcalcification: localized cluster of calcifications with an irregular branching pattern.

- Branching, ductal pattern known as 'casting'
- Grouped in clusters
- Variable density.

14.3.2 ULTRASOUND

US is the investigation of choice for the assessment of breast lumps in younger women. US may also be used for further characterization of a mass or localized density seen on mammography in older women.

US features of a simple cyst:

- Round with thin walls
- Anechoic contents
- Posterior acoustic enhancement.

Complicated cysts on US may have low-level internal echoes and slightly irregular walls due to infection, haemorrhage or cellular and proteinaceous debris.

US features of a benign mass, most commonly fibroadenoma (Fig. 14.9):

- Well-defined hypoechoic mass
- Ovoid in shape with a long axis parallel to the skin.

US features of a carcinoma (Fig. 14.10):

- Focal mass with an irregular infiltrative margin and heterogeneous internal echoes

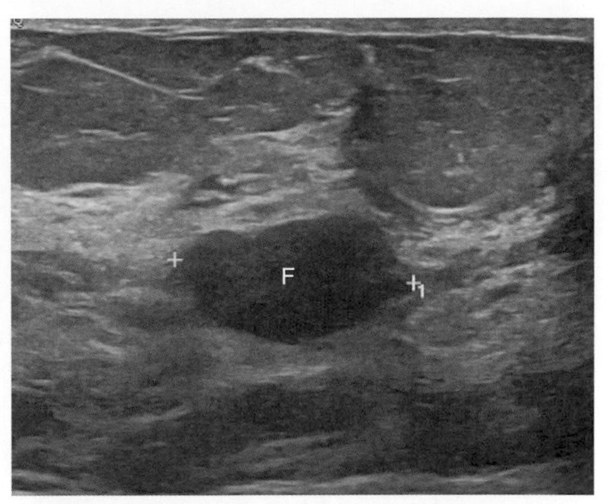

Figure 14.9 Fibroadenoma: US. Lobulated hypoechoic lesion with a homogeneous texture, smooth well-defined margins and the long axis parallel to the skin (F).

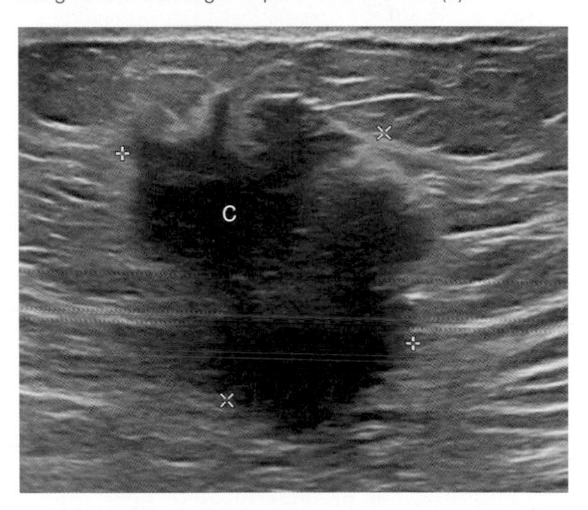

Figure 14.10 Invasive ductal carcinoma: US. Large, irregular, hypoechoic non-shadowing breast mass with the long axis perpendicular to the skin (C).

- Long axis perpendicular to the skin
- Usually firm and non-compressible with a posterior acoustic shadow
- Internal vascularity may be seen in high-grade tumours.

14.3.3 MAGNETIC RESONANCE IMAGING

MRI is most used as a problem-solving tool when mammography and/or US findings are equivocal.

It is also used for screening in young high-risk women and is indicated when histology indicates lobular carcinoma due to high rates of multicentric and bilateral tumour.

MRI features of a malignant lesion include:

- Mass enhancement, i.e. an enhancing space-occupying lesion with a definable margin:
  - Irregular, spiculated margin
  - Rim enhancement with centripetal filling over time
- Non-mass-like enhancement, i.e. diffuse or grouped multifocal enhancement without a defined margin
  - Clumped or heterogeneous enhancement pattern
- Enhancement kinetics showing a washout pattern
  - Early rapid enhancement followed by reduced enhancement with time.

14.3.4 BREAST IMAGING REPORTING AND DATA SYSTEM

The Breast Imaging Reporting and Data System (BI-RADS) was the first of the RADS reporting systems to be developed and has been subsequently revised multiple times by the American College of Radiology.

BI-RADS provides a standardized reporting terminology that can be applied to mammography, US and MRI. Based on findings, breast imaging studies are assigned one of seven assessment categories:

- BI-RADS 0: incomplete: additional imaging or previous images needed
- BI-RADS 1: negative
- BI-RADS 2: benign
- BI-RADS 3: probably benign, less than 2% probability of malignancy
- BI-RADS 4: suspicious, 2–94% probability of malignancy
- BI-RADS 5: highly suggestive, greater than 95% probability of malignancy
- BI-RADS 6: known biopsy-proven malignancy.

These categories provide an evidence-based risk assessment that assists with clinical guidance. For each imaging modality, BI-RADS provides an extensive lexicon to describe the appearance of background breast parenchyma, specific features of a mass/focal lesion, associated features and location. Many of the features used in the BI-RADS lexicon are described above and further details can be found on the companion website.

14.4 STAGING OF BREAST CANCER

Lymph node status at the time of diagnosis is the most powerful predictor of long-term survival of breast cancer. Other less predictive factors include tumour size, histological grade and hormone and HER2/neu receptor status. The techniques for assessing lymph node status include ALND and SLNB (see section 14.2.4). SLNB carries less morbidity than ALND and is used widely in the assessment of lymph node status.

Although metastatic disease is relatively common in breast cancer, this usually consists of undetectable micrometastases at the time of initial diagnosis. The incidence of macroscopically visible metastases at the time of initial diagnosis is low. Despite this, full TNM staging at the time of diagnosis is commonly performed with various protocols, including computed tomography (CT) of the neck, chest, abdomen and pelvis, a radionuclide bone scan and fluorodeoxyglucose (FDG)-positron emission tomography (PET)-CT. Factors relevant in the staging of breast cancer include:

- T: tumour size, extension to the chest wall or skin
- N: regional lymph node groups are axillary, internal mammary and supraclavicular
- M: common sites for metastases from breast cancer include lung, bone, distant lymph nodes (e.g. mediastinum), liver, pleura, adrenal gland, brain and peritoneum.

Specific imaging investigations may be indicated by symptoms, e.g. MRI of the brain for neurological symptoms. Further details of TNM staging of breast cancer may be found on the companion website.

14.5 INVESTIGATION OF NIPPLE DISCHARGE

Causes of nipple discharge include hormonal factors, infection, benign papilloma of a mammary duct, mammary duct ectasia and malignancy. Radiological investigation is particularly indicated for nipple discharge when various clinical factors suggest a greater likelihood of malignancy:

- Age over 60 years
- Discharge is unilateral, from a single duct
- Serous or bloodstained discharge
- Palpable mass.

When imaging is indicated, mammography and US should be performed to exclude any obvious mass or suspicious microcalcification. High-resolution targeted US of the areolar region may also be used to diagnose papilloma or malignancy with visualization of a soft-tissue mass associated with a prominent duct. If mammography and US are negative, MRI is the next investigation of choice.

Galactography (or ductography) is a procedure whereby a mammary duct orifice is gently cannulated and a small amount of contrast material injected, followed by radiographic images of the area of interest. It may be indicated where discharge is from a single duct and other imaging is negative. Findings on galactography include:

- Intraduct papilloma: smooth or irregular filling defect; these may be multiple
- Invasive carcinoma: irregular duct narrowing with distal dilatation.

Galactography is not indicated when discharge is from multiple ducts. In most centres, US, mammography and particularly MRI have superseded galactography.

14.6 BREAST SCREENING IN ASYMPTOMATIC WOMEN

Screening mammography refers to mammographic examination of asymptomatic women to diagnose early-stage breast cancers. Clinical trials have shown that screening mammography is of benefit in reducing mortality from breast cancer, particularly in women aged 50–74 years. In Australia, women in this age group are actively invited to have a free mammogram every 2 years. Women aged 40–49 years and those over 74 may choose to be screened but are not actively recruited. Screening protocols vary from country to country.

Because of multiple factors, including reduced sensitivity of mammography in radiographically dense breasts, screening is generally less effective in younger women and not recommended below the age of 40 years. Exceptions to this include women with significant risk factors, e.g. *BRCA1/BRCA2* gene mutations or a history of chest radiotherapy before the age of 30 years. In these younger women, MRI has greater sensitivity than mammography for breast cancer detection. Annual MRI may be used for screening in high-risk asymptomatic women aged 30–49 years, after which annual mammography is recommended. For women at intermediate risk, i.e. a history of breast or ovarian cancer in a first-degree relative, annual mammography combined with clinical breast examination and US may be recommended.

Screening mammography in average-risk women is performed every 2 years. A dedicated team is essential to the screening process and includes a radiographer, radiologist, surgeon, pathologist and counselling nurse. Mammography is the only validated screening test for breast cancer. Strict quality control over equipment, film processing and training of personnel is essential to provide optimum images and maximize diagnostic efficiency. An abnormality on initial screening leads to recall of the patient and a second stage of investigation comprising any or all of the following:

- US
- Further mammographic views, including magnification
- Clinical assessment
- FNA or core biopsy.

If, after this second stage, a lesion is found to be malignant the patient is referred for appropriate management. About 10% of recalled women will be found to have a breast cancer. The overall rate of cancer diagnosis in screening programmes is about 0.5%.

15 Obstetrics and gynaecology

Ultrasound (US) is the cornerstone of imaging in obstetrics and gynaecology. US is the investigation of choice at all stages of pregnancy. It is used to confirm the viability and dating of early pregnancy and to assess placental position and fetal morphology in later pregnancy. Second- and third-trimester complications such as placental abruption or suspected intrauterine growth retardation (IUGR) are also assessed with US. US is also usually the investigation of choice for most gynaecological disorders, including infertility, pelvic mass, dysmenorrhoea and postmenopausal bleeding.

In obstetrics and gynaecology, transabdominal (TAUS) and/or transvaginal (TVUS) US may be performed. TAUS has a wider field of view and requires a full bladder to visualize the pelvic organs. TVUS utilizes a transvaginal probe and provides better anatomical detail of the uterus and ovaries. TVUS has a smaller field of view and is not appropriate for very young or elderly patients. Apart from these constraints, TVUS is more accurate than TAUS in first-trimester pregnancy and in most gynaecological conditions. Additionally, TVUS can assess the tenderness of pelvic structures analogous to 'Murphy's point probe tenderness' in cholecystitis. TVUS may be used to guide interventional procedures, such as biopsy, cyst aspiration, abscess drainage and ovarian harvest.

Magnetic resonance imaging (MRI) may be used in certain contexts in obstetrics. Fetal MRI may be useful in second- and third-trimester pregnancy for defining complex fetal anomalies. Because of concerns with radiation dose, MRI may also be used as an alternative to computed tomography (CT) in the assessment of maternal abdominal pain, such as investigating acute appendicitis. MRI is used commonly in gynaecology for diverse indications, including suspected endometriosis, the characterization of complex ovarian cystic and solid lesions, the diagnosis and characterization of uterine pathology such as adenomyosis and fibroids and staging of gynaecological malignancies.

Interventional procedures used in gynaecology include recanalization of Fallopian tubes and embolization of uterine fibroids.

15.1 ULTRASOUND IN OBSTETRICS

In industrialized societies, virtually all women will have at least one US scan during pregnancy. US in pregnancy has multiple roles:

- First-trimester US
  - Confirmation of gestation, number and viability

- Accurate assessment of dates
- Diagnosis of ectopic pregnancy
- Nuchal thickness US at 11–14 weeks' gestation as part of non-invasive prenatal testing (NIPT)
- Fetal morphology scan at 19–21 weeks' gestation
- Third-trimester US for a variety of indications, e.g. placenta praevia, suspected IUGR, follow-up of fetal anomalies.

15.1.1 FIRST-TRIMESTER BLEEDING

First-trimester bleeding occurs in around 25% of pregnancies. In most cases it is a solitary event not accompanied by pain and is of no consequence. Initial assessment consists of physical examination, including speculum examination to visualize the cervix. First-trimester bleeding accompanied by severe pain due to uterine contractions and a dilated cervix usually indicates a failed pregnancy. TVUS may be helpful in threatened miscarriage, when bleeding and pain are mild and the cervix is closed. The differential diagnosis includes a normal pregnancy, missed miscarriage, blighted ovum, ectopic pregnancy and trophoblastic disease. The most important factors to establish on US are the presence and appearance of an intrauterine gestational sac.

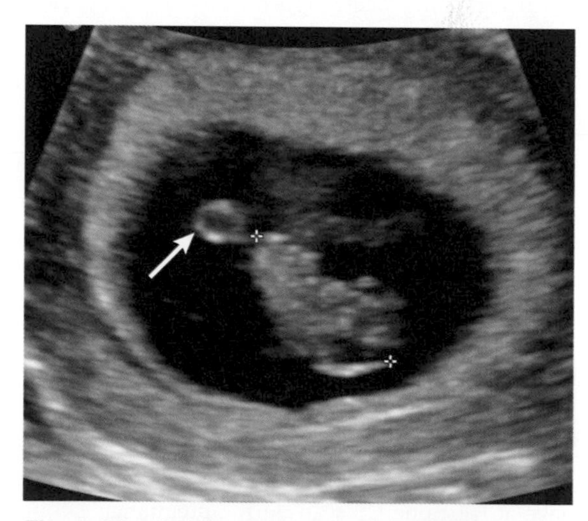

Figure 15.1 Early pregnancy: US. A gestational sac is seen as a round fluid-filled structure in the uterus. It contains a yolk sac (arrow) and a single fetus. Crown–rump length (CRL) measurement (+) provides an accurate estimation of the stage of gestation; in this case 22 mm, indicating 8 weeks and 5 days.

Knowledge of the human chorionic gonadotropin (β-hCG) level may help to clarify the US findings. A gestational sac should become visible on TVUS at a β-hCG level of 1000 mIU/mL (Second International Standard). A yolk sac should become visible when the average diameter of the gestational sac is 8 mm; an embryo should be visible at 16 mm.

Measurement of the length of the embryo (fetal pole) gives the crown–rump length (CRL) (Fig. 15.1). The CRL correlates accurately with gestational age, especially if done at 6–10 weeks. A fetal heartbeat should be visible on TVUS when the CRL is 7 mm.

Signs of a failed pregnancy on TVUS include:

- Gestational sac greater than 25 mm with no fetal pole identified
- Fetal pole greater than 7 mm with no fetal heartbeat identified.

15.1.2 SUSPECTED ECTOPIC PREGNANCY

Clinical diagnosis of ectopic pregnancy is often difficult, with a history of a missed period present in only two-thirds of cases. The classic clinical triad of ectopic pregnancy consists of pain, vaginal bleeding and a palpable adnexal mass. Like most classic triads, all three features occur in a minority of cases. Factors associated with an increased risk of ectopic pregnancy include increasing maternal age and parity, previous ectopic pregnancy and previous Fallopian tube surgery or infection.

Patients with suspected ectopic pregnancy who are haemodynamically unstable should proceed to laparoscopy. For all other patients with suspected ectopic pregnancy, TVUS correlated with serum β-hCG levels is the investigation of choice.

The signs of ectopic pregnancy on TVUS include:

- Empty uterus
- Free fluid in the pelvis
- Direct visualization of the ectopic gestation as a complex adnexal mass (Fig. 15.2)
- On rare occasions, fetal cardiac activity may be seen within the adnexal mass.

Note, however, that an adnexal mass may not be visible and therefore a normal pelvic US examination does not exclude ectopic pregnancy. If a gestational

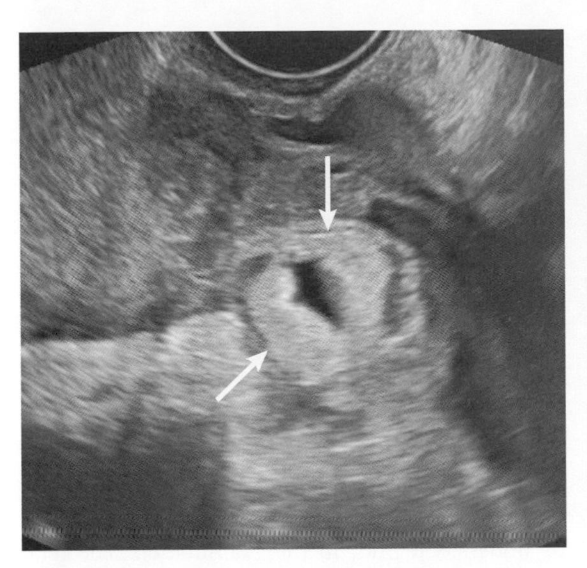

Figure 15.2 Ectopic pregnancy: US. Transvaginal US (TVUS) shows an echogenic adnexal mass (arrows) in a patient with a positive human chorionic gonadotropin (β-hCG) and an empty uterus.

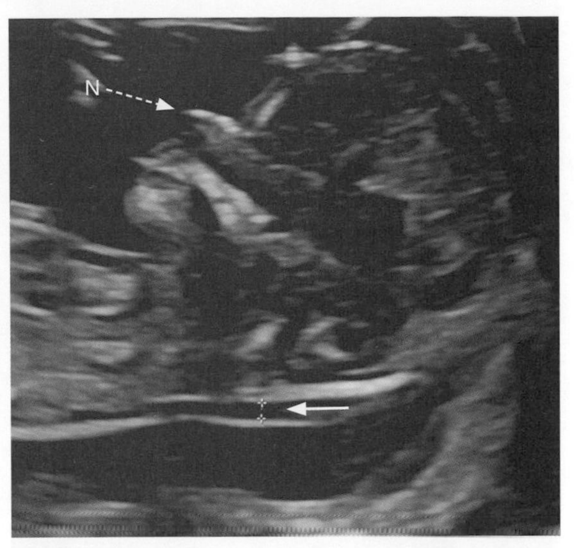

Figure 15.3 Nuchal fold thickness measurement: US. The nuchal fold is seen as a thin hypoechoic layer at the back of the fetal neck (arrow). Also note the presence of the nasal bone (N, dashed arrow), which indicates a reduced risk of aneuploidy.

sac cannot be identified in the uterus with TVUS despite a β-hCG level of 1000 mIU/mL or more, ectopic pregnancy should be suspected.

15.1.3 NUCHAL THICKNESS SCAN AND COMBINED FIRST-TRIMESTER SCREENING

Towards the end of the first trimester, a thin hypoechoic fluid layer can be observed in the posterior neck of the fetus, known as the nuchal translucency (Fig. 15.3). Thickening of the nuchal translucency may be associated with Down syndrome, other types of fetal aneuploidy and an increased risk of fetal demise. Nuchal thickness measurement is performed between 11 weeks 3 days and 13 weeks 6 days of gestation (CRL 45–84 mm) by trained operators using standardized techniques. Combined first-trimester screening refers to a combination of nuchal thickness measurement and maternal hormone levels, specifically β-hCG and pregnancy-associated plasma protein-A (PAPP-A). Further correlating factors in risk assessment are maternal age and the presence or absence of the fetal nasal bone.

A chromosomal abnormality can be confirmed by amniocentesis or chorionic villous sampling (CVS). These tests are invasive and each carries a risk of subsequent miscarriage of about 1%. In general, amniocentesis or CVS is recommended if the risk of aneuploidy as calculated from combined first trimester screening is greater than 1 in 300.

A more modern method for detecting fetal aneuploidy is NIPT. This is a maternal blood test performed after 10 weeks' gestation to detect cell free fragments of fetal DNA. The fetal DNA is from the placental cytotrophoblast and makes up about 10% of cell free DNA in the maternal circulation.

15.1.4 MULTIPLE PREGNANCY

Multiple pregnancy occurs in 1% of pregnancies, with a significantly higher rate for assisted conceptions. It is important to recognize multiple pregnancy as early as possible as there are several associated risks, as well as social implications (Fig. 15.4). Risks to the fetuses include an increased incidence of congenital anomalies, IUGR and low birth weight, and premature labour. Risks to the mother include hyperemesis, cholestasis, antepartum haemorrhage,

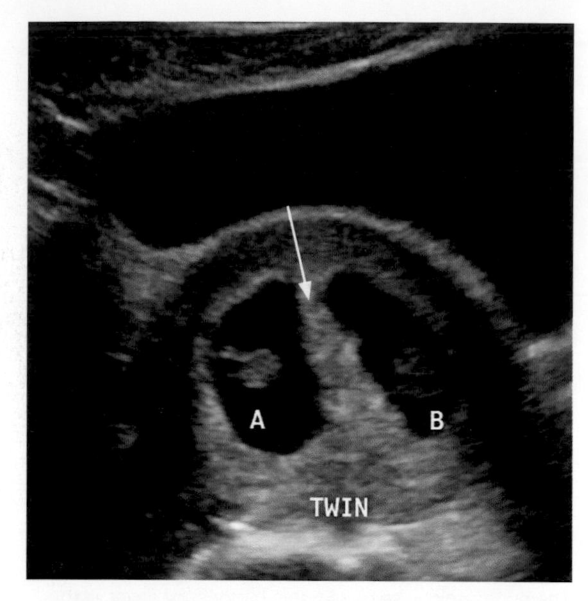

Figure 15.4 Early twin pregnancy: US. Note the two gestational sacs (A, B) separated by a thick membrane (arrow), indicating a dichorionic–diamniotic (DCDA) gestation.

polyhydramnios, hypertension and pre-eclampsia. Twin pregnancy, when recognized on US examination, may be classified as follows:

- Dichorionic–diamniotic (DCDA)
  - May be dizygotic (independent fertilization of two ova) or monozygotic
  - Dizygotic may be different sex; monozygotic are same sex
  - Separating membrane seen between the fetuses
  - Separate placentas may be identified
  - Mortality rate 5–10%
- Monochorionic–diamniotic (MCDA)
  - Monozygotic, therefore same sex
  - Separating membrane between the fetuses may be seen
  - Single placenta
  - Mortality rate 20%
- Monochorionic–monoamniotic (MCMA)
  - Monozygotic, therefore same sex
  - No separating membrane
  - Single placenta
  - Mortality rate 50%.

Because monochorionic twin pregnancies share one placenta they are prone to haemodynamic complications, such as twin–twin transfusion and twin embolization syndrome. As well as these haemodynamic complications, monoamniotic twin pregnancies have further risks, including entanglement and obstruction of umbilical cords.

15.1.5 FETAL MORPHOLOGY SCAN

Obstetric US scan for the assessment of fetal morphology is best performed at 19–21 weeks' gestation. The fetal morphology scan should only be performed when the referring doctor and patient have a clear view of the benefits and limitations of the technique. Potential implications of an abnormal finding should be understood prior to the examination. The fetal morphology scan provides an assessment of gestational age accurate to ±1 week based on several measurements, including:

- Biparietal diameter of the fetal skull (BPD)
- Head circumference (HC)
- Abdomen circumference (AC)
- Femur length (FL).

Placental position is documented, in particular the relationship of the lower placental edge to the internal os, i.e. diagnosis of placenta praevia. If a low-lying placenta is diagnosed on the fetal morphology scan a follow-up scan is performed. The definition of 'low-lying placenta' is variable, but is usually accepted as meaning a lower placental edge within 2 cm of the internal os. Owing to increased growth of the lower uterine segment in later pregnancy, most low-lying placentas will resolve spontaneously.

The amniotic fluid volume is assessed. Low amniotic fluid volume or oligohydramnios may be caused by IUGR secondary to placental insufficiency, chromosomal disorders, congenital infection and severe maternal systemic illness. Severe oligohydramnios may also indicate the presence of renal agenesis or obstruction of the fetal urinary tract. Common causes of increased amniotic fluid volume or polyhydramnios include maternal diabetes, multiple pregnancy, neural tube defect, fetal hydrops and any disorder with impaired fetal swallowing such as oesophageal atresia. In many cases, polyhydramnios is idiopathic, with no underlying cause found.

A detailed assessment of fetal anatomy is performed. Most major fetal malformations can be diagnosed on US at this stage of pregnancy (Fig. 15.5). Fetal MRI may be performed when US findings are equivocal or for specific indications when further clarification is clinically useful (see section 15.1.7).

15.1.6 SECOND AND THIRD TRIMESTER

US may be indicated in later pregnancy for a variety of reasons.

Vaginal bleeding

Second- or third-trimester vaginal bleeding may be due to premature labour or placental problems, including placenta praevia, placental abruption and placenta accreta.

Follow-up of fetal abnormality

In some cases, a fetal abnormality diagnosed at the 19- to 21-week morphology scan may require follow-up. The reasons for this may include monitoring of hydronephrosis or confirmation of an anomaly suspected on an earlier scan (Fig. 15.6).

Suspected intrauterine growth retardation and fetal well-being

Clinical features suggestive of IUGR include small maternal size, slow weight gain, maternal hypertension or a history of complications in previous pregnancies, such as pre-eclampsia. IUGR may be confirmed by various US measurements of the fetus (see sections 15.1.5 and 15.1.6), including BPD, HC, AC, FL and estimation of fetal weight (EFW) based on these parameters. A fetus is defined as being small for gestational age if the EFW is below the 10th centile. The commonest cause of IUGR is placental insufficiency. In such cases, the IUGR is asymmetric, i.e. the abdomen is disproportionately small compared with the head. Symmetrical IUGR (head and abdomen reduced in size to an equal degree) may be caused by chromosomal disorders, including trisomy 13 or 18.

Macrosomia refers to a fetus with an EFW above the 90th centile for gestational age or EFW greater than 4500 g. Macrosomia associated with maternal diabetes carries an increased risk of fetal demise. Macrosomia increases the risk of birth trauma. Management of placental insufficiency and other factors that may impact on fetal well-being is

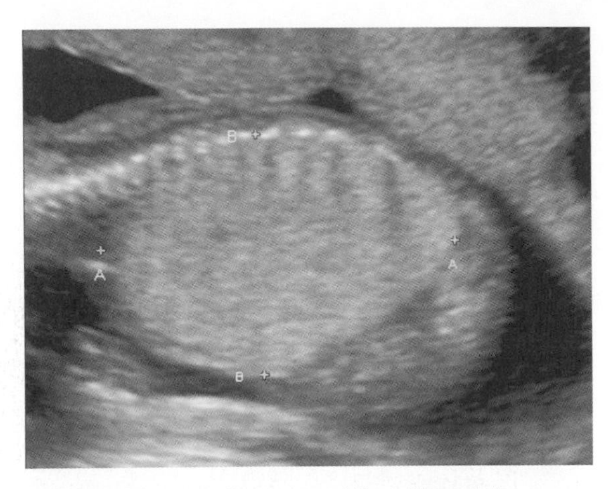

Figure 15.5 Fetal chest mass: US at 19 weeks' gestation. Longitudinal view of the fetus shows a large hyperechoic mass in the chest. The differential diagnosis includes congenital pulmonary airway malformation (CPAM), pulmonary sequestration and diaphragmatic hernia. Subsequently diagnosed as CPAM following delivery.

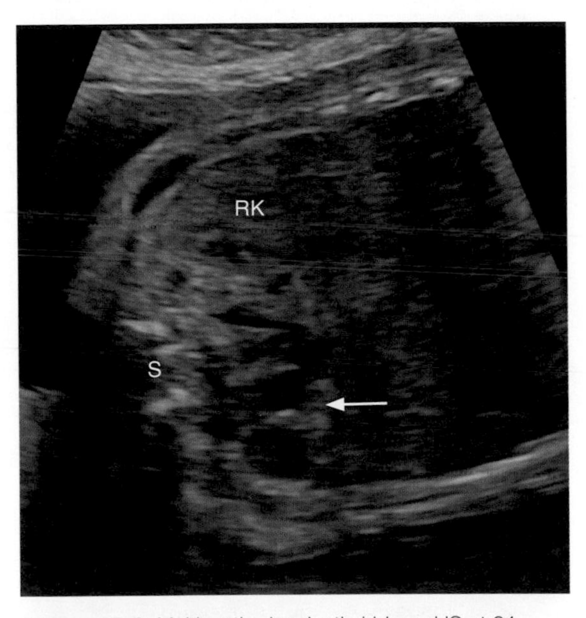

Figure 15.6 Multicystic dysplastic kidney: US at 24 weeks' gestation. There are several non-communicating cysts replacing the left kidney (arrow). Also note right kidney (RK), fetal spine (S).

assisted with assessment of various US parameters, including:

- Amniotic fluid volume
- Doppler analysis of the fetal umbilical artery, ductus venosus and middle cerebral artery
- Doppler analysis of the maternal uterine artery
- Fetal breathing movements
- Fetal limb movements
- Fetal heart rate.

15.1.7 FETAL MAGNETIC RESONANCE IMAGING

Using fast sequences to obtain multiplanar T1- and T2-weighted images, fetal MRI is used increasingly in obstetric practice (Fig. 15.7). Because of small fetal size plus biosafety concerns, fetal MRI is recommended for use after 18 weeks' gestation. It is most indicated when an abnormality is suspected but US findings are equivocal.

Specific areas where fetal MRI may be particularly useful include:

- Brain, e.g. cephalocele, cerebral cortical malformation, posterior fossa abnormality
- Spine, e.g. neural tube defect, sacrococcygeal teratoma
- Head and neck, e.g. lymphatic malformation, congenital cystic mass
- Chest, e.g. congenital diaphragmatic hernia
- Abdomen and pelvis, e.g. anorectal malformation
- Disorders of placentation, e.g. placental accrete.

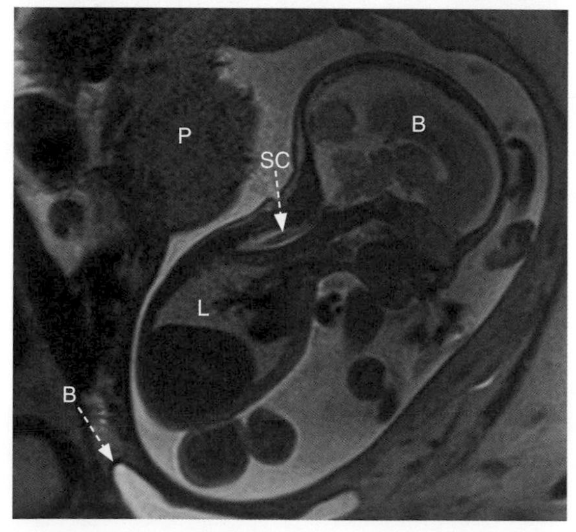

Figure 15.7 Fetal MRI: normal study. T2-weighted image aligned to show the fetus in the sagittal plane. Note the fetal brain (B), lung (L), spinal cord (SC, dashed arrow). Also note maternal bladder (B, dashed arrow), placenta (P).

15.2 PELVIC MASS

US is the investigation of choice for the initial imaging assessment of a pelvic mass. First, US is used to ascertain the organ of origin, usually ovary or uterus. Most solid uterine masses are fibroids (see section 15.4). Most adnexal masses in women are ovarian in origin. Other possible causes of an adnexal mass include pedunculated uterine fibroids, bowel tumours, abscesses or postoperative fluid collection. Ovarian masses may be classified on US as simple cysts, complex cysts or solid. Complex cysts are cysts that are complicated by echogenic fluid contents, multilocularity, soft-tissue septations or nodules, and internal vascularity. Other clinical data may be helpful in diagnosis, such as tumour markers. Cancer antigen 125 (CA-125) is the most commonly elevated tumour marker of ovarian malignancy. Depending on size and specific features, further assessment with MRI may be indicated.

15.2.1 SIMPLE OVARIAN CYST

A cyst is classified as simple on US if it has anechoic fluid contents, a thin wall and no soft-tissue components. Most simple cysts in premenopausal women are follicles (Fig. 15.8). A simple cyst of less than 5 cm in diameter in a postmenopausal woman may be regarded as benign. Cysts larger than 5 cm in diameter may be followed with US; cysts larger than 10 cm may require MRI or specialist assessment. Occasionally, simple cysts may present with acute symptoms due to torsion or haemorrhage ('cyst accident') that require treatment.

15.2.2 COMPLEX OVARIAN CYSTS

Complex ovarian cysts include all cysts that do not fulfil the US criteria for a simple cyst, i.e. cysts with echogenic fluid contents, septations, wall thickening,

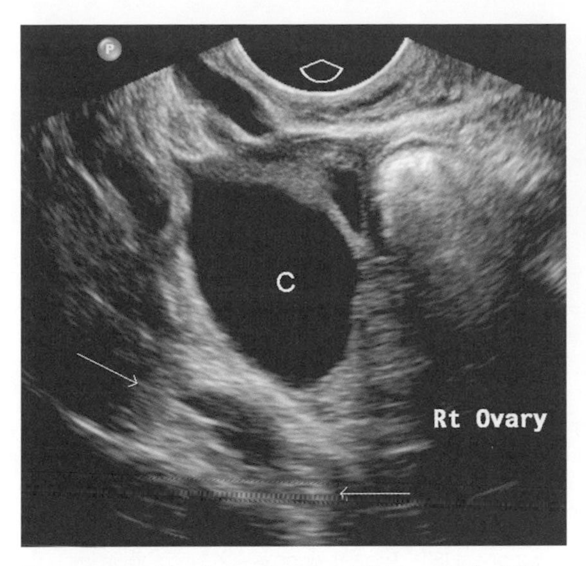

Figure 15.8 Simple ovarian cyst: US. Transvaginal US (TVUS) shows a simple cyst (C) arising on the right ovary and producing typical posterior acoustic enhancement (arrows).

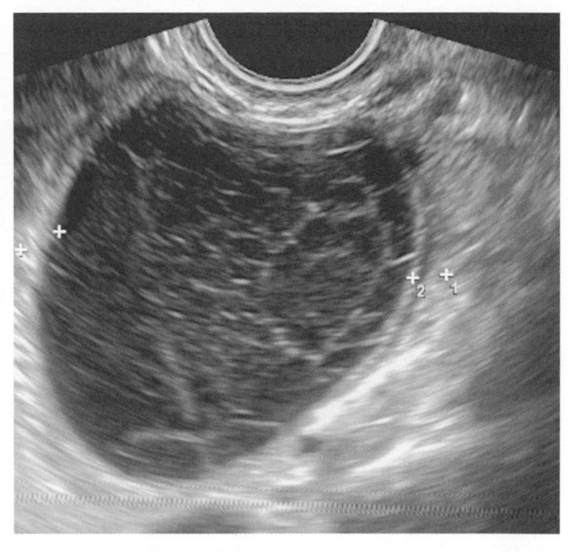

Figure 15.9 Complex ovarian cyst: US. Transvaginal US (TVUS) shows extensive complex echogenicity within an ovarian cyst due to haemorrhage.

papillary projections or internal vascularity. In premenopausal women the differential diagnosis of a complex ovarian cyst is a haemorrhagic follicle with echogenic fluid contents (Fig. 15.9). More complex cystic lesions may be caused by ectopic pregnancy (see section 15.1.2), pelvic inflammatory disease, endometriosis or ovarian torsion.

The most common ovarian tumour in premenopausal women is a mature cystic teratoma or 'dermoid cyst'. The commonly used term 'dermoid cyst' is a misnomer; true dermoid cysts (most common in the head and neck) arise from derivatives of ectoderm, whereas ovarian teratomas derive at least two primitive embryological layers. Mature cystic teratomas contain fat, hair and sometimes teeth, and are bilateral in 10% of cases. They are seen on US as complex cystic or solid lesions with markedly hyperechoic areas owing to fat content (Fig. 15.10). These lesions may be further characterized with MRI (Fig. 15.11). When found incidentally on CT, the presence of fat is usually diagnostic of a mature cystic ovarian teratoma.

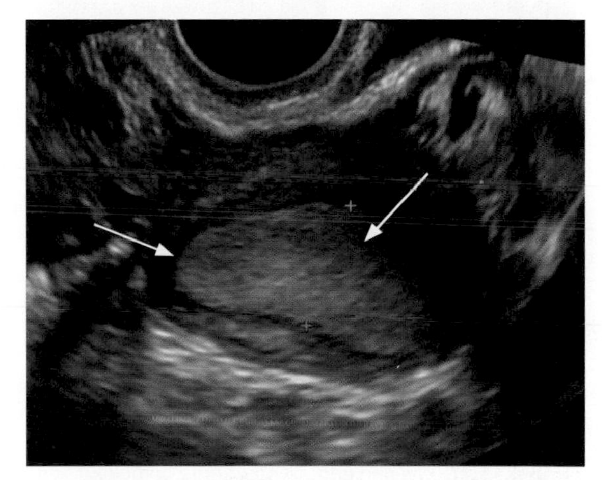

Figure 15.10 Ovarian mature teratoma ('dermoid cyst'). US shows a complex hyperechoic lesion in the right ovary (arrows).

Serous cystadenocarcinoma is the commonest type of ovarian malignancy. These are usually large (>15 cm) and seen on US as multiloculated cystic masses with thick, irregular septations and soft-tissue masses (Fig. 15.12). US may also be used to demonstrate evidence of metastatic spread, such as ascites and liver metastases. Other ovarian tumours seen on US as complex partly cystic ovarian masses include mucinous and serous cystadenoma, mucinous cystadenocarcinoma and endometroid carcinoma.

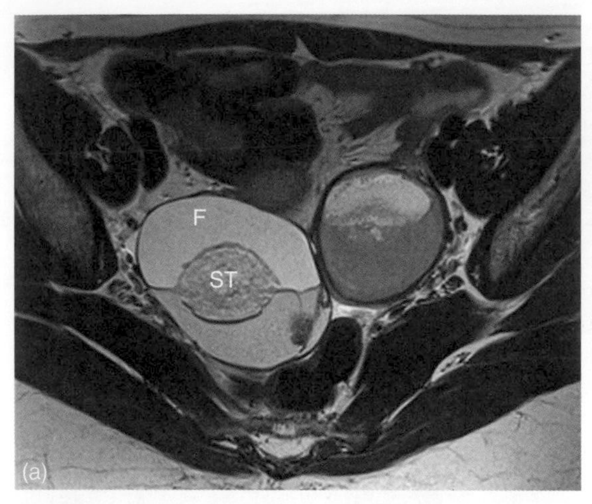

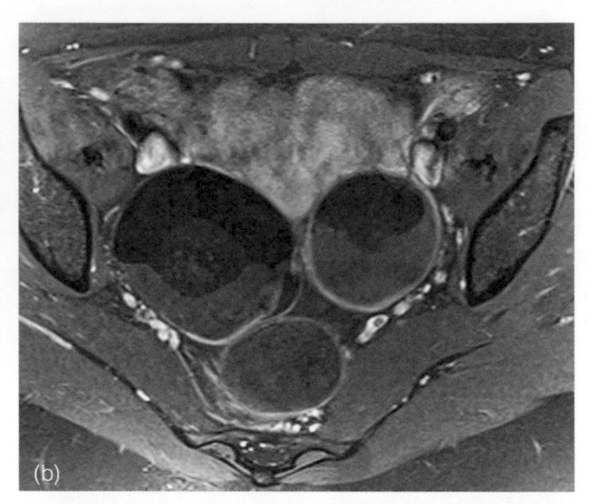

Figure 15.11 Ovarian mature teratoma ('dermoid cyst'), bilateral: MRI. (a) Transverse T2-weighted image shows bilateral complex ovarian lesions. The right-sided lesion shows a fluid–fluid level due to lower density fat (F) 'floating' on complex fluid. This lesion also shows a discrete soft-tissue component (ST). The left-sided lesion also shows fat content. (b) Corresponding transverse T1-weighted fat-saturated contrast-enhanced image shows the fat content as black as a result of fat saturation. Both complex lesions show mild peripheral enhancement.

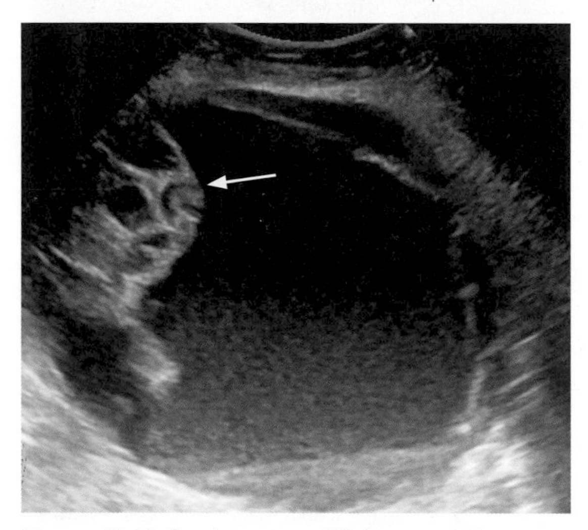

Figure 15.12 Ovarian cancer: US. Large complex multiloculated cystic mass arising from the left ovary. Note that the cyst contents show diffuse low-level echogenicity in keeping with complex fluid, plus an irregular soft-tissue papillary projection (arrow). US appearances consistent with an Ovarian–Adnexal Reporting and Data System (O-RADS) 5 lesion.

15.2.3 SOLID OVARIAN MASSES

Causes of a solid ovarian mass include fibroma and a Brenner tumour. These are seen on US as solid lesions with variable echogenicity, internal vascularity and smooth or irregular margins.

15.2.4 OVARIAN–ADNEXAL REPORTING AND DATA SYSTEM

As a result of multiple factors, including the lethal nature of ovarian cancer, the often non-specific nature of US findings (and reports) of adnexal lesions and the risks of unnecessary surgery, a structured reporting system has been developed. Published in 2020, the Ovarian–Adnexal Reporting and Data System (O-RADS) provides risk stratification categories based on certain imaging features. Each of these categories corresponds to a risk of malignancy and appropriate management recommendations. O-RADS allows for the identification of normal features, including a follicle defined as a simple cyst measuring less than 3 cm or a corpus luteum. It also includes a specific category of 'classic benign lesions' that may be diagnosed confidently on imaging, including mature cystic teratoma, endometrioma and hydrosalpinx.

More recently, an O-RADS lexicon for MRI has been published. MRI is particularly useful in the characterization of adnexal lesions that are indeterminate on US. The presence of solid enhancing tissue in an adnexal lesion is a strong positive predictor for malignancy. MRI is more accurate than US for delineating the nature of fluid in cystic lesions, and it is better able to assess large lesions that may be beyond the field of view of US. Further details of O-RADS for US and MRI may be found on the companion website.

15.3 POLYCYSTIC OVARIAN SYNDROME

Polycystic ovarian syndrome (PCOS) is the most common endocrine disorder in women of reproductive age and is a common cause of chronic anovulation and infertility. PCOS refers to a spectrum of clinical disorders, with the classic triad of oligomenorrhoea, obesity and hirsutism (Stein–Leventhal syndrome) being the best known. The 'Rotterdam criteria' for the diagnosis of PCOS combine clinical features of anovulation and hyperandrogenism with US findings. US criteria are based on examination with TVUS with a high-frequency probe:

- 20 or more follicles measuring 2 9 mm, and/or
- Ovarian volumes of 10 mL or greater.

The diagnostic criteria also include exclusion of other possible aetiologies, such as thyroid disease, hyperprolactinaemia and non-classical congenital adrenal hyperplasia. It is important to note that US should not be used for the diagnosis of PCOS in young women within 8 years of menarche because of the high incidence of normal multifollicular ovaries in this life stage.

15.4 UTERINE FIBROIDS

Uterine leiomyomas, more commonly referred to as fibroids, are benign tumours composed of smooth muscle and fibrous tissue. Fibroids may be:

- Submucosal: projecting into the endometrial cavity
- Intramural: most common location, confined to the myometrium
- Subserosal: lie on the serosal surface of the uterus
- Pedunculated: attached by a stalk of tissue.

They are often multiple and are usually seen on US as masses of variable echogenicity in the smooth muscle wall of the uterus (myometrium). Fibroids are common, occurring in up to 70% of women by menopause. They are usually small, asymptomatic and found incidentally. Occasionally, they may cause symptoms, including pelvic pain, infertility and abnormal vaginal bleeding. Complications include degeneration, haemorrhage and rarely malignant transformation.

Fibroids are usually adequately assessed with US. Occasionally, because of the limited field of view of US, large or multiple fibroids are better assessed with MRI. This is particularly the case when therapy is required. Large symptomatic fibroids may be amenable to treatment with uterine artery embolization.

15.5 ADENOMYOSIS

Adenomyosis is a benign condition characterized by ectopic endometrial tissue within the myometrium. It is most common in women of reproductive age and may be associated with endometriosis and uterine fibroids. Adenomyosis is usually asymptomatic, though it may present with chronic pelvic pain, dysmenorrhoea or menorrhagia or as problems with fertility, including implantation failure with *in vitro* fertilization (IVF). It is usually a diffuse process, most prominently involving the posterior uterus and sparing the cervix. Less commonly, it may be focal with a mass-like lesion (adenomyoma) that may mimic a fibroid on imaging.

US is usually the first investigation in symptomatic women. Findings on US include a bulky heterogeneous myometrium with increased vascularity, linear echogenic striations in the myometrium ('venetian blind' appearance) and an irregular border of endometrium and myometrium. Although US performed in specialist centres may accurately diagnose adenomyosis, it is very operator dependent, and reported sensitivities and specificities are highly variable.

MRI can be used to reliably diagnose adenomyosis and is the investigation of choice (Fig. 15.13). A key anatomical feature of the uterus that is well demonstrated on MRI is the junctional zone. This is

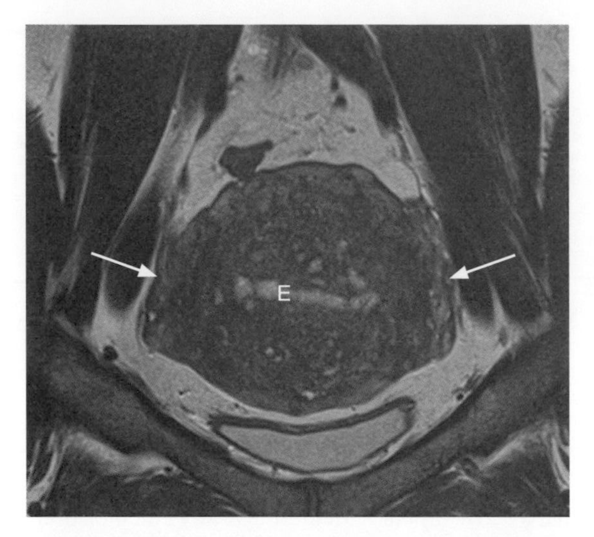

Figure 15.13 Adenomyosis: MRI. Coronal T2-weighted image through the mid-body of the uterus (arrows) shows extensive changes of adenomyosis, including low signal throughout the myometrium with multiple tiny cysts and an irregular outline of the endometrium (E).

a layer of highly compacted smooth muscle cells at the junction of the endometrium and myometrium seen as a low-signal layer on T2-weighted images. Thickening of the junctional zone and irregularity of its outline are key features of adenomyosis. Other features include thickening and heterogeneity of the myometrium and, in the case of focal adenomyosis, a low-signal mass-like lesion in continuity with the junctional zone. MRI may also be used for follow-up after therapy, e.g. with gonadotropin-releasing hormone agonists, particularly in IVF.

15.6 ENDOMETRIOSIS

Endometriosis is a common condition of adolescent girls and young women. It is characterized by the presence of functioning endometrial tissue outside the uterus. Lesions vary from microscopic to several centimetres in size; larger lesions are termed endometriomas. Endometriosis most commonly involves the ovaries and pelvic peritoneum; less common locations include Caesarean section scars in the abdominal wall, small and large bowel, rectum and bladder. A deep infiltrating form with adhesions and fibrosis may involve the pelvis. Symptoms of endometriosis include chronic pelvic pain, which may be cyclical and associated with menstruation, dysmenorrhoea and infertility.

US is highly accurate for the diagnosis of endometriosis involving the ovaries. The typical US appearance of an ovarian endometrioma is a unilocular cyst with homogeneous internal low-level echoes. MRI is

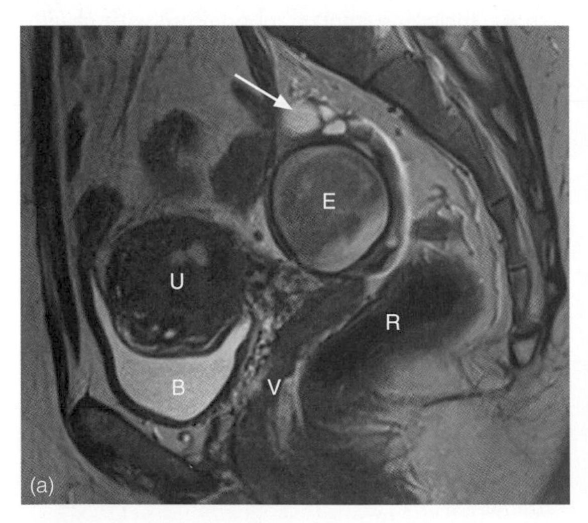

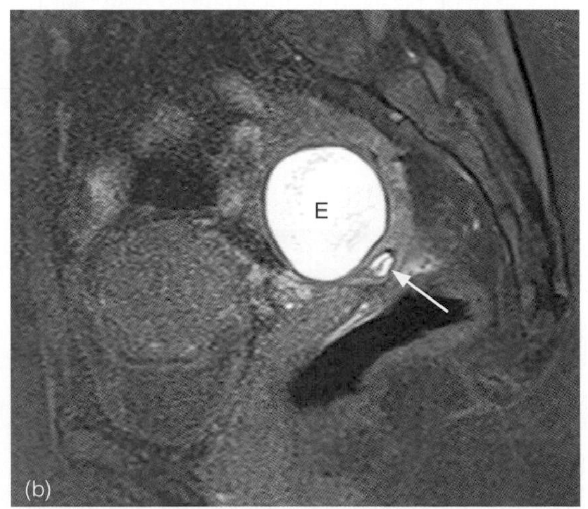

Figure 15.14 Endometriosis: MRI. (a) Sagittal T2-weighted image shows a round ovarian cystic lesion with a low-signal wall and mixed signal contents in keeping with an endometrioma (E). Note: a small follicle in the adjacent distorted ovarian parenchyma (arrows). Also note bladder (B), rectum (R), uterus (U), vagina (V). (b) Corresponding sagittal T1-weighted fat-saturated image shows the typical diffuse high signal of an endometrioma (E). A much smaller second endometrioma is also seen (arrow).

more accurate than US for extraovarian endometriomas and for deep infiltrating disease. A key sequence is T1-weighted imaging with fat saturation (T1FS), on which endometriomas show as high-signal lesions (Fig. 15.14). Deep infiltrating disease is seen on T1- and T2-weighted images as irregular-shaped low signal that distorts anatomical planes and organ interfaces, such as the pouch of Douglas.

15.7 ABNORMAL VAGINAL BLEEDING

15.7.1 PREMENOPAUSAL WOMEN

In non-pregnant premenopausal women, abnormal vaginal bleeding is usually caused by hormonal imbalance and anovulatory cycles (dysfunctional uterine bleeding); it is treated with hormonal therapy. If hormonal therapy does not control the bleeding, endometrial hyperplasia (precursor for endometrial carcinoma) or endometrial polyp are the primary diagnoses (Fig. 15.15). The factors associated with an increased risk of endometrial pathology include age over 35 years, body weight over 90 kg and infertility.

TVUS should be performed to measure endometrial thickness. Endometrial thickness varies with the phase of the menstrual cycle. The ideal time for TVUS is on days 4–6 of the menstrual cycle, when the endometrial echo should be at its thinnest. The likelihood of endometrial hyperplasia is low if the endometrial thickness measured with TVUS is less than 12 mm.

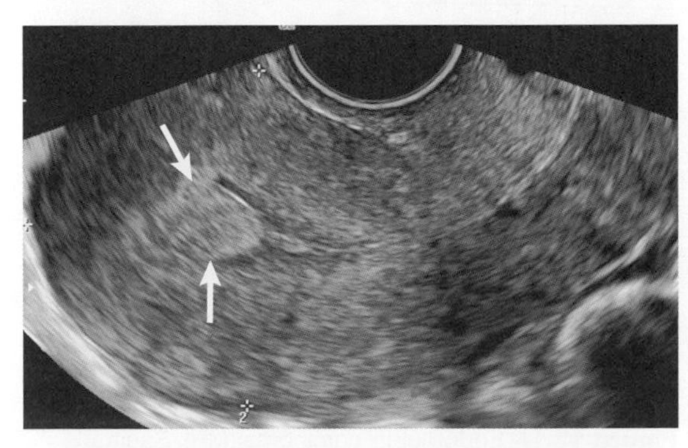

Figure 15.15 Endometrial polyp: US. Longitudinal transvaginal US (TVUS) shows an oval-shaped hyperechoic mass in the endometrial cavity of the uterus (arrows).

Saline infusion sonohysterography is a technique that enhances the accuracy of US assessment of the endometrium:

- A small catheter is placed in the uterus
- Under direct visualization with TVUS, a small volume of sterile saline is injected to distend the uterine cavity.

Saline infusion sonohysterography produces excellent delineation of the two layers of endometrium and allows differentiation of endometrial masses from generalized endometrial thickening.

15.7.2 POSTMENOPAUSAL WOMEN

Postmenopausal bleeding is defined as spontaneous vaginal bleeding that occurs more than 1 year after the last menstrual period. In postmenopausal women, atrophic endometrium is the commonest cause of abnormal vaginal bleeding. If bleeding persists despite a trial of hormonal therapy, TVUS is indicated to assess for endometrial carcinoma. The diagnostic sign of endometrial carcinoma on TVUS is endometrial thickening greater than 5 mm, which in a postmenopausal woman requires further assessment with hysteroscopy and endometrial sampling.

15.8 STAGING OF GYNAECOLOGICAL MALIGNANCIES

Malignancies of the female reproductive system are staged by the International Federation of Gynecology and Obstetrics (FIGO). These classification systems are also converted into the tumour–node–metastasis (TNM) system and published by the American Joint Committee on Cancer (AJCC).

15.8.1 OVARIAN CARCINOMA

Ovarian carcinoma is the leading cause of death from gynaecological malignancy. This is because of the high percentage of late-stage tumours at the time of diagnosis, with over 75% of patients having metastatic disease beyond the ovaries.

Most ovarian tumours are well characterized with US and MRI, including diagnosis of bilateral ovarian involvement. CT is the investigation of choice for pretreatment staging of ovarian cancer. CT is used to search for features relevant to FIGO staging including peritoneal spread, such as ascites and peritoneal masses, liver and pulmonary metastases, pleural effusion, and lymphadenopathy (Fig. 15.16). Further details of the FIGO staging system for ovarian cancer can be found on the companion website.

15.8.2 CARCINOMA OF THE CERVIX

Cervical cancer is the third most common gynaecological malignancy. Mortality from cervical cancer has dramatically decreased over the last 50 years owing to widespread use of the Papanicolaou (pap) smear, and more recently from vaccination against the human papillomavirus (HPV). Histologically, most cervical carcinomas are squamous cell carcinoma. The mode of spread is by local invasion plus involvement of lymph nodes. The FIGO staging system for cervical carcinoma considers the depth of invasion within the cervix and uterus, extension into the pelvis and invasion of local structures, plus the extent and location of lymph node metastases.

Clinical assessment with examination under anaesthetic, colposcopy and hysteroscopy are used for the initial diagnosis and assessment of carcinoma of the cervix. Imaging is used to differentiate stage 1 tumours that can be treated with surgery from more advanced disease. MRI is the investigation of choice for measuring tumour size and assessing the depth of uterine invasion and local tumour extension in the pelvis. Fluorodeoxyglucose (FDG)-positron emission tomography (PET)-CT is the investigation of choice for the detection of distant spread, including retroperitoneal lymphadenopathy, liver metastases and lung metastases. Further details of the FIGO staging system for cervical cancer can be found on the companion website.

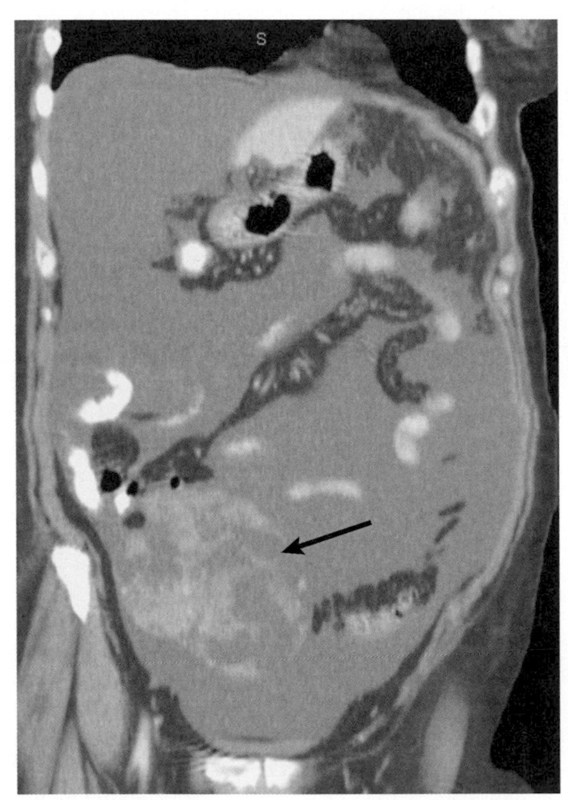

Figure 15.16 Cystadenocarcinoma of the ovary: CT. Coronal reconstruction CT of the abdomen shows a complex partly cystic mass in the right pelvis (arrow). Note: extensive ascites due to peritoneal metastases.

15.8.3 ENDOMETRIAL CARCINOMA

Endometrial carcinoma is the most common gynaecological malignancy. Most tumours are adenocarcinomas, with a peak age of incidence of

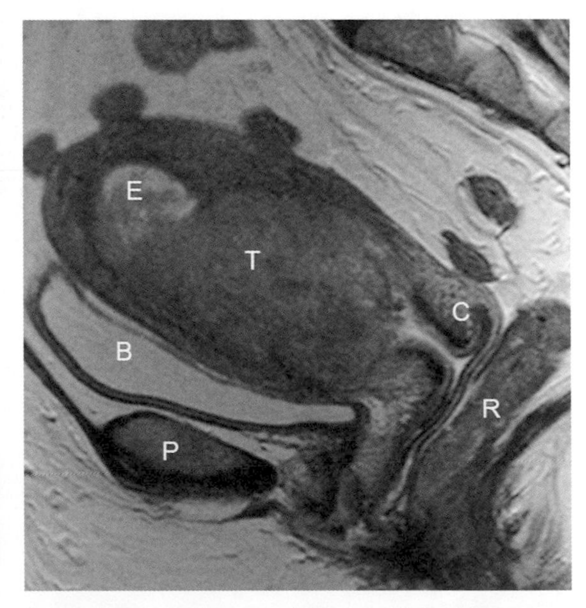

Figure 15.17 Endometrial carcinoma: MRI. Sagittal T2-weighted image shows a large endometrial tumour (T) confined to the body of the uterus. Note: distended endometrial cavity (E) above the tumour, bladder (B), cervix (C), pubic symphysis (P), rectum (R).

55–65 years. The most common clinical presentation of endometrial carcinoma is postmenopausal bleeding (see section 15.7.2). Fifteen per cent of women with postmenopausal bleeding will have endometrial carcinoma. The FIGO staging system for endometrial carcinoma considers the depth and degree of invasion within the uterus plus, with higher stage tumours, pelvic extension, invasion of local structures and distant metastases.

MRI is the investigation of choice for early-stage disease. It is more accurate than US in the assessment of the depth of myometrial invasion, invasion of the cervix and extension through the uterine wall (Fig. 15.17). For later stage disease, FDG-PET-CT is the investigation of choice for detecting distant metastases. Further details of the FIGO staging system for endometrial cancer can be found on the companion website

SUMMARY

Clinical presentation	Investigation of choice	Comment
Pelvic mass	• US • MRI for characterization of complex lesions	O-RADS
PCOS	• TVUS	Specific criteria
Adenomyosis	• US • MRI is the investigation of choice	Junctional zone is a key feature on MRI
Endometriosis	• US: ovarian endometriomas • MRI: non-ovarian and deep infiltrating disease	
Ovarian cancer staging	• US • CT	O-RADS
Cervical cancer staging	• MRI for local extent • FDG-PET	
Uterine cancer staging	• MRI for local extent • FDG-PET	

Abbreviations: FDG, fluorodeoxyglucose; O-RADS, Ovarian–Adnexal Reporting and Data System; PCOS, polycystic ovarian syndrome; TVUS, transvaginal US.

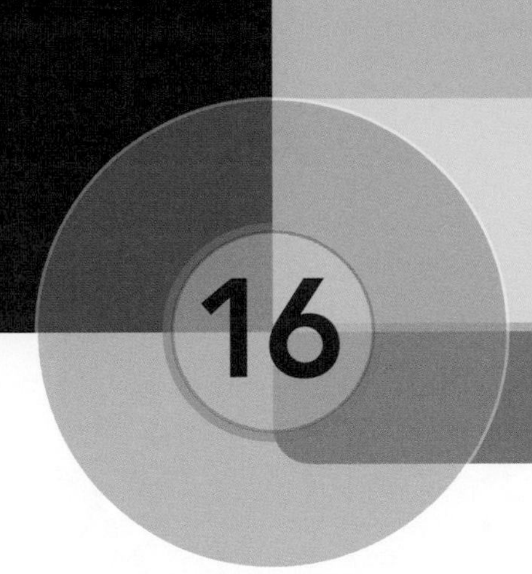

16 Paediatrics

Paediatric radiology is an extremely diverse subject encompassing many subspecialty areas. Many of the topics covered in other chapters of this book, including non-orthopaedic and orthopaedic trauma, bone tumours, central nervous system (CNS) oncology and acute abdomen, are relevant to paediatrics. Highly specialized topics in paediatrics are beyond the scope of a student text and may be referenced elsewhere. These include congenital heart disease, which is imaged with echocardiography and magnetic resonance imaging (MRI), and congenital brain disorders, imaged with MRI. This chapter will discuss some of the more common clinical problems unique to paediatric practice that require imaging.

16.1 NEONATAL RESPIRATORY DISTRESS: THE NEONATAL CHEST

An approach to interpretation of a chest radiograph (chest X-ray, CXR) has been outlined in Chapter 4. Specific features that may be seen on a normal neonatal CXR include:

- Thymus may be prominent
- Heart shadow is often prominent and globular in outline; normal cardiothoracic ratio up to 65%
- Air bronchograms may be seen in the medial third of the lung fields
- Hemidiaphragms normally lie at the level of the sixth rib anteriorly.

The more common causes of neonatal respiratory distress tend to produce quite typical radiographic patterns as described in section 16.2. When assessing a neonatal CXR, the clinical context is paramount; for example:

- Premature infant with respiratory distress: surfactant deficiency disease will be the most likely diagnosis
- Distressed term infant following Caesarean delivery: retained fetal lung fluid will be most likely
- Term delivery with meconium-stained liquor: consider meconium aspiration syndrome.

Finally, it should be remembered that acutely ill neonates may have various tubes and vascular catheters visible on CXR, and it is important to check that these are correctly positioned (Fig. 16.1):

- Endotracheal tube: tip above the carina
- Nasogastric tube: tip in the stomach
- Umbilical artery catheter: tip in the lower thoracic aorta, projected over the lower thoracic vertebral bodies (T6–T10)
- Umbilical vein catheter: tip just above the diaphragm in the lower right atrium.

16.1.1 SURFACTANT DEFICIENCY DISORDER

Also known as respiratory distress syndrome, surfactant deficiency disorder (SDD) is a generalized lung condition of premature infants caused by insufficient surfactant production. Clinical presentation is usually respiratory distress and cyanosis soon after premature birth (earlier than 36 weeks' gestation).

CXR changes of SDD (Figs 16.1 and 16.2):

- Reduced lung volume
- Granular pattern throughout the lungs
- Air bronchograms.

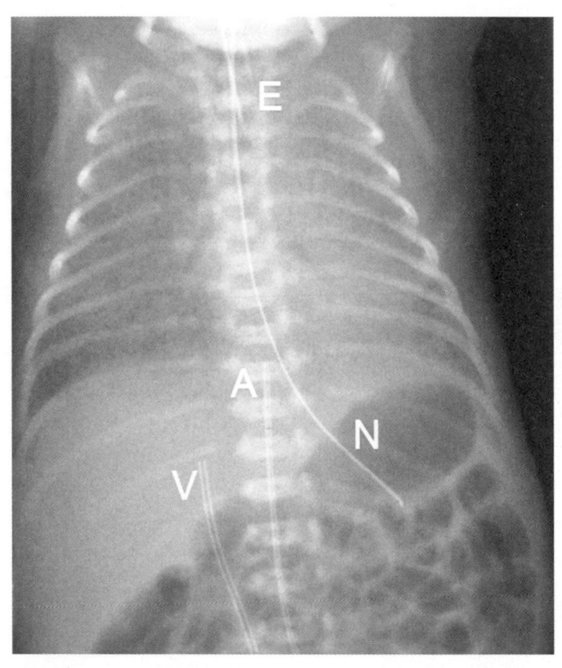

Figure 16.1 Surfactant deficiency disease (SDD) and tube placement. Fine granular opacification throughout both lungs indicating SDD. Note placement of various tubes: umbilical artery catheter tip at T9 (A); endotracheal tube (E) in the mid- to upper trachea; nasogastric tube (N) in the stomach; umbilical venous catheter tip in the liver (V).

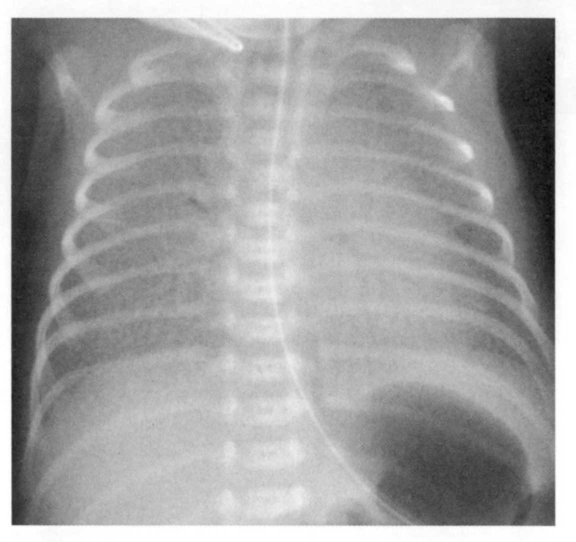

Figure 16.2 Surfactant deficiency disease (SDD). Note a fine granular pattern throughout both lungs with air bronchograms.

Surfactant therapy for SDD usually produces rapid improvement of respiratory distress accompanied by resolution of the radiographic abnormalities. Failure of resolution of the radiographic changes of SDD after a couple of days may imply an additional pathology, such as persistent ductus arteriosus (PDA) or infection. New or worsening airspace

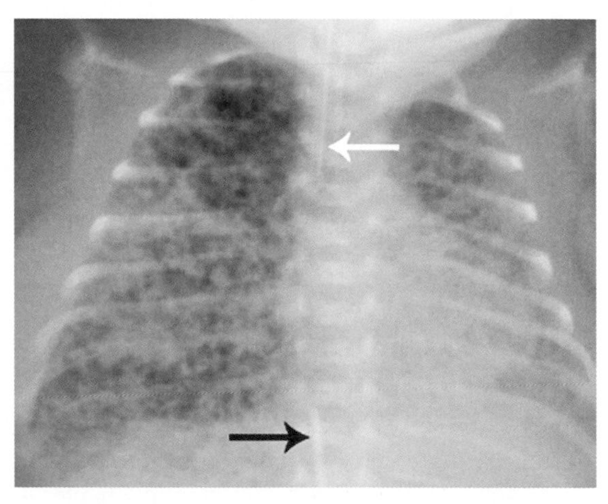

Figure 16.3 Surfactant deficiency disease (SDD) complicated by pulmonary interstitial emphysema. Note the presence of multiple small air bubbles throughout both lungs, more obvious on the right. Also note an endotracheal tube (white arrow) and an umbilical artery catheter (black arrow).

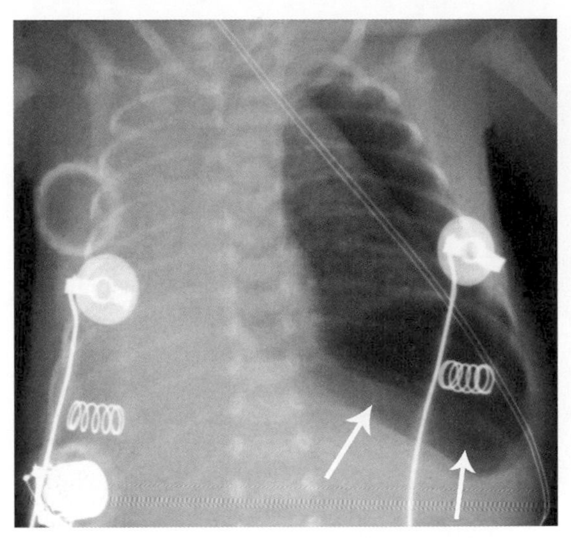

Figure 16.4 Surfactant deficiency disease (SDD) complicated by a left tension pneumothorax. Note the increased volume of the left hemithorax with shift of the mediastinum to the right. Also, as the infant is supine, most of the pneumothorax lies anteriorly and inferiorly, producing lucency of the inferior left chest and upper abdomen (arrows).

consolidation may indicate a pulmonary haemorrhage, which is a recognized complication of surfactant therapy. Other complications of SDD that may be seen on CXR relate to air leaks and include:

- Pulmonary interstitial emphysema (PIE) (Fig. 16.3)
- Pneumothorax (Fig. 16.4)
- Pneumomediastinum.

16.1.2 TRANSIENT TACHYPNOEA OF THE NEWBORN

Also known as retained fetal lung fluid or wet lung syndrome, transient tachypnoea of the newborn (TTN) is a self-limiting condition due to persistence of amniotic fluid in the fetal lungs at birth. TTN usually presents with respiratory distress in a term infant following a prolonged labour or Caesarean section.

CXR signs of TTN (Fig. 16.5):

- Prominent linear pattern, most marked centrally, with thickening of lung fissures
- Small pleural effusions
- Resolution of changes within 24–48 hours.

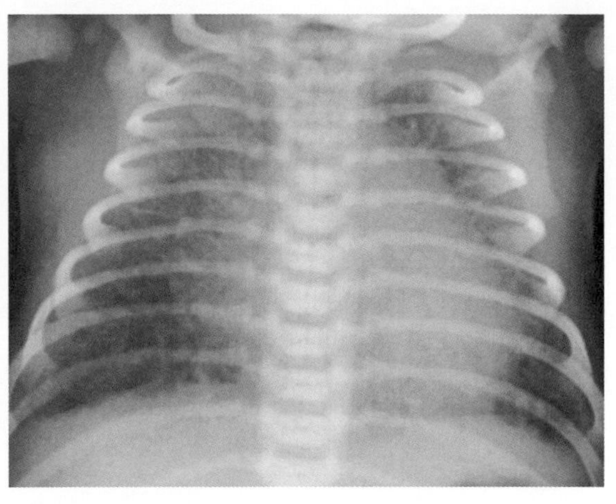

Figure 16.5 Transient tachypnoea of the newborn (TTN). CXR in a term infant born by Caesarean section shows widespread linear opacities throughout both lungs plus small pleural effusions, seen better on the right.

16.1.3 MECONIUM ASPIRATION SYNDROME

Passage of meconium *in utero* may occur in response to fetal distress. Meconium aspiration may be seen in distressed neonates, in association with meconium-stained liquor.

CXR signs of meconium aspiration (Fig. 16.6):

- Increased lung volume
- Dense, patchy opacities in central lungs

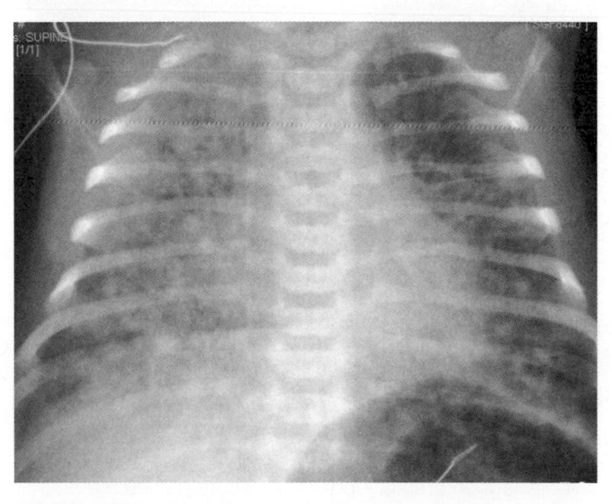

Figure 16.6 Meconium aspiration. Term infant, prolonged labour, heavy meconium staining of the liquor, severe respiratory distress. CXR shows extensive coarse opacity throughout both lungs.

- Small pleural effusions
- Complications:
  - Pneumonia with more extensive consolidation
  - Pneumothorax.

16.1.4 CARDIAC FAILURE

Specific patterns of cardiac enlargement and alterations of the cardiac outline may be seen with congenital heart disease. Suspected congenital heart disease is assessed with echocardiography and MRI. Cardiomegaly on CXR is a feature of cardiac failure, though it is not a reliable sign in neonates. More commonly, signs of cardiac failure on neonatal CXR include alveolar and interstitial opacification bilaterally and pleural effusions (Fig. 16.7). Pleural fluid in neonates commonly extends up the chest wall lateral to the lung, rather than forming a fluid level and meniscus.

16.1.5 NEONATAL PNEUMONIA

Neonatal pneumonia may produce a variety of CXR appearances, including lobar consolidation or patchy widespread consolidation. Dense bilateral consolidation may mimic the appearances of SDD. Correlation of CXR abnormality with clinical findings, particularly the presence of a fever, is important for the diagnosis of neonatal pneumonia.

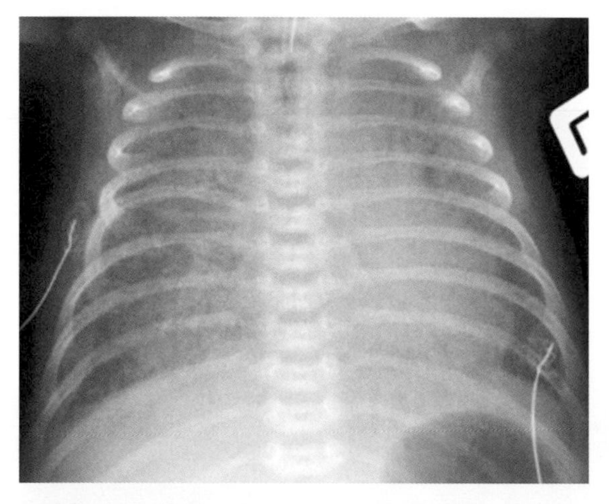

Figure 16.7 Cardiac failure. Term infant with respiratory distress. CXR shows cardiac enlargement, bilateral alveolar and interstitial opacity, and right pleural effusion. Note that, in neonates, pleural fluid tracks lateral to the lung. Subsequent investigations, including echocardiography, revealed total anomalous pulmonary venous drainage.

16.1.6 CHRONIC LUNG DISEASE OF PREMATURITY

Chronic lung disease of prematurity (CLDP) occurs in premature infants, usually born at 23–26 weeks' gestation, and is defined as oxygen dependence extending beyond 36 weeks' corrected gestation. The term CLDP is often used interchangeably with bronchopulmonary dysplasia (BPD). The term BPD has been used in the past to describe a severe chronic lung condition following prolonged respiratory support in premature infants that results in overexpanded airspaces and interstitial fibrosis. With modern management, including antenatal steroids, surfactant administration and more refined oxygen therapy techniques, a new milder form of BPD is described. Although the terminology can be confusing, the incidence of CLDP/BPD increases with low birth weight, premature rupture of membranes, early gestational age and duration of respiratory support, including ventilation or nasal continuous airway pressure.

Radiological changes evolve over time from CXR signs of SSD to the development over several weeks of a 'bubbly' pattern through the lungs, i.e. air-filled 'bubbles' separated by irregular lines. Cardiac enlargement on serial radiographs may signal the development of pulmonary arterial hypertension. Most infants with CLDP survive and CXR changes generally resolve over time, though often with some minor residual pulmonary overexpansion and linear stranding.

16.2 PATTERNS OF PULMONARY INFECTION IN CHILDREN

Most pulmonary infections in children are due to viruses such as respiratory syncytial virus (RSV), influenza, parainfluenza and adenovirus. Viral infections tend to be seasonal and occur in epidemics. Bacterial infections are less common and tend to be sporadic and less seasonal. Bacteria that commonly cause pulmonary infections in children include *Streptococcus pneumoniae, Staphylococcus aureus, Mycoplasma pneumoniae* and, rarely, *Haemophilus influenzae.*

Although there is some overlap in CXR appearances, viruses tend to produce an interstitial pattern while bacteria tend to produce alveolar consolidation. Community-acquired pneumonia caused by *M. pneumoniae* may produce an interstitial or alveolar pattern, or a combination of the two. The most important feature on the CXR of a child with a lower respiratory tract infection is alveolar consolidation. If present, a bacterial aetiology is suspected and antibiotics may be required. If absent, treatment will usually consist of supportive measures without the use of antibiotics.

16.2.1 VIRAL INFECTION

Children with viral lower respiratory tract infection usually present with a history of a couple of days of malaise, tachypnoea and cough. The most common CXR pattern seen with viral pulmonary infection is bilateral parahilar 'infiltration' (Fig. 16.8). This consists of irregular linear opacity extending into each lung from the hilar complexes, with bronchial wall thickening a prominent feature. Hilar lymphadenopathy may increase the amount of hilar opacification. Atelectasis due to mucous plugging and bronchial inflammation may complicate this pattern. Atelectasis may involve whole lobes or may be seen as linear opacities that are transient and migratory on serial radiographs.

Large areas of atelectasis may mimic consolidation; it is important to recognize the lung volume loss associated with atelectasis (collapse) as this will help to differentiate it from consolidation. Consolidation may rarely complicate viral infection and is often due to haemorrhagic bronchiolitis rather than a genuine exudate.

16.2.2 BRONCHIOLITIS

Bronchiolitis is usually caused by RSV, with a peak incidence at around 6 months of age. Affected children present with wheeze, tachypnoea, dyspnoea, cough and, when severe, cyanosis. The usual CXR pattern seen with bronchiolitis is overexpansion of the lungs due to bilateral air trapping. Severe cases may be complicated by atelectasis (Fig. 16.9). When bronchiolitis is recurrent or prolonged, underlying asthma or cystic fibrosis should be considered.

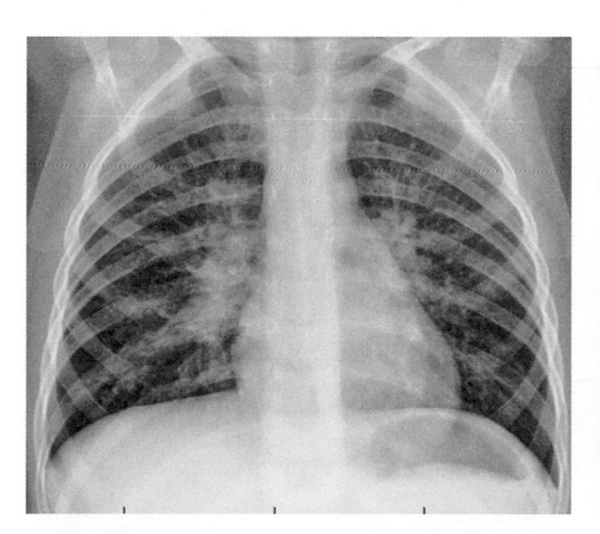

Figure 16.8 Viral lower respiratory tract infection. CXR in a 3-year-old girl shows bronchial wall thickening in the parahilar regions with no focal areas of airspace consolidation.

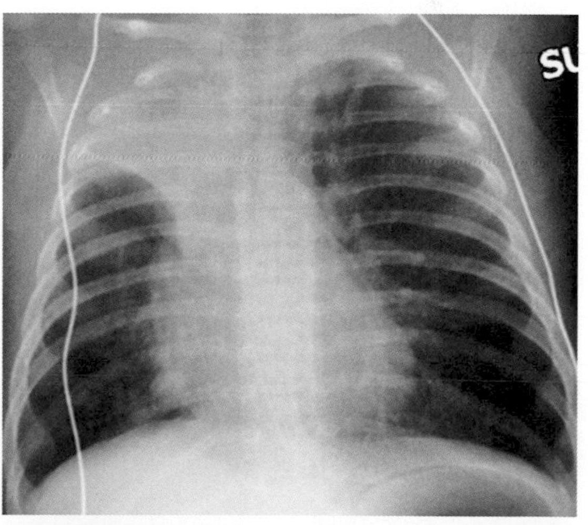

Figure 16.9 Bronchiolitis. CXR in a 3-month-old child with fever and respiratory distress shows overexpansion of the left lung with flattening of the left hemidiaphragm. There is complete collapse of the right upper lobe.

16.2.3 BACTERIAL INFECTION

Children with a bacterial pulmonary infection usually present with abrupt onset of malaise, fever and cough. The typical CXR pattern of bacterial infection is alveolar consolidation, i.e. fluffy opacity with air bronchograms, which may be lobar or patchy in distribution (see Chapter 4).

Round pneumonia is a common CXR pattern of early bacterial infection in children, appearing as a dense round opacity that may be mistaken for a mass (Fig. 16.10). The clinical setting of suspected infection (fever, cough, chest pain) should suggest the diagnosis. Follow-up CXR in 6–24 hours will usually show evolution of the round opacity to a more lobar pattern. Round pneumonia is much less common in adults.

Established cases of bacterial infection are usually easily diagnosed on CXR. Difficulties may arise with early infections, when the consolidation may be extremely subtle.

Overlying structures may obscure certain parts of the lung, so consolidation in these areas may be very difficult to see; in a febrile child with suspected chest infection particular attention should be given to the following review areas:

- Apical segments of the upper lobes, obscured by overlying ribs and clavicle
- Apical segments of the lower lobes, obscured by the hilar complexes
- Lung bases, obscured by the hemidiaphragms
- Left lower lobe, which lies behind the heart.

16.2.4 ASTHMA

Between acute attacks, the CXR of a child with asthma is often normal. 'Baseline changes' that may be seen include overexpanded lungs, thickening of bronchial walls most marked in the parahilar regions and focal scarring from previous infections. During acute asthma attacks the lungs are overinflated as a result of air trapping. Lobar or segmental collapse due to mucous plugging is common (Fig. 16.11). It is important to differentiate collapse from consolidation to avoid the unnecessary use of antibiotics. Other complications of asthma that may be diagnosed on CXR include pneumonia, pneumomediastinum and pneumothorax, and secondary aspergillosis.

16.2.5 CYSTIC FIBROSIS (MUCOVISCIDOSIS)

Cystic fibrosis is an autosomal recessive condition with dysfunction of the exocrine glands and reduced mucociliary function. Pulmonary manifestations are

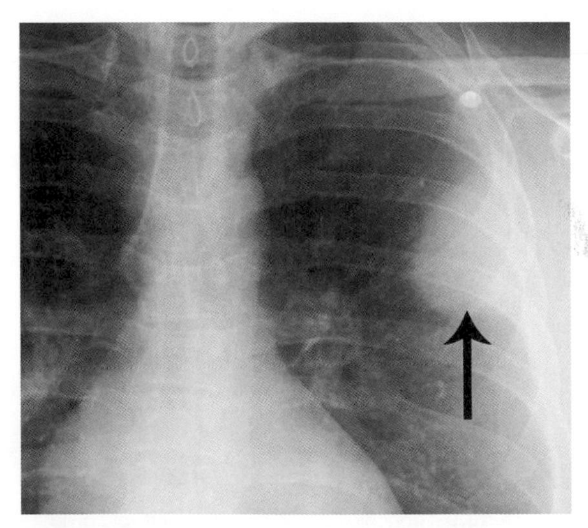

Figure 16.10 Round pneumonia. Round opacity with slightly blurred margins in the left upper lobe (arrow). This resolved rapidly with antibiotic therapy.

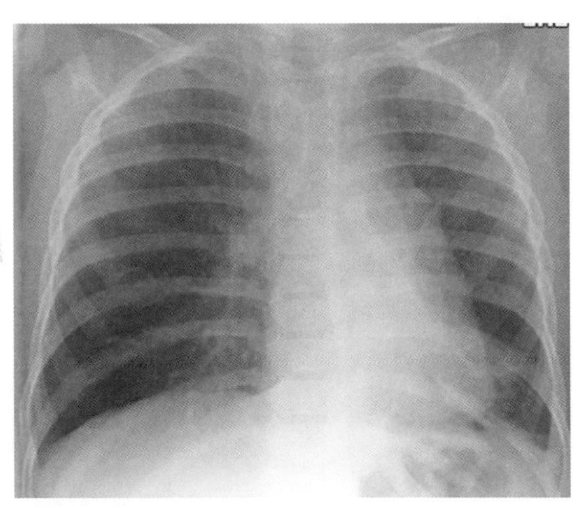

Figure 16.11 Asthma complicated by left lower lobe collapse. Note: reduced volume left lung, triangular opacity behind heart, loss of definition of left hemidiaphragm.

the most common and symptoms include recurrent infections and chronic wet cough. Pancreatic insufficiency leads to steatorrhoea and malabsorption, causing failure to thrive. Meconium ileus may be seen in infants (see section 16.6.5). Complications in older children include recurrent pancreatitis, biliary cirrhosis and meconium ileus equivalent, also known as distal intestinal obstruction syndrome (DIOS).

CXR changes associated with cystic fibrosis (Fig. 16.12):

- Overinflated lungs
- Thickened bronchial walls and bronchiectasis (dilated bronchi)
- Localized finger-like opacities due to mucoid impaction in dilated bronchi
- High incidence of pneumonia producing focal areas of consolidation
- Large pulmonary arteries due to pulmonary arterial hypertension.

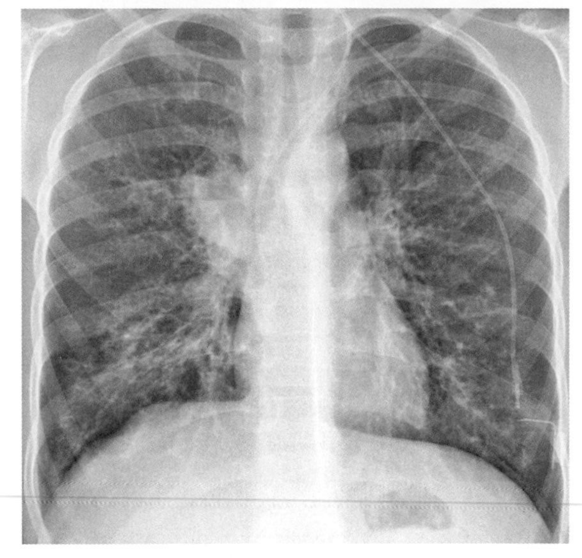

Figure 16.12 Cystic fibrosis. CXR in a 14-year-old girl shows overexpanded lungs with extensive linear densities due to bronchial wall thickening and mucous plugs. Prominence of the right hilum due to lymphadenopathy. Tunnelled central venous catheter inserted via the left internal jugular vein.

16.3 INVESTIGATION OF AN ABDOMINAL MASS

A child with an abdominal mass may present in several ways:

- Hydronephrosis and other congenital masses are frequently diagnosed on obstetric ultrasound (US)
- Detection of a congenital mass at birth by an attending paediatrician
- In older children, an abdominal mass may produce a visible bulge or may be felt by a parent
- Depending on the location there may be specific signs or symptoms, such as jaundice or intestinal obstruction.

Common causes of abdominal masses in children are as follows:

- Benign renal conditions:
  - Hydronephrosis
  - Multicystic dysplastic kidney (MCDK)
  - Polycystic syndromes
- Nephroblastoma (Wilms tumour)
- Neuroblastoma
- Hepatic:
  - Hepatoblastoma
  - Hepatocellular carcinoma
  - Haemangioendothelioma.

The roles of imaging for an abdominal mass are:

- Diagnosis of a mass
- Define the organ of origin
- Characterize margins: well defined or infiltrative
- Characterize contents: calcification, necrosis, cyst formation, fat
- Diagnose complications and evidence of malignancy:
  - Metastases
  - Lymphadenopathy
  - Invasion of surrounding structures
  - Vascular invasion
- Treatment planning
- Guidance of percutaneous biopsy or other interventional procedures, such as nephrostomy
- Follow-up: response to therapy, diagnosis of recurrent tumour.

16.3.1 ULTRASOUND

US is the initial investigation of choice in children for assessing the site of origin of a mass and as guidance for further investigations. Following confirmation of an abdominal mass and development of a differential diagnosis on US, further imaging with MRI, computed tomography (CT) or scintigraphy is usually required for more accurate definition and for staging in the case of malignancy.

16.3.2 MAGNETIC RESONANCE IMAGING AND COMPUTED TOMOGRAPHY

MRI has several advantages in children and, in many centres, is performed in preference to CT for the assessment of an abdominal mass:

- MRI uses no ionizing radiation
- In most cases, MRI provides better definition of relevant structures than CT because of superior soft-tissue definition.

Disadvantages of MRI compared with CT include:

- Relatively long scanning time requiring general anaesthesia in young children
- Inability to accurately image the lungs; CT of the chest is required for accurate staging of tumours that commonly metastasize to the lung.

In centres where MRI has limited availability, CT is used for imaging of abdominal masses in children. CT provides accurate characterization of an abdominal mass and its organ of origin and is highly sensitive for the presence of calcification and fat. The disadvantages of CT include use of ionizing radiation and iodinated contrast material.

A common protocol for the investigation and staging of malignancy in children is a non-contrast-enhanced CT of the chest for accurate assessment of the lungs followed by MRI of the abdomen. Depending on the layout of the medical imaging department this may be done under a single general anaesthetic in young children.

16.3.3 SCINTIGRAPHY

Renal scintigraphy complements US in the assessment of benign renal conditions that may present as an abdominal mass. Renal scanning with ^{99m}Tc-MAG3 or ^{99m}Tc-DTPA (see Table 1.1) provides physiological information, such as differential renal function and diuretic 'washout', as well as anatomical information, such as the level of obstruction (see Fig. 8.1).

Fluorodeoxyglucose (FDG)-positron emission tomography (PET)-CT is increasingly used in staging and follow-up of childhood malignancies. Other scintigraphy studies that may be used in the context of an abdominal mass include bone scintigraphy with ^{99m}Tc-MDP for suspected skeletal metastases and ^{123}I-MIBG in the staging of neuroblastoma (see Table 1.1).

16.3.4 NEPHROBLASTOMA (WILMS TUMOUR)

Nephroblastoma is the most commonly occurring solid intra-abdominal tumour in childhood. Most patients present between the ages of 1 and 5 with an asymptomatic renal mass, though there may be associated haematuria or abdominal pain. Fifteen per cent of nephroblastomas are associated with congenital anomalies, including aniridia in WAGR (Wilms tumour, aniridia, genitourinary abnormalities, range of developmental delays) syndrome, congenital hemihypertrophy and Beckwith–Wiedemann syndrome.

On US nephroblastoma appears as a hyperechoic mass with hypoechoic areas due to necrosis. The mass tends to replace renal parenchyma with progressive enlargement and distortion of the kidney. CT is still commonly used in initial staging rather than MRI, particularly in those patients who may undergo initial surgical management. In patients with more advanced disease who require initial medical management, MRI is the investigation of choice. MRI and CT show a renal mass and distortion of the kidney. The mass shows less intense contrast enhancement than functioning renal tissue. Features of nephroblastoma relevant to staging that can be seen on MRI and CT include lymphadenopathy, vascular invasion (renal vein and inferior vena cava [IVC]), invasion of surrounding structures and peritoneal metastases (Fig. 16.13). Chest CT is more accurate than CXR for the initial diagnosis of pulmonary metastases.

Multiple cancer research cooperative groups have studied the staging and treatment of Wilms tumour. Treatment options include surgery, chemotherapy and radiotherapy. Two staging systems are commonly used; they are based on whether surgery or chemotherapy is the first-line treatment. The National Wilms Tumour Study Group (NWTS) system is a five-stage system based on a surgery-first approach, whereas the Societé Internationale d'Oncologie Pédiatrique (SIOP) system is based on initial treatment with chemotherapy. Both systems are based on anatomy without reference to genetic or molecular markers. Further details of the NWTS and SIOP staging systems for Wilms tumour may be found on the companion website.

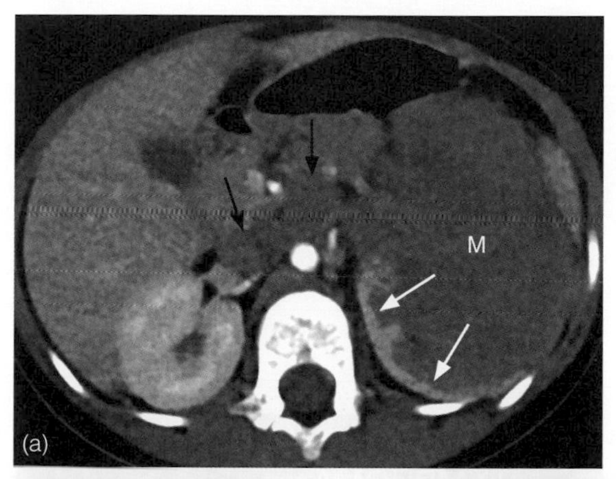

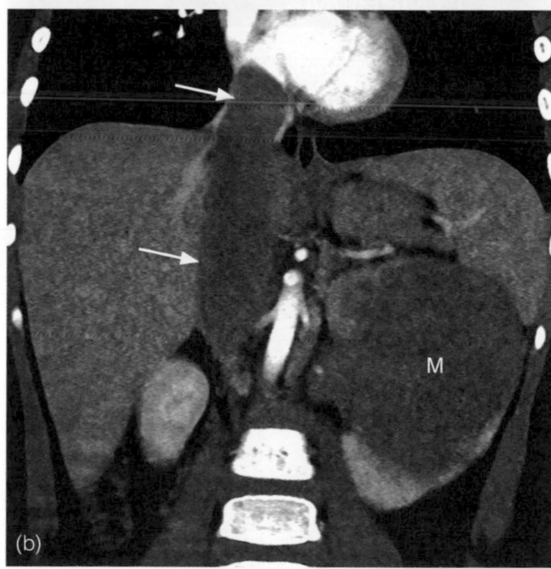

Figure 16.13 Wilms tumour: CT. (a) Transverse image shows a large mass (M) in the left abdomen. A thin rim of distorted peripheral renal tissue confirms that the mass is arising from the left kidney (white arrows). Tumour is also seen extending across the midline in the left renal vein into the inferior vena cava (IVC) (black arrows). (b) Coronal image shows the mass (M) and renal distortion. This image also shows tumour invading the IVC and extending superiorly into the right atrium (arrows).

16.3.5 NEUROBLASTOMA

Neuroblastoma is a malignant childhood tumour arising from primitive sympathetic neuroblasts of the embryonic neural crest. Sixty per cent occur in the abdomen; of these, two-thirds arise in the adrenal gland. Other common abdominal sites of origin of neuroblastoma are the periaortic sympathetic ganglia in the chest and abdomen and the ganglia at the aortic bifurcation. The peak age of incidence is 2 years, with most neuroblastomas occurring before the age of 5. A less common subgroup is congenital neuroblastoma, which occurs in the fetus or during the first neonatal month, and has a better prognosis because of its tendency to spontaneously regress.

US shows a mass with a heterogeneous texture due to areas of necrosis, haemorrhage and calcification. MRI (or CT) shows a heterogeneous mass with displacement or invasion of the kidney. Calcification is seen on CT in most cases. Neuroblastoma tends to spread across the midline, encasing or displacing the aorta. Other complications seen on MRI or CT include invasion of the surrounding structures, extension into the spine, lymphadenopathy and liver metastases (Fig. 16.14). Further staging is performed with chest CT for pulmonary metastases and bone scintigraphy with ^{99m}Tc-MDP. Scintigraphy with ^{123}I-MIBG may also be used for staging and to assess response to therapy in patients with advanced disease.

The staging of preoperative neuroblastoma has evolved over the last decade to a system that is highly reliant on imaging features. The International Neuroblastoma Risk Group Staging System

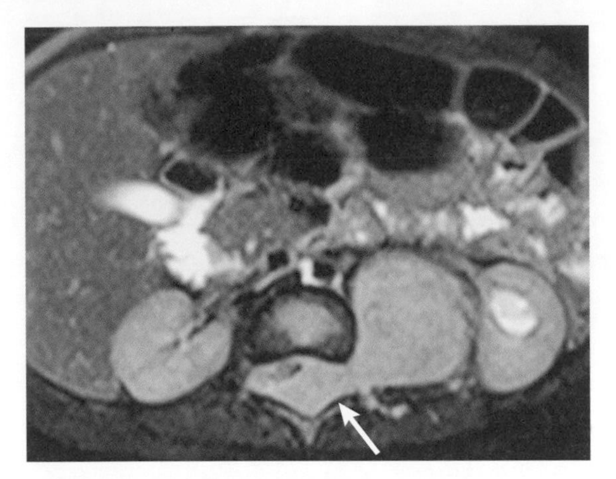

Figure 16.14 Neuroblastoma: MRI. Transverse T2-weighted fat-saturated image shows a tumour medial to the left kidney, displacing it laterally. Tumour can be seen invading the spinal canal (arrow).

(INRGSS) stages preoperative neuroblastoma into four groups based on multiple factors, including the presence of one or more specific image-defined risk factors (IDRFs). Over 20 IDRFs are defined and include extension between anatomical spaces (e.g. abdomen to chest), encasement of blood vessels or nerves, tracheobronchial compression and invasion or infiltration of structures (e.g. the spinal canal or skull base). A full list of IDRFs and details of INRGSS staging of preoperative neuroblastoma may be found on the companion website.

16.3.6 HEPATOBLASTOMA

Hepatoblastoma is the most common hepatic tumour in children. Hepatoblastoma has an increased incidence in Beckwith–Wiedemann syndrome, hemihypertrophy and biliary atresia. There is no association with cirrhosis. Most hepatoblastomas occur under the age of 3 years. α-Fetoprotein is elevated in most cases. US of hepatoblastoma shows a well-circumscribed mass of higher echogenicity than surrounding liver. MRI or CT shows a hepatic mass with areas of necrosis, calcification, and occasionally fat. Hepatoblastoma may be complicated by vascular invasion, seen on MRI or CT as a filling defect within an enlarged portal vein, hepatic vein or IVC.

16.3.7 HEPATOCELLULAR CARCINOMA

Hepatocellular carcinoma is uncommon in children, with an increased incidence in chronic liver diseases, such as cirrhosis, biliary atresia or tyrosinaemia. US shows an ill-defined hypoechoic mass in the liver. MRI or CT may show a solitary hepatic mass or multiple confluent masses.

16.3.8 HAEMANGIOENDOTHELIOMA

Haemangioendothelioma is a highly vascular, benign, multicentric liver tumour that may be associated with cutaneous haemangiomas. It usually presents in infancy with hepatomegaly, cardiac failure or acute haemorrhage. US shows multiple discrete hyperechoic masses in the liver. MRI or CT shows multiple hepatic masses with occasional calcification.

16.4 LEUKAEMIA AND LYMPHOMA

The three most common types of malignancy in children are leukaemia (33%), CNS tumours (25%) and lymphomas (10%). Leukaemia and lymphoma are classified according to the 2016 World Health Organization (WHO) classification of tumours of haematopoietic and lymphoid tissues. These malignancies also occur in adults and many of the comments below may be applied to older patients.

16.4.1 LEUKAEMIA

Leukaemia is a group of haematological neoplasms characterized by excess production of abnormally differentiated haematopoietic cells or immature lymphoblasts. These cells reside in the bone marrow and often in the peripheral circulation. The classification of leukaemia is complex and includes many uncommon subtypes. Modern categorization is more focused on molecular features, which guide specific therapies. The most common types are classified on two features:

1. Degree of proliferation and differentiation of abnormal cells and an associated reduction

in normal blood cells and platelets: acute or chronic
2. Type of cell lineage: lymphoblastic or myeloid.

Acute lymphoblastic leukaemia (ALL) is the most common type in children, followed by acute myeloid leukaemia (AML). Chronic myeloid leukaemia (CML) is uncommon in children and chronic lymphocytic leukaemia (CLL) is almost exclusively a disease of older adults.

The main role for imaging in childhood leukaemia is the assessment of treatment complications (see section 16.4.3). Imaging may also be used in certain instances where leukaemia is associated with specific presentations, e.g. neurological symptoms from intradural spinal disease or cough and shortness of breath as a result of pulmonary leukaemic infiltrates.

16.4.2 LYMPHOMA

Lymphoma is a group of malignancies arising from lymphocytes (B, T and natural killer [NK]) and lymphoblasts. Although the classification of lymphoma is complex, the principal division is into Hodgkin lymphoma (HL) and non-Hodgkin lymphoma (NHL). HL is characterized by the presence of Reed–Sternberg cells and is common in children, usually presenting with lymphadenopathy. Burkitt lymphoma is the most common type of NHL in children. NHL may present with nodal or extranodal disease that can occur virtually anywhere in the body.

All imaging modalities may be used in lymphoma depending on the type and site of clinical presentation. HL, Burkitt lymphoma and most other types of NHL are staged with FDG-PET-CT; this modality is also used for the assessment of response to therapy and restaging (see Fig. 1.13). The Lugano staging classification is the most widely used system. The designation of limited and advanced disease is based on imaging and clinical factors, including:

- Extent of nodal and extranodal disease
- Presence of disease on one or both sides of the diaphragm
- Involvement of the spleen
- Absence (A) or presence (B) of systemic symptoms: fever, night sweats, unexplained weight loss.

Further details of the Lugano staging classification of lymphoma may be found on the companion website.

16.4.3 TREATMENT-RELATED COMPLICATIONS

Complications related to treatment of malignancy are many and varied. Some common complications are related directly to therapy at specific sites, e.g. radiation-induced pneumonitis or white matter disease due to radiotherapy and/or chemotherapy. Chemotherapeutic agents may cause toxicities in multiple organs, including heart, lung and brain. A particular consideration in the treatment of leukaemia and lymphoma is immunosuppression. This may result from chemotherapeutic regimes or steroid therapy. Haematopoietic stem cell transplant (HSCT) is commonly used both as a primary treatment and to replace bone marrow function, which is destroyed by other therapies. HSCT may be associated with prolonged neutropenia, leading to various opportunistic infections and non-infectious inflammatory conditions, including:

- *Pneumocystis jiroveci* pneumonia (PJP) (Fig. 16.15)
- Invasive aspergillosis: lungs, paranasal sinuses, brain

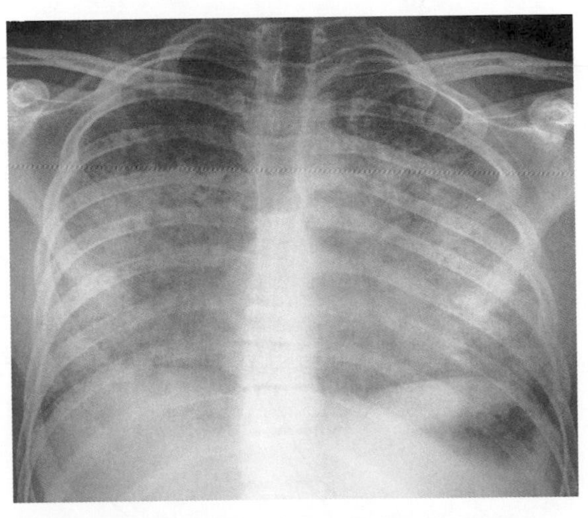

Figure 16.15 Pneumocystis pneumonia: CXR. Dry cough and shortness of breath in an immunosuppressed 15-year-old girl following bone marrow transplant. Note the extensive bilateral alveolar opacification.

- Candidiasis: lungs, oesophagus
- Tuberculosis (TB): chest, abdomen, skeleton
- Neutropenic colitis.

Imaging assessment of treatment-related complications depends on the clinical presentation and includes a range of investigations: MRI of the brain and CT of the paranasal sinuses, chest and abdomen.

16.5 URINARY TRACT DISORDERS IN CHILDREN

16.5.1 URINARY TRACT INFECTION

Urinary tract infection (UTI) is one of the most common indications for imaging in paediatrics. UTI is more common in young children. UTI in infants occurs with equal incidence in boys and girls and usually presents with signs of generalized sepsis, including fever, vomiting and anorexia. In children older than 1 year UTI is more common in girls. Clinical presentation in preadolescent children is usually more specific for UTI with fever, frequency and dysuria. Flank pain may indicate pyelonephritis. Most UTIs in children are caused by Gram-negative bacteria, most commonly *Escherichia coli*.

Roles of imaging in the investigation of a child with UTI:

- Diagnose underlying urinary tract abnormalities, e.g. hydronephrosis, posterior urethral valves
- Diagnose and grade vesicoureteric reflux (VUR)
- Differentiate cystitis (UTI confined to the bladder) from pyelonephritis (UTI involving one or both kidneys)
- Document renal damage
- Establish a baseline for subsequent evaluation of renal growth
- Establish prognosis and guide management.

ULTRASOUND

US of the renal tract is the initial investigation of choice for children with UTI. US is performed to detect abnormalities of the urinary tract that may predispose the child to the development of recurrent UTI. Most children with uncomplicated UTI have a normal US examination; in most of these cases, no further imaging is required. In patients in whom US is abnormal, the more common findings include hydronephrosis, neurogenic bladder (usually associated with congenital neurological abnormalities such as spina bifida) and renal duplex. Depending on the results of US as well as the clinical situation, further imaging may be performed to diagnose VUR, document renal function and diagnose renal scars.

MICTURATING CYSTOURETHROGRAM

A micturating cystourethrogram (MCU), also known as a voiding cystourethrogram (VCU), is performed primarily to diagnose VUR and grade its severity as follows (Fig. 16.16):

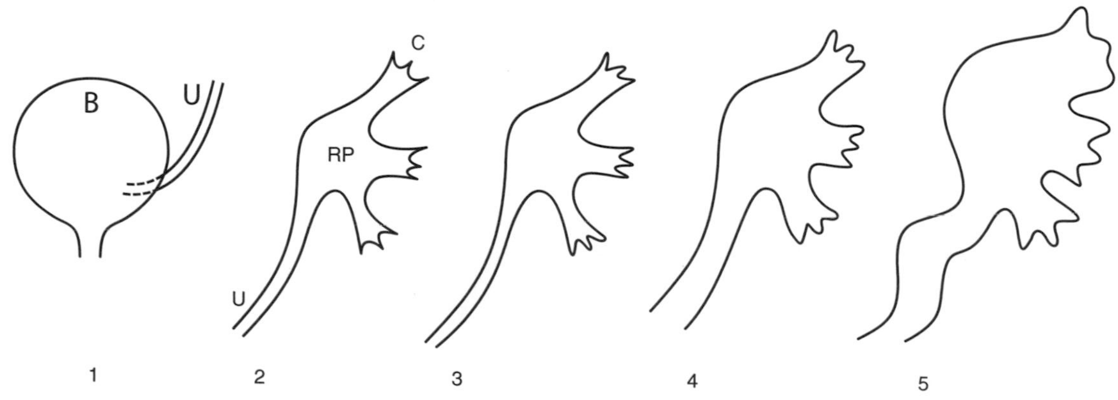

Figure 16.16 Schematic diagram illustrating the five grades of vesicoureteric reflux (VUR). For orientation, note the following labels: bladder (B), calyces (C), renal pelvis (RP), ureter (U).

- Grade 1: reflux into a non-dilated ureter
- Grade 2: reflux into a non-dilated collecting system
- Grade 3: reflux into a mildly dilated collecting system (Fig. 16.17)
- Grade 4: reflux into a moderately dilated collecting system
- Grade 5: reflux into a grossly dilated collecting system with a dilated, tortuous ureter.

MCU may be performed radiographically or with scintigraphy; both methods involve catheterization of the child. Radiographic MCU provides more precise anatomical imaging of the urinary tract, including the urethra, and may therefore be helpful in diagnosing underlying anomalies such as posterior urethral valves in males. When moderate to severe VUR is diagnosed, or in the presence of underlying urinary tract anomalies, further imaging assessment with scintigraphy may be required.

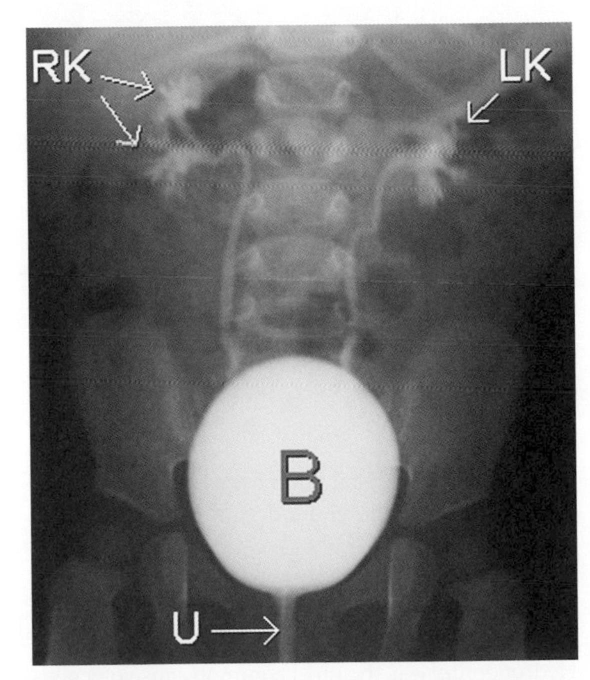

Figure 16.17 Vesicoureteric reflux (VUR). Micturating cystourethrogram in an infant girl shows contrast material filling the bladder (B) and outlining the urethra (U). There is bilateral grade 3 VUR. Note the reduced number of calyces on the left (LK) compared with the right (RK), indicating reflux into the lower moiety of a duplex collecting system.

SCINTIGRAPHY

Scintigraphy with ^{99m}Tc-MAG3 or ^{99m}Tc-DTPA may be performed to differentiate obstructive from non-obstructive hydronephrosis and to quantify the differential renal function. The differential renal function is expressed as the percentage of overall renal function contributed by each kidney.

Scintigraphy with ^{99m}Tc-DMSA (see Table 1.1) is much more sensitive than US for the documentation of renal scars. DMSA is taken up by cells of the proximal convoluted tubule and retained in the renal cortex. Cortical scars show on DMSA scans as focal areas of reduced tracer uptake, with irregularity of the outline of the kidney. DMSA scans are also used to diagnose pyelonephritis, which is seen as focal areas of reduced tracer uptake in an acutely febrile child.

GUIDELINES FOR IMAGING CHILDREN WITH URINARY TRACT INFECTION

In most cases, imaging is not required following a single UTI in children older than 1 year. Indications for imaging in UTI include:

- Any UTI under 1 year of age
- Recurrent UTI
- Atypical organism, e.g. *S. aureus*
- Bacteraemia
- Lack of response to antibiotics
- Abdominal mass
- Renal impairment and electrolyte derangement
- Abnormal voiding.

Recommendations may also be made as to the use of the various imaging modalities:

- US as the first-line investigation in all:
  - MAG3 scan if obstruction suspected on US
- MCU for children younger than 1 year, especially when US shows hydronephrosis
- DMSA for young boys and recurrent UTI in others:
  - May also be used to make the specific diagnosis of pyelonephritis if this will alter management
- More aggressive investigation for recurrent or complicated cases.

16.5.2 RENAL DUPLEX

Renal duplex is a single kidney with two separate collecting systems. (The term 'renal duplication' should be reserved for patients with two separate kidneys on one side.) The part of the kidney drained by each collecting system of a duplex kidney is referred to as a moiety. The term 'duplex kidney' refers to a range of anomalies, including a bifid renal pelvis, two separate ureters that unite above the bladder or two ureters that drain separately into the bladder (complete ureteric duplication).

With complete ureteric duplication the ureter draining the upper moiety usually inserts inferior and medial to the ureter from the lower moiety (Weigert–Meyer rule) (Fig. 16.18). The upper moiety ureter may enter the inferior bladder or may have an ectopic insertion. Possible sites of ectopic ureteric insertion include the bladder neck, urethra, vagina or perineum in females and the prostatic urethra and ejaculatory system in males. Regardless of the site of insertion, the upper moiety ureter is prone to obstruction. Ureterocele may also complicate the bladder or ectopic insertion of the upper moiety ureter (Fig. 16.19). Ureterocele is a cyst-like expansion of the distal end of the ureter projecting into the bladder. The ureter draining the lower moiety is prone to VUR.

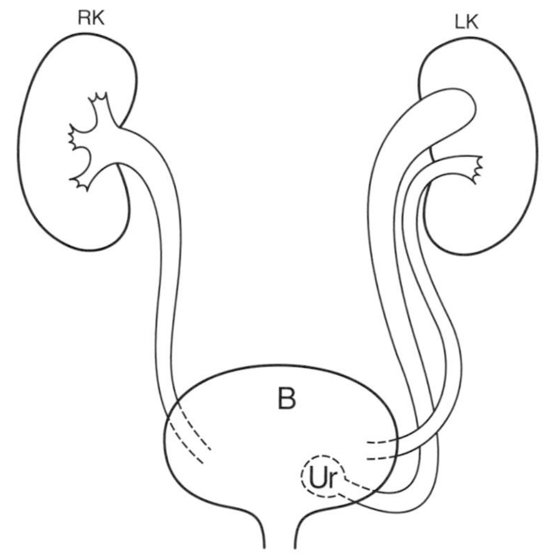

Figure 16.18 Schematic diagram illustrating the potential problems of a duplex renal collecting system. For orientation, note the right kidney (RK), left kidney (LK) and bladder (B). The ureter from the upper moiety implants lower than that from the lower moiety and is sometimes complicated by ureterocele (Ur) and obstruction. The ureter from the lower moiety implants higher and is prone to reflux.

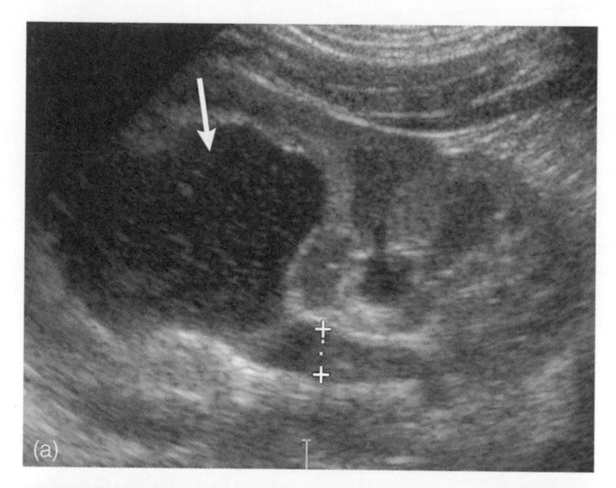

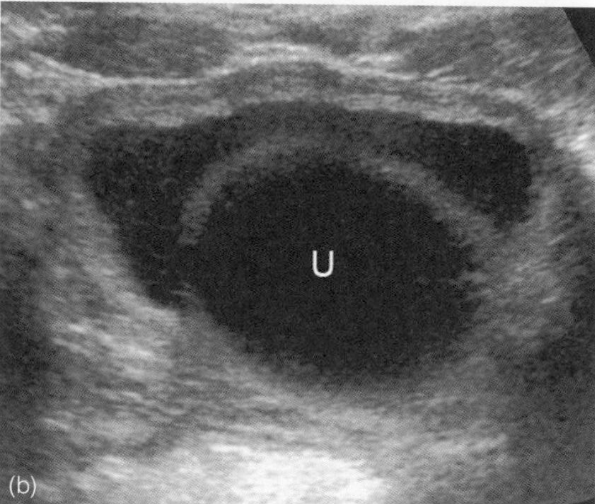

Figure 16.19 Duplex collecting system: US. (a) Longitudinal image of the kidney shows a dilated upper moiety collecting system (arrow), a dilated upper moiety ureter (+) and a normal lower moiety. (b) Transverse image of the bladder shows a ureterocele (U) at the insertion of the upper pole ureter.

16.5.3 HYDRONEPHROSIS

Hydronephrosis is the most common cause of a neonatal abdominal mass. Hydronephrosis may also present with UTI or may be detected on prenatal (obstetric) screening US. Widespread use of obstetric US screening has led to a significantly increased incidence of prenatal diagnosis of hydronephrosis.

Common causes of hydronephrosis in children include:

- Pelviureteric junction (PUJ) obstruction
- Vesicoureteric junction (VUJ) obstruction
- VUR
- Primary megaureter
- Duplex kidney with obstruction of the upper pole moiety ureter.

The roles of imaging of hydronephrosis are to:

- Document the severity of urinary tract dilatation
- Differentiate obstructive from non-obstructive causes
- Define the level of obstruction
- Diagnose underlying anatomical anomalies.

ULTRASOUND

US is the initial imaging modality of choice in the investigation of hydronephrosis.

Signs of hydronephrosis on US include:

- Dilated renal pelvis and calyces
- Underlying anomalies such as ureterocele or a duplex collecting system
- PUJ obstruction: round, dilated renal pelvis (Fig. 16.20)
- VUJ obstruction: dilated ureter can be followed down to the bladder
- Chronic hydronephrosis may cause thinning of the renal cortex.

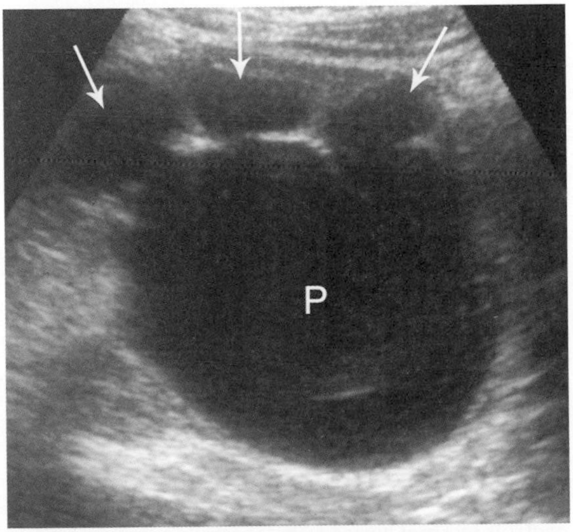

Figure 16.20 Hydronephrosis due to pelviureteric junction (PUJ) obstruction: US. Longitudinal image shows a markedly dilated renal pelvis (P) communicating with dilated calyces (arrows).

SCINTIGRAPHY

Diuretic scintigraphy with ^{99m}Tc-MAG3 or ^{99m}Tc-DTPA is used to differentiate mechanical urinary tract obstruction from non-obstructive causes of hydronephrosis. Furosemide is injected after the renal collecting system is filled with isotope. The rate of 'washout' of isotope is then assessed. With mechanical obstruction such as PUJ obstruction, isotope continues to accumulate in the collecting system following diuretic injection (see Fig. 8.1). Isotope is rapidly washed out of the dilated collecting system in cases of non-obstructive hydronephrosis, such as VUR. Scintigraphy is also used to quantify differential renal function and to show the level of obstruction at either the PUJ or VUJ. VUR is suspected when scintigraphy shows a non-obstructive hydronephrosis. In such cases, MCU may be indicated to confirm and grade VUR.

16.5.4 MULTICYSTIC DYSPLASTIC KIDNEY

MCDK is replacement of the kidney with multiple cysts of varying size with absence of the ipsilateral ureter and hypoplasia of the ipsilateral renal artery. There is associated congenital abnormality of the contralateral kidney in 30% of cases – usually PUJ obstruction. The natural history of MCDK is involution; many adults diagnosed with a solitary kidney were probably born with MCDK. Bilateral MCDK is incompatible with life.

US is the investigation of choice for suspected MCDK. US shows that the kidney has been replaced by a lobulated collection of variably sized non-communicating cysts (Fig. 16.21). MCDK is often diagnosed prenatally on obstetric US (see Fig. 15.6). Scintigraphy with ^{99m}Tc-MAG3 or ^{99m}Tc-DTPA may be used to confirm MCDK by showing the absence of renal function on the affected side.

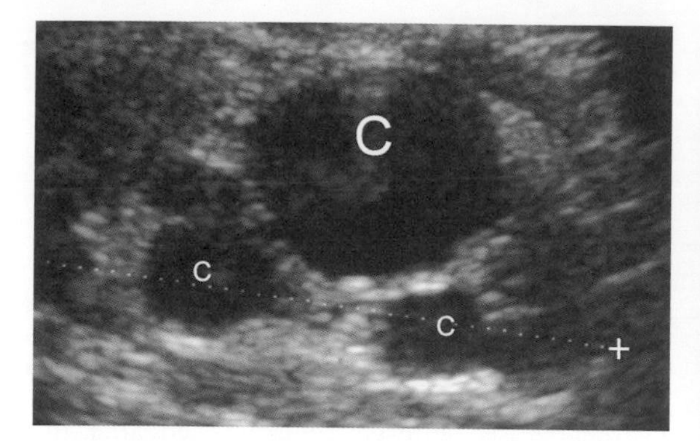

Figure 16.21 Multicystic dysplastic kidney (MCDK): US. Longitudinal image of the left kidney replaced by a collection of non-communicating cysts (C).

16.5.5 POLYCYSTIC RENAL CONDITIONS

Polycystic renal conditions are classified according to genetic inheritance, pathological findings and clinical presentation.

Autosomal recessive polycystic kidney disease (ARPKD) refers to a spectrum of disorders with associated liver disease. Infantile and juvenile forms are described. In the infantile form, renal disease tends to be more severe, with less hepatic involvement and higher mortality; in the juvenile form, liver disease is the dominant feature. US in ARPKD shows symmetrically enlarged hyperechoic kidneys (Fig. 16.22).

Autosomal dominant polycystic kidney disease (ADPKD) usually presents in middle age with enlarged kidneys and hypertension. US in adults with ADPKD shows enlarged kidneys containing multiple cysts of varying size. ADPKD may occasionally present in childhood with bilateral enlarged kidneys, which may be asymmetrical. On US examination, the kidneys are of increased echogenicity owing to multiple cysts that are too tiny to be seen individually. Occasionally, separate small anechoic cysts are seen.

Various hereditary syndromes, including tuberous sclerosis and von Hippel–Lindau disease, may be associated with renal cysts.

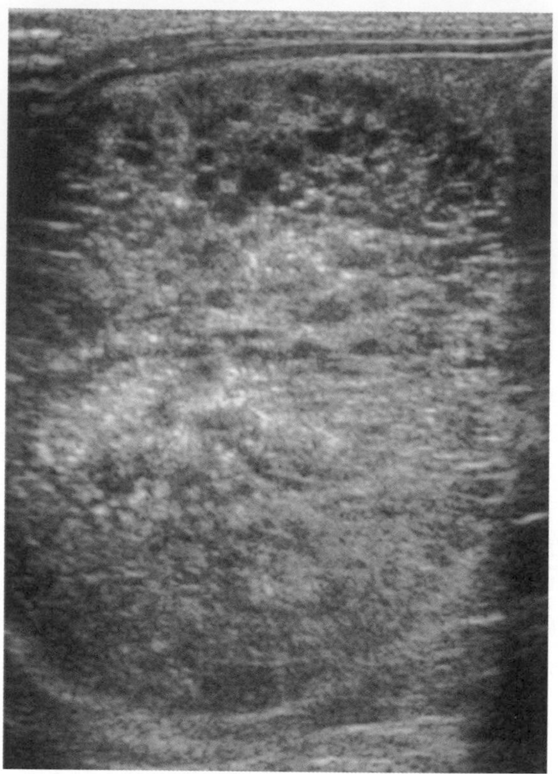

Figure 16.22 Autosomal recessive polycystic kidney disease (ARPKD). US in a 3-day-old girl shows marked enlargement of the kidneys. Transverse view of the kidney shows loss of the normal parenchymal pattern and innumerable tiny cysts.

16.6 NEONATAL GUT OBSTRUCTION AND/OR BILE-STAINED VOMITING

Neonatal gut obstruction with or without bile-stained vomiting is a common clinical problem with a wide differential diagnosis. Historically, abdomen radiograph (abdomen X-ray, AXR) is the investigation of choice for most neonates with suspected gut obstruction. For some causes, such as duodenal obstruction, AXR alone may be sufficient for diagnosis. In other conditions, such as malrotation, the AXR may be normal. Contrast studies, such as upper gastrointestinal series and contrast enema, are often required for the diagnosis of neonatal gut obstruction, particularly malrotation and large bowel disorders.

16.6.1 DUODENAL OBSTRUCTION

The causes of congenital duodenal obstruction include:

- Duodenal atresia: most common
- Duodenal stenosis or web
- Annular pancreas: rare congenital anomaly whereby pancreatic tissue encircles and constricts the second part of the duodenum.

Thirty per cent of patients with duodenal atresia have Down syndrome. Anomalies that may be associated with duodenal atresia include oesophageal atresia, imperforate anus, renal anomalies and congenital heart disease. Duodenal atresia may be diagnosed on prenatal US with visualization of a fluid-filled 'double bubble' in the fetal abdomen due to a dilated stomach and duodenal cap.

Signs of duodenal atresia on AXR (Fig. 16.23):

- Classic 'double bubble' sign due to gas in the distended stomach and duodenal cap
- Absence of gas in the distal bowel
- Occasionally, gas in the gallbladder may produce a third bubble.

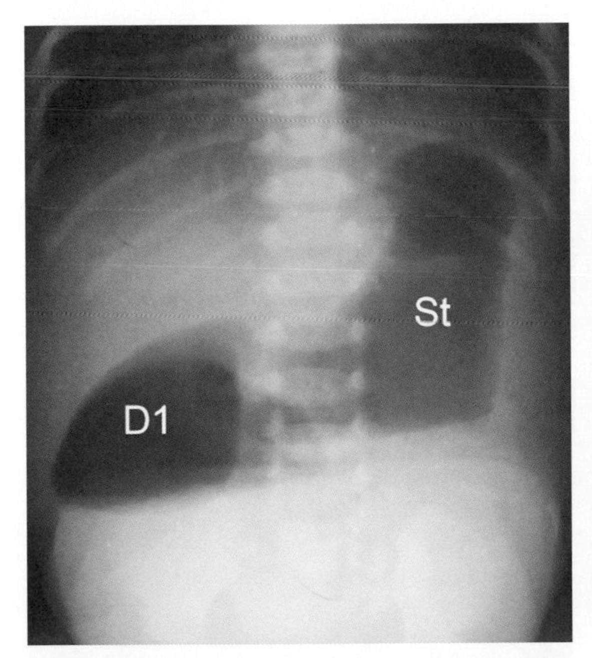

Figure 16.23 Duodenal atresia. AXR shows the characteristic 'double bubble' due to gas filling the stomach (St) and first part of the duodenum (D1). Gas is unable to pass more distally due to atresia of the second part of the duodenum.

16.6.2 SMALL BOWEL ATRESIA

Atresia of the small bowel most commonly occurs in the proximal jejunum. AXR shows a few dilated small bowel loops in the left upper quadrant and absent bowel gas distally. Occasionally, because of small bowel perforation, widespread abdominal calcification due to meconium peritonitis may be seen.

16.6.3 ANAL ATRESIA (IMPERFORATE ANUS)

The absence of an anus indicates anal atresia, which is classified as either a low or a high anomaly. The key anatomical feature in the classification of anal atresia is the levator sling:

- Low anomaly: bowel ends below the levator sling
- High anomaly: bowel ends above the levator sling; this is usually associated with a fistula into the vagina or posterior urethra.

Lateral and frontal abdominal radiographs are performed to classify anal atresia by assessing the relationship of the most distal part of the bowel to the pelvic floor (Fig. 16.24). Gas in the bladder or

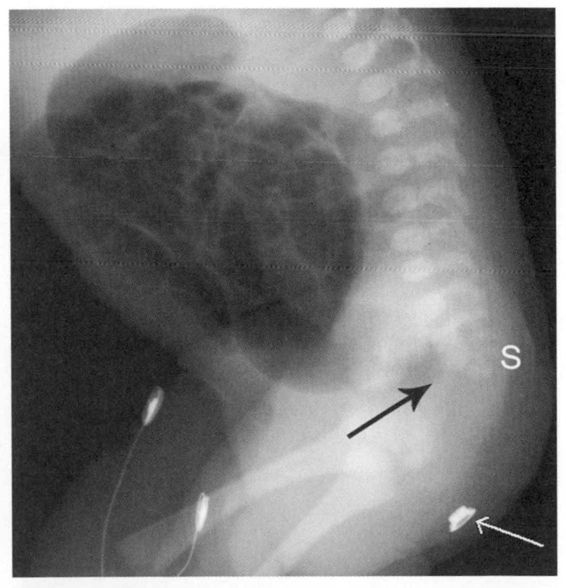

Figure 16.24 Anorectal atresia. Lateral radiograph showing the high termination of the distal large bowel (black arrow), marker placed on the perineum (white arrow) and failure of formation of the distal sacral segments (S).

vagina indicates the presence of a fistula. Associated sacral anomalies may also be seen, including failure of sacral segmentation or sacral agenesis. US of the perineum may be used to determine the distance between the anal dimple on the perineal surface and the distal bowel end and thus aid in surgical planning.

16.6.4 HIRSCHSPRUNG DISEASE

Hirschsprung disease refers to an aganglionic segment of distal large bowel. Distal colonic aganglionosis occurs during embryological development as a result of the arrest of normal craniocaudal migration of neuroblasts. The most common form of Hirschsprung disease is a short distal aganglionic segment, which causes distal large bowel obstruction. Normally innervated bowel proximal to the aganglionic segment is dilated. Hirschsprung disease usually presents in neonates with failure to pass meconium in the first 48 hours of life. In older children it may be a cause of chronic constipation.

AXR in Hirschsprung disease may show dilated bowel loops (Fig. 16.25). Contrast enema is definitive when it shows an abrupt transition from a narrow distal aganglionic segment to dilated normally innervated bowel. Total colonic aganglionosis occurs in 5% of cases; this may be very difficult to diagnose with imaging because of a lack of a transition point. Diagnosis of Hirschsprung disease is confirmed with biopsy.

16.6.5 MECONIUM ILEUS

Meconium ileus is due to viscous meconium impaction within the distal ileum and occurs in association with cystic fibrosis. Obstetric US may show polyhydramnios and hyperechoic contents in fetal small bowel.

Signs of meconium ileus on AXR (Fig. 16.26):

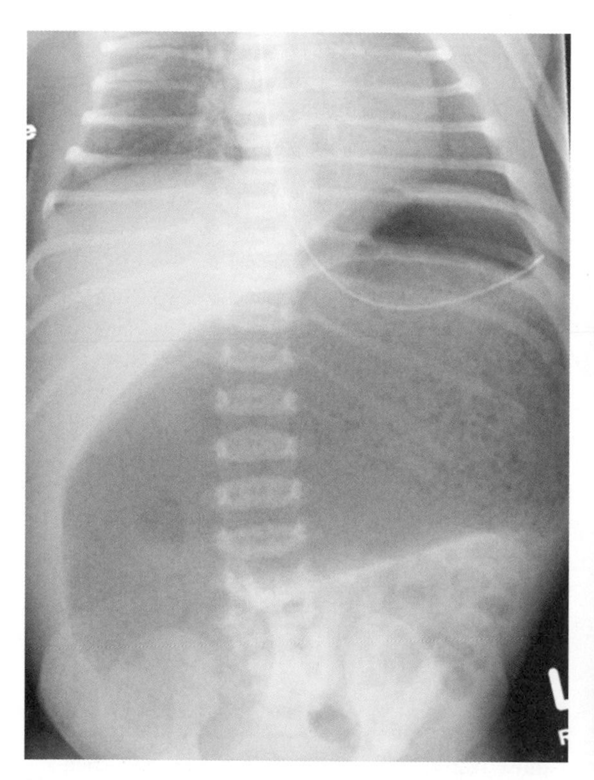

Figure 16.25 Hirschsprung disease. AXR in an infant with abdominal distension shows marked dilatation of the transverse colon. The stomach can be seen pushed upwards with a nasogastric tube *in situ*.

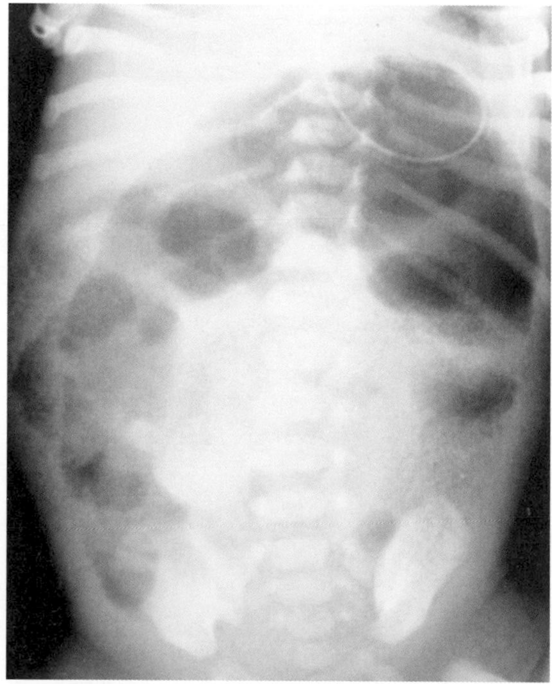

Figure 16.26 Meconium ileus. AXR shows distended large bowel with a characteristic 'soap bubble' appearance on both sides of the abdomen.

- 'Soap bubble' appearance in the right lower quadrant due to complex retained meconium in the distal small bowel
- Dilated small bowel loops of variable calibre with no fluid levels on the erect view.

Contrast enema shows a small colon (microcolon) plus a large distal ileum with filling defects due to meconium. Contrast enema may be therapeutic in that it may disimpact the viscous meconium.

16.6.6 MECONIUM PLUG SYNDROME

Meconium plug syndrome refers to inspissated meconium causing distal large bowel obstruction. It is not related pathologically to meconium ileus. AXR usually shows non-specific dilated small bowel loops. Contrast enema shows a dilated rectum with large filling defects in the colon and is often therapeutic.

16.6.7 MALROTATION AND MIDGUT VOLVULUS

Small and large bowel from the second part of the duodenum to the distal transverse colon are formed from the embryological midgut in several stages:

- Up to the sixth week of gestation: the midgut lies within the abdominal cavity
- From the sixth to the 10th week of gestation: the midgut develops outside the abdominal cavity (physiological herniation)
- During the 10th week of gestation: the midgut returns to the abdominal cavity.

During these various stages of embryological development, the midgut rotates through 270°. This rotation produces the final normal orientation of the small bowel mesentery and bowel loops:

- Junction of the fourth part of the duodenum with the jejunum (duodenojejunal flexure) lies to the left of the midline
- Proximal small bowel loops lie to the left
- Caecum lies in the right lower quadrant.

Malrotation refers to a wide spectrum of anatomical variants, the common feature being abnormal rotation of the midgut. Anatomical variations seen with malrotation include:

- Duodenojejunal flexure in an abnormal position, usually to the right of the midline (key feature)
- Colon to the left of the midline
- Caecum in the left upper quadrant
- Transverse colon lying posterior to the superior mesenteric artery
- Peritoneal (Ladd) bands: fibrous bands that cross the duodenum and may cause compression
- Internal paraduodenal hernia
- Shortened small bowel mesenteric attachment.

The anatomical variations seen in malrotation may produce clinically significant complications, including volvulus of the small bowel and duodenum and intestinal obstruction due to Ladd bands or paraduodenal hernia. These complications lead to two types of clinical presentation:

1. Common: severe bile-stained vomiting in neonates
2. Uncommon: intermittent vomiting, nausea and abdominal pain in older children.

Imaging investigation of suspected malrotation consists of a contrast study of the upper gastrointestinal tract (GIT), and occasionally AXR. AXR in a child with malrotation is often normal, particularly if performed when the child is asymptomatic. In the symptomatic child, AXR may show non-specific signs, such as dilatation of the duodenum. Upper GIT contrast study is usually definitive in the diagnosis or exclusion of malrotation. The key finding in malrotation is malposition of the duodenojejunal junction to the right or in the midline. As well as examining the upper GIT, contrast material may be followed through the small bowel to the caecum and colon. Other signs of malrotation that may be seen on the contrast study include (Fig. 16.27):

- Duodenal obstruction
- Proximal jejunum lying in the right abdomen
- 'Corkscrew' appearance of small bowel loops
- Abnormally high caecum on follow-through films.

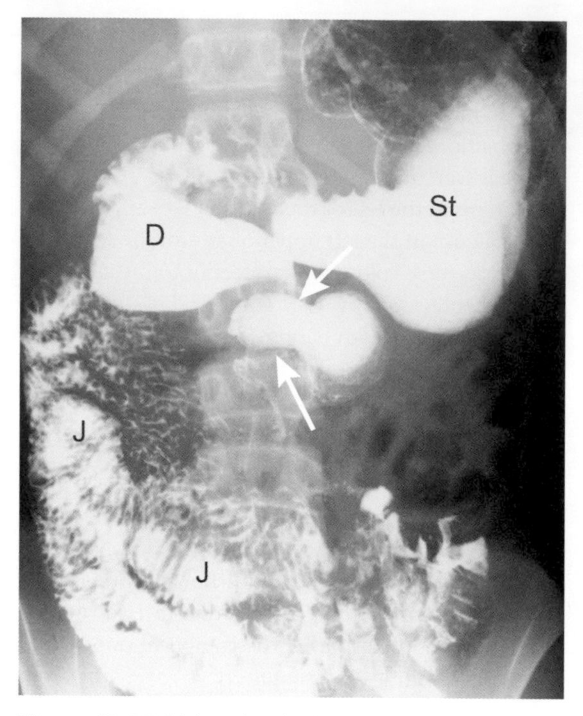

Figure 16.27 Malrotation: barium study. Note: normally located stomach (St), duodenum (D) does not pass across the midline to the left, 'corkscrew' configuration of the proximal small bowel (arrows), jejunum (J) located abnormally on the right.

16.7 OTHER GASTROINTESTINAL TRACT DISORDERS IN CHILDREN

16.7.1 OESOPHAGEAL ATRESIA AND TRACHEO-OESOPHAGEAL FISTULA

During early embryological development the foregut develops into a ventral respiratory component (lungs and trachea) and a dorsal digestive component (oesophagus and stomach). Congenital foregut malformations due to failure of complete separation of the dorsal and ventral foregut components occur in 1:3000 live births. Congenital foregut malformations are classified as shown in Fig. 16.28. With the widespread use of obstetric US, oesophageal atresia and tracheo-oesophageal fistula (TOF) may be suspected prenatally. Findings on obstetric US may include polyhydramnios and the absence of a normal fluid-filled fetal stomach.

Most cases of oesophageal atresia and TOF may be diagnosed with radiographs (CXR and AXR) of the neonate. Radiographic findings depend on the type of malformation (Fig. 16.29):

- Air in a blind-ending upper oesophageal pouch posterior to the trachea, best seen on a lateral view
- Nasogastric tube curled in a pouch
- Air in the GIT implies a distal fistula

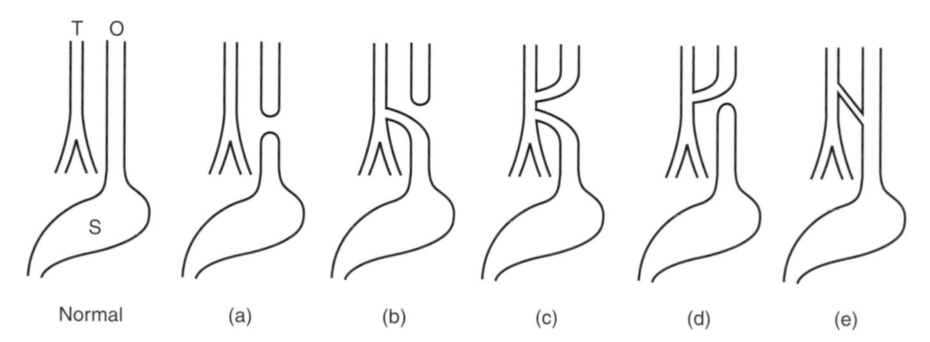

Figure 16.28 Schematic diagram illustrating the classification and relative incidences of oesophageal atresia and tracheo-oesophageal fistula (TOF). Note the normal orientation of the trachea (T), oesophagus (O) and stomach (St). (a) Oesophageal atresia with no fistula: 9%. (b) Oesophageal atresia with distal fistula: 82%. (c) Oesophageal atresia with proximal and distal fistulae: 2%. (d) Oesophageal atresia with proximal fistula: 1%. (e) Fistula without oesophageal atresia ('H'-type fistula): 6%.

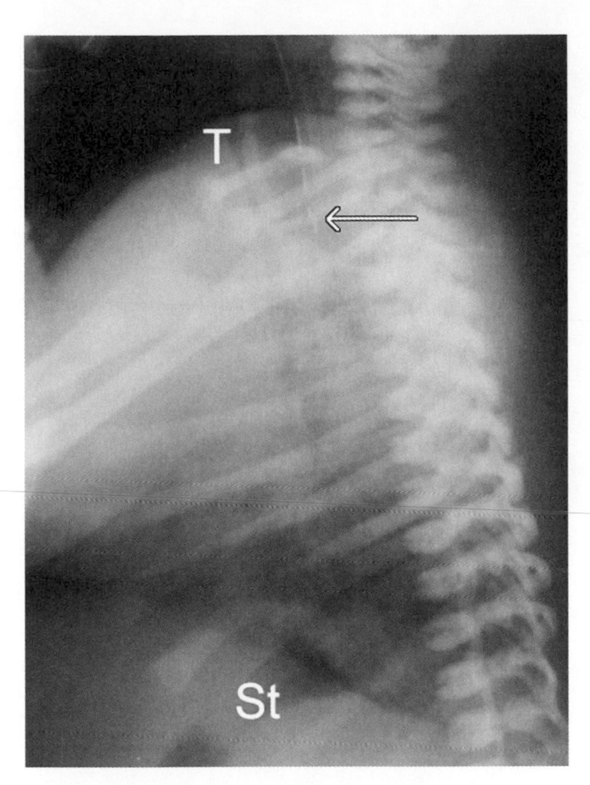

Figure 16.29 Oesophageal atresia and tracheo-oesophageal fistula (TOF). Lateral view shows a nasogastric tube in the blind-ending upper oesophageal segment (arrow). Gas in the stomach (St) indicates the presence of a fistula from the trachea to the distal oesophagus. Also note that the trachea (T) is narrowed as a result of tracheomalacia, which is commonly associated with oesophageal atresia.

- Gasless abdomen is seen with oesophageal atresia without fistula, or a proximal TOF
- Signs of aspiration pneumonia on CXR.

Contrast studies are usually not needed except for the diagnosis of 'H'-type TOF.

In this uncommon variant, the oesophagus is formed normally with no oesophageal atresia; however, a thin fistula forms between the upper oesophagus and trachea. Plain films are often normal, apart from possible signs of aspiration pneumonia. Contrast studies are usually required for demonstration of the fistula, with water-soluble contrast material being injected through a feeding tube placed in the upper oesophagus.

Associated anomalies occur in approximately 25% of cases of oesophageal atresia and TOF. These are part of a constellation of associated anomalies known as the VACTERL association, including:

- Vertebral anomalies: congenital scoliosis, spina bifida
- Anal anomalies: anal atresia
- Cardiac anomalies: ventricular septal defect (VSD), atrial septal defect (ASD), PDA
- Tracheo-oeophageal anomalies: TOF, oesophageal atresia
- Renal and radial anomalies: MCDK and renal agenesis; radial dysplasia
- Limb anomalies: polydactyly, oligodactyly

Because of these associations, all patients with a TOF should have a renal US and an echocardiogram. Radiographs of the chest and abdomen may demonstrate vertebral anomalies. A right-sided aortic arch is seen in 5% of cases. It is important to diagnose a right-sided aortic arch preoperatively, as the surgical approach to TOF may have to be altered.

16.7.2 HYPERTROPHIC PYLORIC STENOSIS

Hypertrophic pyloric stenosis refers to progressive gastric outlet obstruction due to idiopathic hypertrophy of the circular muscle fibres of the pylorus. Clinical presentation is usually at around 6 weeks of age, with forceful non-bile-stained vomiting leading to dehydration and hypokalaemic hypochloraemic metabolic alkalosis. Palpation of a pyloric muscular mass in the right upper quadrant of an infant with a typical clinical history is classic but not common.

US is the investigation of choice and is highly sensitive and specific. US signs of pyloric stenosis indicate pyloric enlargement and obstruction and include (Fig. 16.30):

- Thickened pylorus seen as a rim of hypoechoic thickened muscle with a hyperechoic centre producing a target appearance
- US measurements indicating hypertrophic pyloric stenosis:
    - Total pyloric diameter greater than 13 mm
    - Pyloric muscle thickness greater than 3 mm
    - Pyloric length greater than 16 mm
- Distended stomach

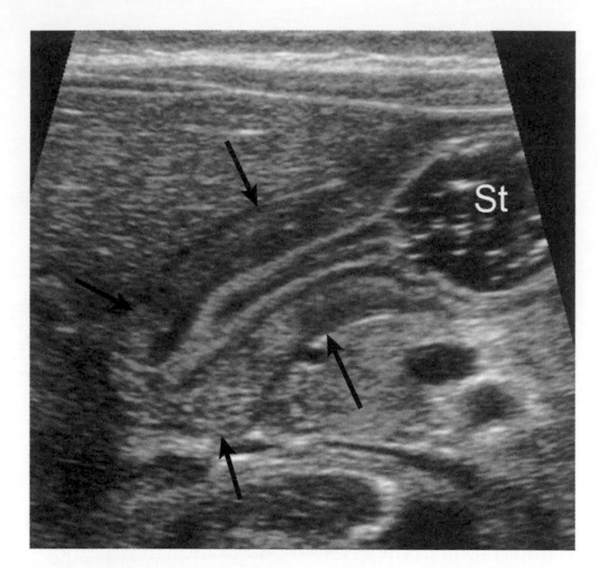

Figure 16.30 Pyloric stenosis: US. Thickening and elongation of the pylorus (arrows), with failure of passage of fluid from the stomach (St).

- Lack of passage of gastric contents through the thickened pylorus on real-time scanning.

16.7.3 INTUSSUSCEPTION

Intussusception refers to prolapse or telescoping of a segment of bowel (referred to as the intussusceptum) into the lumen of more distal bowel (the intussuscepiens). The most common form of intussusception is ileocolic, i.e. prolapse of the distal small bowel into the colon. Intussusception occurs most commonly in young children, usually from 6 months to 2 years of age, with a peak incidence at around 9 months. At this age intussusception is usually regarded as idiopathic, although enlarged lymph nodes secondary to viral infection are thought to be responsible in most cases. In older children, a lead point should be suspected, such as a Meckel diverticulum, mesenteric cyst or lymphoma. (Intussusception may also occur in adults with underlying causes, including benign small bowel tumours such as lipoma, a Meckel diverticulum or a foreign body.) The clinical presentation of intussusception includes vomiting, colicky abdominal pain, listlessness and occasionally a palpable abdominal mass. Blood-stained stool ('redcurrant jelly') may be seen late and suggests bowel ischaemia. Imaging in suspected intussusception consists of US and occasionally AXR.

ULTRASOUND

US of intussusception shows a multilayered mass that consists of hypoechoic and hyperechoic concentric rings as a result of layers of oedematous bowel wall and mesentery (Fig. 16.31). In older children or adults, US may occasionally show a lead point, such as lymphoma or a duplication cyst.

ABDOMEN RADIOGRAPH

Signs of intussusception on AXR (Fig. 16.32):

- 'Target' lesion in the right upper quadrant owing to a swollen hepatic flexure seen end-on with layers of peritoneal fat within and surrounding the intussusception
- Meniscus sign due to air outlining the intussusceptum
- Relatively gasless right side of the abdomen

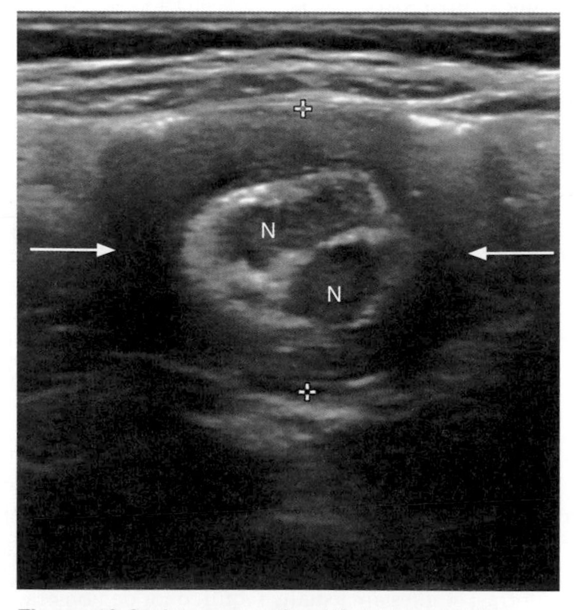

Figure 16.31 Intussusception: US. Intussusception seen as a target-like appearance on US (arrows). This consists of a hypoechoic periphery due to oedematous bowel wall, with a more complex hyperechoic centre due to mesenteric fat. Oval hypoechoic lymph nodes (N) within the mesenteric fat are probably the lead point for the intussusception.

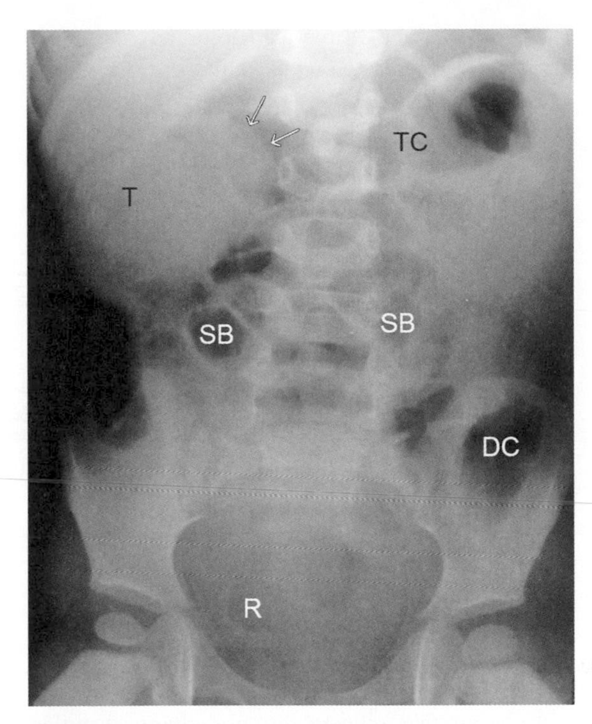

Figure 16.32 Intussusception. AXR shows a normal rectum (R) and descending colon (DC) with a few moderately distended loops of small bowel (SB). A round soft-tissue opacity (arrows) is seen projecting into the transverse colon (TC). This is the leading edge of the intussusception. Also note a target-shaped 'mass' (T) in the right upper abdomen that is due to multiple thickened layers of bowel seen 'end-on'.

- Small bowel obstruction
- Free air indicates intestinal perforation.

REDUCTION

Intussusception is a surgical emergency and early involvement of radiological and surgical teams is mandatory. Non-surgical treatment of intussusception, known as 'reduction', consists of pushing the intussusceptum back into its normal position. Reduction is most commonly performed under fluoroscopic screening using barium or gas introduced via an enema tube. Some centres use US-guided liquid reduction.

Gas reduction is now widely used and has several advantages:

- Relatively quick and clean
- Highly effective
- Low complication rate.

Contraindications to radiological reduction:

- Shock: the child must be adequately hydrated prior to attempting reduction
- Intestinal perforation, as indicated by clinical signs of peritonism and/or visualization of free air on AXR
- Duration of symptoms longer than 12 hours or small bowel obstruction make radiological reduction more difficult and decrease the likelihood of success but are not of themselves absolute contraindications.

Recurrent intussusception occurs in 5-10% of cases and should lead to repeat enema reduction. Surgery is indicated for multiple recurrences or a suspected pathological lead point.

16.8 SKELETAL DISORDERS IN CHILDREN

16.8.1 NON-ACCIDENTAL INJURY

Non-accidental injury (NAI) refers to injury of a child as a result of intentional physical abuse by another person. NAI is encountered most in young children, particularly those aged less than 1 year of age. Clinical presentation may include symptoms and signs of a specific skeletal injury or non-specific symptoms such as apnoea, seizures, lethargy or difficulty feeding. Diagnosis relies on recognition of suspicious features, including:

- Nature of the injury not consistent with the clinical history:
    - May include brain injury, subdural haematoma (SDH), rib fractures and metaphyseal fractures
- Bruises or other evidence of injury to multiple body parts
- Burns
- Injuries inconsistent with the child's stage of development
- Multiple fractures at different stages of healing
- Fractures at unusual sites, such as the sternum or scapula.

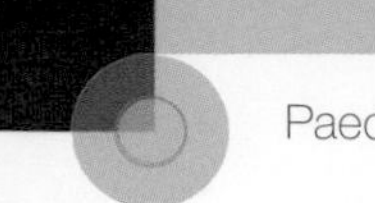

Imaging findings are often crucial to the diagnosis of NAI. Radiographs of the affected areas plus a skeletal survey (radiographs of the ribs, skull and long bones) are important in the diagnostic work-up.

Patterns of skeletal injury suggestive of NAI (Fig. 16.33):

- Long bones:
  - Periosteal new bone formation related to prior fractures
  - Metaphyseal or epiphyseal plate fractures ('corner' fractures)
  - Spiral diaphyseal fractures
- Ribs:
  - Posterior rib fractures
  - Up to 80% of rib fractures are occult and may only become visible with healing
- Skull:
  - Multiple/complex fractures
  - Depressed fractures, especially in the occipital bone
  - Wide fractures, i.e. more than 5 mm.

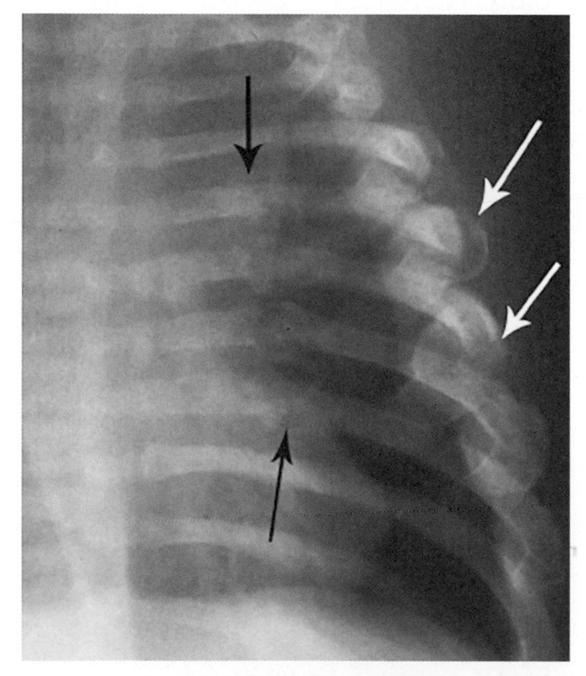

Figure 16.33 Non-accidental injury. CXR shows multiple posterior (black arrows) and lateral (white arrows) rib fractures.

Soft-tissue injuries may also occur in NAI, including hepatic, splenic and renal trauma.

Brain injuries are common. SDH in infants is unusual in accidental injury and is commonly associated with severe shaking of the child. SDHs may be multiple and different ages. Retinal haemorrhage can also occur from violent shaking. The differential diagnosis of NAI includes accidental injury, birth-related trauma and conditions causing abnormally fragile bones, such as osteogenesis imperfecta. Radiologists play an important role in dating injuries for child protection services.

16.8.2 DEVELOPMENTAL DYSPLASIA OF THE HIP

Developmental dysplasia of the hip (DDH) occurs in 1 or 2 per 1000 births. Girls are more commonly affected than boys, with a ratio of 8:1. The left hip is more commonly involved than the right. Previously known as congenital hip dislocation, the term DDH more accurately reflects the underlying disorder, which is dysplasia of the acetabulum. Acetabular dysplasia may lead to varying degrees of hip joint subluxation, dislocation and dysfunction. Risk factors for the development of DDH include family history, breech presentation, neuromuscular disorders and foot deformities. Early diagnosis is essential to prevent long-term complications, including worsening dysplasia, abnormal gait and premature osteoarthritis. Conservative measures, such as splinting for a few weeks, are usually successful in all but the most severe cases.

US is the investigation of choice for suspected DDH in infants (Fig. 16.34). US has several advantages, including:

- Lack of ionizing radiation
- Cartilage structures are seen well, including the femoral head, hyaline acetabular cartilage and fibrocartilaginous labrum
- Reproducible measurements of the angle of the acetabular roof and the position of the femoral head may be taken and used in follow-up examinations
- Dynamic real-time US is used to assess hip stability
- Position of the hip in a splint may be confirmed.

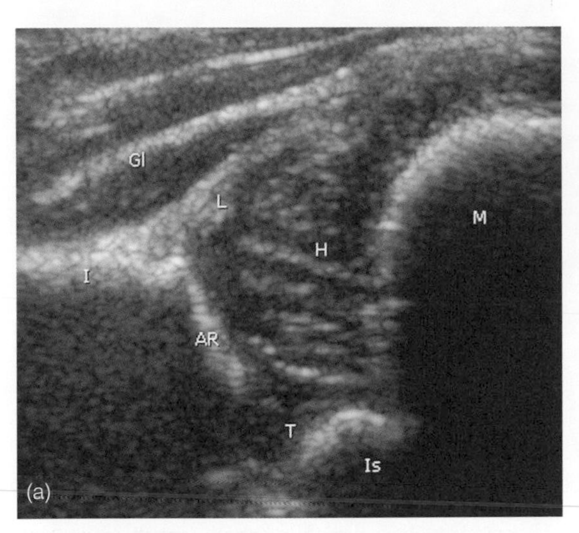

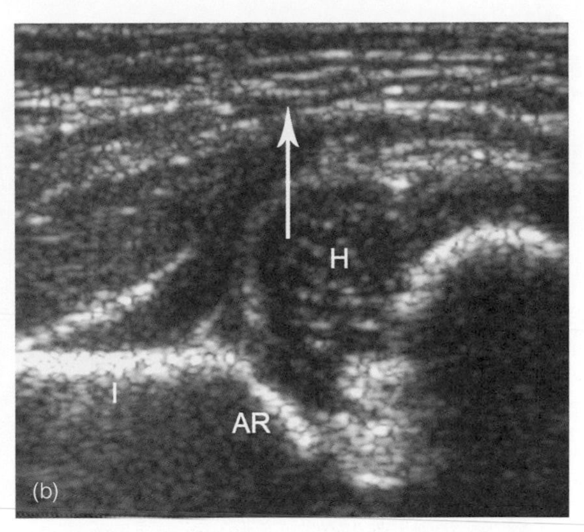

Figure 16.34 Developmental dysplasia of the hip (DDH): US. (a) Coronal image of a normal infant hip showing the following: acetabular roof (AR), gluteal muscles (Gl), femoral head (H), lateral wall of the ileum (I), ischium (Is), femoral metaphysis (M), triradiate cartilage (T). (b) Coronal image of DDH showing a shallow angle between the acetabular roof and ileum plus displacement of the femoral head out of the acetabulum (arrow).

Radiography has limited accuracy in infants as most of the essential structures such as the femoral head and acetabular rim are composed of cartilage and cannot be seen. Radiographic assessment is used in children over 9 months of age.

In severe cases, including those who do not respond to splinting, MRI or arthrogram may be indicated for further assessment of the internal structures of the hip joint, including the fibrocartilaginous labrum. The choice of modality usually reflects local availability and expertise.

Children with missed DDH usually present with late walking or a limp. In cases of missed DDH, permanent acetabular dysplasia and delayed femoral head ossification may occur with long-term complications, including limp, early and severe osteoarthritis and tearing of the acetabular labrum.

16.8.3 OSTEOMYELITIS

Osteomyelitis refers to infectious inflammation of bone. Osteomyelitis may occur at any age, though it is more common in young children, with over 50% of cases occurring before the age of 5 years. The common sites of involvement are the metaphyses of long bones and the growth centres (metaphyseal equivalents) in the pelvis, mandible and spine. Osteomyelitis is usually due to haematogenous spread from the skin, respiratory tract or a UTI. Less commonly, osteomyelitis may be due to direct penetration, especially of the calcaneus or distal toes. Most common organisms causing childhood osteomyelitis are *S. aureus*, β-haemolytic *Streptococcus* and *S. pneumoniae*. (In adults, osteomyelitis is often caused by compound fractures, adjacent soft-tissue infection, diabetes or intravenous drug use.) The clinical presentation of osteomyelitis in children is variable, though it usually consists of pain, local tenderness and fever. In younger children, symptoms may be less specific, such as the development of a limp, an unwillingness to use the affected limb, lethargy and poor feeding in neonates.

RADIOGRAPHY

Radiographs are often the first investigation performed, though they are generally normal at the time of initial presentation. Radiographic signs of osteomyelitis usually develop over a few days and include:

- Soft-tissue swelling

- Bony lucency that progresses to frank destruction
- Subperiosteal new bone formation, termed periosteal reaction; this is usually visible after symptoms have been present for 7–10 days.

A Brodie abscess is a type of chronic circumscribed osteomyelitis, most common in the lower extremity and seen radiographically as a focal lucency with marginal sclerosis.

MAGNETIC RESONANCE IMAGING

MRI is the investigation of choice when osteomyelitis is suspected clinically and radiographs are normal or equivocal (Fig. 16.35). The advantages of MRI for the investigation of suspected osteomyelitis in children include:

- MRI uses no ionizing radiation
- MRI is usually positive at the time of presentation
- Whole-body short TI (inversion time) inversion recovery (STIR) images are often included for two reasons:
    - Localization of symptoms is often difficult in children
    - Osteomyelitis may occasionally be multifocal
- MRI is usually able to differentiate conditions such as Ewing sarcoma or Langerhans cell histiocytosis (LCH), which may mimic osteomyelitis clinically or radiographically.

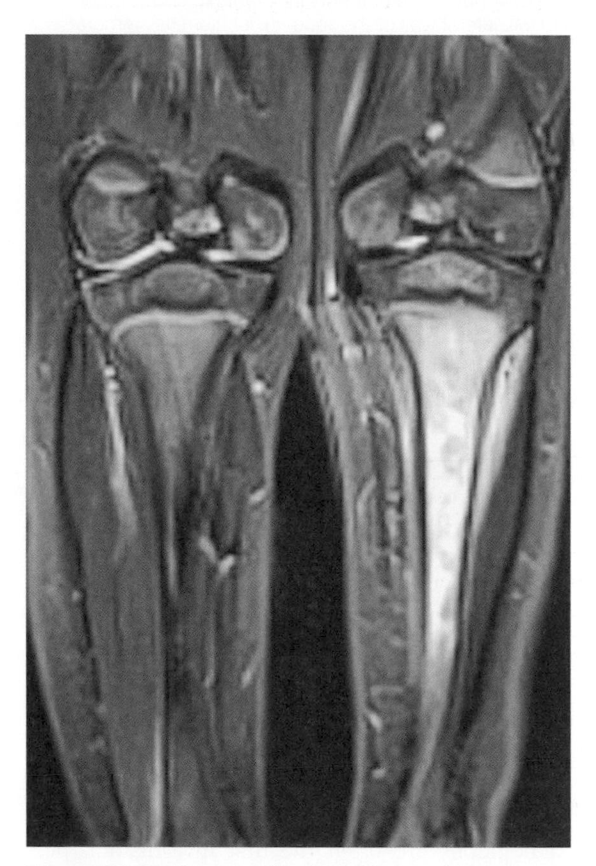

Figure 16.35 Osteomyelitis: MRI. Limp and fever in a 2-year-old boy. Coronal short TI (inversion time) inversion recovery (STIR) image of the legs shows extensive high signal in the marrow cavity of the left tibia. Oedema is also seen in adjacent soft tissue with no evidence of a soft-tissue mass.

Bone scintigraphy with ^{99m}Tc-MDP will be positive within 24–72 hours of infection and is used when MRI is unavailable. Depending on local expertise, US may also be used.

16.8.4 SEPTIC ARTHRITIS OF THE HIP

Septic arthritis of the hip most commonly presents before the age of 3 years. It is usually due to haematogenous spread from skin or is of unknown cause. *Staphylococcus aureus* and β-haemolytic *Streptococcus* are the most common pathogens. Radiographs are insensitive and early scintigraphy may be negative.

US is the investigation of choice to diagnose the presence of a hip joint effusion (Fig. 16.36). Diagnostic aspiration of the hip joint may be performed safely under US guidance.

16.8.5 TRANSIENT SYNOVITIS (IRRITABLE HIP)

Transient synovitis is a benign self-limiting hip disorder. The peak age of incidence is 4–10 years, with boys more commonly affected than girls. The clinical presentation usually suggests the diagnosis of transient synovitis and consists of a limp that develops rapidly over 1–2 days, often following a history of a recent viral illness and mild fever. Transient synovitis

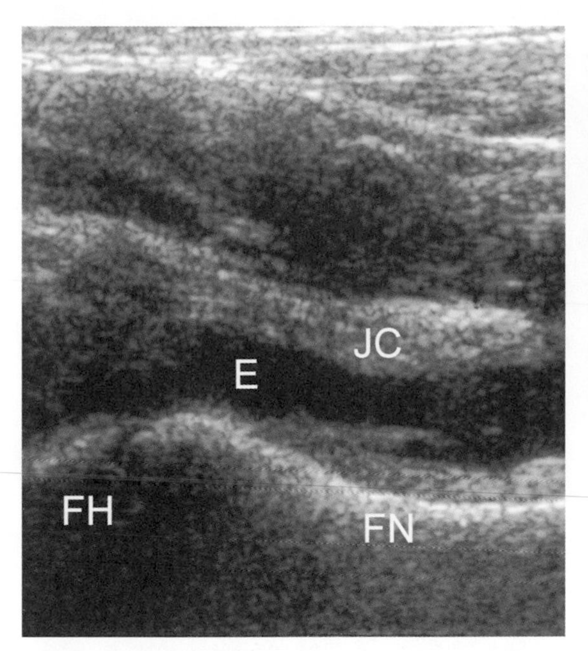

Figure 16.36 Hip joint effusion: US. US image obtained with the probe parallel to the femoral neck (FN) with the round surface of the femoral head (FH) seen medially. The effusion is seen as anechoic fluid (E) elevating the joint capsule (JC).

usually settles with analgesia. Radiographs are performed to exclude fracture and other hip pathologies and are usually normal. US often demonstrates a non-specific joint effusion.

16.8.6 PERTHES DISEASE

Perthes disease refers to avascular necrosis of the proximal femoral epiphysis. Perthes disease has a peak age of incidence of 4–7 years; 10% of cases are bilateral. Radiography of the hips is the initial investigation of choice.

Early radiographic signs of Perthes disease:

- Reduced size and sclerosis of the femoral epiphysis with joint space widening
- Subchondral fracture producing a linear lucency deep to the articular surface of the femoral head.

Radiographs may be normal at the time of initial presentation. In such cases, MRI may show signs of ischaemia of the femoral head prior to development of visible irregularity or collapse.

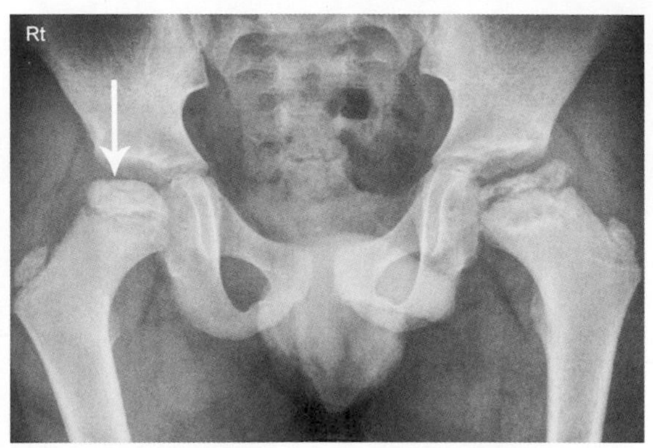

Figure 16.37 Perthes disease. Advanced changes of Perthes disease on the left with flattening, irregularity and sclerosis of the femoral epiphysis, widening of the metaphysis and widening of the hip joint. There are much subtler early changes on the right with slight irregularity and flattening of the femoral head (arrow).

Late radiographic signs of Perthes disease (Fig. 16.37):

- Delayed maturation of the femoral head
- Fragmentation and flattening of the femoral head (coxa plana)
- Cyst formation and widening of the femoral neck (coxa magna).

16.8.7 SLIPPED CAPITAL FEMORAL EPIPHYSIS

Slipped capital femoral epiphysis (SCFE) refers to posteromedial slip of the capital femoral epiphysis, producing acute onset of hip or groin pain and a limp. It represents a Salter–Harris type 1 injury (see Chapter 13). SCFE occurs most commonly in adolescent boys; 20% of cases are bilateral. Obesity is a risk factor. Avascular necrosis of the femoral head develops in approximately 10% of cases. Radiographic signs of SCFE are best appreciated on a lateral projection, where the slip of the femoral head is well seen.

Signs on the anteroposterior (AP) film may be more difficult to appreciate and a 'frog leg' AP film improves detection. Signs include:

- Widening and irregularity of the femoral growth plate
- Reduced height of the epiphysis (Fig. 16.38).

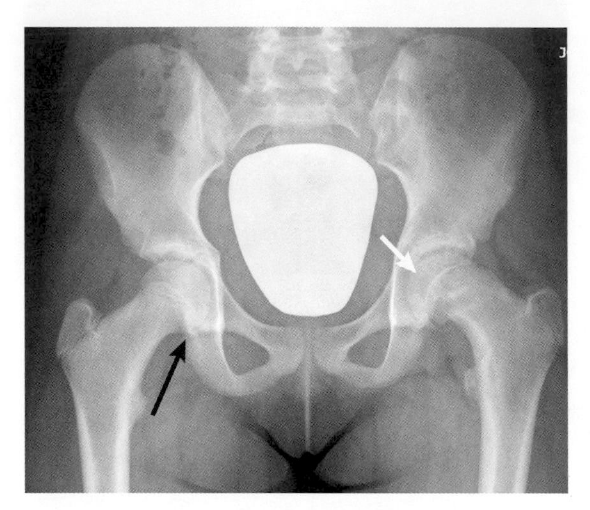

Figure 16.38 Slipped capital femoral epiphysis (SCFE). Slip of the left capital femoral epiphysis (white arrow). Note the normal metaphyseal overlay sign on the right side producing a white triangle where the lower corner of the femoral metaphysis overlays the acetabulum (black arrow). This appearance is lost on the left as a result of the metaphysis being pushed laterally.

16.8.8 LANGERHANS CELL HISTIOCYTOSIS

LCH describes a spectrum of disorders, the common feature being histiocytic infiltration of tissues and aggressive bone lesions. LCH may be subclassified as restricted or extensive LDH. Extensive LDH refers to visceral organ involvement with or without bone lesions. Visceral involvement may produce organ dysfunction and failure. Skin rash and diabetes insipidus are common. Restricted LCH refers to monostotic bone or polyostotic bone lesions, or isolated skin lesions. The monostotic bone lesion of LCH occurs in children with a peak age of incidence of 5–10 years, though it may also be seen in older patients. Clinical presentation may be with local pain or pathological fracture (see Fig. 13.9). Radiographically, LCH produces focal, well-defined, lytic skeletal lesions in the skull, spine and long bones.

SUMMARY

Clinical presentation	Investigation of choice	Comment
Neonatal respiratory distress	CXR	
Pulmonary infection	CXR	
Cystic fibrosis	CXR	
Abdominal mass	• US for initial assessment • CT/MRI for further characterization and staging	
Urinary tract infection	US	• MAG3 scintigraphy for suspected obstruction • MCU ± DMSA in selected cases
Hydronephrosis	• US • MAG3 scintigraphy	
Neonatal gut obstruction/bile-stained vomiting	AXR	Contrast studies in selected cases, e.g. suspected malrotation or Hirschsprung disease
Oesophageal atresia and tracheo-oesophageal fistula	CXR and AXR	
Hypertrophic pyloric stenosis	US	
Intussusception	US	Imaging-guided reduction unless contraindicated
Non-accidental injury	Radiography (skeletal survey)	
Developmental dysplasia of the hip	US	Radiography in older children (>6–9 months)
Osteomyelitis	MRI	Radiography at the time of presentation often negative
Acutely painful hip (suspected septic arthritis or transient synovitis)	US	
Perthes disease	Radiography	MRI if radiography negative
Slipped capital femoral epiphysis	Radiography	
Langerhans cell histiocytosis	Radiography	CT/MRI in complex areas, e.g. temporal bone

DMSA, see Table 1.1; MAG3, see Table 1.1; *Abbreviation*: MCU, micturating cystourethrogram.

Index

Note: page numbers in *italics* indicate figures and tables.

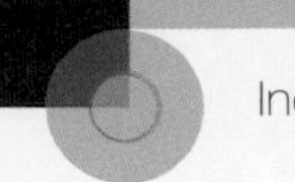

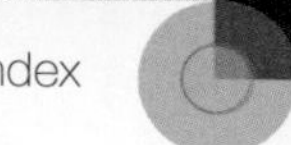

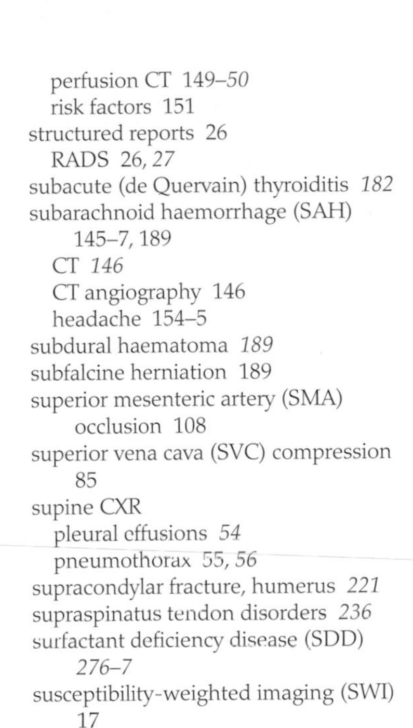